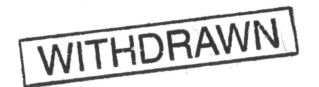

EPIDEMIOLOGY OF SPORTS
INJURIES by D J. CAINE,
C G. CAINE & K J. LINDNER

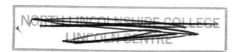

# EPIDEMIOLOGY OF SPORTS INJURIES

**Dennis J. Caine, PhD**
Western Washington University

**Caroline G. Caine, PhD**
Western Washington University

**Koenraad J. Lindner, PhD**
University of Hong Kong

Editors

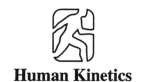

**Human Kinetics**

**Cataloging-in-Publication Data**

Epidemiology of sports injuries / [edited by] Dennis Caine, Caroline
     Caine, Koenraad J. Lindner.
          p.     cm.
     Includes bibliographical references (p.   ).
     ISBN 0-87322-466-3
     1. Sports injuries--Epidemiology.   I. Caine, Dennis John, 1949-
          II. Caine, Caroline, 1945-      .   III. Lindner, Koenraad J., 1941-

RA645.S68E65   1996
617.1'027--dc20

95-39000
CIP

ISBN: 0-87322-466-3

The chapters presented in this book are the result of the Epidemiology of Sports Injuries Symposium held April 7-9, 1994 at the Human Kinetics Conference Facilities in Champaign, Illinois.

Developmental Editor: Rodd Whelpley
Assistant Editors: Kent Reel, Ann Greenseth, Henry Woolsey
Editorial Assistants: Andrew Starr, Jennifer Hemphill, Coree Schutter
Copyeditors: Denelle Eknes, June Waldman
Proofreader: Jim Burns
Production Manager: Kris Ding
Text Designer: Judy Henderson
Typesetting and Text Layout: Sandra Meier
Layout Artist: Tara Welsch
Cover Designer: Jack Davis
Illustrator: Craig Ronto
Printer: BookCrafters

Printed in the United States of America

10  9  8  7  6  5  4  3  2  1

**Human Kinetics**
P.O. Box 5076, Champaign, IL 61825-5076
1-800-747-4457

*Canada*: Human Kinetics, Box 24040, Windsor, ON N8Y 4Y9
1-800-465-7301 (in Canada only)

*Europe*: Human Kinetics, P.O. Box IW14, Leeds LS16 6TR, United Kingdom
(44) 1132 781708

*Australia*: Human Kinetics, 2 Ingrid Street, Clapham 5062, South Australia
(08) 371 3755

*New Zealand*: Human Kinetics, P.O. Box 105-231, Auckland 1
(09) 523 3462

# Contents

# Contributors

**David G. Addiss**, MD, MPH
Division of Parasitic Diseases
Centers for Disease Control and Prevention
Atlanta, Georgia

**M.J.L. Alexander**, PhD
Health, Leisure and Human Performance Institute
University of Manitoba
Winnipeg, Manitoba

**Hubert A. Allen**, MS
Baltimore, Maryland

**Steven J. Anderson**, MD
Department of Pediatrics
University of Washington School of Medicine
Seattle, Washington

**Caroline G. Caine**, PhD
College of Fine and Performing Arts
Western Washington University
Bellingham, Washington

**Dennis J. Caine**, PhD
Department of Physical Education, Health and
   Recreation
Western Washington University
Bellingham, Washington

**Michael A. Clark**, PhD
Institute for the Study of Youth Sports
Michigan State University
East Lansing, Michigan

**Andrew L. Dannenberg**, MD, MPH
Johns Hopkins Injury Prevention Center
Johns Hopkins University
Baltimore, Maryland

**Andrea Ferretti**, MD
Orthopedics and Traumatology
University of Rome

**James G. Garrick**, MD
Center for Sports Medicine
Saint Francis Hospital
San Francisco, California

**Deborah A. Goebert**, MS
Pacific Basin Rehabilitation Research and
   Training Center
Honolulu, Hawaii

**Peter A. Harmer**, PhD, A.T.C.-R.
Department of Exercise Science-Sports Medicine
Willamette University
Salem, Oregon

**Lawrence E. Hart**, MB.BCh, MSc, FRCPC, FACP,
   FACR, Dip. Sport Med.
Associate Professor
Department of Medicine
McMaster University
Hamilton, Ontario

**G. Harley Hartung**, PhD
Cardiology Service, Department of Medicine
Tripler Army Medical Center
Hawaii

**Warren B. Howe**, MD
Team Physician
Western Washington University
Bellingham, Washington

**Rey Jaffet**, MS, A.T.C.
Head Athletic Trainer
Florida International University
Miami, Florida

**Barry D. Jordan**, MD
Medical Director
New York State Athletic Commission
New York, New York
and Assistant Professor of Neurology and Public
   Health
Cornell University Medical College
New York, New York

**Kathleen Knutzen**, PhD
Department of Physical Education, Health and
   Recreation
Western Washington University
Bellingham, Washington

**Melinda Larson**, MS, A.T.C.
Assistant Athletic Trainer, Instructor
Whitworth College
Spokane, Washington

**Koenraad J. Lindner**, PhD
Physical Education and Sports Science Unit
The University of Hong Kong

**V. Patteson Lombardi**, PhD
Department of Biology
University of Oregon
Eugene, Oregon

**Bert R. Mandelbaum**, MD
Santa Monica Orthopedic and Sports Medicine
     Group
Santa Monica, California

**Nicholas Mohtadi**, MD, MSc, FRCSC, Dip. Sport
     Med.
Clinical Associate Professor
University of Calgary Sport Medicine Centre
Department of Surgery (Orthopaedic)
Faculties of Medicine and Kinesiology
University of Calgary
Calgary, Alberta

**William J. Montelpare**, PhD
Health Studies Program
Brock University
St. Catharines, Ontario

**Craig K. Moore**, MD
Family Practice and Sports Medicine
Bellingham, Washington

**Frederick Mueller**, PhD
Department of Physical Education, Exercise, and
     Sport Science
University of North Carolina at Chapel Hill
Chapel Hill, North Carolina

**Robert Nebergall**, DO
Tulsa Orthopedic Surgeons
Tulsa, Oklahoma

**Arthur J. Pearl**, MD
Orthopaedic Surgeon
Fort Pierce, Florida

**Robert L. Pelletier**, DPE
School of Human Kinetics
University of Ottawa
Ottawa, Ontario

**Arlene Peters**, MS
Dept. of Physical Education, Exercise and Sport
     Science
University of North Carolina at Chapel Hill
Chapel Hill, North Carolina

**Willy Pieter**, PhD
London, England

**Alex Poole**, BA, BASc, MD
University of Calgary
Calgary, Alberta

**Ralph K. Requa**, MSPH
Saint Francis Hospital
San Francisco, California

**Frederick P. Rivara**, MD, MPH
Director, Harborview Injury Prevention and
     Research Center
George Adkins Professor of Pediatrics
University of Washington
Seattle, Washington

**Benjamin D. Rubin**, MD
North Tustin Sports Medicine Center
Santa Ana, California

**Andrew Rudawsky**, MS, PT, A.T.C.
U.S. Men's National Team Athletic Trainer
U.S. Soccer House
Chicago, Illinois

**William A. Sands**, PhD
Department of Exercise and Sport Science
University of Utah
Salt Lake City, Utah

**Vern Seefeldt**, PhD
Department of Health Education, Counseling
     Psychology, and Human Performance
Michigan State University
East Lansing, Michigan

**Charles A. Soma**, MD
North Shore Orthopaedic Surgery and Sports
     Medicine
Wailuku, Maui, Hawaii

**Diane C. Thompson**, MS
Epidemiologist
Harborview Injury Prevention and Research
     Center
University of Washington
Seattle, Washingtion

**Robert S. Thompson**, MD
Director, Department of Preventive Care
Group Health Cooperative of Puget Sound
Seattle, Washington

**Stephan Walk**, MS
Institute for the Study of Youth Sports
Michigan State University
East Lansing, Michigan

**Diane S. Watanabe**, MA, ATC
Santa Monica Orthopaedic and Sports Medicine
   Group
Santa Monica, California

**John Weaver**, MD
Family Practice and Sports Medicine
Bellingham, Washington

**Randall R. Wroble**, MD
Orthopaedic Surgeon
Sportsmedicine Grant
Columbus, Ohio

**Eric D. Zemper**, PhD
Exercise Research Asssociates of Oregon
Eugene, Oregon

**John Zvijac**, MD
Department of Orthopaedics and Rehabilitation
Division of Sports Medicine
University of Miami School of Medicine
Coral Gables, Florida

# Preface

Some years ago, before we met each other, we were all interested in the study of injuries affecting young athletes in selected athletic endeavors. Our early investigations, first individually and later jointly, centered on a concern about needless injuries, which then led to a more general interest in the epidemiology of sports injuries. Sports injury epidemiology is the study of the distribution and determinants of varying rates of injuries in human populations for the purpose of establishing procedures to prevent their occurrence. The epidemiologic approach to sports injury research, although still relatively new, has already resulted in rule changes, equipment standards, improved coaching techniques, and better conditioning of athletes.

The purpose of *Epidemiology of Sports Injuries* is to review integratively and comprehensively the distribution and determinants of injury rates as reported in the literature, and further to suggest measures for injury prevention and directions for further research. Our book provides the first global, state-of-the-art account of the epidemiology of injuries across a broad spectrum of sports. While some attempts to provide this information have been made for selected sports, these reviews usually did not strive to identify and track down all the literature available; nor did they consistently provide insights into how past research was found, evaluated, and integrated.

The contributors to this volume sought and synthesized sports injury data through a common methodological approach and participated in the book's quality control. The authors of each chapter met during a three-day symposium at the conference facilities at Human Kinetics and presented their findings to their peers. Prior to the symposium, the first draft of each chapter was critiqued by the editors for form, content, application of methodology, and uniform terminology. Dialogue among symposium participants resulted in uniform strategies for an evidence-based approach to organizing and interpreting the literature, and this approach has been applied across the chapters.

A unique feature of *Epidemiology of Sports Injuries* is its organization. All of the sport-specific chapters are laid out with the same basic headings so that the reader can easily find common information across chapters. The discussion in each chapter is amply illustrated with tables to make it easy to examine injury factors between studies within a sport and between sports. Most significantly, the reader is apprised of the level of evidence behind the data so that he or she can decide how much confidence to place in suggested injury prevention measures which have arisen from this literature.

*Epidemiology of Sports Injuries* is organized around three foci: an introduction, 24 sport-specific chapters, and two culminating chapters. The introductory chapter, "The Epidemiologic Approach to Sports Injuries," provides the reader with a knowledge base from which to interpret and evaluate the epidemiologic information provided in subsequent chapters. A proposed model depicting the epidemiology of sports injuries is introduced. The main part of the book consists of the sport-specific chapters themselves. We have included chapters on as many sports as possible in this part, including athletic endeavors like dance and adult recreational fitness which are non-competitive in nature. Most epidemiologic data have been generated from research on competitive sports. However, in some sport-specific chapters, such as "Bicycling" and "Ocean Sports," most data reviewed are from non-competitive settings. We have invited researchers whose interests and expertise lie within a given sport or sport group to author a chapter on that particular subject.

The book culminates in two chapters which apply practical aspects of sports injury epidemiology: "Suggestions for Injury Prevention" and "Suggestions for Further Research." The "Suggestions for Injury Prevention" chapter identifies injury prevention measures which are generic across sports. "Suggestions for Further Research" identifies directions for further research which are applicable across sports. The intent of this latter chapter was to get at the methodological problems which seem systemic to sports epidemiology studies and to suggest ways to ensure better controlled studies in the future.

The information in this book will benefit physicians, physical therapists, athletic trainers, sports scientists, sports governing bodies, coaches, parents, and reference librarians. Physicians, physical therapists, and athletic trainers will find *Epidemiology of Sports Injuries* helpful in identifying problem areas in which appropriate preventive measures can be initiated to reduce the incidence and severity of injuries. Some sports scientists, as well as health care professionals, will find the information in this book useful as a basis for continued epidemiologic study of injuries in various sports, while others may find it useful as a course text. We are optimistic that sports governing bodies and coaches may use this information as an informed basis for the design and conduct of various sports as well as for the development of injury prevention programs related to such factors as exposure, training techniques, equipment modifications, and rules.

Reliable and accurate data on sports injuries may also help potential sports participants and parents (on behalf of their children) to make better informed decisions about which sports to take up, and the levels of expertise and competition for which to aim. Most optimistically, we hope that the *Epidemiology of Sports Injuries* will be a welcome addition to libraries as THE source on sports injury statistics. If our book stimulates the development of more and better-informed professionals with regard to sports injury epidemiology and to the importance of continued research in sports injuries, then our efforts will have been well rewarded.

Dennis J. Caine
Caroline G. Caine
Koenraad J. Lindner

# Acknowledgments

An edited text like *Epidemiology of Sports Injuries* would be inconceivable without the contributions and support of a great many people. To begin, I would like to express my deep gratitude to Rainer Martens, Human Kinetics' C.E.O., for his readiness to merge our ideas on *Epidemiology of Sports Injuries*, and for his being such an important source of motivation and support throughout the research and writing of this text. I would also like to thank Rainer for sponsoring the book symposium by providing conference facilities.

Two of the Human Kinetics staff deserve special mention. I would like to thank Michelle Watson of the conference division for her assistance with the symposium planning and her diligence and charm in accommodating all on-site symposium needs. Rodd Whelpley, developmental editor for *Epidemiology of Sports Injuries*, could always be depended on for clear editorial suggestions. But Rodd has been more than a developmental editor—through this process, he became a friend and colleague.

The researching, writing, identifying and recruiting the contributing authors, and editing this book required both monetary and human resources. My thanks to the Department of Physical Education, Health and Recreation and the Bureau for Faculty Research at Western Washington University, and to the University of New Brunswick, for providing some of these resources.

The time required to research and write rigorous scientific overviews of the sports injury literature, combined with a readiness to sacrifice personal time and resources to attend and participate in the book symposium, required more than a professional willingness on the part of the contributing authors. I am truly grateful to all the authors of *Epidemiology of Sports Injuries* for believing in the importance of this project and for committing their time, energy, and resources to seeing it through.

Thanks most especially to my co-editors, Caroline Caine and Koenraad Lindner. The editorial process for this book has been far more than one person could reasonably handle. For fifteen years of instructive collaboration on scholarly projects, the most recent being *Epidemiology of Sports Injuries*, my thanks go to Koenraad. He has been my mentor and friend and I truly owe much to his patience and guidance in the area of scholarly writing and research. *Epidemiology of Sports Injuries* would not have been possible without the collaboration, love, and support of my wife, Caroline. We have worked closely together on every phase of this project, including conceptualization, research and writing, bringing authors on board, editing, as well as the planning and administration of the book and the symposium. Caroline's editorial experience and facility with words enabled our work to reach its final form. But more than that, our book reflects the camaraderie in probing joint ideas and the challenge of questioning individual ideas which only close friends can do well, and Caroline is that friend.

Dennis J. Caine

# 1

# The Epidemiologic Approach to Sports Injuries

*Caroline G. Caine, Dennis J. Caine, and Koenraad J. Lindner*

What do we know about sports injuries? From the vast medical and sports medicine literature we know many facts—but we lack integrated answers. For instance, we know from several studies on gymnasts that they are likely to experience specific types of injuries, but the studies differ so much in such factors as definition, design, and training and competitive levels that finding bottom line answers about what injuries and gymnasts are most likely at risk is at best difficult. Like piecing together a jigsaw puzzle, one works to find a relationship among all the pieces of information, hoping to consolidate the picture eventually. However, if some pieces are formed from a different premise—defined differently—than other pieces, then the resulting picture could look quite Cubist! Whereas in the art world this would evoke stimulating discourse and conjecture, subjective interpretation is not the goal of sports medicine research.

Parents are not interested in conjecture. They want to know if a particular sport is safe for their children. How likely is their son to be hurt in football or their daughter injured in soccer? Indeed, athletes of all ages and everyone who works with them, whether they are parents, sports medicine personnel, sports governing bodies, or coaches, need to know answers to questions such as the following: Is the risk of injury greater in some sport activities or levels of activity than in others? What types of injuries are most common in a given sport? What is the average time lost from injury and what is the risk of permanent impairment? Are some athletes more injury prone than others? Are particular physical or psychological characteristics associated with greater risk of injury? How can injury be predicted or prevented? How effective are the preventive measures that are implemented? These are all questions that sports medicine personnel and coaches should be prepared to respond to, and the information should be made readily available to them. Answers to these questions are basic to informed decision making about which sports to take up and what levels of expertise and competition to aim for.

Sports medicine personnel also need injury information when they are asked to take care of a team or to monitor a special sports event. Furthermore, they need to be able to tell patients or parents about more than the risk of musculoskeletal injury. Metabolic injuries such as heat stress, hormonal changes that affect mineral balance, and even the risk of sudden death during exercise are also important aspects to share with patients and parents. More important, sports medicine personnel, instructors, and participants all need to know how to prevent injury and adverse changes to the body before any rigorous sport or fitness program is initiated.

Unfortunately, the answers to these questions are difficult, often impossible, to find for two reasons. First, many answers are obscured by the volume of information provided in the enormous research literature. Second, a lot of the information simply does not answer the questions asked because of differing definitions of injury, weak study designs, insufficient numbers of subjects, and other limitations. Some of these questions, especially those dealing with risk factors and preventive measures, have simply not been adequately addressed. Until we can extract the numerous messages buried in the literature, we cannot claim to know very much about sports injuries. To find answers to these important questions, we also need to identify where we need to go from here in terms of further research.

That is what this book is about—extracting the knowledge contained in all English language sports injury studies since 1975 in order, for the first time, to bring you as close as possible to an integrated answer. In each sport-specific chapter an epidemiologic picture has been systematically developed from the available data in prospective cohort, retrospective cohort, case-control, and cross-sectional studies and from case series, case reports, and literature reviews. From this picture, it became possible to suggest preventive measures that seemed reasonable, given the level of evidence available (i.e., ways of using the *known*), and to suggest needed areas for further research (i.e., directions for seeking the still *unknown*).

A unique feature of our book is the approach taken to reviewing the literature. Most past reviews have attempted to synthesize the results and conclusions of selected publications on a given topic. Data are typically discussed on a study-by-study basis. Our reviews, or "overviews" as Sackett et al. (22) would express it, strive to identify and report comprehensively—across studies rather than study by study—all the epidemiologic injury literature on each sport reviewed since 1975. Some chapters integrate information from even earlier studies and include foreign publications. We felt, especially in view of the many reports to review, that the results of the overview would be untrustworthy unless the review processes were systematized and made as rigorous as the methodology required of primary researchers. The overview is thus perceived as a study itself in which the reviewer posits a research problem, gathers data on it (in the form of previous articles), then analyzes them and draws conclusions (22). In this regard, many strategies that have been proposed for assessing clinical literature reviews (17, 22) or developing integrative research reviews of the social science literature (4) were used as a basis for formulating the overviews in this text. Where appropriate, data are displayed in table format to facilitate a discussion of data across studies rather than on a study-by-study basis. Unfortunately, study design limitations and the associated variability of injury data across studies prevented the application of a statistical strategy for assembling the results of the studies into a single estimate, as in meta-analysis. However, within the limitations of the current body of sports injury literature, we have reduced an enormous amount of data on athletic injuries acquired through hundreds of independent research endeavors, and delivered an epidemiologic picture of injuries across a broad spectrum of sports.

## Sports Injury Epidemiology

What is epidemiology? Epidemiology is the study of the distribution and determinants of varying rates of diseases, injuries, or other health states in human populations for the purpose of identifying and implementing measures to prevent their development and spread. The initial development of the theory and methods of epidemiology focused on applications to infectious and communicable diseases. However, in his classic paper on "The Epidemiology of Accidents," Gordon (7) recognized that injuries conformed to certain biological laws, as do infectious diseases, and therefore could be studied by the application of basic epidemiologic principles. Application of epidemiologic concepts and methods to the characterization and prevention of accidental injury followed. By the early 1960s epidemiologic techniques were also being applied to sports injury problems (8). This marked a transition from the clinical series, which emphasized a particular sport, type of injury, anatomic site, or clinical experience (27).

The epidemiologist in sports medicine is concerned with quantifying injury occurrence (*how much*) with respect to *who* is affected by injury, *where* and *when* injuries occur, and *what* is their outcome, for the purpose of explaining *why* and *how* injuries occur and identifying strategies to control and prevent them (5). The study of the distribution of varying rates of injuries (i.e., who, where, when, what) is referred to as descriptive epidemiology, and the study of the determinants of an exhibited distribution of varying rates of injuries (i.e., why and how) is referred to as analytical epidemiology. The components of the two interrelated types of epidemiologic research—descriptive and analytical—are shown in Figure 1.1 as they relate to prevention and are discussed below with the purposes of highlighting their various contributions to the epidemiologic picture and preparing the reader with some basic understandings that will help with the interpretation of the chapters to follow.

### Descriptive Epidemiology

Descriptive epidemiology is by far the most common type of epidemiologic research that has been published in the sports injury literature. In descriptive epidemiology the researcher attempts to quantify the occurrence of injury. The most basic measure of injury occurrence is a simple count of injured persons. However, frequency data alone

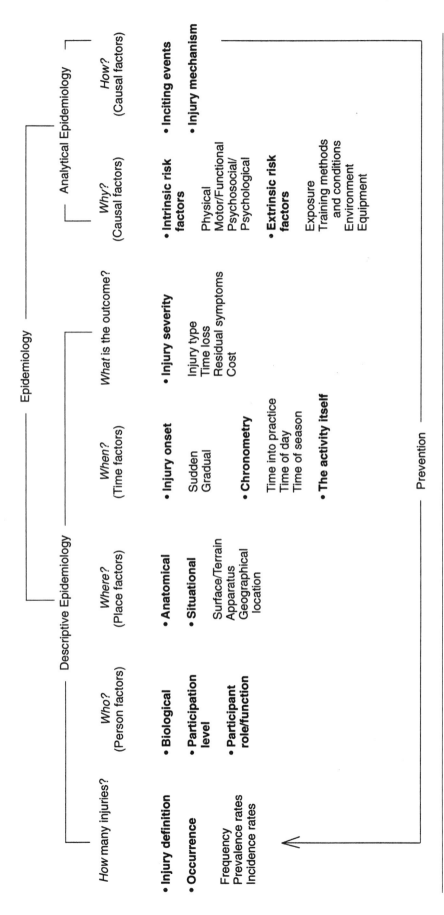

**Figure 1.1**  Epidemiology of sports injuries.

have very limited epidemiologic utility (9) and should not be confused with rates. To investigate the distribution of injuries it is necessary to know the size of the source population from which the injured individuals were derived, or the population at risk. An injury rate may be derived when the number of injured persons is divided by the population at risk for the problem (18). For gymnastic injuries, for instance, the injured gymnasts represent the numerator and all the gymnasts who might be injured represent the denominator.

The two most commonly reported rates in the sports injury literature are *incidence* and *prevalence* (18). Prevalence rates pertain to the total number of cases, new or old, that exist in a population at risk at a specific period of time. Incidence rates pertain to the number of new injuries that occur in a population at risk over a specified period of time. Thus, prevalence is a static measure and incidence rate is dynamic (10). Relative to incidence rates, prevalence rates have been infrequently reported in sports injury literature. Most prevalence studies reviewed in this book reported prevalence rates for specific injury conditions, such as chronic brain injury among retired boxers, spondylolysis among competitive gymnasts, or digital ischemia among high school and college baseball players. A comparison of the characteristics of prevalence and incidence rates is shown in Table 1.1.

Two types of incidence rates reported in the literature are *case rates* and *athlete rates*. Athlete rates are determined by dividing the total number of athletes injured by the total number of athletes participating. A difficulty in comparing athlete rates is that some athletes may be injured more

than once. In the more frequently reported case rates, the numerator is typically the total number of reported injuries that occur during the study period, and the denominator refers to everyone in the population who is exposed to the possibility of injury or injury condition counted in the numerator. In practice, case rates are generally multiplied by a constant $k$ (i.e., some power of 10) to provide numbers that are neither extremely large nor extremely small and to make comparisons easier (32). In the epidemiologic literature on sports injuries these rates are often presented as injuries per 100 athletes, which is analogous to the rate per 100,000 used for reporting disease rates. For example, if there are 16 injuries among 32 soccer players over the study period, the case rate would be 16/32 (or 0.5) x 100 = 50 injuries per 100 participants. In sports, incidence rates are usually expressed as a rate per season, rate per practice, rate per game, and so forth (20).

Unfortunately, the common practice of reporting athletic injuries as a rate per 100 participants can lead to questionable conclusions, particularly when results from different sports, or even from different studies within the same sport, are compared (32). Meaningful comparison of these rates can be compromised because of the varying exposure of participants to the risk of injury (i.e., denominator data). For example, a sidelined or second team player who sees little or no contact during a game is not at the same risk of sustaining injury as a healthy first team player. In addition, the number of practices and games varies considerably from one sport to another and often varies from one team to another, or even from one year to another in a given sport.

More precise methods for quantifying exposure have been introduced in some of the more recent literature and include reporting the number of injuries as a rate per $k$ athlete-exposures (an athlete-exposure is defined as one athlete participating in one practice or game in which there is the possibility of sustaining an athletic injury), per $k$ time-exposures (one time-exposure is defined as one athlete participating in one minute, hour, or day of activity in which there is the possibility of sustaining an athletic injury), or per $k$ element-exposures (one element-exposure is defined as one athlete participating in one element of activity in which there is the possibility of sustaining an athletic injury). Examples of exposure elements include vaults, pitches, bike trips, climbs, and dives. The logistics of acquiring the appropriate data are usually a major factor in determining what the unit of risk will be (26).

**Table 1.1   Characteristics of Incidence and Prevalence**

|  | Incidence | Prevalence |
| --- | --- | --- |
| Numerator | New injuries occurring during a time period among a group initially free of injury | All injuries counted on a single survey or examination of a group |
| Denominator | All susceptible people present at the beginning of the period | All people examined/ interviewed, including injured and uninjured |
| Time | Duration of the (study) period | Single point |
| How measured | Cohort study | Cross-sectional study |

*Note.* Adapted from Fletcher et al., 1988.

Another difficulty that may arise in comparing incidence rates from different studies is the injury definition employed. A review of the sports injury epidemiology literature reveals that no common operational definition exists. Definitions include such criteria as presence of a new symptom or complaint, decreased function of a body part or decreased athletic performance, cessation of practice or competition activities, and consultation with medical or training personnel (28). Clearly, if injury is defined differently across studies, a meaningful comparison of injury rates is compromised because of different criteria for determining numerator values. Other sources of bias may also compromise the comparability of injury rates, even when rates are similarly defined. For example, psychological factors may determine when players with the same injury return to play or whether they seek care from sports medicine personnel. In addition, the impact of some injuries on performance may be sport or position specific. For example, contrast the impact of a wrist sprain on the continued performance of a gymnast versus a distance runner, or on a goalie versus a forward in soccer. Who determines an injury has occurred and who records the injury information are other potential sources of bias. Awareness of the differences in injury definition and the potential sources of bias in injury determination is important in interpreting and comparing study results reported in the chapters that follow.

Having addressed the *how much* (injury rates) of descriptive epidemiology, we now direct your attention to the distribution of varying rates of injury (see Figure 1.1). "Injury distribution" relates to person factors (*who*), place factors (*where*), time factors (*when*), and injury outcome (*what*), and these provide the descriptive characteristics of injuries. Person factors may be expressed in terms of biological characteristics of the participants, participation level, and the participant's role or function in the organization. In the sports injury literature the distribution of injury rates has been expressed in terms of such categorical variables as age and gender. Variables such as maturity and rate of growth have also been categorized for the purpose of expressing and comparing injury rates, although infrequently. Other approaches to categorizing rates, based on biological characteristics, have been found in the literature but are expressed as percentages and not as rates. These include hormonal status, personality and behavioral traits, nutritional habits, stress management, and body composition. As might be expected, injury rates are most often categorized according to the way in which participants are organized for sports (e.g., amateur or recreational, high school or college, and a variety of competitive level classifications). In addition to participation level, injury rates have been reported according to function in the organization, such as by player position on a team or position in a dance company.

The *where* of injury distribution involves identifying the place on the body (anatomical) as well as the environmental or situational location. Environmental and situational factors include surface or terrain on which the activity takes place, apparatus, such as balance beam or parallel bars in gymnastics, and the geographical location and environment, taking into account indoor versus outdoor tracks, relative sea level, air quality, and climate. The studies reviewed in this book generally report data related to place factors as percent values. For example, studies reporting on injury location—the most commonly reported place factor—might report that 35% of injuries involved the ankle, 15% the knee, and so forth. What is important to remember with percentages is that the numerator is a frequency of injury associated with one portion of the data set (e.g., ankle injuries) and the denominator is the total frequency of injuries, and not the population at risk (20).

As Figure 1.1 indicates, the next characteristic of injury distribution is the *when* of injury occurrence. These time factors are expressed as onset of injury, chronometry of injury, and the activity engaged in at the time injury occurred. The reader will find a paucity of data on time factors across chapters in this book, and most data are presented as a percent of total injuries derived from frequency data.

There are two broad categories of injury onset that differ markedly in their etiology (15). Injuries that occur suddenly are often termed sudden impact or acute injuries and are associated with a macrotraumatic event. Examples of sudden impact injuries are fractures and sprains. Injuries that develop gradually and worsen over time are often referred to as gradual onset, overuse, or chronic injuries and are associated with repetitive microtrauma. Examples of these injury types include stress fractures and tendinitis. An injury history may actually involve both categories of injury onset, such as when an acute injury is superimposed on a chronic mechanism. However, this third injury category was not often distinguished in the epidemiologic literature on sports injuries reviewed for this book.

Examples of chronometry include time into practice, time of day, and time of season when injury occurs. The *when* of injury, expressed in terms of the activity itself, requires explanation. Activity at the time of injury may be expressed in general terms such as during practice or competition. Or, it may be reported for more specific aspects of the activity such as a rodeo event (e.g., steer wrestling, calf roping) or phase of play in volleyball (e.g., blocking and spiking). The reader needs to be careful not to confuse percentages (which are often reported in these regards) with injury rates. More injuries may occur in association with a given activity simply because more time (i.e., exposure) is spent participating in the activity. For example, in women's collegiate gymnastics 79% of injuries occurred in practice and 21% in competition. However, when rates were calculated the risk of injury was almost three times greater during competition (16).

We next direct your attention to injury outcome related to severity—or the *what* of injury. Injury severity can span a broad spectrum from abrasions to fractures, to those injuries that result in severe permanent functional disability (i.e., catastrophic injuries) or even death. In the epidemiologic literature on sports injuries, injury severity is typically indicated by one or more of the following: injury type, time loss, residual symptoms, and financial costs. With the exception of injury type, however, there is a paucity of data on injury severity and most data are presented as frequency data or as a percent of total injuries.

A breakdown of injury types is reported in most epidemiologic studies of sports injuries. Occasionally, these are combined with "location" data to provide more specific information on injuries. Although injury type is generally reported in well-recognized medical terms such as sprain or strain, you will encounter some ambiguities in reporting injury types throughout the literature. For instance, some studies may list "back pain" among the types of injury. Not only is it debatable whether the injury should be included in injury types or in injury locations, but it is equally ambiguous whether the injury was an inflammation, strain, muscle tear, or something else altogether. Comparison of injury severity data across studies is further limited by the absence of such indicators as "grade" or "degree" of injury, where applicable.

Although absence from work or school has been suggested as a meaningful indicator of time loss caused by injury (11, 25), most studies reporting time loss have used days lost from practice or competition as a measure of injury severity. These time loss data are often categorized (e.g., 1-2 days, 3-6 days) indicating degree of severity. Although the use of days lost from practice/competition may be among the more precise representations of injury severity in the literature (24), this approach is not without problems (12, 24). For example, subjective factors, such as personal motivation, peer influence, or coaching staff reluctance/encouragement, may determine if and when players return to play (24).

Perhaps the most important question one can ask related to injury severity concerns residual effects—or how permanent impairment affects the remainder of the players' lives (12). If residual symptoms are slight, they may cause the individual to modify his or her sporting level. In some cases, however, functional limitations resulting from injury may preclude further participation in sport (25). Activities of daily living may also be affected. In extreme cases, serious physical damage may result in permanent, severe functional disability such as quadriplegia (3) or death. Unfortunately, the reader will find a paucity of epidemiologic data reviewed in this book that pertain to the residual effects of injury. Most data reported were obtained from injury surveillance systems like the National Center for Catastrophic Sports Injury Research, the National Collegiate Athletic Association, and the National Electronic Injury Surveillance System. These surveillance systems report frequency, percent, and/or rate data for catastrophic and fatal injuries.

Assessment of the cost of sports injuries has also been suggested as an important measure of injury severity (11, 25). Financial costs may be either direct or indirect (25). Direct costs are those incurred in conjunction with medical treatment (e.g., treatment, medication, X rays), and indirect costs are those associated with the loss of productivity because of increased morbidity and mortality levels. Although there have been attempts to estimate these costs for a few selected sports/activities, comparison of results has been hampered by differences in health care and wage compensation systems (25).

In summary, descriptive epidemiology addresses the distribution of varying rates of injury in a specified population in relation to how many injuries occur as well as to whom, where and when they occur, and what is the outcome. In practice, the distributions of injuries have been typically reported as frequency data or as percent of total injuries. Descriptive data provide a background against which causes of injury can be probed. However, good descriptive data have led directly to suggestions for injury prevention that, once implemented, have helped to control and prevent the occurrence of severe sports injuries such as eye injuries in hockey and spinal injuries in football.

## Analytical Epidemiology

The epidemiologic approach is rooted in the assumption that injuries do not happen purely by chance (5), so an important part of sports injury epidemiology is the identification of factors that contribute to the occurrence of athletic injury. What complicates this process, however, is that many factors may play a role before the actual occurrence of the injury event. These factors (i.e., the *why*), as indicated in Figure 1.1, are commonly referred to as risk factors and have been classified as either intrinsic or extrinsic (13). Intrinsic factors are individual biological and psychosocial characteristics predisposing a person to the outcome of injury. Intrinsic factors might include (a) physical characteristics such as age, gender, somatotype, previous injury, malalignment of the lower extremities, body fat, and body size; (b) motor/functional characteristics such as strength, endurance, speed, balance, and flexibility; and (c) psychosocial/psychological characteristics such as stressful life events, anxiety, locus of control, and self-concept.

Extrinsic risk factors are factors that have an impact on the sport participant "from without." Extrinsic factors might include (a) exposure to risk in relation to playing or practice time, position on a team, level of competition, skill level, event, and phase of play or match; (b) training methods or conditions such as the coach's qualifications, individual skill, and fitness development sequencing; (c) environmental factors such as type and condition of playing surface, weather conditions, time of day of practice or performance, and time into the performance or competitive season; or (d) sport-specific equipment such as protective equipment, shoes, or clothing.

Risk factors should be seen as hypotheses (i.e., *proposed* answers to the question why injuries occur) until they have been substantiated as defensible injury predictors through correlational or experimental research. What complicates the identification and quantification of risks is that in many situations factors interact. Causes of injury usually don't lie in a single intrinsic or extrinsic factor, but in combinations of them. In a recent article, Meeuwisse (15) proposed a model that accommodates a multifactorial assessment of causation in athletic injuries. In his model intrinsic factors are viewed as factors that predispose the athlete to react in a specific manner to an injury situation.

However, once the athlete is predisposed, extrinsic or "enabling" factors may facilitate manifestation of injury. Meeuwisse (15) suggests that intrinsic and extrinsic factors may interact to make the athlete more susceptible to injury (i.e., to make the athlete "an accident waiting for a place to happen").

Much of the published analytical sports injury literature suffers from insufficient information and absence of appropriate analyses for detecting multifactorial risks. Where such analyses have been applied, statistical assumptions and power standards have often been violated, especially with respect to determining appropriate sample sizes (29). In addition, exposure patterns in injured and uninjured athletes have not been consistently identified as a basis for determining reasons for injury occurrence in study populations with representative prevalence of injury. Finally, risk factors may interact differently with the categories of injury onset (15), a possibility that was not accounted for in the analytical research reviewed. We therefore urge the reader, armed with this information, to be alert to the limitations of the risk factor analyses reviewed in the sport-specific chapters that follow. These analyses should be viewed as initial steps in the important search for predictor variables and may provide interesting characteristics for manipulation in other experimental or quasi-experimental designs.

Having addressed the *why* of analytical epidemiology, we now direct your attention to the *how* of injury (see Figure 1.1). Although risk factors may render the athlete more susceptible to injury, they are usually not sufficient for an injury to occur. Continuing with his model of the multifactorial assessment of causation in athletic injuries, Meeuwisse (15) suggests that the final element in the web of causation involves an inciting event and injury mechanism (i.e., the *how*). An inciting event is more obviously (or visually) related to injury than a risk factor and may be viewed as a precipitating factor associated with the definitive onset of an injury. For example, the inciting event for an anterior shoulder dislocation in a football quarterback may be a tackle during the windup phase of a throwing maneuver, and the injury mechanism could be an abduction/external rotation force. The quarterback may have been predisposed to this injury by his history of previous shoulder dislocation (i.e., intrinsic risk factor) and an enabling factor such as wet field conditions, which resulted in the athlete slipping and being tackled (15). Other examples of inciting events include blocking, kicking, and collision (i.e., with ball, sideline obstruction). In the literature, inciting events are often referred to as "activities" (19) or "actions" (2, 31) occurring at the time of injury. An injury mechanism characterizes the force that causes injury and may be identified as either direct impact, indirect force, torsion, stretch, impingement, overuse, shearing, or other spontaneous or insidious force (19).

With the exception of data reported by various injury surveillance systems, there are very limited data pertaining to inciting events and injury mechanisms presented in the literature. Most inciting event data are presented as frequency data or percent of total injuries. Data on injury mechanisms, on the other hand, tend to be most often reported with reference to specific injuries that have occurred. A difficulty in reporting injury mechanisms in the literature is that the magnitude and direction of the injury-causing forces cannot be reliably documented in field studies (12). Thus, the more general aspects of injury mechanisms, or inciting events, tend to be reported.

In summary, analytical epidemiology is concerned with the identification of injury determinants in a specified population. A model was reviewed that accommodates a multifactorial assessment of causation in sports injuries and that clarifies the relationship of intrinsic and extrinsic risk factors, inciting events, and injury mechanisms. Most risk factors discussed in the sport-specific chapters of this book should be viewed as hypothetical because they have not been substantiated as defensible injury predictors through correlational or experimental research.

## Prevention

Once the analytical evidence points to an association between certain risk factors and injury, thereby establishing a degree of predictability for those participants who are likely to sustain injury, the next step in epidemiologic research is to seek ways to prevent or reduce the occurrence of such injury (i.e., intervention). Testing the suggested preventive measure to determine its effectiveness is an extension of the analytical epidemiologic process and fulfills the ultimate goal of epidemiology—prevention. The effectiveness of injury prevention measures should be tested prior to recommending their general implementation (14).

The effectiveness of a preventive measure can most reliably be determined by employing an intervention study (also known as experimental study or clinical trial) in which subjects are randomly assigned to treatment and control groups (9). Two general types of intervention studies are preventive trials and therapeutic trials (9). A therapeutic trial is conducted among subjects with a particular injury to determine the ability of an agent or procedure (e.g., taping, bracing) to diminish symptoms or prevent recurrence of that injury. A preventive trial involves the evaluation of whether an agent or procedure reduces the risk of incurring injury among those free from injury at enrollment in the study. Meeuwisse (14) has described two strategies that may be adopted in this latter regard: removal of the risk factor known to cause injury and modification of the risk factors in which more than one factor has been correlated with an injury, so as to reduce injury.

In practice, there has been very little research designed to determine the effectiveness of injury prevention measures, particularly those designed to reduce risk of injury in otherwise uninjured groups. Ethical, cost, and feasibility issues no doubt combine to preclude experimental research (as in disease epidemiology). Yet, with the exception of therapeutic studies, there has also been very little quasi-experimental research designed to test the effectiveness of preventive measures. Most injury prevention strategies have emerged from clinical practice and descriptive epidemiologic research and have not been tested to determine their effectiveness.

Although not scientifically tested, however, many of the implemented preventive measures have helped to reduce sports injuries, including such catastrophic injuries as blindness in hockey and paralysis in football. Evidence for these results has typically been derived from comparisons of descriptive data and/or clinical series gleaned from periods before and after the implementation of the preventive measure. Although the institution of a preventive strategy on the basis of intuition may still prevent injury (14), the most reliable suggestions for prevention are believed to emerge from experimental or quasi-experimental research.

## Study Designs

Based on the information provided in the foregoing discussion about the components of epidemiology, the authors of the sport-specific chapters attempted to organize, analyze, and evaluate the available data in their respective subject areas according to the relative strengths of descriptive and analytical data. Sports injuries are described in the literature through a variety of study designs, including case reports, case series, cross-sectional, case-control, and prospective and retrospective cohort studies. A full discussion of epidemiologic methodology is beyond the scope of this book and detailed descriptions about epidemiologic methodology can be found in several publications (6, 9, 20, 23, 29, 30). However, we have attempted in Table 1.2 and in the discussion that follows to provide the reader with sufficient information to distinguish between design types and their major strengths and weaknesses, as well as their relationship to the discussion of Figure 1.1.

Intervention study, also referred to as experimental study or randomized controlled trial (RCT), is generally acknowledged as the strongest design in clinical epidemiology because it reduces problems of bias and confounding that affect the power of nonrandomized designs (5, 6, 29). In this design, risk factors are controlled by randomly assigning subjects (or teams) to one of two exposure groups: a treatment group and a control group. Control group members differ from the experimental group only in their nonexposure to the preventive measure. Groups are typically followed prospectively to determine any differences in injury occurrence that may be attributed to the intervention agent or procedure. This study design is thus capable of generating both descriptive and analytical data. In practice, intervention studies, particularly preventive trials, have been infrequently used to study a proposed means of prevention or a hypothesized cause of injury.

Well-conducted cohort studies are the next best design to experiments because they can be conducted to minimize the effects of selection and measurement biases, as well as known confounding biases (6). The strongest of these designs, the prospective cohort design, consists of subjects assembled at baseline and measured on variables believed to be related to injury (i.e., risk factors). The group is then followed prospectively for a period of time during which the occurrence of injury and (ideally) exposure is monitored and recorded. After follow-up is completed injury data may be analyzed for both descriptive and analytical results. In practice, most prospective cohort studies have been descriptive in nature and have not attempted to identify injury determinants or test the effectiveness of preventive agents or measures.

Sometimes the research question may require an immediate answer, which the prospective cohort design cannot provide. In this case, the retrospective cohort study may be used. Like the prospective cohort design, subjects are assembled at baseline and measured on variables that are believed to be related to injury (i.e., risk factors). Unlike the prospective design, these cohorts have already been exposed to the risk of injury prior to the study, and injuries have already been incurred by some of them sometime in the past. Thus, data are collected retrospectively and subsequently analyzed for both descriptive and analytical results.

In practice, the retrospective design appears frequently in the literature, and like the prospective design, it can be used to generate both descriptive and analytical data; however, it has been used most often as a descriptive study design. It is often used in conjunction with other study designs, for example prospective and cross-sectional studies, to collect injury history information.

In the case-control design, a case group or series of injured athletes and a control group of uninjured athletes are selected. Information regarding prior exposure to risk factors is then established retrospectively. Any difference in the distributions of these variables between the two groups would indirectly suggest potential risk factors for injury. Thus, the primary purpose of this design is to generate analytical data. In practice, the case-control study has been the least frequently used design to study the association between risk factors and sports injury occurrence (29).

In cross-sectional designs the investigator collects information on injury status and risk factors at one point in time. Most cross-sectional studies have been descriptive in nature and have attempted to generate prevalence rate estimates for particular injury types, or for proportions of various injury types and locations. Some cross-sectional studies have assumed an analytical posture but have met with limited success in providing evidence for a cause-and-effect relationship because they provide no direct evidence of the sequence of events (6).

As indicated in Table 1.2, all of the foregoing observational designs possess some degree of fallibility, yet they effectively estimate three kinds of risk or rate values—absolute risk of injury (prospective cohort), relative risk of injury (retrospective cohort and case-control designs), and prevalence rate at a given time (cross-sectional studies) (29). As denominator-based designs they possess greater strength than numerator-based designs, which provide only frequency data.

Case reports and case series are numerator based; they describe what has happened to an individual or a group of individuals who share a common eventuality, such as incurring injury. Unlike denominator-based studies, case reports and case

**Table 1.2    A Comparison of Study Designs Used in Sports Injury Research**

| Study design | Strengths | Weaknesses |
| --- | --- | --- |
| Randomized controlled trial (RCT) | • Provides the strongest epidemiologic evidence of a cause-effect relationship.<br>• Investigator controls randomized grouping.<br>• Investigator controls exposure to or exclusion from a potentially beneficial agent or experience.<br>• Most statistical tests rest on the assumption of random allocation.<br>• Confounding variables can be balanced between groups, thus allowing comparable groups.<br>• Blindness can be maintained. | • Costs time and money.<br>• Some bias through self-selection, if volunteers are used.<br>• Subject to considerations of feasibility and ethics. |
| Prospective cohort | • Easier and less costly to administer than RCT.<br>• Data collection moves forward in time thereby establishing a sequence of events between risk factor(s) and injury.<br>• Injury rates can be calculated because the design involves both numerator and denominator populations.<br>• Investigator controls selection of subjects and measurements.<br>• Confounding variables can be balanced between groups, thus allowing for comparable groups.<br>• Can evaluate a range of potential risk factors simultaneously. | • Requires large sample sizes.<br>• Time consuming and expensive relative to other analytical designs.<br>• Because of lack of randomization some statistical tests cannot be used.<br>• May be difficult to achieve or maintain blindness.<br>• Large sample sizes and follow-up periods are needed for studying rare sports injuries.<br>• Susceptible to subject mortality. |
| Retrospective cohort | • Injury rates can be calculated because the design involves both numerator and denominator populations.<br>• Easier and less costly to administer than prospective cohort design.<br>• Can evaluate a range of potential risk factors simultaneously. | • Relies on adequacy of records.<br>• Selection and recall bias.<br>• Difficult to establish sequence of events between risk factor(s) and injury (especially for gradual onset injuries) because data are collected from past records or from recall.<br>• Confounding variables are likely. |
| Case-control | • Relatively less time consuming and less costly than cohort and RCT designs.<br>• Applicability for studying rare sports injuries, or situations in which considerable time has elapsed between exposure and outcome.<br>• Fewer subjects are needed for this design than for cross-sectional study design.<br>• Relative sizes of injured and uninjured samples of subjects can be balanced to improve the power of the study.<br>• Can evaluate a range of potential risk factors simultaneously. | • Relies on adequacy of records.<br>• Selection and recall bias.<br>• Difficult to establish sequence of events between risk factor(s) and injury (especially for gradual onset injuries).<br>• Confounding variables are likely.<br>• May be difficult to find appropriate control group after selection of cases.<br>• Limited to one outcome variable.<br>• Does not yield prevalence or incidence; however, relative risk can be estimated.<br>• Inefficient design for studying rare risk factors unless the study is very large or the attributable risk percent is high (i.e., the risk factor is characteristic of those who are injured). |
| Cross-sectional | • Data collection can be completed in a relatively short period of time.<br>• Investigator controls selection of subjects and measurements.<br>• No one is subjected to a potentially rewarding or harmful agent or experience.<br>• Several risk factors may be studied simultaneously.<br>• Prevalence rates can be determined. | • Only injuries actually present at the time of the survey are registered; thus data are not representative of all injuries in the population.<br>• Does not establish sequence of events between risk factor(s) and injury.<br>• Cannot test etiologic hypotheses.<br>• Cannot always control group size, resulting in inferior statistical power.<br>• Does not yield incidence rates.<br>• Not feasible for rare conditions. |
| Case series/case report | • Relatively easy to carry out, because most of the data collection relies on clinical records.<br>• Provides an estimate of relative frequency of injuries.<br>• Provides an estimate of morbidity load on a clinic. | • Lack of adequate comparison group (i.e., population at risk).<br>• Reported injuries do not necessarily represent complete injury picture.<br>• Cannot be used to identify high-risk athletes or to detect factors that increase the risk of injury. |

series provide no information on the population at risk and therefore cannot be used to generate incidence rates or to test hypotheses on the cause of injury. However, these numerator-based designs can provide descriptive information on the relative frequencies as they apply to the *who, when, where,* and *what.* They are also important designs for identifying the presence or coming of a new disease or condition (injury) and can lead to the formulation of hypotheses concerning possible risk factors (9).

## Organization of the Sport-Specific Chapters

Our text is an outgrowth of the early pioneering work of the Research Committee for the American Orthopedic Society for Sports Medicine (21) and represents the first account of the epidemiologic picture on injuries across a spectrum of sports. With the exception of this introductory chapter and the two concluding chapters, which generalize suggestions for injury prevention and further research across sports, the 24 sport-specific chapters follow the same outline and approach to reviewing the literature. By following the same outline, authors molded their discussions into a common presentation that contributed to a uniform language and conceptualization of data across the chapters. Authors generally distinguished between design types in the tables and discussion to avoid any inappropriate inferences.

A brief orientation to the components of the outline, which every sport-specific chapter follows, is presented below. Depending on the availability of data in each sport-specific body of literature, some chapters include additional subsections, such as injury rates in practice versus competition and reinjury rates. It was not possible to organize the chapters precisely according to the epidemiologic process presented in Figure 1.1 because some elements (e.g., inciting factors) could not be categorically addressed because of paucity of data. Chapter length had to be restricted to stay within the publisher's allotted total number of pages, which limited some authors. Great effort has been made, however, to arrange all of the available information in an efficient and consistent manner as outlined below.

### 1. Introduction

Each sport-specific chapter begins with an introduction in which authors generally provide the reader with the following information:

- A statement of the research problem (what is being reviewed, who is the population of interest, and what is the purpose)
- A brief description of the search methods that were used for the research review
- An indication of the time period addressed by the computer search(es) and key words used to guide the search
- A succinct comment on the limitations of the studies reviewed to alert the reader to the level of evidence associated with the data gleaned from the research

### 2. Incidence of Injury

### 2.1 Injury Rates

Availability of data permitting, injury rate information is shown in the tables by level of competition or age. Information related to injury rates would typically be derived from prospective and retrospective data. The following information, when available, has been included in the tables:

- Study design
- Data collection methods
- Duration of study
- Number of participants
- Number of injuries
- Injury rates

### 3. Injury Characteristics

### 3.1 Injury Onset

In this section authors comment briefly on injury onset that is typical of injuries in their sport-specific chapter. In some sports, there were sufficient data to illustrate the proportion (%) of, say, chronic to acute injuries.

### 3.2 Injury Type

Information related to injury types is typically derived from prospective and retrospective studies and represented in a table as percent of the total number of injuries. However, in some sports a number of relatively large case series and cross-sectional studies have been conducted that provide useful data on injury types. These data may appear in some of the chapters and are usually reported as a percent of the total number of injuries. Where appropriate, injury mechanism (i.e., how injury occurs) is briefly discussed with reference to various injury types.

### 3.3 Injury Location

Information related to injury location, or anatomical site, is typically derived from prospective and retrospective studies and presented as a percent of the total number of injuries. Similar to Section 3.2, data from studies with other design types (i.e., cross-sectional or case series) may also appear in the tables and discussion if these are reported as a percent of the total number of injuries.

3.3.1 Head/Spine/Trunk

3.3.2 Upper Extremity

3.3.3 Lower Extremity

Information related to specific injury types occurring in the above body regions is typically derived from case reports, case series, and cross-sectional data on injuries. In some chapters, however, the literature search resulted in so many case reports on same or similar injuries that some authors elected to refer the reader to them rather than to present them in the tables. As in Section 3.2, where appropriate, injury mechanism with reference to specific injury locations is briefly discussed in some of the chapters.

4. Injury Severity

Depending on availability of data, this section provides an opportunity to discuss injury severity in terms of time loss, catastrophic injury, and/or clinical outcome or residual symptoms. The discussion of these indicators of injury severity is based on data derived from all studies regardless of research design and often includes comments on injury mechanism.

5. Injury Risk Factors

The discussion of risk factors purports to answer "why injury occurs." In the absence of analytical data, which is the present reality in most of the sports injury literature, many authors ruminate about the role of injury risk factors that may have arisen from the descriptive data reviewed in Sections 1 through 4 or other pertinent research (e.g., biomechanical). Throughout the discussion, an attempt has been made to identify the level of evidence underlying each proposed risk factor so the reader can judge how much weight to assign to the findings as they presently stand.

5.1 Intrinsic Factors

5.2 Extrinsic Factors

6. Suggestions for Injury Prevention

This section is organized under the following subheadings suggested by Adrian's "Action Model to Evaluate and Reduce Risk of Catastrophic Injuries" (1). Most of the sport-specific chapters were able to adhere to this structure.

6.1 Players

6.2 Sport

6.3 External Environment

6.4 Health Support System

Authors attempted to limit their discussions of proposed suggestions for injury prevention to those gleaned from the data presented throughout their chapters, particularly from Section 5 on "Injury Risk Factors." However, since most of the epidemiologic literature on sports injuries is descriptive in nature, it follows that most of the suggestions for injury prevention that are gleaned from the literature are unfortunately not derived from an analytical evaluation of risk factors. Even fewer injury prevention suggestions will have been evaluated as to their effectiveness in preventing injury.

7. Suggestions for Further Research

This is an important section because informed decisions regarding injury prevention depend ultimately on quality research. The section begins with a discussion of the authors' suggestions about injury definition, study population, study design data collection methods, and research team. This is followed by suggestions for further research, which are presented in paragraph or table format, whichever works best for the individual chapter, and are generally derived from the preceding chapter sections, from injury rates to injury prevention.

## Concluding Comment

The epidemiology of sports injuries is still emerging. Although still in its infancy in some sport disciplines, as a field of research endeavor it is perhaps in its adolescence. As such, the epidemiology of sports injuries has grasped the principles of what is expected of it, but is yet grappling somewhat self-consciously with its awkwardness and clumsy mistakes. We are confident, however, that sports injury epidemiology will continue to scrutinize its present limitations and will ultimately attain the poise of a mature discipline. In that vein, this book represents both the product of the current state of sports injury epidemiology and a part of the process that may enable it to one day provide definitive answers.

## References

1. Adrian, M. Action model to evaluate and reduce risk of catastrophic injuries. In: Adams, S; Adrian, M.J.; Bayless, M.A., eds. Catastrophic injuries in sports: avoidance strategies. 2nd ed. Indianapolis: Benchmark Press; 1987:243-249.

2. Big Ten Injury Reporting System. Am. J. Sports Med. 16:S169-S221; 1988.

3. Cantu, R.C. Catastrophic injuries in high school and college athletes. Surg. Rounds Orthop. 2(11):62-66; 1988.

4. Cooper, H.M. Integrating research. A guide for literature reviews. 2nd ed. Newbury Park, CA: Sage Publication; 1988.

5. Duncan, D.F. Epidemiology. Basis for disease prevention and health promotion. New York: Macmillan; 1988.

6. Fletcher, R.H.; Fletcher, S.W.; Wagner, E.H. Clinical epidemiology: the essentials. 2nd ed. Baltimore: Williams & Wilkins; 1988.

7. Gordon, J.E. The epidemiology of accidents. Am. J. Public Health. 39:504-515; 1949.

8. Haddon, W.; Ellison, A.E.; Carroll, R.E. Skiing injuries. Public Health Rep. 77: 975-985; 1962.

9. Hennekens, C.H.; Buring, J.E. Epidemiology in medicine. Boston: Little, Brown; 1987.

10. Hunter, R. E.; Levi, M. Vignettes. In: Noyes, F.R.; Albright, J.P., eds. Sports injury research. Am. J. Sports Med. 16:S25-S37; 1988.

11. Keller, C.S.; Noyes, F.R. The medical aspects of soccer epidemiology. Am. J. Sports Med. 16:S105-S112; 1988.

12. Lindenfeld, T.N.; Noyes, F.R.; Marshall, M.T. Components of injury reporting systems. In: Noyes, F.R.; Albright, J.P., eds. Sports injury research. Am. J. Sports Med. 16:S69-S80; 1988.

13. Lysens, R.; Steverlynck, A.; van den Auweele, Y.; Lefevre, J.; Renson, L.; Claessens, A.; Ostyn, M. The predictability of sports injuries. Sports Med. 1:6-10; 1984.

14. Meeuwisse, W.H. Predictability of sports injuries. What is the epidemiological evidence? Sports Med. 12(1):8-15; 1991.

15. Meeuwisse, W.H. Assessing causation in sport injury: a multifactorial model. Clin. J. Sports Med. 4:166-170; 1994.

16. National Collegiate Athletic Association 1993-94 Men's and Women's Gymnastics Injury Surveillance System. Kansas City: NCAA Report; 1994.

17. Oxman, A.D.; Guyatt, G.H. Guidelines for reading literature reviews. Can. Med. Assoc. J. 138:697; 1988.

18. Powell, K.E.; Kohl, H.W.; Caspersen, C.J.; Blair, S.N. An epidemiological perspective on the causes of running injuries. Physician Sportsmed. 14(6):100-114; 1986.

19. Powell, J.W. National high school athletic injury registry. Am. J. Sports Med. 16: S134-S166; 1988.

20. Powell, J.W. Epidemiologic research for injury prevention programs in sports. In: Mueller, F.O.; Ryan, A.J., eds. Prevention of athletic injuries: the role of the sports medicine team. Philadelphia: Davis; 1991.

21. Research Committee for the American Orthopedic Society for Sports Medicine. Sports injury research. Am. J. Sports Med. 16 (Suppl. 1); 1988.

22. Sackett, D.L.; Haynes, R.B.; Guyatt, G.H.; Tugwell, P. Clinical epidemiology. A basic science for clinical medicine. 2nd ed. Boston: Little, Brown; 1991.

23. Schootman, M.; Powell, J.W.; Torner, J.C. Study designs and potential biases in sports injury research. The case-control study. Sports Med. 18(1):22-37; 1994.

24. Thompson, N.; Halpern, B.; Curl, W.W.; Andrews, J.R.; Hunter, S.C.; McLeod, W.D. High school football injuries. Am. J. Sports Med. 16:S97-S104; 1988.

25. Van Mechelen, W.; Hlobil, H.; Kemper, C.G. Incidence, severity, aetiology and prevention of sport injuries. A review of concepts. Sports Med. 14(2):82-89; 1992.

26. Wade, C.E. What is the question? In: Noyes, F.R.; Albright, J.P., eds. Sports injury research. Am. J. Sports Med. 16(Suppl. 1):38-42; 1988.

27. Wallace, R.B. Application of epidemiologic principles to sports injury research. In: Noyes, F.R.; Albright, J.P., eds. Sports injury research. Am. J. Sports Med. 16(Suppl. 1):22-24; 1988.

28. Wallace, R.B.; Clarke, W.R. The numerator, denominator, and population-at-risk. In: Noyes, F.R.; Albright, J.P., eds. Sports injury research. Am. J. Sports Med. 16(Suppl. 1):55-56; 1988.

29. Walter, S.D.; Hart, L.E. Application of epidemiological methodology in sports and exercise science research. In: Pandolf, K.B.; Holloszy, J.O., eds. Exercise and sports science reviews (Number 18). Baltimore: Williams & Wilkins; 1990:417-488.

30. Walter, S.D.; Sutton, J.R.; McIntosh, J.M.; Connelly, C. The aetiology of sport injuries. A review of methodologies. Sports Med. 2:47-58; 1985.

31. Yale Athletic Reporting System. Am. J. Sports Med. 16:S167-S168; 1988.

32. Zemper, E.D. Epidemiology of athletic injuries. In: McKeag, D.B.; Hough, D.; Zemper, E.D., eds. Primary care sports medicine. Dubuque, IA: Brown & Benchmark; 1993:63-73.

# 2

# Adult Recreational Fitness

*Ralph K. Requa and James G. Garrick*

## 1. Introduction

It is generally accepted that one can enhance health by regularly engaging in almost any type of fitness activity. Adults are encouraged to increase their levels of physical activity to benefit their cardiovascular health as well as their general fitness, physical appearance, and mental attitude. And whereas attention is directed toward the safety of exercise from a cardiac-risk standpoint, substantially less has been written about the musculoskeletal (injury) consequences of many common recreational/fitness activities.

Thus, for many of the activities that take place regularly in health and fitness facilities across the country, it is difficult to weigh the potential benefits against the risks of participation, for the risks have not been measured. Enthusiasts, physicians, and fitness professionals alike could benefit from information about the relative risks of using stationary bicycles, free weights, weight machines, and stair climbers and of participating in some of the newer variations of established fitness activities, such as step- and low-impact aerobics.

The omission of comparative risk is in large part the result of few investigations into the injury consequences of participation in many adult fitness activities. For some, such as running, skiing, cycling, and aerobic dance, there is information available (1-8). Many popular activities, however, take place in unsupervised, unstructured settings and have largely escaped study.

Comparisons between studies, even if each is well done, are difficult due to differing study populations and injury definitions. A single prospective approach that follows a large group of participants through a variety of exposures allows comparisons to be made; whatever definitional, population, case ascertainment, and classification biases exist should at least be constant across activities.

A large group of adult fitness participants were followed, using consistent methods and definitions of injury, in order to document the consequences of adult fitness activities in active exercisers. Physicians prescribing exercise or fitness enhancement programs for their adult patients may find such information useful.

### 1.1 Sample

Participants were recruited from 15 San Francisco Bay Area fitness clubs and exercise studios through fitness personnel and direct in-facility recruitment. The focus of the study was the active recreational participant. In order to participate, volunteers had to engage in aerobic dance for at least three sessions of at least 45 minutes each week or perform more than one major fitness activity for at least four times a week in sessions of at least 45 minutes.

As an inducement to sign up and continue to participate, those that continued to participate for the full 12 weeks were eligible to enter a drawing, held at the close of the study, for prizes consisting of pairs of shoes and sports-gear bags.

Prospective documentation of injuries occurring in a large group of recreational participants has several clear advantages over surveillance of a single sport or activity. Beginning with a large group of active adults makes it possible to examine a wide variety of both organized and unorganized recreational activities. More importantly, injury rates arising from these various activities can be meaningfully compared.

This population may not be typical of all adult recreational athletes. The members of this population were relatively young, healthy, and able to pay for club memberships. Because of club memberships, some activities that take place outside organized fitness facilities may be less frequent (e.g., cycling, hiking, tennis, golf, etc.) than in an active population not characterized by fitness club membership. At the same time it seems unlikely that the nature of this group's participation in outside activities would be radically different from that of nonclub members.

Because the study was not based on a season or period of time when participants were beginning a new activity, it also avoided the period in which the highest injury rates are often observed. To the extent that this is true, the overall injury rates may better reflect on-going activities rather than start-up activities, and they may be somewhat lower than would otherwise be the case.

The sample was voluntary; participants had to agree to take part in the study and also to be interviewed on a regular basis. This favors cooperative people who were willing to report on their experience. This sample might also have tended to favor those with some interest in sports injuries, perhaps those who already had experienced an injury. The extent to which this may have skewed the selection of the entire sample is unknown but seems unlikely to have had a major effect, given that the rates of previous injury are not particularly high.

The participants had to state that they met the participation rule noted above, so it is likely their activity levels may be somewhat higher than a group selected with no activity level requirement. In addition, because of the weekly phone calls, anecdotal evidence suggests that activity levels, particularly for the less active, may have been encouraged. More than one participant apologized for their levels of participation in one week or another.

How well the sample represents typical active recreational participants is unknown.

## 1.2 Data Collection

In addition to fulfilling these activity level criteria, participants agreed to a weekly telephone contact to document both athletic activities and injuries. Trained telephone interviewers phoned the volunteers and recorded all recreational and sports activity for the week, the amount of time involved, and any injuries that occurred.

Enrollment data included age, gender, prior physical activity, history of orthopaedic limitations, and previous injuries. Weekly data collected included nature and duration of physical activity and any injury or complaint. For an injury or complaint, the onset, severity, location, description, treatment, time-loss days, and relation of exercise activity to injury were recorded.

## 1.3 Data Validation

To evaluate the validity of injury information acquired by telephone, the first 35 injuries reported and classified by the interviewers were examined in detail. Ten participants were either seen by a physician (and thus were by definition correctly classified) or their injuries were obvious (e.g., minor contusion). The 25 other injured participants were interviewed in person by an athletic trainer. In 22 of 25 cases the anatomic/pathologic classifications were completely unchanged; in the remaining 3 the athletic trainer was able to glean additional detail through face-to-face conversations. A "forearm strain," for example, upon examination was further classified as a wrist flexor strain. There were no significant discrepancies between the diagnostic codes assigned by the telephone interviewers versus the athletic trainer. The athletic trainer talked to about three quarters of the participants (> 300) reporting injuries or complaints over the telephone and reviewed all of the injury forms. At the request of the interviewers, the athletic trainer also met with 12 injured participants whose symptoms could not be satisfactorily resolved over the telephone.

Using telephone interviewers to gather the major part of the injury information suggests the possibility of a certain lack of precision in injury classification. In fact an initial comparison suggests just the opposite. We found no anatomic/pathologic "errors," which suggests that the general accuracy of the data is acceptable. We encouraged each individual to continue participation in the study for 12 weeks although some elected to withdraw before that time.

## 1.4 Definition of Injury and Severity

Injury and injury severity were defined by the impact that they had on a person's activity level (see Table 2.1).

A given injury may have varying levels of severity at different times. There were four levels of severity ranging from a significant complaint (one that does not interfere with a participant's activities) to an injury that renders a participant unable to do his or her fitness activities and, in addition, interferes with daily living (e.g., requires the use

**Table 2.1   Injury Definition**

| Level | Time lost? | Description |
|-------|-----------|-------------|
| Level I | No | Injury or pain *not* affecting sport and fitness activities |
| Level II | Yes | Injury or pain resulting in *modifying* duration or intensity of sport and fitness activities |
| Level III | Yes | Injury or pain resulting in *missing* part or all of any sport and fitness activity |
| Level IV | Yes | Injury or pain resulting in *missing* part or all of any sport and fitness activity and in alterations in daily life (e.g., crutches) |

of crutches). Whether medical care was sought is also a measure of severity and was noted. In addition to recording the number of days of activity affected at each level of severity for each injury, each injury was also assigned an overall level of severity equal to the highest level attained throughout its course.

To provide some comparison between our study and others, we can place some injury rates in a similar context by comparing time-loss injuries among our runners using a similar definition to that used by Koplan and associates (4). They noted that more than one third of their sample cited an injury that at least diminished mileage over a year of running. Our definition of time-loss injuries, those which altered or stopped participation, was similar. The rate of time-loss injury among our participants who ran was 10.79/1,000 hours or 43.3/100 study-person-years, slightly higher than that noted by Koplan et al. Our study participants may have differed from runners selected from participants in a road race, since we required our subjects to engage in more than one major fitness activity. Few participated regularly in road races. Whether this had an effect on their rate of injury is not known. Even so, the comparison shows that the rates obtained from recreational runners with our methodology did not differ substantially from those obtained over 10 years ago from a completely different technique, a questionnaire survey of 10K-race participants.

Our definition of injury distinguished between an action of the participant due to an injury (e.g., altered or missed activity due to a flare-up of a chronic condition) versus an action taken simply as a result of the participant's choice (e.g., stopped

or modified an activity due to fear of injury). Missing or altering sports participation had to be due to a new injury or flare-up on an old injury to qualify as a reportable time-loss injury event.

The easy availability of multiple activities, as well as variations within activities such as aerobic dance, means that these data should be viewed from a somewhat different perspective than one employs when looking at the conventional, single-sport epidemiologic study. Here, it was normal for the participants' athletic activities to vary from week to week. Unlike members of a football or gymnastic team, the participants in this investigation were neither rigidly supervised or coached, nor were they held accountable for performing specific athletic tasks. With a myriad of different activities available, these tasks could be altered according to the participant's health or preferences on any given day.

In the traditional sport environment, *time loss* means the inability to perform the tasks associated with the activity (e.g., the inability to run, throw, or catch the football) and some sort of *time loss* is usually reflected in the definition of an *injury*. In this group, because of the mixed activities, the inability to perform a specific task because of an injury may have meant only the cessation or alteration of that one activity. Applying the definition of an injury and accounting for time loss becomes somewhat more complicated with many activities involved. Indeed, the common pattern of engaging in specific activities only one, two, or three times throughout the week reduces the possibility of having a one-day time-loss injury. While this type of participation presents challenges from the standpoint of precisely accounting for participation and time loss, it may well have benefited the participants.

## 2. Incidence of Injury

### 2.1 Injury Rates

The sample was taken from 1,089 recreational athletes who filled out an initial enrollment form. Eighteen elected not to participate when first contacted by telephone, 32 were disqualified (had a current injury, too few workouts per week, enrolled too late to participate, had moved out of the area, etc.), and 53 were never enrolled (lived out of town, could not be reached by phone, etc.) leaving 986 who were enrolled. Subjects engaged in 10,582 weeks of activity, for an average of 10.7 weeks per participant (Table 2.2).

**Table 2.2  Total Hours of Participation by Type of Activity**

| Activity/sport | Activity-specific person-totals | Hours |
|---|---|---|
| For entire population | 6,650 | 60,629.40 |
| Aerobic dance | 999 | 13,599.94 |
| Class - dance - other | 119 | 980.82 |
| Class - yoga | 39 | 416.67 |
| Class - other | 165 | 1,076.63 |
| Cycles | 566 | 3.386.77 |
| Cross-country skiing exercise equipment | 39 | 214.72 |
| Rowing machines | 153 | 566.50 |
| Stair climbing | 651 | 5,423.72 |
| Treadmills | 279 | 1,100.50 |
| Other cardiovascular equipment | 12 | 31.00 |
| Free weights | 528 | 8,459.35 |
| Cybex™ | 211 | 1,329.38 |
| Nautilus™ | 272 | 2,141.42 |
| Pyramid™ | 9 | 36.78 |
| Universal™ | 42 | 135.97 |
| Bodymaster™ | 8 | 53.90 |
| Polaris™ | 79 | 335.83 |
| Gravitron™ | 74 | 115.53 |
| Weight work, misc | 23 | 195.10 |
| Individual-cycling | 254 | 2,164.65 |
| Individual-roller skating | 30 | 143.25 |
| Individual-running | 413 | 4,818.18 |
| Individual-skiing - Alpine | 157 | 2,182.32 |
| Individual-walking | 474 | 3,982.52 |
| Individual-all other | 668 | 3,799.12 |
| Team-basketball | 98 | 1,310.68 |
| Team-racquetball | 58 | 428.58 |
| Team-tennis | 104 | 1,163.33 |
| Team-other | 126 | 1,036.25 |

The various forms of aerobic dance were the most popular activity, with over 13,000 hours. Free weights, stair climbing, and stationary bicycles (mostly Life Cycles) were also very popular. Stairmaster and Life Cycles were the most popular specific pieces of exercise equipment used. Running represented the most hours for individual activities outside the fitness facilities. Within the general category of aerobic dance, the original form of aerobic dance (now often referred to as *high impact*) was the favorite, followed by *step* and *low impact* aerobics. The participants averaged seven to eight different activities each. Some accumulated as many as 25 different activities throughout the study period.

## 2.2 Injury Rates

The rates for all injuries (time loss and complaints) and time-loss injuries were 7.83 and 5.92/1,000 hours of activity, or 2.33 and 1.76 injuries per year, based on the observed average hours per week (5.73 hours/week × 52). Time loss injuries (≥ Level II) made up about three quarters of all injuries or complaints. Among time-loss injuries, one quarter (23.7%) altered participation, almost two thirds (64.9%) stopped participation, and 11.4% stopped participation and altered the activities of daily life.

## 2.3 Injury Rates by Major Categories of Activity

Team/competitive activities had the highest overall and time-loss rates of injury, followed by individual recreation, strength exercise equipment, dance/aerobic dance, and aerobic fitness exercise equipment, that is, cardiovascular exercise equipment (exercise bicycles, NordicTrac, etc; Figure 2.1).

The rates for time-loss injuries and complaints in activity categories with more than 250 hours (Figure 2.2) were highest for team sports (basketball); intermediate for running and aerobic dance; and lowest for exercise cycling, exercise walking, and calisthenics. Injury rates varied by the form of aerobic dance; dance-style aerobics (jazz, funk) had higher rates compared to other forms of aerobics (all injuries = 19.47 vs. 4.98, $p < .05$; time-loss injuries = 12.03 vs. 3.81, $p < .05$).

Individual recreation activities varied and included everything from mountaineering, jogging, swimming, and walking to wind surfing and scuba diving. Competitive activities such as lacrosse, rugby, squash, water polo, and Frisbee were included, but each had fewer than 250 hours of participation. Rugby and lacrosse stood out among team sports as both had rates of about 60/1,000 hours activity for all and 30/1,000 hours activity for time-loss injuries. Together their rates were 3 to 4 times higher than the combined team-sport rates ($p < .05$), although together they had fewer than 175 hours of participation.

## 2.4. Age and Gender

The majority of our participants were in their 20s and 30s. Fewer than 20 were under age 20 (17 years was the youngest). The median age was 32, although over 150 participants were in their 40s and almost 60 were over 50 years of age (76 was the oldest). There were slightly more women in our sample (58%, 568) than men (42%, 418).

Rates for complaints appear relatively constant for males and females across age groups (Figure

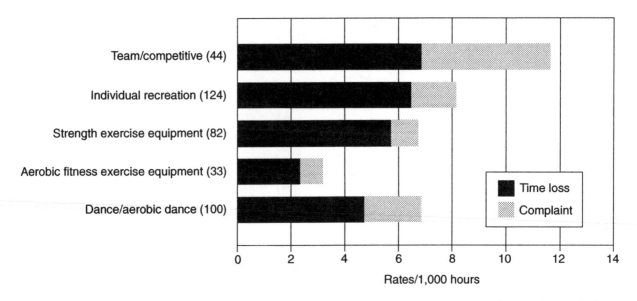

**Figure 2.1**   Injury rates and time loss by category.

2.3). Rates for injuries were indistinguishable in age 29 and under, but for ages 30 to 39, the male rate was 64% higher (8.43 vs. 5.15, $p < .05$). While the rates appear to decrease slightly for males beyond the 30 to 39 group, staying higher than the females, there were no significant differences beyond ages 30 to 39.

### 2.5 Reinjury Rates

#### 2.5.1 History

A condition of enrollment was that an existing injury did not significantly interfere with participation, although an existing stable limitation did not preclude participation. Almost 75% of the participants had one or more "previous significant injuries" (70.6%, 696 of 986). Two or more sites were checked by 43%, and almost 1 in 10 checked five or more locations (83 participants). Ten anatomic areas were each checked "yes" for a previous injury more than 5% of the time (Figure 2.4). The knee was the clear leader, with almost one third of the participants indicating a previous injury to that area.

#### 2.5.2 Previous Injury

Rates were calculated for injuries to the five most common specific areas, comparing those with and without a history of injury to that particular location of the body. Rates of occurrence for these five locations for both groups can be seen in Figure 2.5. Those who gave a positive history of injury for a particular area were about twice as likely to sustain

an injury during the study than those with a negative history. This appears to be true for both complaints and time-loss injuries. These differences are significant, $p < .05$, with the exception of those occurring to the lower leg and time-loss injuries at the ankle.

Looking at specific activities in this way is more difficult because relatively few injuries occur to any single area in any one activity. Running is one exception; it had over 71 injuries, and many occurred to a single area, the knee. Those with a positive history of previous injury to the knee had a threefold higher rate of time-loss knee injury during the study (5.88 vs. 1.83, $p < 0.05$). However, because the rates of complaint were similar (1.96 vs. 2.13), the overall rate was only 2 times higher for those with a positive history (7.83 vs. 3.96, $p < .05$) (see Figure 2.6).

## 3. Injury Characteristics

### 3.1 Injury Onset

Onset will be described in relation to type and location of injury after we have discussed injury type.

### 3.2 Injury Type

The five most common types of injury are listed in Table 2.3.

#### 3.2.1 Type by Severity

The percentage of each type of injury that resulted in time loss varied from 69% for "pain-ache" injuries to 90% for strains. Another measure of

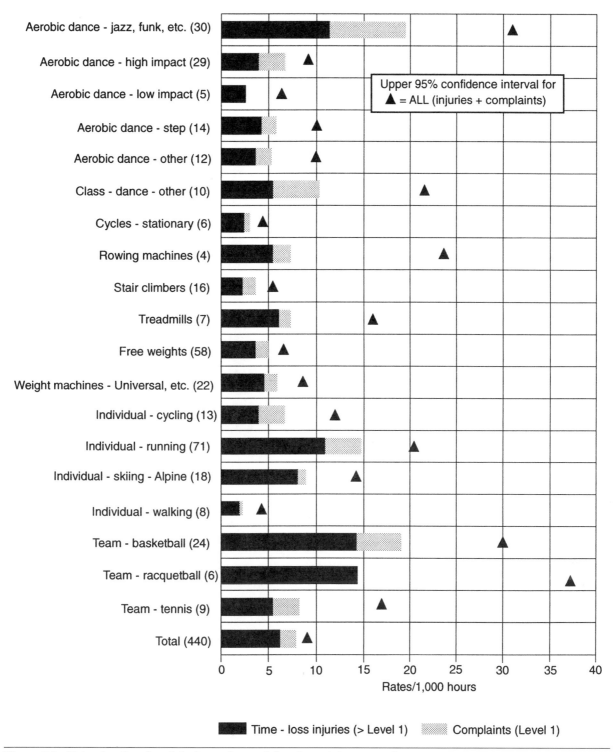

**Figure 2.2**    Rates for time-loss injuries and complaints in activity categories.

severity is the need for medical care, that is, whether an injury resulted in the participant consulting a physician. While only 2% of the strain and 3% of the pain-ache classifications resulted in a physician visit, the figure rose to more than one in four for sprains (28%).

### 3.2.2 Type by Activity

Activity groups differed somewhat in their injury rates by type of injury (Figure 2.7). Team/competitive sports led in every category except for pain-ache, where it ranked third. Individual recreation were second highest in other, pain-ache, and

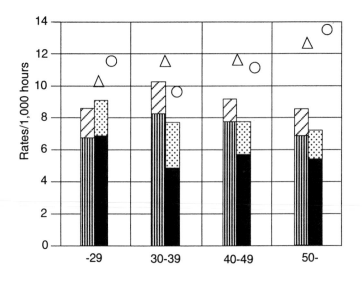

**Figure 2.3**    Rates for complaints and injuries by age groups and gender.

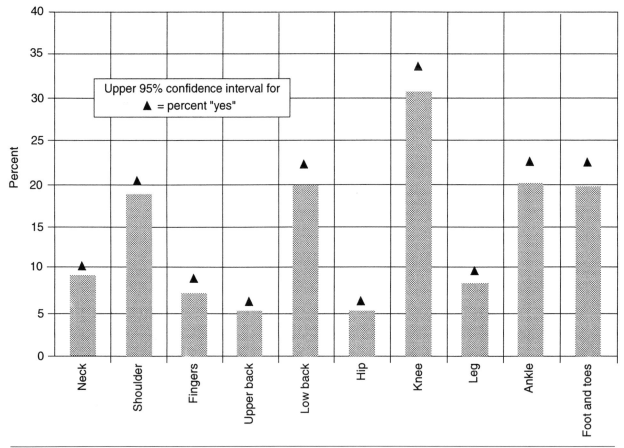

**Figure 2.4**    Percent of anatomic areas with positive history of previous injury (greater than 5%). $N = 986$. *Note.* Each area is independent; survey participants checked as many areas as they wished.

contusion categories, whereas strength exercise equipment activities were second highest in strain/inflammation and sprain categories. Aerobic fitness exercise equipment activities ranked lowest in all but the pain-ache and contusion categories, where it ranked next to lowest. Dance and aerobic dance was intermediate for most types of injury, but led in the rate of pain-ache.

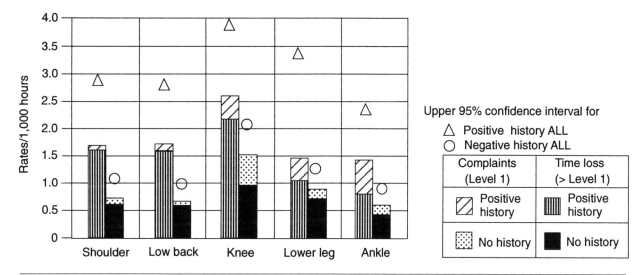

**Figure 2.5**  Time-loss and complaint rates by history of previous injury.

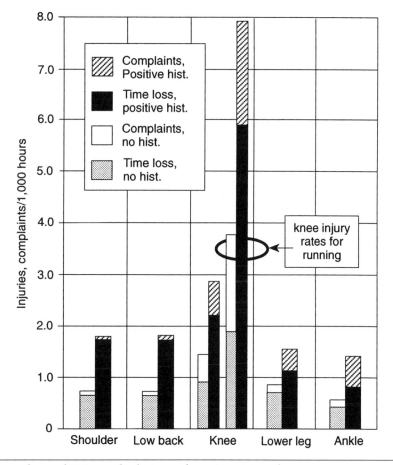

**Figure 2.6**  Time-loss and complaint rates by history of previous injury for runners.

### 3.2.3 Type by Onset

Comparing the injuries in terms of their onset, over 80% of the sprains and contusions, just over half of the strains, and about one quarter of the inflammations and pain-aches were acute.

## 3.3 Injury Location

### 3.3.1 Percent Comparison of Injury Locations

The knee led all other areas with almost 25% of the injuries (Figure 2.8). The shoulder, lower back,

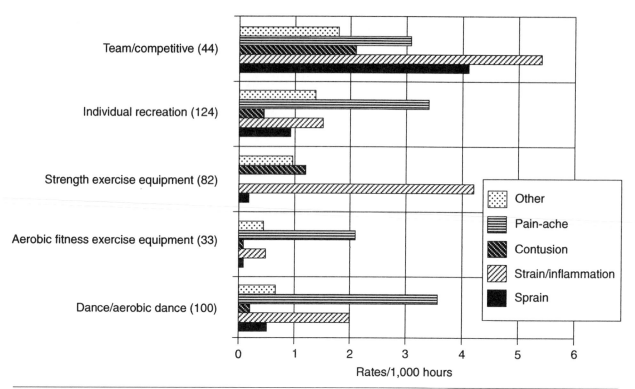

**Figure 2.7**   Injury rates for activity groups by type of injury.

**Table 2.3   Top Five Types of Injuries Account for 85.3% of All Injuries**

|  | Total | Time loss (> Level I) | | MD/DO/ DPM reported | | Acute | |
|---|---|---|---|---|---|---|---|
|  | # | # | % | # | % | # | % |
| Sprain | 47 | 38 | 80.9 | 13 | 27.7 | 38 | 80.9 |
| Strain | 84 | 76 | 90.5 | 2 | 2.4 | 46 | 54.8 |
| Inflammation | 77 | 60 | 77.9 | 10 | 13.0 | 17 | 22.1 |
| Pain-ache | 211 | 146 | 69.2 | 6 | 2.8 | 55 | 26.1 |
| Contusion | 29 | 23 | 79.3 | 3 | 10.3 | 25 | 86.2 |
| Total | 448 |  |  |  |  |  |  |

lower leg, and ankle each made up about 10% while the upper extremity-other category (forearm, wrist, hand, and fingers), hip, and thigh each contributed about 5% to 7%. The remaining areas each made up less than 5% of the injuries.

### 3.3.2 Location

Grouping the parts of the lower leg distal to the ankle into a single foot & toes category makes it one of the six most common injury sites (Table 2.4).

### 3.3.3 Location by Severity

The percent of injuries by location that resulted in time loss varied from 65% to 92%; percentage of those consulting a physician ranged from 6% to 11%. The ankle was the location most often associated with a physician visit, yet least likely to result in time loss. Conversely, the low back most often resulted in time loss, yet (after the lower leg) was least likely to require physician care.

### 3.3.4 Location by Onset

The ankle suffered from an acute episode almost two out of three times (60.9%); conversely, the foot and toe area sustained a much smaller proportion of acute injuries (21.7%).

### 3.3.5 Upper Extremity Injuries, Lower Extremity Injuries, and Spine/Trunk Injuries

Collapsing anatomic location into three categories allows a simpler comparison to be made with activity groups. Injuries to the lower extremity made up almost two thirds of the injuries (65.9%). The upper extremity region contained slightly over one in five injuries (21.7%), while the spine/trunk region made up the remaining 12.4%.

Lower extremity injuries were most frequent in team/competitive activities, least frequent in

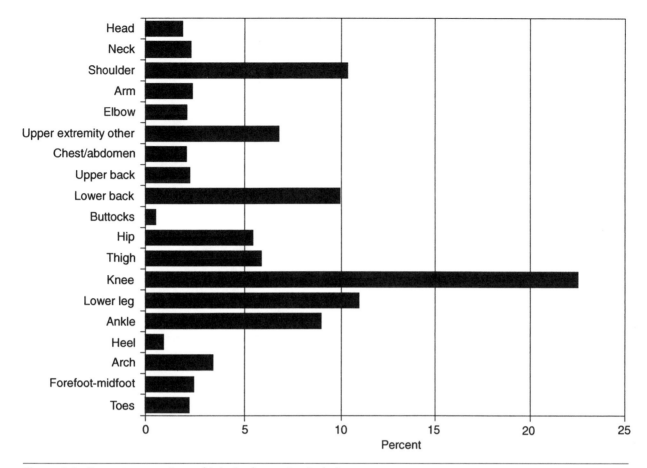

**Figure 2.8**   Percent comparison of injuries by anatomical site.

**Table 2.4   Top Six Locations of Injury Account for 69.7% of All Injuries**

| | Total | Time loss (> Level I) | | MD/DO/ DPM reported | | Acute | |
|---|---|---|---|---|---|---|---|
| | # | # | % | # | % | # | % |
| Shoulder | 54 | 47 | 87.0 | 5 | 9.3 | 22 | 40.7 |
| Low back | 51 | 47 | 92.2 | 3 | 5.9 | 18 | 35.3 |
| Knee | 115 | 82 | 71.3 | 11 | 9.6 | 39 | 33.9 |
| Leg | 54 | 43 | 79.6 | 3 | 5.6 | 17 | 31.5 |
| Ankle | 46 | 30 | 65.2 | 5 | 10.9 | 28 | 60.9 |
| Foot & toes | 46 | 30 | 65.2 | 4 | 8.7 | 10 | 21.7 |
| Total | 366 | | | | | | |

strength exercise equipment and aerobic fitness exercise equipment, and intermediate in dance/ aerobic dance (Figure 2.9). Upper extremity injuries were most frequent in team/competitive and strength exercise equipment categories and much less frequent in the remaining three groups. The rate of injuries to the spine/trunk appeared to follow the overall rates, highest in team/competitive and lowest in the aerobic fitness exercise equipment group.

### 3.4. Nature of Injury Onset

Injury onset has been discussed above with respect to type and location of injury. As common sense would suggest (and as we saw), the onset of the injury varied according to the nature of the injury.

In a similar fashion onset also varied according to the cause and mechanism of injury (Figure 2.10). Gradual onset injuries were more likely when the cause of injury involved equipment and customary activities; falls, collisions, and cutting maneuvers/ lateral movements favored acute injuries.

Mechanism of injury also showed a definite relationship to injury onset (Figure 2.11). A mechanism noting a preexisting condition, overuse/intensity, or customary activity injury was much more likely to be gradual in onset. On the other hand, twisting/stretching or a direct blow was more likely to result in an acute episode.

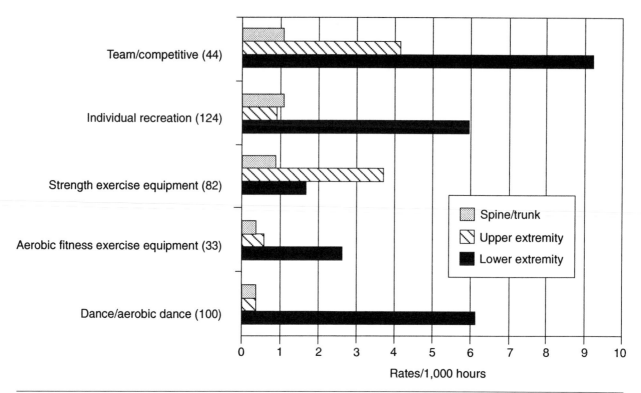

**Figure 2.9**   Injury and complaint rates by body region.

### 3.5 Injury Cause

There were a great variety of causes cited by the participants for their injuries. The majority of both males and females related that there were no special or unusual events associated with the injury, rather they arose out of normal activities ("customary activity"). Changes of activity or mistakes in choosing activity levels, falls, equipment, collisions, and movements of various sorts were all cited as causes. Only collisions seemed to have any gender relationship.

### 3.6 Injury Mechanism

Once again, the mechanism of injury most often cited was customary activity. Preexisting conditions, overuse/too much intensity, twisting or stretching, and direct blows were all noted at approximately the 10% level. Only direct blows seemed to vary by gender, and males mentioned it a bit less than twice as often as females.

## 4. Injury Severity

### 4.1 Time Loss

Injury severity as measured by time loss varied somewhat by category of activity, as we noted

above. The percent time-loss injuries to total injuries demonstrated this because the individual recreation (78%) and strength exercise equipment (86%) groups had higher percents versus the others (60-70%; Figure 2.12). The activity group with the highest overall rate, the team/competitive, had the highest rate of both time-loss and non-time-loss injuries, although it had one of the lowest percentages of time-loss injury to total.

### 4.2 Catastrophic Injury

As far as we know, our group had but one injury in this category, resulting in major permanent disability. One cyclist was hit by a car, suffering a head injury that produced impairment. At the close of the study, there had been significant improvement, but the rehabilitation process was not complete. It was predicted, however, that there would be permanent and significant gait and mental sequelae.

### 4.3 Clinical Outcome/Medical Care

Overall almost 1 in 10 participants with injuries and complaints (9.5%) sought medical attention from an MD, DO, or podiatric physician (DPM)

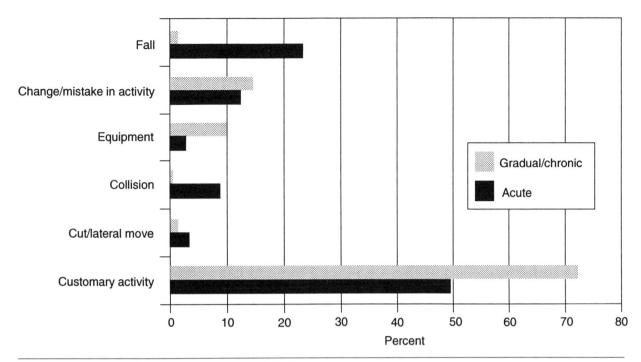

**Figure 2.10**   Causes of injury.

while another 5.9% (28 participants) were seen by other health workers such as chiropractors, acupuncturists, physical therapists, or nurses. Team/competitive, individual recreation, and strength exercise equipment had from 12% to 15% of injuries and complaints seeking physician care; for dance/aerobic dance and aerobic fitness exercise equipment, the rate was less than 5%.

# 5. Injury Risk Factors

The medical community is playing an increasingly active role in encouraging fitness enhancement. Whether by threats (the dangers of high cholesterol or LDL, osteoporosis, or cardiovascular disease) or promises (enhanced competitive performance or lowered body fat), at least some portion of organized medicine appears to be encouraging the fitness movement. At the same time, such support might be applied more thoughtfully if it were possible to better predict the injury consequences of participation. It is useful to attempt to identify risk factors and suggest what might be done to alter these factors.

## 5.1 Intrinsic Factors

### 5.1.1 Physical Characteristics

***5.1.1.1 Previous Injury.***   Significantly, history of a previous significant injury to a particular area (knee, shoulder, ankle, etc.) appeared to roughly double the risk of sustaining a subsequent injury. This is particularly important because knowledge that a previous injury is a risk factor for reinjury suggests potential methods of injury prevention. The physician, fitness leader, or therapist may intervene by instituting appropriate rehabilitation and by promoting recreational activities with lower risks of reinjury.

***5.1.1.2 Age.***   The injury rates did not seem to vary greatly by age. Although the 30 to 39 age group had the highest injury rates, this trend was only shown in the males.

***5.1.1.3 Gender.***   Although males in the 30 to 39 age group had a significantly higher rate of injury, this is primarily due to their participation in the higher risk team/competition activities. In addition to contact sports, which did contribute injuries to the male injury rate (some from relatively few hours of participation), basketball was also a significant contributor.

## 5.2 Extrinsic Factors

### 5.2.1 Competitive Versus Recreational

Generally the rates of injury were highest for team and competitive sports compared to endeavors engaged in more for recreation. Many noncompetitive activities also were engaged in at lower levels of intensity than were the competitive activities, such as basketball, lacrosse, racquetball, rugby,

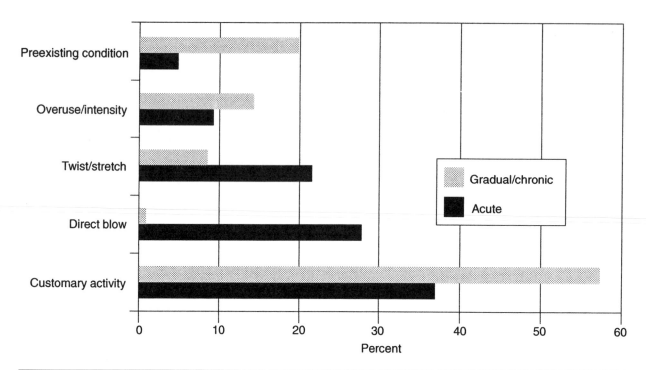

**Figure 2.11**    Mechanism of injury in gradual/chronic and acute injuries.

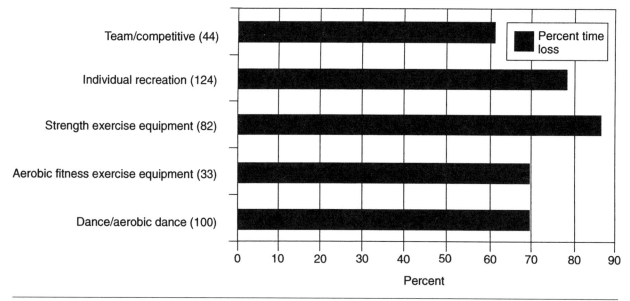

**Figure 2.12**    Percent of time-loss injuries to total injuries in various activities.

and so on, so it is difficult to separate the degree of competition from the intensity of play.

### 5.2.2 Team Versus Individual

Although generally the rates of injury were highest for team and competitive sports it is impossible to say whether it was the team-versus-solo aspect of activity rather than the intensity that was actually influencing the rates of injury. Except for running,

which resembled team activities in overall injury rates, most individual activities had relatively low rates of injury as did most forms of dance, aerobic dance, and working with exercise equipment of both the cardiovascular and weight variety.

### 5.2.3 Characteristics of the Activity

In addition to an activity's solo-versus-individual character or its competitiveness or intensity, it is clear that what actually goes on in a particular sport or pastime strongly influences the patterns and severity of injury. Some sports are clearly lower extremity sports and so are their injury patterns. However, because an activity may represent a particular package of characteristics, it is often difficult to see the contribution of a single element. Situations that allow comparisons, where men and women play in similar sports or where there are similar activities by participants of varying ages, are not always present in the team and competitive sports. However, for individual activities participation is often not restricted to discrete categories.

## 6. Suggestions for Injury Prevention

### 6.1 Players

Injuries occurred about twice as frequently to those with a history of a previous injury, suggesting ways that the risks of sustaining injuries in recreational activities might be altered. Avoiding more hazardous recreational activities is one important way. Certainly the recreational athlete with a previous injury should engage in a suitable rehabilitation program, one aimed at eliminating any lack of strength or flexibility resulting from a past injury. It is hoped that rehabilitation would reduce the risks of reinjury to an area shown to be vulnerable.

### 6.2 Sport

Relatively low rates of injury were found for most recreational sports activities, even using a sensitive definition of injury that included minor as well as major problems. Overall, the rate for injuries that caused an alteration in participation was less than two per person per year, based on the level of activity observed in the study.

While most individual activities appear to be relatively benign, running had a higher risk of injury than did many team/competitive sports. Most aerobic fitness activities (exercise cycling, step climbing, aerobic dance, etc.) carried low rates of injury, as did most weight activity, both free and machine. As might be expected, adults participating in a competitive contact sport, such as basketball, fared worse.

### 6.3 External Environment

In an active adult population, the majority of the injuries seen will be of the nonacute variety, suggesting the external environment is not, at least in an obvious sense, hazardous. While it is recognized that many (if not the majority) of the injuries will be gradual onset or overuse in nature, conceptually the injury prevention model is often that of the acute injury. We need to consider injury prevention strategies in light of the demonstrated prevalence of gradual onset, chronic, acute exacerbations of chronic injuries, and reinjuries in the active adult population.

### 6.4 Health Support System

In a parallel way, since the majority of the injuries seen by professionals will be of the nonacute variety, the health support system must learn to cope better with these sorts of subtle, long-lasting problems. The acute-injury model is still strong in the minds of many health care professionals and participants. It is easy to fail in treating these injuries when we become frustrated from unrealistic expectations based on the acute injury recovery model. Both injury treatment and prevention strategies need to recognize these realities.

## 7. Suggestions for Further Research

### 7.1 Definitions

The issue of injury definitions is difficult, particularly for recreational activities where there are rarely medical personnel on site. Time-loss and medical-utilization data give information that can be compared to other studies because they are understood and commonly used. Collecting more detailed and sophisticated data should not preclude the collection of standard types of data as well. There are operational difficulties in applying a definition, and of course, there are great variations in time loss experienced and medical care utilized by different persons for the same injury. Whatever definition is employed should serve the purposes of the study and provide as much comparison as possible with previous work.

### 7.2 Study Population

It is critical that the population sampled, the process, and the resultant sample be thoroughly described. It is regrettable that samples are often obtained by less than ideal methods; however, no selection process is ideal and at the very least researchers should fully and openly share with their readers their sampling methods (or lack thereof) and the resultant characteristics of the sample obtained.

## 7.3 Research Design

A prospective cohort approach following a large group of participants in recreational activity, through a variety of exposures, has several advantages. Selecting the group in advance helps to minimize recall bias.

Applying consistent methods and definitions of injury allows reasonable comparisons to be made between activities; whatever definitional, population, case ascertainment, and classification biases exist should at least be constant across activities.

Although rigorously monitoring subjects via telephone calls as described is somewhat expensive, particularly compared to simple questionnaire methods, it offers the advantages we have outlined.

By our definition *activity* is impure when compared to an organized team sport. (All participants in this study were required to engage in a variety of recreational activities.) This approach is very useful, however, when the interest is in multisport participation or where there is no organized structure to participation (no leagues, no registration) to identify participants.

## 7.4 Data Collection

Weekly monitoring by trained callers helps to reduce memory errors because the information is collected shortly after the event. Injury information must be collected at some interval after the event, of course, but because of the frequent telephone contacts, little time had generally elapsed after an injury before the initial information was collected. Standard weekly calls documented any time loss and medical care sought more or less as they occurred.

## 7.5 Research Team

Training is a key issue with any data gathering effort. This study depended primarily upon telephone interviewers to gather and code the information, and much effort was spent hiring, training, testing, and devising procedures and definitions that could be written up and distributed to the team. Even so, questions continued to arise throughout the data collection effort.

Whether team members are working at different times, as in our case, or in different locations, an efficient working environment and standardized office procedures must be established. After the initial weeks of training and testing for reliability, first daily, then regular weekly meetings were held to go over active cases to make sure that all callers were coding the events consistently. Because there were morning and evening shifts, locations for notes and ways to exchange problem cases for review were established.

## Acknowledgments

We wish to express a heartfelt thanks to our interviewers Pamela Turner, Francine Cohen, Heidi Harrison, Alicia Head, and Jim Taylor; to our database supervisor Constance Foester-Bourges; and to our field supervisor, Bernetta Schadewald, ATC. Without their skill, dedication, and persistence, this study would not have been possible.

We also gratefully acknowledge the financial support provided by AVIA Athletic Footwear, Inc. We particularly wish to thank Todd Miller and Dan Richards for their constant interest and encouragement.

## References

1. Bouter, L.M.; Knipschild, P.G.; Volovics, A. Personal and environmental factors in relation to injury risk in downhill skiing. Int. J. Sports Med., Vol. 10, 298-301; 1989.

2. Burns, T.P.; Steadman, J.R.; Rodkey, W.G. Alpine skiing and the mature athlete. Clinics In Sports Medicine, 10(2):327-342; 1991.

3. Garrick, J.G.; Requa, R.K. Aerobic dance: a review. Sports Medicine, Vol. 6, 169-179; 1988.

4. Koplan, J.P.; Powell, K.E.; Sikes, R.K.; Shirley, R.W.; Campbell, C.C. An epidemiologic study of the benefits and risks of running. JAMA 248(23):3118-3121; 1982.

5. Macera, C.A. Lower extremity injuries in runners. Advances in prediction. Sports Medicine, 13(1):50-57; 1992.

6. Macera, C.A.; Pate, R.R.; Powell, K.E.; Jackson, K.L.; Kendrick, J.S.; Craven, T.E. Predicting lower-extremity injuries among habitual runners. Archives of Internal Medicine, 149(11):2565-2568; 1989.

7. Thompson, D.C.; Thompson, R.S.; Rivara, F.P. Incidence of bicycle-related injuries in a defined population. AJPH, Vol. 80, 1388-1390; 1990.

8. Walter, S.D.; Hart, L.E.; McIntosh, J.M.; Sutton, J.R. The Ontario cohort study of running-related injuries. Arch Intern Med, Vol. 149, 2561-2564; 1989.

# 3

# Alpine and
# Cross-Country Skiing

*Charles A. Soma, Bert R. Mandelbaum,*
*Diane S. Watanabe, and Steve Hanft*

## 1. Introduction

Skiing and other snow sports have enjoyed remarkable popularity and experienced rapid
growth during the past 25 years. Alpine and cross-
country skiing share the characteristics of exposure
to injury from high speed impact (collisions), torsional loads (twisting falls), and the environment
(exposure). Both sports are characterized by a
predominance of torsional injuries to the lower
extremities and impact injuries to the upper
extremities.

This chapter reports the results of an epidemiologic review of the skiing injury literature. The
intent of the review is to describe the quantitative
aspects of injury statistics affecting Alpine and
cross-country skiers, to identify potential injury
risk factors, to suggest possible injury prevention
strategies, and ultimately to make recommendations for further research. It is important to focus
our limited research resources on identifying those
factors most likely to reduce the morbidity of skiing injuries.

Data collection focused on the English language
literature; however, foreign publications, which
have been reviewed or translated elsewhere, have
been included. Data was collected using the following procedures:

- Ancestry approach, that is, retrieval of research cited and published research in reviews such as clinical or research reports and
  literature reviews and
- Computer searches using the Medline system, covering the time period from 1975 to
  the present. The medical subject headings

used to identify literature were sports, athletic injuries, and accidents. Key words used
to cross-reference within the headings were
skiing, cross-country, and alcohol. It is assumed that another reviewer using these
methods would arrive at similar conclusions.

The majority of ski injury studies available are
case series or retrospectively reported injury data
from ski patrol or hospital records. A number of
ongoing, prospective ski injury studies, specifically
the works of Johnson of Vermont (18-25), Lystad
of Norway (31), and Matter of Switzerland (33),
provide information from which more significant
epidemiologic observations are possible. The limitations of the various retrospective studies include
recall bias and underreporting when injured skiers
were treated outside the research facilities. The
citations from case series provide information
about the details and characteristics of a given type
of injury, but these studies are less useful in determining incidence of injury in the skiing population.

## 2. Incidence of Injury

### 2.1 Injury Rates

#### 2.1.1 Alpine Skiing

A comparison of prospective and retrospective
population studies of injuries in Alpine skiing is
shown in Table 3.1.

A review of these data suggests that current injury rates overall are declining and that injuries
occur at the rate of about 3.2 injuries per 1,000

**Table 3.1   Alpine Skiing: Incidence of Injury**

| Author/year | [1]Study design | Duration | Sample | Study locale | Incidence of injury |
|---|---|---|---|---|---|
| Tapper, 1978 | P | 4 years 1972-1976 | 4,227 injuries 2,000 controls | USA | 3 injuries/1,000 skier days 50% advanced and expert skiers |
| Carr et al., 1981 | P | 6 years 1972-1978 | 1,711 injuries 998 controls | USA | Overall 4.2 injuries/1,000 skier days UE[3] 1.06 injuries/1,000 skier days |
| Johnson & Ettlinger, 1982 | P | 9 years 1972-1981; 771,690 skier days | 3,171 injuries 1,268 controls | USA | Mean days between injuries: 1972 → 1981 206 → 284 Significant trends ($p < .1$): Twist injuries (spiral fx, ankle sprains) ↓79% $R^2$ = .92   p = .005 Bending injuries (boot top fracture) ↓57% $R^2$ = .29   p = .1 MCL, Grade I ↓57% $R^2$ = .49   p < .025 Spine injuries ↓45% |
| Lystad, 1985 | P | 1 year 1981-1982; 156,000 skier days | 143 total injuries 51 LEER[2] (16 did not have bindings tested) 92 non-LEER 126 controls | Norway | 0.91 injuries/1,000 skier days |
| Matter et al., 1987 | P | 15 years; dates not specified | 17,246 | Switzerland | Total skied: 2.5 million vertical km/year Rescue transports per 10,000 km of vertical skiing distance 1972: $4/10^4$km 1986: $1/10^4$km |
| Johnson et al., 1993 | P | 18 years 1972-1990; 2,032,000 skier days | 6,671 injuries (6,139 skiers) 2,083 controls | USA | Rate of all injuries decreased 48% over 18 yrs ($R^2$ = .50, P < 0.01) |
| Eriksson, 1976 | R | 1 year 1973-1974 | 885 injuries | Sweden | None |
| Young et al., 1976 | R | 8 years 1966-1973 | 4,458 injuries 659 controls | USA | Begin: 4.2 injuries/1,000 skier days End: 2.8 injuries/1,000 skier days |
| Sherry & Fenelon, 1991 | R | 27 years 1962-1988 (7 years of missing data) | 22,261 injuries | Australia | 1962: 10.9 injuries/1,000 skier days 1988: 3.22 injuries/1,000 skier days Annual decline 2.8% for 1962-1988 (95% CI 2.5-3.1) |
| Young & Lee, 1991 | R | 2 years 1987-1989; 552,500 skier days | 1,885 injuries (1,762 skiers) | USA | 3.25 injuries/1,000 skier days |
| Shealy, 1993 | R | 2 years 1988-1990 | 21,817 injuries 2,318 controls | USA | 2.66 injuries/1,000 skier days |

[1]Study design: P = prospective study; R = retrospective study.

[2]LEER = lower extremity equipment-related injuries.

[3]UE = upper extremity.

skier days for skiers of average ability. The most current prospective surveys of Alpine skiing-related injuries have reported incidence rates for most types of injuries to be in decline, attributed to improved grooming, preparation, education, and equipment. Although most authors use injuries per 1,000 skier days to report incidence, a more useful unit of injuries per 10,000 kilometers of vertical feet skied (33) has been used in a European study. In other epidemiologic studies, the sample population of skiers was estimated from number of lift tickets sold. This method may produce inconsistencies due to varied distances that each skier completed during a day. Use of the unit of injuries per 10,000 kilometers of vertical skiing distance may be a more effective method to eliminate this exposure bias.

### 2.1.2 Cross-Country Skiing

A comparison of injury rates derived from population injury studies in cross-country skiing is shown in Table 3.2. A perusal of the available data, particularly Sherry and Asquith (50), suggests that for cross-country skiing injury rates are lower than Alpine skiing rates, averaging less than one injury per 1,000 skier days.

## 2.2 Reinjury Rates

### 2.2.1 Alpine Skiing

An important injury characteristic not often addressed in the injury studies is the extent of reinjury. This is an important area of investigation because it is believed that previous injury is a risk factor for subsequent injury at the same site (30, 43). Of the studies that reported either reinjury rates (15) or a history of previous injuries (3), the following generalizations can be made:

- Minor injury reporting rates may be severely underestimating actual incidence (3).
- Expert skiers are at significant risk for reinjury in their competitive career following surgical repair of a ligamentous knee injury (particularly anterior cruciate legiment repair) (15).

### 2.2.2 Cross-Country Skiing

Although no incidence of reinjury associated with cross-country skiing has been reported in the literature, chronic overuse-type injuries are considered, including chronic lower extremity compartment syndromes in the competitive cross-country skier (13) and stress fractures in cross-country skiers (38).

## 3. Injury Characteristics

### 3.1 Injury Onset

### 3.1.1 Alpine skiing

The ski injury literature is replete with discussions of mechanism of injury as it relates to ski equipment and binding release capabilities. Alpine skiing injuries tend to be acute onset injuries related to specific traumatic incidents involving either a twisting fall, impact with an obstacle, or collisions with other skiers.

### 3.1.2 Cross-Country Skiing

Acute injuries in cross-country skiing are more frequently the result of impact with the snow surface or obstacles, producing a higher proportion of upper extremity injuries. Chronic overuse injuries, including anterior compartment syndromes (13), stress fractures (38), and back pain are prevalent among cross-country skiers (12, 50). Exposure and hypothermia accounted for 20% of medically treated cross-country skiing injuries in one series (16).

**Table 3.2  Cross-Country Skiing: Incidence of Injury**

| Author/year | [1]Study design | Duration | Sample | Study locale | Incidence of injury |
|---|---|---|---|---|---|
| Renstrom & Johnson, 1989 | Literature review | N/A | N/A | N/A | Injuries/1,000 skier days: Garrick 1.5-2.0 Westlin .50 Sherry .49 Eriksson .20 |
| Sherry & Asquith, 1987 | R | 2 years 1984-1985 180,118 skier days | 88 injuries | Australia | Cross-country: 0.49 injuries/1,000 skier days Alpine: 3.50 injuries/1,000 skier days |

[1]Study design: P = prospective study; R = retrospective study.

## 3.2 Injury Type

### 3.2.1 *Alpine Skiing*

The trend over the period shows a shift from ankle sprains and fractures (pre-1970) to tibial shaft fractures (in the 1970s to early 1980s) to severe knee sprains (1980s to present) in Alpine skiing injuries (2-6, 8, 9, 11, 17, 19-24, 28, 33, 40, 46, 47, 49, 52, 58, 59, 63-65). The cited papers include both retrospective and prospective analyses of injury data (listed in Table 3.3), and both types of work support the following observations:

- Among Alpine skiers, knee sprains are the most common injury in all studies to date.
- Fractures as a proportion of total injuries are decreasing among Alpine skiers over the period 1970-1993.
- Lower extremity injuries among Alpine skiers occur as a result of torsion; upper extremity injuries are mainly due to impact.

**Table 3.3   Alpine Skiing: Injury Type**

| Author/year | [1]Study design | Injury type | |
|---|---|---|---|
| Carr et al., 1981 | P | Lower extremity:<br>  22% knee sprain<br>  7% ankle sprain<br>  2.5% ankle fracture | Upper extremity:<br>  9.5% ulnar colateral sprain<br>  4.6% shoulder soft tissue<br>  2.3% shoulder dislocation |
| Lystad, 1985 | P | Sprain 28%<br>Fracture 24%<br>51/143 LEER[2]<br>  8.5% boot-top contusion<br>  34% fracture<br>  58% sprain | |
| Kristiansen & Johnson, 1990 | P | 15.3% of all injuries were fx (871 fxs) | |
| Eriksson, 1976 | R | Cross-country skiers 12% fracture<br>Alpine skiers 50% fracture<br>Tibia fractures: 23% adults, 48% children | |
| Johnson & Pope, 1977 | R | Spiral fracture 42%<br>Boot top/transverse or oblique fracture 51% | |
| Johnson et al., 1979 | R | Sprains of MCL<br>  Grade I: 65%<br>  Grade II/III: ≈30% | |
| Edlund, 1980 | R | Ligament sprains | |
| Sherry, 1984 | R | Sprain 37%<br>Fracture 22%<br>Dislocation 6% | |
| Higgins & Steadman, 1987 | R | ACL tear location<br>  80% proximal, 3% combined, 7% middle, 10% distal | |
| Young & Lee, 1991 | R | Sprain 54%<br>Fracture 10%<br>Dislocation 4% | |
| Paletta et al., 1992 | R | Of 75 skiers with ACL injuries, 31 (41%) had associated meniscal tear.<br>Of those 31:<br>  25 (81%) had lateral meniscus injury (p < .05)<br>  8 (26%) had medial meniscus injury<br>Of 75 nonskiers with ACL injury<br>  37 (49%) had meniscal tear<br>  26 (35%) had lateral tear<br>  28 (37%) had bilateral tear | |
| Shealy, 1993 | R | Sprain 48%<br>Fracture 19% → 13.5% | |

[1]Study design: P = prospective study; R = retrospective study.

[2]LEER = lower extremity equipment-related injuries.

- The incidence of bending-type lower extremity fractures in Alpine skiing is decreasing (23, 26).
- The incidence of lacerations has decreased since the advent of ski brakes for Alpine skis.
- Severe anterior cruciate ligament (ACL) sprains comprise 25% to 30% of all knee injuries in skiing and have become the most common severe injury related to snow sports (18, 22).

### 3.2.2 Cross-Country Skiing

Cross-country skiing is performed at lower speeds than Alpine skiing, and subsequently less kinetic energy is involved, producing less severe injuries. Not surprisingly, the incidence of acute traumatic injuries is lower, while overuse injuries from high intensity training on or off the snow occur more frequently than in Alpine skiing. As shown in Table 3.4

- among cross-country skiers, overuse injuries are common;
- acute cross-country skiing injuries have a similar distribution of injury types to those in Alpine skiing; and
- the majority of knee injuries involve the medial collateral ligament (MCL) with very few injuries to the anterior cruciate ligament.

**Table 3.4   Cross-Country Skiing: Injury Type**

| Author/ year | [1]Study design | Injury type | | |
| --- | --- | --- | --- | --- |
| Orava et al., 1985 | C | 37 stress fractures 3 femoral neck fractures 2 femur fractures | | |
| Sherry & Asquith, 1987 | R | Sprain 45% Fracture 19% Dislocation 5% Concussion 3% | | |
| Steinbrück, 1987 | R | | Cross-country | Alpine |
| | | Sprain | 15% | 38% |
| | | Fracture | 22% | 22% |
| | | Dislocation | 7% | 2% |
| | | Tendon rupture | 18% | 23% |
| Pigman & Karakla, 1990 | R | Sprain 27% 60% of knee injuries were MCL | | |
| Frost & Bauer, 1991 | C | 10 hip fractures | | |

[1]Study design: P = prospective study; R = retrospective study; C = case series.

## 3.3 Injury Location

### 3.3.1 Head/Spine/Trunk

#### 3.3.1.1 Alpine Skiing.
As shown in Table 3.5, injuries to the head, spine, and trunk comprise roughly 10% to 15% of all injuries in Alpine skiing (31, 61, 64). Injuries to the head were mainly concussions or lacerations. Injuries to the spine and trunk were combined by most authors, and made up between 2.5% (26) and 7% (58) of all injuries.

A case series of 11 skiing-related spinal injuries over a 7-year period in Canada revealed a predominance of thoracolumbar burst fractures (10 of 11 cases). Skiers were injured when landing incorrectly from a jump or skiing out of control into trees. One third of these fractures resulted in paralysis, and two thirds had an associated major injury of the extremities, thorax, abdomen, or head (44).

#### 3.3.1.2 Cross-Country Skiing.
As shown in Table 3.6, a review of the studies addressing cross-country skiing injuries shows that head, neck, and trunk injuries comprise between 5% (50) and 17% (38) of all injuries. Overuse injuries to the spine and trunk were more frequent than traumatic injuries (38, 55), attributed to the repetitive hyperextension of the spine during the cross-country skiing stride. A large number of the injuries sustained by cross-country skiers are attributable to cross-training techniques (running or working on exercise equipment) (38).

### 3.3.2 Upper Extremity

#### 3.3.2.1 Alpine Skiing.
As shown in Table 3.5, upper extremity injuries account for 13% (64) to 36% (49) of all injuries in Alpine skiing. Injury to the ulnar collateral ligament of the thumb, termed *gamekeeper's thumb*, is the most common skiing injury of the upper extremity, accounting for between 10% and 17% of all injuries (7, 64). The thumb is vulnerable to injury from impact with the snow during a fall, rupturing the ulnar collateral ligament and rendering the thumb unstable (56).

Shoulder trauma (fractures and dislocations) accounted for 5% to 10% of all Alpine skiing injuries (22, 27, 49, 64). The most common mechanisms for anterior shoulder dislocations were falls onto the affected shoulder (60%), falls onto the flexed elbow (20%), and an external rotation/abduction torque applied to the arm when a ski pole is caught in bushes (16%; 27).

#### 3.3.2.2 Cross-Country Skiing.
As shown in Table 3.6, upper extremity injuries account for 7% (38) to 25% (50) of cross-country skiing injuries. The

**Table 3.5   Alpine Skiing: Injury Location**

| Author/ year | [1]Study design | Injury location | | |
|---|---|---|---|---|
| Johnson et al., 1980 | P | ↓41% overall | p > 0.1 | NS |
| | | ↓25% upper body | p > 0.1 | NS |
| | | ↓56% LEER | p < 0.02 | |
| | | ↓71% LE non-ER | p < 0.1 | NS |
| | | ↓72% fx tibia | p < .025 | |
| | | ↓28% knee sprain | p > 0.1 | NS |
| | | ↓50% all LE | p > 0.03 | NS |
| Carr et al., 1981 | P | Upper extremity 25.5% Lower extremity 40% | | |
| Lystad, 1985 | P | Lower extremity 43% Upper extremity 29% Head 14% | | |
| Matter et al., 1987 | P | | 1972 | 1986 |
| | | Upper extremity | 17% → | 35% |
| | | Lower extremity | | 50% |
| | | Head/trunk | 9% → | 3% |
| Kristiansen & Johnson, 1990 | P | Upper extremity 6.5% Lower extremity 7.4% Trunk 7% Spine 2.5% | | |
| Johnson et al., 1993 | P | Regression analysis of incidence changes: ↓89% ankle sprains ↓70% knee sprains (I/II) ↑209% ACL tears ↓88% tibial fracture ($R^2$ = .81, p < .01) | | |
| Eriksson, 1976 | R | Lower extremity 72% Upper extremity/trunk 20% Head 3.1% | | |
| Johnson et al., 1979 | R | MCL = 86.2% of all ligament injuries of knee ACL = 6/306 (2%) PCL = 6/306 (2%) Both = 1% | | |
| Edlund, 1980 | R | Knee ligament injuries include MCL 98% ACL 13% PCL 4% | | |
| Sherry, 1984 | R | Upper extremity 36% Lower extremity 42% Head/neck 17% | | |
| Sherry & Fenelon, 1991 | R | Significant changes   Knee ↑3.8% per yr   p = .001   Tibia fx ↓11.3% per yr   p = .001   Ankle ↓9.0% per yr   p = .001 | | |
| Young & Lee, 1991 | R | Upper extremity 40% Lower extremity 45% Back/chest 5% Head 9% | | |
| Paletta et al., 1992 | R | Knees   80% of lateral meniscal tears   (LMT) in posterior horn Of 25 LMT   40% partial thickness   20% bucket handle | | |
| Shealy, 1993 | R | | 1980 | 1990 |
| | | Total | | |
| | | Lower extremity | 51% | 46% |
| | | Upper extremity | 18% | 19% |
| | | Head | 15% | 13% |

[1]Study design: P = prospective study; R = retrospective study.

**Table 3.6   Cross-Country Skiing: Injury Location**

| Author/ year | [1]Study design | Injury location | | |
|---|---|---|---|---|
| Orava et al., 1985 | C | Upper extremity 7% Lower extremity 85% Trunk 8% | | |
| Sherry & Asquith, 1987 | R | Upper extremity 25% Lower extremity 41% Trunk 5% Head 9% | | |
| Steinbrück, 1987 | R | | Cross-country | Alpine |
| | | Upper extremity | 48% | 19% |
| | | Lower extremity | 34% | 77% |
| | | Trunk | 15% | 4% |
| | | Head | 3% | 0.4% |
| Westlin, 1976 | R | Upper extremity 25% Lower extremity 61% Trunk 9% Head 5% | | |
| Pigman & Karakla, 1990 | R | Upper extremity 18% Lower extremity 62% Trunk 18% Head 2% | | |
| Frost & Bauer, 1991 | C | 4 femoral neck fractures 6 trochanteric fractures | | |

[1]Study design: P = prospective study; R = retrospective study; C = case series.

pattern of injury to the shoulder and ulnar collateral ligament of the thumb was similar to that found in Alpine skiing. Shoulder problems (impingement syndromes, rotator cuff tears) represented 7% of all overuse injuries among a large group of Finnish cross-country skiers, due to the repetitive motion involved in ski-poling (38).

### 3.3.3 Lower Extremity

**3.3.3.1 Alpine Skiing.**   As shown in Table 3.5, injuries to the lower extremity account for 40% to 70% of skiing-related trauma (3, 8, 14, 21, 22, 28, 31, 33, 47, 48, 58, 63, 65). Knee sprains, tibia fractures, and ankle sprains and fractures are by far the most common injuries in this group. Over the period of the ongoing Vermont injury study (1972-1990), several trends are notable: ankle sprains have decreased 89%, MCL sprains have decreased 70%, tibia fractures have decreased 88%, and ACL tears have increased 209% (20-22). Fractures of the lower extremity were responsible for 7.4% of all injuries in this study population (26). As a reference point for the consideration of the current incidence rates, an earlier review (covering the period

1972-1978) of this study population revealed that MCL tears from a valgus/external rotation mechanism accounted for 86% of all knee injuries (19).

Descriptions of the injury mechanism of ACL sprains have been the focus of much recent work (9, 15, 17, 22, 34, 39, 48). Five modes of injury to the ACL are cited. They include hyperextension, external rotation/valgus, "phantom foot," "boot induced," and "combined loading."

Feagin et al. reported a mechanism involving hyperextension of the knee, resulting from sudden deceleration as a skier hits the "crud line" in spring skiing conditions (9). In this case, a narrow intercondylar notch effectively guillotines the ACL producing the tear.

The external rotation/valgus forces produced when the outside edge of a ski catches the snow and rotates the ski outward can tear the MCL, medial meniscus, and finally the ACL (19).

In the phantom-foot mechanism, injury is sustained when the skier is off balance and shifts body weight to the downhill ski to regain control. When the ski recovers its inside turning edge, it rotates the knee violently, tearing the ACL as the ski carves a sharp, inward turn (18).

The boot-induced mechanism occurs when a skier is airborne (after a jump) and off balance with weight shifted rearward. Upon landing, the tail of the ski contacts the snow and the center of pressure of the snow against the ski moves forward until the section of the ski under the boot comes into contact with the snow. The force is then transmitted up the boot, forcing the tibia forward and stretching or tearing the anterior cruciate ligament (23).

In the combined-loading mechanism, injuries are sustained when skiers are in a compression mode with weight on the tails of the skis. With skis tracking ahead, the quadriceps' eccentric contraction forces the already stretched ACL to tear (34).

### 3.3.3.2 Cross-Country Skiing.

As shown in Table 3.6, lower extremity injuries account for 34% to 85% percent of cross-country skiing injuries (10, 16, 41, 42, 45, 50, 55). Lower extremity injuries result from torque applied to the leg when the ski tracks either twist or catch on an object, and the load is dissipated upon a sprain of the ankle or knee, or (rarely) a fracture of the tibia or ankle. A case series of 10 hip fractures from falls on a hard snow surface while cross-country skiing was presented (10).

A series of overuse injuries in cross-country skiers revealed 85% occur in the lower extremities

and a high number (79%) are the result of non-skiing (cross-training) activities. In this category are a variety of documented overuse conditions, including medial tibial stress syndrome, iliotibial band friction syndrome, chronic hamstring strain, patellofemoral stress syndrome, and greater trochanteric bursitis (38). Stress fractures of the tibia and metatarsals from overuse (38, 57) are not uncommon. Anterior tibial tendon ruptures and bilateral compartment syndromes of the leg (13, 29) have also been documented.

## 4. Injury Severity

### 4.1 Time Loss

A useful measure of injury severity is the duration of restriction from athletic performance. One can assume that the proportion of fractures in skiing approaches 15% (26) and that the treatment and immobilization required for such injuries is approximately 8 to 12 weeks. Johnson reported on the treatment of tibial shaft fractures sustained during Alpine skiing and showed an average time-to-union of between 9.1 weeks (patients 16 years or under) to 16.7 weeks (patients over 16 years; 23). For injuries of lesser degree, such as minor sprains accounting for 45% to 65% (19) of all injuries, a period of several days to a few weeks was usually required for a complete functional recovery.

ACL tears have become the single most important Alpine skiing injury in terms of disability and the costs of care. Higgins et al. reviewed the treatment of 27 world-class skiers with ACL tears (15). For this group, the average return to recreational skiing after surgery (ACL repair) was 5.4 months; 90% were racing again 9.1 months following surgery (15). Current treatment for an acute ACL tear is surgical reconstruction using a patellar tendon autograft procedure, followed by a 6-month functional rehabilitation program to facilitate a full return to sport (39).

### 4.2 Catastrophic Injury

A catastrophic injury is either fatal or has extreme consequences, such as paralysis, irreversible loss of mental function, loss of limb, or loss of the use of a limb. Catastrophic injuries occur infrequently in skiing, as shown in Table 3.7. Always a shocking tragedy, the death of downhill racer Ulrike Meier in the 1993-94 World Cup race season comes to mind when speaking of such injuries.

**Table 3.7   Catastrophic Skiing Injuries: Incidence of Injury**

| Author/year | [1]Study design | Duration | Sample | Study locale | Incidence of injury |
|---|---|---|---|---|---|
| National Ski Areas Association, 1994 | R | 1979-1993 14 years | 1990-1993 (2 seasons) 23 paraplegics 13 quadriplegics 30 head injuries 105 deaths | USA | 1979-1993 1.01 serious injuries/ million skier visits |
| Sherry & Clout, 1988 | R | 32 years 1956-1987; 33,000,000 skier days | 29 deaths | Australia | .87/million skier days .24 trauma .45 cardiac-related .18 hypothermia |

[1]Study design: P = prospective study; R = retrospective study.

The National Ski Areas Association (NSAA) has published annual reports since 1979, revealing an average rate of 1.01 catastrophic injuries per 1,000,000 skier visits; these include severe spinal injuries, head injuries, serious internal injuries, and deaths due to skiing as reported throughout the United States. From the 1990-1991 through the 1992-1993 ski season, 23 paraplegics, 13 quadriplegics, 30 head injuries, and 105 deaths were attributed to ski injuries (36).

A multicenter review of 29 skiing-related deaths over 32 years revealed that myocardial infarction, trauma to the head and neck, and hypothermia are the leading causes of death in the skiing population (51). The majority of the traumatic deaths occurred in men, whose average age was 28 years. This group has been identified as "risktakers" by Shealy, as compared to victims of fatal highway accidents, noting their similar age and sex (47, 48).

In a series of 19 cases of hypothermia during 2 seasons in Australia, 60% of the victims were under age 14; among the adult victims, alcohol intake was involved in a significant number (54). Another extended review of death due to skiing recorded a total of six deaths over 62 years of the Vasa cross-country long distance race in Sweden, giving a rate of 1 per 285,000 hours of activity (45).

# 5. Injury Risk Factors

## 5.1 Intrinsic Factors

### 5.1.1 Alpine Skiing

Some evidence suggests an increased risk of injury, especially for the less severe knee injuries, among beginner or low ability skiers (2, 5, 11, 14, 19-23, 47, 64). Beginners' injury rate was 2 to 9 times that of experienced skiers in European studies (14). Tibia fractures account for 12% of injuries in skiers under age 13, but only 4% of injuries to adult skiers (2). Skiers under age 11 have the same incidence of injury as adults, but those between 12 and 16 years are more prone to injury (2, 11). Grade I medial collateral ligament sprains are significantly more likely to occur in skiers of female sex, low weight, and inexperience (4, 5, 19-23, 49). However, females do not sustain tibia fractures at higher rates than males (20, 23).

### 5.1.2 Cross-Country Skiing

Risk factors cited in the cross-country skiing literature include skiing technique, suggesting that new, aggressive double-poling and V-skating methods are leading to an increase in soft tissue and bony stress injuries (13, 45). One investigator found no association between skiing technique or ski type in the development of chronic compartment syndrome in a group of 10 patients (29).

## 5.2 Extrinsic Factors

### 5.2.1 Alpine Skiing

The study of lower extremity torsional injuries and the reduction of these types of injuries via equipment modifications have been remarkable in recent years. Equipment design and function contribute a great deal to the safety of the sport, and dramatic injury pattern shifts have occurred with the development of multimode release bindings and modern midcalf-height boots (22, 32). Modern release bindings have played a major role in the reduction of most lower leg injuries in Alpine skiing, but the Vermont group has shown that the quality and function of modern bindings is apparently not related to Grade III ACL sprains (18). It is believed that the modern Alpine ski and boot, and the way that today's skiers use them, are more closely related to Grade III ACL injuries.

Most injuries in skiing are the result of a fall. Some Grade III ACL sprains, however, occur without a fall. Initial ski industry engineering standards for binding release settings were developed in an effort to reduce tibial fractures (31). The problem may be that the threshold for MCL rupture and tibial fracture may be higher than for ACL rupture in some injury modes and that consequently ACL rupture occurs prior to binding release. Engineers in this field are working to develop ski boots that release from the foot during loads that could produce ACL injury while retaining support during aggressive skiing. The difficulty lies in programming the equipment to recognize the difference between the two situations.

Another equipment-related factor in Alpine skiing injuries is the ski-pole grip, which can induce a hyperextension/abduction injury to the thumb (56). Injuries to the thumb in skiing account for 10% to 17% of all injuries (3, 20). While use of the ski strap has been shown not to increase the risk of gamekeeper's thumb, those using a grip with a broad superior plate are indeed more likely to suffer such an injury. This large-size grip is however recommended to prevent penetrating injury from the handle of the pole.

Injury rates peak in midafternoon to late afternoon, indicating that fatigue is a significant risk factor in skiing injuries (64).

### 5.2.2 Cross-Country Skiing

Extrinsic factors involved in cross-country injuries include the ski-pole grip as just mentioned, the skiing environment (e.g, hypothermia, frostbite, avalanches), and the ski binding/boot combination.

In comparison to Alpine ski bindings, cross-country ski bindings do not typically provide firm heel fixation, contributing to a lower incidence of torsional injuries to the lower extremities (16, 41, 50, 56). Interlocking heel plates of some cross-country ski bindings have been implicated in the higher incidence of ankle and tibia fractures in skiers using such bindings. Typically the injuries are of a low-energy character, responding well to standard therapeutic techniques (16, 45, 50).

Renstrom and Johnson noted that a significantly higher percentage of those with twisting injuries had ridge/groove heel plates (45). They proposed that injuries to the ankle in the cross-country skier were related to the height of the cross-country ski boot (45).

## 6. Suggestions for Injury Prevention

### 6.1 Alpine Skiing

Injury prevention strategies are at the center of attention in the field of ski injury research. A few of the ideas being considered to reduce injuries include

- Equipment modification: Softening of the radical sidecut of Alpine skis for recreational skiers to reduce the effect of oversteer in the phantom-foot mechanism of ACL injury, and development of conditional support systems in ski boots to allow for a breakaway type of release in certain load bearing situations.
- ACL awareness training: ACL tears remain a common disabling injury among Alpine skiers. Consequently, prevention of ACL tears has become the focus of current investigative work in the field. The NSAA sponsored the establishment of an ACL injury-awareness training program for ski area employees beginning in the 1993-1994 season. This experimental program was designed and produced in conjunction with the Vermont Safety Research Group. The program includes live and video presentations on the avoidance of high-risk behavior, recognition of potentially dangerous situations, and development of personal strategies for responding to these potentially dangerous situations. The evaluation of this program is ongoing and may result in such a program for the general skiing population in the future[1].
- Conditioning: The emphasis of conditioning in all sports has gained increasing popularity. Conditioning has been supported as one method of reducing the chance of injury to the anterior cruciate ligament. Little information is available to substantiate such contentions, but it appears that some benefit is derived by the well-conditioned skier.

---

[1]For more information on this program, please contact Carl Ettlinger at Vermont Safety Research, P.O. Box 85, Sandhill Road, Underhill Center, Vermont 05490 (phone 802-899-4738).

- Ski-racing technique: With the recent advances in ski-racing technology and critical technical analysis, racecourse performance has improved but perhaps at the expense of safety. The best high speed gliding technique occurs when the pressure to the ski-edge is applied more posteriorly on the ski, resulting in the least amount of snow resistance. This technique offers less control as a side effect of increasing speed due to the point on the ski at which edge pressure is applied. As tail weighting is the key to improved gliding mechanics, it has taken over as the technique of choice for high speed or downhill racing; however, it places the racer at increased risk for anterior cruciate ligament sprains (25, 34). Lunging across the finish line while "sitting back on the tails" certainly places the racer at risk, and this practice should be discouraged. Additionally, the removal of jumps from the racecourse should reduce ACL tears by the boot-induced mechanism described earlier in this chapter.
- Prophylactic bracing: The use of prophylactic or functional knee braces to decrease knee ligament injuries continues to be controversial. The use of functional knee braces in those patients with ACL tears and functional instability remains popular. However, there has been no objective study to show any significant decrease in mechanical instability under physiologic loading while using such a brace (62). Only during the application of very low forces have these braces been found to be effective. They cannot be relied upon to protect the knee with an injured or weakened anterior cruciate ligament.

## 6.2 Cross-Country Skiing

- Clothing/nutrition/hydration: Layered clothing appropriate for subzero wear is the best defense against hypothermia. Accessories such as masks, insulated or heated undergarments, and glove liners are readily available in most skiing resorts. Adequate nutritional and liquid replenishment are the key factors allowing the cross-country skier to participate and to compete without undue risk of exposure-related illness (51, 54). Alcohol consumption should be discouraged; alcohol produces vasodilatation and promotes heat loss, increasing the risk of exposure-related illness.

- Training progressions: Where overuse injuries are known to occur, specific attention should be paid to training progressions. Avoiding extreme changes in exercise intensity, duration, or both is the cornerstone of any program designed to reduce injuries, as cross-training is integral to the fitness programs of most competitive cross-country skiers. The consistent practice of a multisport training regimen for the recreational skier would certainly be of significant benefit.
- When addressing overuse injuries in general, one must employ treatment designed to relieve the inciting stresses (e.g., improved technique and rest), apply modalities to control pain and swelling (NSAIDS, ice, compressive wrapping), and gradually reinstitute activity as pain and mobility permit. By adhering to these guidelines, the rate and severity of overuse injuries should be reduced to the lowest possible level.

# 7. Suggestions for Further Research

## 7.1 Alpine Skiing

The group from Vermont has contributed a great deal of knowledge about how to decrease skiing-related injuries. Its current focus involves the implementation of a ski injury prevention program, initially among employees of ski resorts. Analysis of this program in the next few years may lead to its subsequent implementation among recreational skiers.

Equipment-related research continues in the laboratories of ski equipment manufacturers around the world. Refinements of ski equipment might include

- ski boots that release the foot when loaded in a rapid anterior direction;
- ski side-cut dampening to decrease oversteer;
- electronic or computerized release bindings; and
- protection for the thumbs on the ski-pole grip to reduce ulnar collateral ligament injuries to the thumb.

More rigorous epidemiologic study should focus on the severity and outcome of the treatment of skiing-related injuries and include more analysis of work time lost, medical/social expenditures, and the skier's ability to return to skiing at the same level of proficiency.

Stratification of the injured skier in terms of experience, age, level of fitness, and risk-taking behavior would be useful in targeting injury-prevention programs to the appropriate target audiences.

Long-term evaluation of injury-prevention programs (such as ACL awareness training) should include a control population, making risk calculation and cost analysis a more valid and useful tool. Because ACL injuries are the most common severe injury in snow sports (18, 22), further investigation could better define the problem and reduce its recurrence. Information from a well-structured outcome study examining surgical technique, rehabilitation protocol, postoperative bracing, and patient education could optimize treatment and reduce dependence on anecdotal information.

## 7.2 Cross-Country Skiing

Reduction of overuse injuries and prevention of catastrophic injuries due to exposure are the most important goals. Future research should focus on effects of cyclical progressions of training designed to reduce the incidence of stress fractures and other overuse injuries, during both winter skiing and off-season training. Preparation of the cross-country skier for harsh trail conditions (53) could further reduce catastrophic injuries and deaths associated with cross-country skiing.

# References

1. Bernhard, C. Skiskador i statistik. Nordisk Medicin 1:386-388; 1939.
2. Blitzer, C.M.; Johnson, R.J.; Ettlinger, C.F.; et al. Downhill skiing injuries in children. Am. J. Sports Med. 12:142-147; 1984.
3. Carr, D.; Johnson, R.J.; Pope, M.H. Upper extremity injuries in skiing. Am. J. Sports Med. 9:378-383; 1981.
4. Criqui, M.H. The epidemiology of skiing injuries. Minn. Med. 60:877-880; 1977.
5. Edlund, G.; Gedda, S.; Hemborg, A. Knee injuries in skiing: a prospective study from northern Sweden. Am. J. Sports Med. 8(6):411-414; 1980.
6. Ellison, A.E. Skiing injuries. Clinical Symposia 29:3-38; 1977.
7. Engkvist, O.; Balkfors, B; Lindsjö, U. Thumb injuries in downhill skiing. Int. J. Sports Med. 3:50-55; 1982.
8. Eriksson, E. Ski injuries in Sweden: a one year survey. Ortho. Clin. North Amer. 7:3-9; 1976.
9. Feagin, J.A.; Lambert, K.L.; Cunningham, R.R.; Anderson, L.M.; Riegel, J.; King, P.H.; Van Generen, L. Considerations of the anterior cruciate ligament injury in skiing. Clin. Orth. Rel. Res. 216:13-18; 1987.
10. Frost, A.; Bauer, M. Skiers hip—a new clinical entity? J. Ortho. Trauma 5:47-50; 1991.
11. Garrick, J.G.; Requa, R.K. Injury patterns in children and adolescent skiers. Am. J. Sports Med. 7(4):245-248; 1979.
12. Frymoyer, J.W.; Pope, M.H.; Costanza, M.C.; Rosen, J.C.; Goggin, J.E.; Wilder, D.G. Epidemiological studies of low-back pain. Spine 5:419-423; 1980.
13. Gertsch, P.; Borgeat, A.; Wälli, T. New cross-country skiing technique and compartment syndrome. Am. J. Sports Med. 15:612-613; 1987.
14. Hauser, W.; Asang, E.; Müller, B. Injury risk in alpine skiing. Skiing trauma and safety: fifth international symposium. ASTM STP 860:338-348; 1985.
15. Higgins, R.W.; Steadman, J.R. Anterior cruciate ligament repairs in world class skiers. Am. J. Sports Med. 15:439-447; 1987.
16. Hixson, E.G. Injury patterns in cross country skiing. Physician Sportsmed. 9:45-53; 1981.
17. Howe, J.; Johnson, R.J. Knee injuries in skiing. Clin. Sports Med. 1:277-288; 1982.
18. Johnson, R.J. Prevention of cruciate ligament injuries. In Feagin, J.A. ed. The crucial ligaments. New York: Churchill Livingstone; 1988:349-356.
19. Johnson, R.J.; Pope, M.H.; Weisman, B.E.M.E.; White, B.F.; Ettlinger, C. Knee injury in skiing. Am. J. Sports Med. 7:321; 1979.
20. Johnson, R.J.; Ettlinger, C.F. Alpine ski injuries: through the years. Clin. Sports Med. 1:181-197; 1982.
21. Johnson, R.J.; Ettlinger, C.F.; Campbell, R.J.; Pope, M.H. Trends in skiing injuries: analysis of a 6-year study (1972-1978). Am. J. Sports Med. 8:106-113; 1980.
22. Johnson, R.J.; Ettlinger C.F.; Shealy, J.E. Skier injury trends—1972-1990. Skiing trauma and safety: ninth international symposium. ASTM STP 1182:11-22; 1993.
23. Johnson, R.J.; Pope, M.H. Tibial shaft fractures in skiing. Am. J. Sports Med. 5:49-62; 1977.
24. Johnson, R.J.; Pope, M.H.; Weisman, G.; et al. Knee injury in skiing. Am. J. Sports Med. 7:321-327; 1979.
25. Joubert, B. What makes a great downhill racer? Skiing 37:218-228; 1984.
26. Kristiansen, T.K.; Johnson, R.J. Fractures in the skiing athlete. Clin. Sports Med. 9:215-224; 1990.
27. Kuriyama, S.; Fujimaki, E.; Katagiri, T.; Uemura, S. Anterior dislocation of the shoulder joint sustained through skiing: arthographic findings and prognosis. Am. J. Sports Med. 12(5):339-346; 1984.
28. Lamont, M.K. Ski injury statistics: what changes? Skiing trauma and safety: eighth international symposium. ASTM STP 1104:158-163; 1991.
29. Lawson, S.K.; Reid, D.C.; Wiley, J.P. Anterior compartment pressures in cross-country skiers: a comparison of classic and skating skis. Am. J. Sports Med. 20:750-753; 1992.
30. Lysens, R.J.; deWeerdt, W.; Nieuwboer, A. Factors associated with injury proneness. Sports Medicine 12:281-289; 1991.

31. Lystad, H. A one year study of alpine ski injuries in Hemsedal, Norway. Skiing trauma and safety: fifth international symposium. ASTM STP 860:314-325; 1985.

32. Margreiter, R.; Raas, E.; Lugger L.J. The risk of injury in experienced alpine skiers. Ortho. Clin. North Amer. 7(1):51-54; 1976.

33. Matter, P.; Ziegler, W.J.; Holzach, P. Skiing accidents in the past 15 years. J. Sports Sci. 5:319-326; 1987.

34. McConkey, J.P. Anterior cruciate ligament rupture in skiing—a new mechanism of injury. Am. J. Sports Med. 14:160-164; 1986.

35. Meeuwisse, W.H. Predictability of sports injuries: what is the epidemiological evidence? Sports Med. 12:8-15; 1991.

36. National Ski Areas Association (NSAA) News Release. Lakewood, Colorado: NSAA Publications; 1994.

37. Oh, S. Cervical injury from skiing. Int. J. Sports Med. 5:268-271; 1984.

38. Orava, S.; Jaroma, H.; Hulkko, A. Overuse injuries in cross-country skiing. Brit. J. Sports Med. 19:158-160; 1985.

39. Paletta, G.A., Jr.; Levine, D.S.; O'Brien, S.J.; Wickiewicz, T.L.; Warren, R.F. Patterns of meniscal injury associated with acute anterior cruciate ligament injury in skiers. Am. J. Sports Med. 20:542-547; 1992.

40. Paletta, G.A., Jr.; Warren, R.F. Knee injuries and alpine skiing. Sports Med. 17:411-423; 1994.

41. Pigman, E.C.; Karakla, D.W. Skiing injuries during initial military nordic ski training of a U.S. Marine Corps battalion landing team. Milit. Med. 155:303-305; 1990.

42. Pigman, E.C.; Volcheck, G.W.; Grice, G.P. Profiles with two different types of NATO ski bindings. Milit. Med. 155:354-356; 1990.

43. Powell, K.; Koho, H.W.; Casperson, C.J.; et al. An epidemiological perspective on the causes of running injuries. Physician Sportsmed. 14:111-114; 1986.

44. Reid, D.C.; Saboe, L. Spine fractures in winter sports. Sports Medicine 7:393-399; 1989.

45. Renstrom, P.; Johnson, R.J. Cross-country skiing injuries and biomechanics. Sports Medicine 8:346-370; 1989.

46. Sandelin, J.; Kiviluoto, O.; Santavirta, S. Injuries of competitive skiers in Finland: a three year survey. Ann. Chir. Gynaecol. 69(3):97-101; 1980.

47. Shealy, J.E. Comparison of downhill ski injury patterns—1978-81 vs. 1988-90. Skiing trauma and safety: ninth international symposium. ATSM STP 1182:23-33; 1993.

48. Shealy, J.E. Death in downhill skiing. In Schroeder, R.J.; Green, K.A.; Hoersch, et al, eds. Ski trauma and safety. Proceedings of the fifth international sympo-sium. Philadelphia: ASTM Publications; 1985:111-114.

49. Sherry, E. Skiing injuries in Australia. Med. J. Aust. 142:530-531; 1984.

50. Sherry, E.; Asquith, J. Nordic (cross-country) skiing injuries in Australia. Med. J. Aust. 146:245-246; 1987.

51. Sherry, E.; Clout, L. Deaths associated with skiing in Australia: a 32 year study of cases from the Snowy Mountains. Med. J. Aust. 149:615-618; 1988.

52. Sherry, E.; Fenelon, L. Trends in skiing injury type and rates in Australia: a review of 22,261 injuries over 27 years in the Snowy Mountains. Med. J. Aust. 155:513-515; 1991.

53. Sherry, E.; Henderson, A. Hazards of cross-country skiing. Aust. Fam. Phys. 16:851; 1987.

54. Sherry, E.; Richards, D. Hypothermia among resort skiers: 19 cases from the Snowy Mountains. Med. J. Aust. 144:457-461; 1986.

55. Steinbrück, K. Frequency and aetiology of injury in cross-country skiing. J. Sports Sciences 5:187-196; 1987.

56. Stener, B. Displacement of the ruptured ulnar collateral ligament of the metacarpophalangeal joint of the thumb. J. Bone Joint Surg. 44B:869; 1962.

57. Stuart, M.J. Traumatic disruption of the anterior tibial tendon while cross-country skiing. A case report. Clin. Ortho. 281:193-194; 1992.

58. Tapper, E.M. Ski injuries from 1939-1976: the Sun Valley experience. Am. J. Sports Med. 6:114-121; 1978.

59. Ungerholm, S; Engkvist, O.; Gierup, J.; Lindsjö, U.; Balkfors, B. Skiing injuries in children and adults: a comparative study from an 8-year period. Int. J. Sports Med. 4:236-240; 1983.

60. Westlin, N.E. Factors contributing to the production of skiing injuries. Ortho. Clin. North Amer. 7:45-49, 55-58; 1976.

61. Weston, J.T.; Moore, S.M.; Rich, T.H. A five-year study of mortality in a busy ski population. J. Forensic Sci. 22(1):222-230; 1977.

62. Wojtys, E.M.; Loubert, P.V.; Samson, S.Y.; et al. Use of a knee brace for control of tibial translation and rotation. A comparison in cadavers of available models. J. Bone Joint Surg. 72A:1323-1329; 1990.

63. Young, L.R.; Lee, S.M. Alpine injury pattern at Waterville Valley. Ski trauma and safety, 8th intl. symposium. ASTM STP 1104:125-132; 1991.

64. Young, L.R.; Oman, C.M.; Crane, H.C.; et al. The etiology of ski injuries: an eight year study of the skier and his equipment. Ortho. Clin. North Amer. 7:13-29; 1976.

65. Yvars, M.; Kanner, H.R. Ski fractures of the femur. Am. J. of Sports Med. 12(5):386-390; 1984.

# 4

# American Football

*Frederick Mueller, Eric D. Zemper, and Arlene Peters*

## 1. Introduction

Over the past 20 years, football, like a number of other sports, has shown a significant increase in the number of participants. In 1992 there were 1,500,000 high school and junior high school players and 75,000 college and university athletes (68, 69). Since 1971 the number of high school participants has increased by 25% (300,000 players), while participation at the college level has remained steady at approximately 75,000 players. With this increased number of athletes playing football, we would expect there to be an increase in the total number of injuries each year, and an increased number of football injuries has been documented (57). Of course, this translates into an increased burden on the health-care system. Knowledge of the variables influencing and contributing to the incidence of football-related injuries is important to all those involved in the game. Such information allows for the comprehensive detection and prevention of football-related injuries, making the game safer and more enjoyable for everyone.

To better educate players, coaches, athletic trainers, physicians, and sport administrators about the likelihood of injury, it is necessary to identify the causal and influential factors and mechanisms contributing to the risk of injury in the game of football. The purpose of this chapter is to document and describe football injury research studies of players at the high school and college levels. In comparing, contrasting, and evaluating this injury research literature, the goal is to give a detailed picture of the injury situation in football.

We undertook a search of the available research literature on football injuries since 1971, utilizing our personal resources as well as searches of Medline and Sport Discus and using football (injury or accident) and language-English for the on-line search request. Football is one of the few sports that does have a sizeable body of published literature on injuries, and we retrieved a large number of titles. However, relatively few published studies can be considered true epidemiologic studies, prospective or even retrospective. Most of the studies in the published literature are reports of one or two cases of an unusual nature or a case series of football injuries seen in a particular hospital or clinic. These types of studies provide no information on the population from which the injured athletes were drawn, and therefore can provide no information on football injury rates. With a few exceptions, we did not include such case reports or case series in the literature reviewed in this chapter in order to make the reviewing task more manageable and to keep the focus on true epidemiologic data. For similar reasons, we did not include studies involving data collection methods such as review of insurance claims because they provide no data on the population at risk, and it should be obvious that not all injuries result in insurance claims.

While reviewing these studies, it became clear that injury rates were calculated differently across different studies and the definition of a reportable injury varied widely. Any attempt to compare across studies, therefore, was very difficult and, in most cases, meaningless unless they happened to be using similar rates and definitions. Those reporting high school data tended to report their injury distributions as a percentage of the total number of injuries recorded or as the number of injuries per 100 players. At the collegiate level most researchers reported their results as injuries per 1,000 athlete-exposures (A-E), in which one A-E is one athlete participating in one game or practice where he is exposed to the possibility of being injured.

Although the rate of injuries per 100 players is frequently used in the literature, it does not take into account the varying number of games and practices across teams, or that all players are not involved in every practice or game. This can result in some very misleading comparisons, even if two studies report rates per 100 players (104, 108). Reporting injury rates per 1,000 A-E compensates for these differences and allows for more direct comparisons between studies, assuming the studies used similar definitions of a reportable injury. These problems in making comparisons across studies should be kept foremost in the reader's mind while considering the results from the various studies summarized in this chapter.

## 2. Incidence of Injury

### 2.1 Injury Rates

The relatively high number of injuries seen in football is the result of several factors. First, the dramatic increase in participation has produced an increase in the total number of injuries (57). Second, the inherently violent nature of the game, the physically demanding aspects of the game, and the speed, strength, and size of the players combine to make football a high risk sport (102).

The total injury rates found in various studies of high school and college football teams are presented in Tables 4.1 and 4.2, respectively. From these two tables a few observations can be drawn:

• The rate of injuries at the high school level as a percent of the players on the team (essentially an injury rate per 100 players), which was most often reported at the high school level, ranged from 11.8 to 81.1. For the reasons mentioned previously, trying to make comparisons across these studies using this type of "rate" carries very little validity. The wide range of results probably stems largely from the variety of definitions of a reportable injury used in the various studies and whether medically trained individuals were recording the data. Among studies with similar injury definitions, the range was 48.8 to 81.1.

• The one study that reported an injury rate per 1,000 A-E (4) reported a rate of 8.1 injuries per 1,000 A-E, which was similar to the values reported in Table 4.2 for college teams. Because this study reported the same type of rate and used the same definition of a reportable injury, a direct comparison with the college studies is possible.

• In the college level studies (Table 4.2) the injury rates per 1,000 A-E all fall within the range of 6.1 to 11.1 (for those studies that used the same injury definition of missing one day or more). The older studies tended to have the higher rates and the more recent studies the lower rates, indicating a possible trend toward slightly decreasing injury rates over the past 15 years.

• It is apparent from a comparison of the results in Tables 4.1 and 4.2 that when a common injury rate is reported and a common injury definition is used, as most studies at the college level did (Table 4.2), direct comparisons between studies are much easier. This is contrasted with the situation in Table 4.1 in which the high school reports tended to use a less rigorous type of injury rate and a wide variety of definitions of a reportable injury.

**Table 4.1   A Comparison of Injury Rates in High School Football**

| Study | Type | Duration | Reportable injury definition | # subjects/ # teams | # injuries | Inj. per 100 players | Inj. per 1,000 A-E |
|---|---|---|---|---|---|---|---|
| Alles et al., 1979 | P[a] | 1975-77 | Time loss ≥ 1 day | 2,674[b]/53 | 1,696[b] | 63.4[b] | 8.1 |
| Blyth and Mueller, 1974 | P | 1969-72 | Time loss ≥ 1 day | 8,776/43 | 4,287 | 48.8 | |
| Garrick and Requa, 1978 | P | 1973-75 | Time loss ≥ 1 day | 624/8 | 506 | 81.1 | |
| Hoffman and Lyman, 1988 | P (games only) | 1986 | Prevent from continuing play | 1,180/14 | 139 | 11.8[b] | |
| NATA, 1987 | P | 1986 | Time loss ≥ 1 day | 6,544/105 | 4,292 | 65.6[b] | 8.2[b] |
| Olson, 1979 | P | 1970-78 | Time loss ≥ 2 days or 1 game | 3,300/? | 465 | 14.1 | |
| Prager et al., 1989 | P | 1982-85 | Time loss ≥ 2 days | 598/4 | 251 | 42.1 | |

[a]P = prospective cohort study.

[b]These figures were not presented in the original article, but were calculated based on data provided in the article.

**Table 4.2  A Comparison of Injury Rates in College Football**

| Study | Type | Duration | Reportable injury definition | # subjects/ # teams | # injuries | Inj. per 100 players | Inj. per 1,000 A-E |
|---|---|---|---|---|---|---|---|
| Alles et al., 1979 | P[a] | 1975-77 | Time loss ≥ 1 day | 13,416[b]/148 | 12,432[b] | 92.7[b] | 11.1 |
| Buckley and Powell, 1982 | P | 1975-80 | Time loss > 7 days | 28,419/309 | 7,190[b] | 25.3 | 3.1 |
| Canale et al., 1981 | P | 1975-79 | Time loss ≥ 1 day | 265/1 | 283 | 46.6 | |
| Clarke and Miller, 1977 | P | 1975-76 | Time loss > 7 days | ?/38 | | | 7.1 |
| NCAA, 1990 | P | 1984-89 | Time loss ≥ 1 day | ?/408 | 19,243 | | 6.4 |
| Whiteside et al., 1985 | P | 1972-83 | Unable to function in usual capacity | 2,730/1 | 2,186 | 80.1[b] | |
| Zemper, 1989b | P | 1986-88 | Time loss ≥ 1 day | 8,325/80 | 3,744 | 45.0 | 6.1 |

[a]P = prospective cohort study.

[b]These figures were not presented in the original article, but were calculated based on data provided in the article.

## 2.2 Reinjury Rates

The rate of reinjury to football players appears to be a neglected area of research in the literature. This area warrants further research because it appears that prior injury may be a risk factor for further injury. What little information is available comes from three of the studies reviewed here. In a 4-year study Blyth and Mueller (10) found that 60% of high school players with a prior injury had another injury, whereas only 40% of players without any prior injury had a new injury. The NATA study (64) documented that over 10% of the injuries reported in the 1986 study of high school players were reinjuries to a previously hurt area and that 4% of those injuries were directly related to the prior injuries. Although this study indicated a rate of 65 injuries per 100 players, it was noted that only 37% of the players in the study were injured at least once, implying that a considerable proportion of the players were injured more than once, though not necessarily to the same body part. At the collegiate level, Zemper (104, 105) noted that although there was an injury rate of 45 per 100 players, only 33.2 players out of 100 incurred at least one injury, implying that the remaining injuries were recurrent injuries or new injuries to a different body part in a player who had been injured previously.

## 2.3 Injury in Practice and Competition

The authors of many studies discuss whether practices or games are more dangerous or carry a higher risk. However, most studies make comparisons based on a percentage breakdown of injuries occurring in practices and games, and conclude that because more injuries (or a greater percentage) occur in practices, they are riskier for a player than games. For instance, the 1986 NATA high school study (64) states that 62% of the recorded injuries occurred in practices and only 38% in games. When considering this type of data, it must be remembered that a percentage breakdown of total injuries is *not* a *rate* and therefore has no relation to estimating risk. Because a team has at least five or six times as many practices as games, and usually more players participate in practices than games, it would be expected that the total *number* (or percentage) of injuries would be higher in practices. This type of information has its importance; as the NATA summaries correctly point out, more injuries occur in practices in high school, where there is less likely to be adequate medical coverage. This is a situation that needs to be addressed. But this does not mean that an individual player is at a greater *risk* of injury in practices. Among the few studies that correctly address this issue are the collegiate studies done by the NCAA (67) and by Zemper (104, 105), in which injury *rates* are calculated separately for practices and for games, and a *relative risk* can therefore be calculated based on these rates. The NCAA study (67) provides a practice injury rate of 3.99 per 1,000 A-E and a game injury rate of 35.45 per 1,000 A-E, from which a relative risk of 8.9 can be calculated. This indicates that an individual player is 8.9 times as likely to be injured in a game as he is in a practice, even though the NCAA data also show that the majority (57%) of the injuries occur in practice. The data from Zemper (105) show a practice rate of 3.79 per 1,000 A-E and a game rate of 32.11 per 1,000 A-E, so the game injury rate in this study is 8.5 times higher than the practice rate.

## 3. Injury Characteristics

### 3.1 Injury Onset

Given that football is a collision sport, it would be expected that most football injuries are acute, as opposed to overuse or gradual onset injuries. None of the studies reviewed here directly addressed this issue, so no conclusions or comparisons can be drawn. The only hint along these lines comes from some unpublished data from Zemper on college football, which indicates that over a 4-year period only 5% of 4,559 reported injuries (that kept a player out for one day or more) were overuse or gradual onset injuries.

### 3.2 Injury Type

A review of the literature summarized in Table 4.3 indicates that at both the high school and college levels the three most commonly occurring types of injuries in the game of football are sprains (ligaments), strains (muscles), and contusions. This result was fairly consistent across all the studies, including the only two college level studies that provided a breakdown of injuries by type. The great discrepancies seen in the percentages of sprains and strains reported by Lackland (52) raise

the question of how these two injury types were defined in this particular study, but also may reflect other differences between this and other studies, such as definitions of a reportable injury and methods of reporting and collecting data.

Information about injury type and location is important because it allows all parties involved in the game of football to pay particular attention to these areas so that effective training, conditioning, preventive, and rehabilitative measures can be developed and employed.

### 3.3 Injury Location

#### 3.3.1 Head/Spine/Trunk

The head (skull and brain) is particularly susceptible to injury because it cannot be conditioned to accept trauma, and once injured is further susceptible to injury (5, 22, 35, 50). Cantu (22) describes three principles to understand how biomechanical forces produce head injury: (a) Coup injuries occur when the head in a resting state is struck by another object producing maximal brain injury beneath the point of cranial impact; (b) contra-coup injuries occur when the head collides with a nonmoving object producing maximal brain injury opposite the side of cranial impact; and (c) direct injuries to the brain tissue may occur in the presence of a skull fracture when the bone displaces at the moment of impact.

**Table 4.3  A Percent Comparison of Injury Types**

| | | High school | | | | | | | | College | |
| --- | --- | --- | --- | --- | --- | --- | --- | --- | --- | --- | --- |
| | | Culpepper and Niemann, 1983 | Hale and Mitchell, 1981 | Lackland et al., 1982 | Blyth and Mueller, 1974 | Hoffman and Lyman, 1988 | NATA, 1987 | Olson, 1979 | HS range | Whiteside et al., 1985 | Zemper, 1989b |
| Injury type | # injuries | 1,877 | 885 | 528 | 4,287 | 139 | 4,292 | 465 | | 2,186 | 3,744 |
| | Study type | CS[a] | CS | CS | P[a] | P | P | P | | P | P |
| | # participants | ? | ? | ? | 8,776 | 1,180 | 6,544 | 3,300 | | 2,730 | 8,325 |
| Abrasion | | 0.2 | — | 2.8 | — | 3.6 | — | — | 0.2-3.6 | — | 0.2 |
| Concussion | | 1.0 | 4.7 | — | 5.4 | 6.5 | 5.7 | 9.0 | 1.0-9.0 | 6.9 | 5.4 |
| Contusion | | 24.8 | 30.1 | 22.3 | 26.8 | 26.6 | 28.8 | 14.4 | 14.4-30.1 | 15.5 | 15.2 |
| Dislocation | | 2.1 | 5.4 | — | 2.1 | — | — | 7.8 | 2.1-7.8 | 1.1 | 1.9 |
| Fracture | | 11.0 | 9.4 | 12.9 | 10.6 | 8.6 | 6.6 | 24.1 | 6.6-24.1 | 3.8 | 6.8 |
| Laceration | | 0.4 | — | — | 5.8 | — | — | — | 0.4-5.8 | — | 1.3 |
| Sprain | | 32.2 | 25.4 | 54.4 | 25.5 | 21.6 | 28.2 | 8.17 | 8.2-54.4 | 42.0 | 32.1 |
| Strain | | 12.4 | 21.0 | — | 16.2 | 8.6 | 21.3 | — | 8.6-21.3 | 9.0 | 18.6 |
| Tear (tendon) | | 3.8 | — | — | 2.0 | — | — | — | 2.0-3.8 | — | 5.6 |
| Other | | 12.3 | 3.2 | 7.6 | 5.6 | 24.5 | 9.4 | — | 3.2-24.5 | 21.8 | 12.9 |

[a]CS = case series, P = prospective cohort study.

Cantu (22) also lists several other types of head injuries that may occur as a result of football. These include intracranial hemorrhage: (a) epidural hematoma, (b) subdural hematoma, (c) intracerebral hematoma, and (d) subarachnoid hematoma; and malignant brain edema syndrome.

In both coup and contra-coup injuries, shearing forces (a force applied parallel to a surface) appear to be the major type of stress generated by an applied force. Two less severe types of stress are also generated by an applied force. These include compressive and tensile (negative pressure) stresses (22).

Head injuries also may occur as the result of an indirect (glancing) blow to the head resulting in impulsive loading in which the head is set into motion (22). Concussions may occur when "the skull is put into motion before the contained brain" (74).

Many definitions of a concussion exist in the literature, but there does seem to be some consensus that concussions are either transient or protracted and are the result of traumatically induced alterations, impairments, and dysfunction of mental (neural) function with manifested signs and symptoms including one or more of the following: loss of awareness, amnesia, dizziness, headaches, blurred vision, double vision, loss of equilibrium, feelings of deja vu, and visual and auditory hallucinations (14, 22, 35, 50).

A review of the literature indicates that cerebral concussions are the most frequently occurring types of head injuries in the game of football at the high school and college levels (3, 13, 22, 54, 104, 106). As shown in Table 4.3, concussions account for at least 5% of all reported football injuries, or at least one out of every 20 injuries.

The high incidence of cerebral concussion in the game of football is compounded by the fact that athletes appear to be susceptible to more severe head injury following an initial concussive event in which symptoms from the prior injury persist. In the literature this has been labeled as the second impact syndrome (22, 81). Furthermore, studies have shown that players suffering an initial concussion are four times more likely to sustain a second concussion compared with a player with no prior concussion (22, 35). The study of high school players by Gerberich et al. (35) involved only loss of consciousness injuries in arriving at their finding of four times greater risk for a subsequent injury. A recent study of college football players by Zemper (109) showed that players with a history of cerebral concussion (of any severity) any time during the previous 5 years were six times

as likely to suffer a new concussion as those with no history. Albright et al. (3) documented that 26 of 78 players with an initial head injury had a subsequent head injury during their collegiate career, and these were more severe than the initial injury. In the same vein, Cantu (22) stressed that athletes are less likely to suffer subsequent concussions if they have fully recovered from the initial cerebral concussion.

There appears to be some controversy in the literature concerning the mechanisms involved in cervical neck/spine injuries occurring in football. Hyperflexion, hyperextension, and axial loading have all been proposed as the primary mechanism contributing to cervical injuries.

Injuries to the cervical spine traditionally have been attributed to hyperflexion and/or hyperextension mechanisms (23, 32, 33, 79, 82). Hyperflexion, in which the head is driven downward (as seen in head butting), may be the more dangerous and frequent mechanism involved in cervical spine injuries (33, 55). In a retrospective analysis conducted by Maroon (55) seven neck injuries involved hyperflexion as the primary mechanism of injury. Five of the seven players injured were involved in the process of tackling.

Schneider et al. (82) suggested that cervical spine injuries documented in their study resulted from hyperextension (shear forces) when the face mask was impacted, driving the posterior rim of the helmet against the back of the neck and providing a "guillotine" effect. This suggestion led Schneider et al. (82) to recommend that the rim of the helmet be cut higher to prevent its impact on the neck. However, this suggestion has been refuted, since more dangerous hyperextension occurs to the upper cervical spine when the helmet is cut high. A reduction in force is seen when the posterior rim of the helmet is allowed to make contact with the back of the neck and even further loading conditions are evident when the posterior rim of the helmet makes contact with the shoulder pads (23).

Axial loading occurs when the neck is slightly flexed, cervical lordosis is straightened, and the spine is converted into a segmented column. When a load is applied to the top of the helmet, as in spearing, force is transmitted down the straightened cervical spine, and an axial load is created and transmitted to the spinal structures. This results in the spine being compressed and crushed, and fractures and/or dislocations will occur (96).

Injuries to the cervical spine can be divided into four categories: (a) sprains, (b) strains, (c) fractures, and (d) dislocations (7). Torg (95) further categorized spinal injuries into five groups according to their severity. Group I is made up of mild sprain and strain injuries that improve with or without treatment, and includes *burners* or *stingers* (pinched cervical nerve syndrome). Group II is made up of moderate injuries and includes compression fractures, degenerative spine changes, and brachial plexus axonotmesis. Group III is made up of more severe neck injuries and includes unstable lesions with fractures, dislocations, and/or subluxation without neurologic deficit. Group IV is made up of very severe injuries including fracture-dislocations with neurologic deficit. Group V is made up of catastrophic disabling injuries, which include permanent quadriplegia or death. We will discuss the latter group in section 4.2—Catastrophic Injuries.

Lateral flexion (stretching, bending, or traction of the cervical nerve roots) has been identified as a mechanism of injury in cervical neck/spine injuries. This mechanism results in brachial plexus injuries, commonly called burners or stingers. These occur when a player receives a forceful blow to the head from the side with simultaneous depression of the opposite shoulder. Injury also may result from head extension or by depression of the shoulder while the neck and head are fixed.

A review of the literature indicates that brachial plexus injuries associated with a prickly burning sensation in the shoulders, and pain and weakness in the neck, arms, and hands, are the most commonly observed neck injuries (33, 54, 87). Robertson et al. (77) in a study of collegiate football players indicated that approximately 50% of the players on the team experienced at least one and sometimes more injuries of the plexus during a season. Furthermore, players with repeated incidence of this type of injury were at higher risk of developing further weakness and neurological dysfunction. Dolan et al. (32) report that a collegiate football team may experience an average of six stingers during a single game with as many as five or six major neck injuries, including fractures, disk or ligament disruptions, or persistent neuropathies, during one football season. Albright et al. (3) indicated that the majority (55%) of the neck injuries suffered by collegiate players were of a soft tissue or skeletal nature with sprains being the most common type of injury (64% with a mean time loss of 5.5 days). When reviewing high school incidence rates, Albright et al. (2) found that 32% of college freshman players demonstrated evidence of prior neck injury sustained during their high school football careers.

### 3.3.2 Upper Extremities

Injuries to the upper extremities commonly occur in the game of football. The most frequently reported cases appear to be the shoulders, hands, and fingers. The frequent occurrence of these injuries is not surprising considering that the hands and fingers are minimally protected by padding and are under constant trauma through blocking and tackling, and although the shoulder is protected by pads, it is often the initial contact point in tackling and blocking. The hand may be particularly vulnerable to injury because it is used often in direct contact against the headgear, the face mask, the shoulder pads, and the opponent's body. Injuries to the fingers also may occur as players grasp the opponent's belts, jerseys, and pads while tackling and blocking.

### 3.3.3 Lower Extremities

Football, a violent collision and contact sport, puts some of the greatest demands on the lower extremity because it is the major weight-bearing area of the body and is usually fixed to the ground. Additionally, football players are required to make severe running, cutting, and jumping moves, all adding to the stress placed on the lower body. The knee is particularly vulnerable to injury because it is minimally protected by padding and is often in an exposed position (20, 73, 90).

Because knee motion is limited to internal and external rotation as the leg straightens (extension) and bends (flexion), injury may occur when the joint is stressed into awkward and unusual positions, usually as the result of direct contact from other players. Noncontact injuries often involve unnatural twisting motions and drills that prevent the natural rotation of the knee joint. Such injuries are commonly seen in cutting maneuvers when the foot is fixed to the ground, causing damage to the anterior cruciate ligaments, the collateral ligaments, menisci, and patella (30, 90, 99).

A review of Tables 4.4 and 4.5 demonstrates that, at the high school and college levels, the knee is the most frequently injured body part in the lower extremity. Among the most common knee injuries in football are ligament injuries (grade I, grade II, and grade III sprains), of which the medial collateral ligament is the most commonly sprained (31). The frequent occurrence of knee sprains is a concern because a significant percentage of these injuries may require surgical intervention and result in significant time loss from active participation (31, 47). Additionally, injury to the medial collateral ligament often increases the likelihood of further injury to the supporting structures of the knee, particularly damage to the anterior cruciate ligament (70). Other common knee injuries include medial femoral condyle fractures, epiphyseal fractures, anterior and posterior cruciate damage, meniscus injuries, and patellofemoral arthritis (8, 45, 58, 63, 100).

A review of Tables 4.4 and 4.5 shows that injuries to the lower extremities also commonly occur in the ankle, toe, hip, quadriceps, and hamstring. According to Rishel et al. (76), most ankle injuries are inversion sprains that result in tears to the lateral ligament structures. Damage to these ligaments leads to ankle instability, making the athlete more susceptible to recurrent ankle injuries.

Injuries to the toe, particularly the metatarsal-phalangeal joint (bunion joint of the big toe), also are significant lower extremity injuries commonly seen in football players. This injury is referred to as turf-toe (100).

A 5-year retrospective study conducted by Heiser et al. (40) demonstrated that injuries to the hamstring may also be common among collegiate football players, highlighting the need for an evaluation and rehabilitation program to prevent and lessen the frequency and severity of hamstring strains. The study revealed that, prior to a strengthening and rehabilitation program, 7.7% of the players reported hamstring strains, with 31.7% sustaining one or more recurrent injuries. Players utilizing a Cybex II program reported only a 1.1% hamstring injury rate with no recurrent injuries being reported.

## 4. Injury Severity

Injury severity for our purposes is broken down into two broad categories. The first is the common time-loss injury from which the athlete recovers in a matter of hours, days, or occasionally weeks, and which usually is measured by number of days before return to unrestricted activity. The second category is the catastrophic injury resulting in some form of permanent disability. This latter category also includes fatalities.

**Table 4.4  A Percent Comparison of Injury Location**

| Injury type | | | High school | | | | | | | | College | | |
|---|---|---|---|---|---|---|---|---|---|---|---|---|---|
| | | Culpepper and Niemann, 1983 | Hale and Mitchell, 1981 | Lackland et al., 1982 | Blyth and Mueller, 1974 | Hoffman and Lyman, 1988 | NATA, 1987 | Olson, 1979 | | Canale et al., 1981 | Whiteside et al., 1985 | Zemper, 1989b |
| | # injuries | 1,877 | 885 | 528 | 4,287 | 139 | 4,292 | 465 | | 283 | 2,186 | 3,744 |
| Injury type | Study type | CS[a] | CS | CS | P[a] | P | P | P | HS | P | P | P |
| | # participants | ? | ? | ? | 8,776 | 1,180 | 6,544 | 3,300 | range | 265 | 273 | 8,325 |
| Head | | 7.6 | 4.0 | 6.6 | 10.3 | 10.1 | 11.8 | 9.0 | 4.0-11.8 | 5.7 | 6.9 | 7.3 |
| Spine/trunk | | 9.4 | 7.0 | 8.6 | 12.4 | 18.0 | 10.0 | 5.4 | 5.4-18.0 | 14.7 | 11.2 | 14.3 |
| Neck/spine | | — | 2.0 | 2.5 | 2.6 | 4.3 | — | 0.8 | 0.8-4.3 | 4.8 | 7.2 | 5.3 |
| Trunk (torso) | | — | - | - | - | - | 10.0 | — | —-10.0 | — | — | — |
| Back | | 4.9 | 5.0 | 1.9 | 4.7 | 6.5 | — | 2.3 | 1.9-6.5 | 4.2 | 4.0 | 4.5 |
| Chest/rib | | 3.4 | — | 4.2 | 3.1 | 3.6 | — | 2.3 | 2.3-4.2 | 2.4 | — | 2.4 |
| Abdomen | | 0.7 | — | — | — | 2.9 | — | — | 0.7-2.9 | — | — | 0.3 |
| Groin | | 0.4 | — | — | 2.0 | 0.7 | — | — | 0.4-2.0 | 3.3 | — | 1.8 |
| Upper extremities | | 34.8 | 33.0 | 31.8 | 24.4 | 15.1 | 24.3 | 25.7 | 15.1-34.8 | 13.2 | 5.4 | 21.7 |
| Shoulder | | 13.3 | 10.0 | — | 8.3 | 3.6 | 9.7 | 9.3 | 3.6-13.3 | 8.7 | 5.4 | 12.0 |
| Arm (upper & lower) | | 3.4 | 4.0 | 15.3 | 3.8 | 3.6 | — | 1.9 | 1.9-15.3 | 0.3 | — | 0.8 |
| Elbow | | 3.4 | 3.0 | 2.3 | 2.4 | 2.2 | — | 1.6 | 1.6-3.4 | 1.2 | — | 1.9 |
| Wrist | | 2.9 | — | 3.0 | 1.9 | 0.7 | 14.6 | 4.7 | 0.7-14.6 | 3.0 | — | 0.8 |
| Hand/finger | | 11.8 | 16.0 | 11.2 | 8.0 | 5.0 | — | 8.2 | 5.0-16.0 | — | — | 6.2 |
| Lower extremities | | 48.3 | 46.0 | 53.0 | 49.0 | 49.7 | 49.1 | 55.9 | 46.0-55.9 | 48.9 | 42.0 | 55.3 |
| Pelvis/hip | | 2.4 | 3.0 | 4.9 | 2.7 | 1.4 | 17.9 | — | 1.4-17.9 | 2.1 | — | 3.0 |
| Knee | | 22.2 | 13.0 | 17.2 | 19.3 | 14.4 | 14.6 | 36.5 | 13.0-36.5 | 20.1 | 22.6 | 19.7 |
| Leg (upper & lower) | | 8.6 | 18.0 | 9.1 | 8.8 | 20.2 | — | 7.8 | 8.6-20.2 | 14.1 | — | 14.1 |
| Ankle | | 10.9 | 12.0 | 18.8 | 15.3 | 11.5 | 16.6 | 9.7 | 9.7-18.8 | 10.8 | 19.4 | 15.4 |
| Foot/toe | | 4.2 | — | 3.0 | 2.9 | 2.2 | — | 1.9 | 1.9-4.2 | 1.8 | — | 3.1 |
| Other | | 0.2 | 10.0 | 0.0 | 3.9 | 7.1 | 4.8 | 3.9 | 0.0-10.0 | 16.9 | — | 1.3 |

[a]CS = case series, P = prospective cohort study.

**Table 4.5   A Rate Comparison of Injury Location (Injury Rate/1,000 Athlete-Exposures)**

| Injury location | | High school | College | | |
|---|---|---|---|---|---|
| | | Alles et al., 1979 | Alles et al., 1979 | Buckley and Powell, 1982 | Zemper, 1989b |
| | # injuries | 1,696 | 12,432 | 7,190 | 3,744 |
| | Study type | P[a] | P | P | P |
| | # participants | 2,674 | 13,416 | 28,419 | 8,325 |
| Head | | 0.62 | 0.78 | 1.7 | 0.44 |
| Spine/trunk | | 0.63 | 0.49 | 0.9 | 0.87 |
|   Neck/spine | | — | — | — | 0.32 |
|   Trunk (torso) | | 0.63 | 0.49 | 0.9 | — |
|   Back | | — | — | — | 0.27 |
|   Chest/rib | | — | — | — | 0.15 |
|   Abdomen | | — | — | — | 0.02 |
|   Groin | | — | — | — | 0.11 |
| Upper extremities | | 1.59 | 1.75 | 2.5 | 1.32 |
|   Shoulder | | 0.67 | 1.07 | 1.4 | 0.73 |
|   Arm (upper & lower) | | 0.92 | 0.68 | 1.1 | 0.05 |
|   Elbow | | — | — | — | 0.12 |
|   Wrist | | — | — | — | 0.05 |
|   Hand/finger | | — | — | — | 0.37 |
| Lower extremities | | 4.61 | 6.20 | 8.1 | 3.34 |
|   Pelvis/hip | | — | — | — | 0.18 |
|   Knee | | 1.95 | 3.16 | 3.1 | 1.19 |
|   Leg (upper & lower) | | 1.19 | 1.30 | 2.4 | 0.85 |
|   Ankle | | 1.47 | 1.74 | 2.6 | 0.93 |
|   Foot/toe | | — | — | — | 0.19 |
| Other | | 0.40 | 0.00 | 0.2 | 0.08 |

[a]P = prospective cohort study.

## 4.1 Time Loss

Few of the articles reviewed for this chapter had more than a minimal mention of time loss in relation to injuries. Blyth and Mueller (10) found in 4 years of covering football injuries in 43 North Carolina high schools that 18.1% of the reported injuries kept a player out for one day, 47.2% for 2 to 6 days, and 34.7% for 7 or more days. At the collegiate level, Buckley (15) found in 5 years of NAIRS data from the late 1970s that the total reportable injury rate (time loss of 1 day or more) was 10.1/1,000 athlete-exposures, whereas injuries severe enough to cause more than 7 days of time loss occurred at a rate of 2.7/1,000 A-E. More recently, data on college football from Zemper (105) (3 years) and the NCAA (67) (6 years) found injury rates of one day or more duration to be 6.1 and 6.4/1,000 A-E, respectively.

Data on college football injuries during the 1988 to 1990 seasons collected by Zemper (unpublished) included the number of days lost for each of 3,363 injuries reported. For injuries that kept a player out for 1 to 2 days the rate was 1.7/1,000 A-E

(27.6% of the total number of injuries), for 3 to 4 days 1.3/1,000 A-E (20.9%), 5 to 6 days 0.8/1,000 A-E (12.2%), 7 to 9 days 0.7/1,000 A-E (10.4%), and for 10 or more days 1.8/1,000 A-E (28.9%). For the 3,363 injuries there were a total of 48,730 days lost, with an average of 14.6 days lost per injury.

## 4.2 Catastrophic Injury

Catastrophic injuries are defined as injuries that result in death or some type of permanent disability. The nonfatal injuries generally include permanent paralysis (quadriplegia, paraplegia, or hemiplegia) caused by spinal cord damage or brain trauma (e.g., subdural hematoma).

### 4.2.1 Spinal Cord

Reference to Table 4.6 indicates that during the 16-year period from 1977 to 1992 a total of 155 football players had incomplete neurological recovery from cervical cord injuries (62). One hundred and twenty-seven of these injuries were to high school players, and 20 to college players. The remaining

**Table 4.6  Football Fatalities and Catastrophic Injuries (1970-1992)**

| Year | High school | | | College | | |
|------|---------------------|-----------------------|----------------------|---------------------|-----------------------|----------------------|
|      | Direct fatalities | Indirect fatalities | Incomplete recovery | Direct fatalities | Indirect fatalities | Incomplete recovery |
| 1970 | 23 | 12 | — | 3 | 2 | — |
| 1971 | 15 | 7 | — | 3 | 2 | — |
| 1972 | 16 | 10 | — | 2 | 1 | — |
| 1973 | 7 | 5 | — | 0 | 3 | — |
| 1974 | 10 | 5 | — | 1 | 3 | — |
| 1975 | 13 | 3 | — | 1 | 3 | — |
| 1976 | 15 | 7 | — | — | 2 | — |
| 1977 | 8 | 6 | 10 | 1 | 0 | 2 |
| 1978 | 9 | 8 | 13 | 0 | 1 | 0 |
| 1979 | 3 | 8 | 8 | 1 | 1 | 3 |
| 1980 | 9 | 4 | 11 | 0 | 0 | 2 |
| 1981 | 5 | 6 | 6 | 2 | 0 | 2 |
| 1982 | 7 | 7 | 7 | 0 | 3 | 2 |
| 1983 | 4 | 6 | 11 | 0 | 3 | 1 |
| 1984 | 4 | 3 | 5 | 1 | 0 | 0 |
| 1985 | 4 | 1 | 6 | 1 | 1 | 3 |
| 1986 | 11 | 7 | 3 | 1 | 1 | 0 |
| 1987 | 4 | 4 | 9 | 0 | 3 | 0 |
| 1988 | 7 | 10 | 10 | 0 | 0 | 1 |
| 1989 | 4 | 9 | 12 | 0 | 2 | 2 |
| 1990 | 0 | 3 | 11 | 0 | 3 | 2 |
| 1991 | 3 | 3 | 1 | 0 | 1 | 0 |
| 1992 | 2 | 8 | 4 | 0 | 1 | 0 |
| Totals | 183 | 142 | 127 | 17 | 36 | 20 |

*Note.* Figures are updated annually to include new cases investigated after publication. Catastrophic injuries are defined as those involving some disability (monoplegia, hemiplegia, paraplegia, quadriplegia) at the time of injury, including complete or incomplete neurological recovery. In this table incomplete recovery was the result of cervical cord injuries. Direct fatalities and injuries are defined as those resulting directly from participating in the game of football. Indirect fatalities are defined as those resulting from systemic failure as a result of exertion while participating in the game of football or by a complication secondary to a nonfatal injury.

8 injuries were to players participating at other levels (sandlot and professional). Although the 1988, 1989, and 1990 data suggest an increase in cervical cord injuries, the 1991 data show the most dramatic reduction since the beginning of the study in 1977. In 1991 there was only one cervical cord injury with incomplete neurological recovery at the high school level and none at the college level.

Table 4.7 illustrates the incidence rates of spinal cord injuries for both high school and college participants. The incidence rates per 100,000 participants are low in both high school and college. Based on the 16 years covered in this table, the high school incidence is 0.59 per 100,000 participants and the college incidence is 1.66 per 100,000 participants.

When comparing cervical cord injuries in offensive and defensive players, it appears to be safer playing offensive football. From 1977 to 1992, 113

of the 155 players (73%) with cervical cord injuries were playing defense with only 24 of the injuries occurring on the offensive side of the ball. A majority of the defensive players were injured as a result of tackling, which clearly is the most dangerous activity in the game of football. Past yearly reports by Mueller et al. have revealed that defensive backs were injured at a higher rate than other positions.

### 4.2.2 Fatalities

Table 4.6 shows that after a slight rise in the number of football fatalities during the 1986 season, the 1990 data revealed the elimination of direct football fatalities (62). That was the first time in 59 years that there have been no direct football fatalities.

Since 1960 most of the direct fatalities have been caused by head and neck injuries. The authors of the Annual Survey of Football Injury Research, Dr. Mueller and Mr. Schindler, are convinced that

**Table 4.7  Direct Football Fatalities and Catastrophic Injury Incidence per 100,000 Participants (1970-1992)**

| Year | High school | | College | |
| | Fatality incidence | Catastrophic incidence | Fatality incidence | Catastrophic incidence |
| --- | --- | --- | --- | --- |
| 1970 | 1.92 | — | 4.00 | 0.00 |
| 1971 | 1.25 | — | 4.00 | 0.00 |
| 1972 | 1.33 | — | 2.67 | — |
| 1973 | 0.58 | — | 0.00 | — |
| 1974 | 8.83 | — | 1.33 | — |
| 1975 | 1.08 | — | 1.33 | — |
| 1976 | 1.00 | — | 0.00 | — |
| 1977 | 0.53 | 0.77 | 1.33 | 2.67 |
| 1978 | 0.60 | 1.00 | 0.00 | 0.00 |
| 1979 | 0.23 | 0.62 | 1.33 | 4.00 |
| 1980 | 0.69 | 0.85 | 0.00 | 2.67 |
| 1981 | 0.38 | 0.46 | 2.67 | 2.67 |
| 1982 | 0.54 | 0.54 | 0.00 | 2.67 |
| 1983 | 0.30 | 0.85 | 0.00 | 1.33 |
| 1984 | 0.30 | 0.38 | 1.33 | 0.00 |
| 1985 | 0.30 | 0.46 | 1.33 | 4.00 |
| 1986 | 0.77 | 0.23 | 1.33 | 0.00 |
| 1987 | 0.30 | 0.69 | 0.00 | 0.00 |
| 1988 | 0.46 | 0.77 | 0.00 | 1.33 |
| 1989 | 0.27 | 0.80 | 0.00 | 2.66 |
| 1990 | 0.00 | 0.73 | 0.00 | 2.66 |
| 1991 | 0.20 | 0.07 | 0.00 | 0.00 |
| 1992 | 0.07 | 0.27 | 0.00 | 0.00 |

*Note.* Fatality incidence and catastrophic incidence are based on 1,500,000 junior and senior high school players and 75,000 college players.

current rules eliminating the head in blocking and tackling, the helmet research conducted by the National Operating Committee on Standards for Athletic Equipment (NOCSAE), excellent physical conditioning, proper medical supervision, and a good data collection system have played primary roles in reducing fatalities and serious head and neck injuries in football. This is illustrated by the increase in both head and cervical spine fatalities during the decade from 1965 to 1974. This time period was associated with blocking and tackling techniques that involved the head as the initial point of contact. In the decade from 1975 to 1984 there was a reduction in head and cervical spine injuries that was associated with the 1976 rule change eliminating the head as the initial contact point in blocking and tackling. There is no doubt that the 1976 rule change has made a difference, and that a continued effort should be made to keep the head out of the fundamental skills of football. These data illustrate the importance of data collection and analysis in making changes in the game

of football that help reduce the incidence of serious injuries.

A majority of the indirect fatalities are heat related (62). A continuous effort should be made to eliminate heat stroke deaths associated with football. There have been 46 heat stroke deaths from 1970 to 1992, and since 1974 there has been a dramatic reduction in these deaths with the exception of 1978 when there were four. There was one heat stroke death in 1992. All coaches, trainers, and physicians should continue their efforts toward eliminating athletic fatalities that result from inappropriate physical activities in hot weather.

## 4.3 Clinical Outcome/Residual Symptoms

Very little work on long-term outcome of football injuries currently can be found in the literature; it is an area that needs attention in the future. The only example of this type of research found in this survey was a long-term follow-up study of 23 high school athletes that followed the relationship between knee injuries and the development of knee osteoarthritis. Moretz (60) showed that 39% of the injured football players suffered knee injuries and that half of them showed significant degenerative changes and/or functional disability of their knees.

# 5. Injury Risk Factors

## 5.1 Intrinsic Factors

### 5.1.1 Physical Characteristics

There is evidence in the literature that lower extremity injuries may be the result of lower body strength imbalances and other leg deficiencies. According to Darden (30), 80% of all knee injuries occur to the weaker of the two legs, with as many as 88% of injuries occurring to athletes with leg length inequalities. Furthermore, athletes with insufficient ligament stability as a result of poor muscular support are prone to hyperextensive knee injuries.

Other researchers have provided evidence to dispel the theories of muscle imbalances and ligament instabilities as predisposing factors for lower extremity injury. In a prospective blind study conducted by Grace et al. (36) on high school football players, no relationship was found between isokinetically measured thigh-muscle imbalances and the increased likelihood of knee joint injuries. In a similar vein, Kalenak et al. (48) reported that selective strengthening and stretching activities, to correct for joint instability in loose-jointed college football players, did not reduce the incidence of knee injuries. Furthermore, tight-jointed and loose-jointed football players had similar knee ligament rupture incidence rates. In one other study, it was shown that ligament laxity (flexibility) tests were ineffective in predicting knee injuries in collegiate football players (59).

There does seem to be some agreement in the literature about the importance of overall lower extremity strength, conditioning, and maintenance. Athletes with poor muscle strength, particularly in the quadriceps, hamstring, and gastrocnemius muscles, are more prone to injury caused by the lack of support these muscles provide to the surrounding structures of the knee and other joints (30, 91, 99). It also has been postulated that athletes with tight heel cords may be more susceptible to lower extremity injury (98).

A review of the literature demonstrates that much research is needed in regard to the relationship size, age, weight, and height play in the overall picture of lower extremity injury. In one study it was shown that players with a greater mean height and weight showed a higher incidence of knee-joint injuries (36). However, from the way the data was analyzed, it was not evident whether the explanation for this could have been that taller, heavier players, who tend to be older, could have been receiving more exposure to the possibility of being injured because they were first string players.

Neck injuries in football can lead to serious problems, and it is clear from the literature that players with neck injuries are at a higher risk for future injuries to this area. In a study conducted 20 years ago, prior to several rule changes regarding blocking and tackling aimed at reducing head and neck injuries, Albright et al. (2) found that one third of college freshman football players demonstrated evidence of prior neck injury sustained during their high school football careers. Similar trends were evidenced for back injuries and head injuries. Albright found that after an initial injury, the chances of a player suffering subsequent head or neck trauma increased to 42% with a 67% chance that the injury would occur in some subsequent season. It also appears that players with long, thin, and poorly developed necks are at a higher risk of sustaining a neck injury (87).

Brachial plexus injuries are the most commonly observed neck injuries, and Robertson et al. (77) found that approximately 50% of the players on a college team experienced at least one and sometimes more injuries of the brachial plexus. Players with this type of neck injury are felt to be at a high risk of developing further weakness and neurological dysfunction.

## 5.2 Extrinsic Factors

### 5.2.1 Exposure

The inherently violent nature of the game of football (full contact drills and activities) combined with all the physically demanding aspects of the game (running, jumping, diving, tackling, blocking, and cutting maneuvers) make it easy to understand why and how football players are so prone to injury.

A review of the literature reveals several factors that contribute to the incidence of injury among players at different positions. (See Tables 4.8 and 4.9 for a comparison of injuries by player positions.) First, there appears to be a direct relationship between the amount of contact a player gives or receives and the incidence of injury. Whiteside et al. (102) state that the offensive and defensive line players are at greatest risk for injury because they are involved in contact on every play. In their study, offensive and defensive line players sustained 47% of the total number of time-loss injuries and illnesses with the offensive line exhibiting the largest percentage (29%).

Powell (73) states that the high incidence of injury to offensive and defensive linemen may be due to the fact there are more linemen on the field at any one time than other players. When adjusting for each individual player at his position, running backs evidenced the greater incidence of injury with 9.3 injuries per 100 games. Offensive and defensive linemen combined incurred 8.0 injuries per 100 games.

Further review of the literature indicates that the style of play exhibited by any particular team may also be a factor as to which players are going to be most prone to injury. As for practice situations, a study by Cahill et al. (17) revealed that contact activities were 4.7 times more likely to produce an injury than controlled activities. Mueller and Blyth (61) also found that limited contact practices yielded significantly lower rates of injury compared with practices with regular contact.

An interesting finding in the literature is that football players in high school will play more than one position on both offense and defense (72). It then would seem that high school athletes are at a greater risk for injury than collegiate players because of these higher exposure rates and resulting

**Table 4.8   A Comparison of Injury by Player Position in High School Football**

| Player position | Type of study Type of rate # injuries | Culpepper and Nieman, 1983 Case series % of inj. 1,877 | Blyth and Mueller, 1974 Prospective % of inj. 4,287 | Olson, 1979 (Time-loss > 7 days) Prospective % of inj. 465 | Prager, 1989 Prospective % of inj. 251 | % of injuries range | NATA, 1987[a] Prospective Inj. per 100 games 4,292 |
|---|---|---|---|---|---|---|---|
| **Offense** | | | | | | | |
| End | | — | — | 12.8 | — | —-12.8 | 3.4[b] |
| Tackle | | 11.6 | 5.7 | 8.2 | 19.5[c] | 5.7-19.5 | — |
| Guard | | 7.8 | 7.1 | 1.9 | 9.6[c] | 1.9-9.6 | — |
| Center | | 4.3 | 3.6 | 2.3 | 5.2[c] | 2.3-5.2 | — |
| Quarterback | | 8.7 | 6.1 | 3.9 | 6.4 | 3.9-8.7 | 6.9 |
| Running back | | 19.6 | 21.1 | 26.1 | 15.9 | 15.9-26.1 | 9.3 |
| Flanker/wide receiver | | 7.2 | 3.3 | — | 2.0 | 2.0-7.2 | 2.9 |
| Tight end | | 5.2 | 4.7 | — | 6.4 | 4.7-6.4 | 4.2 |
| Totals | | 64.4 | 51.6 | 55.2 | 65.0 | 51.6-65.0 | 26.7 |
| **Defense** | | | | | | | |
| End | | 4.7 | 9.2 | 8.2 | — | 4.7-9.2 | — |
| Lineman | | 5.5 | 16.7 | 17.9 | — | 5.5-17.9 | 4.7 |
| Defensive back | | 9.2 | 10.6 | 16.3[d] | 7.2 | 7.2-16.3 | 3.4 |
| Linebacker | | 9.0 | 11.4 | — | 13.1 | 9.0-13.1 | 5.1 |
| Halfback/cornerback | | — | — | — | — | — | — |
| Safety | | — | — | 1.6 | 2.0 | 1.6-2.0 | — |
| Totals | | 28.4 | 47.9 | 44.0 | 22.3 | 22.3-47.9 | 13.2 |
| Kicker/punter | | — | — | 0.8 | 1.6 | 0.8-1.6 | — |
| Other | | 7.2 | 0.2 | — | 11.1 | 0.2-11.1 | — |
| Totals | | 7.2 | 0.2 | 0.8 | 12.7 | 0.2-12.7 | — |

[a]Game-related injuries only.

[b]Listed as injuries to offensive line.

[c]No differentiation made between offensive and defensive linemen.

[d]Listed as injuries to defensive backfield.

fatigue factors. However, no conclusions were drawn from this finding.

In a prospective study on a group of collegiate football players, Derscheid et al. (31) showed that there was a relationship (although small) between player position and the risk of reinjuring the knee. Defensive team members, particularly linebackers, middle guards, and defensive tackles, appeared to be at higher risk for knee injury.

Some studies have shown that the largest proportion of knee injuries occurs in practice and scrimmage situations. Cahill et al. (18) states that nearly 55% of knee injuries occur in nongame-related activities compared with nearly 44% during games. These results are supported by Derscheid et al. (31), who found knee injuries were more than three times as likely to occur in spring practices, with their greater frequency of scrimmages, compared with the fall, when rates were based on player exposures. Keeping in mind the difference between the percentage or proportion of total injuries and an injury rate based on amount of expo-

sure, one can postulate that the greater number of injuries during practices and scrimmages is linked to the greater number of hours involved in training and practice (exposure time), as well as the larger numbers of players involved in these situations.

### 5.2.2 Training Methods

The lack of a well-rounded full year conditioning and rehabilitative program also may be viewed as a potential risk factor. A conditioning program with emphasis on stretching and strength training should be implemented at both the high school and college levels. Rehabilitative programs need to focus on reconditioning athletes to full strength before they return to practice and competition. Additionally, the lack of adequate preparticipation examinations, improper injury recognition, screening, and evaluation may all be considered potential risk factors (99).

An 8-year study of high school football varsity players demonstrated that preseason conditioning

**Table 4.9  A Comparison of Injury by Player Position in College Football**

| Player position | Type of study Type of rate # injuries | Canale, 1981 Prospective % of total injuries 283 | Whiteside, 1985 Prospective % of total injuries 2,186 | NCAA ISS, 1984 Prospective Per 1,000 athl.-exp. 3,218 | NCAA ISS, 1985 Prospective Per 1,000 athl.-exp. 3,002 | Zemper, 1989b Prospective Per 1,000 athl.-exp. 3,744 |
|---|---|---|---|---|---|---|
| **Offense** | | | | | | |
| End | | 7.8[a] | 28.9[a] | 0.81 | 0.81 | 0.30[b] |
| Tackle | | — | — | 1.03 | 0.52 | 0.22 |
| Guard | | — | — | 1.13 | 0.57 | 0.23 |
| Center | | — | — | 0.46 | 0.46 | 0.18 |
| Quarterback | | 5.9 | 1.3 | 0.58 | 0.58 | 0.26 |
| Running back | | 21.6 | 14.3[c] | 1.88 | 0.95 | 0.43 |
| Slotback/wingback | | — | — | 0.16 | 0.16 | 0.06 |
| Flanker/wide receiver | | 7.8 | 6.3 | 1.03 | 1.03 | 0.48 |
| Tight end | | 3.9 | — | — | — | — |
| Totals | | 47.0% | 50.8% | 7.08 | 5.08 | 3.02 |
| **Defense** | | | | | | |
| End | | 11.8 | — | — | — | — |
| Lineman | | 17.6 | 17.9 | 2.17 | 0.43 | 0.23 |
| Defensive back | | 21.6 | 14.0[d] | — | — | — |
| Linebacker | | 2.0 | 14.6 | 2.04 | 0.68 | 0.32 |
| Halfback/cornerback | | — | — | 1.36 | 0.69 | 0.29 |
| Safety | | — | — | 0.82 | 0.82 | 0.15 |
| Totals | | 53.0% | 46.5% | 6.39 | 2.62 | 0.99 |
| Special teams | | — | — | 0.39 | 0.39 | — |
| Kicker/punter | | — | 2.7 | 0.11 | 0.11 | — |
| Other | | — | — | 0.05 | 0.05 | — |
| Totals | | — | 2.7% | 0.55 | 0.55 | — |

[a]Listed as injuries to the offensive line.

[b]Adjusted for number of players at each position (e.g., rate for offensive tackles is 0.44 per 1,000 A-E and for centers is 0.18, but because there are two tackles and one center playing at a time, the adjusted rates are 0.22 and 0.18, respectively.

[c]Listed as injuries to the offensive backs.

[d]Listed as injuries to the defensive backs.

of the total body decreased the incidence of early season knee injuries, decreased the total number of knee injuries throughout the season, and decreased the severity of injuries. Linemen experienced greater benefits from the preseason conditioning program, with a 61% reduction in knee injuries, with improvements also being seen in flexibility and agility (16). In a follow-up study, Cahill et al. (18) demonstrated that even with the reduction of direct supervision in a preseason total body conditioning program, the incidence and severity of knee injuries were still decreased.

The incidence of football injuries may be a direct reflection of the coaching staff and their coaching philosophies and practices. A football program directed by incompetent and inexperienced personnel is more likely to suffer and promote a large number of football injuries. It is, therefore, primarily the coaches' responsibility to properly educate, prepare, condition, and train their athletes with regard to proper playing techniques. Additionally, a program using faulty and inadequate equipment and playing surfaces provides further factors contributing to the increased incidence of football-related injuries (44).

Differences in physical maturity between the players on the field may cause an unfair and unsafe playing environment. Much of the increased frequency of football-related injuries is the result of pitting players of varying size, strength, speed, and agility against each other (101).

### 5.2.3 Environment

Fixation of the foot through rigid cleating has been shown to be a primary factor in the production of lower extremity injuries, particularly of the knee and ankle (10, 20, 94). In a study conducted by Torg et al. (94) it was demonstrated that the conventional football shoe with seven 3/4 inch cleats caused the foot to become excessively fixed to the ground and uncompliant to any movement forces. In contrast, a soccer-style shoe with multiple, shorter cleats reduced foot fixation and resulted in fewer and less severe knee injuries. On the basis of these results, Torg et al. (94) recommended replacing the conventional football shoe with shoes of the following specifications: (a) synthetic molded soles, (b) minimum of 15 cleats per shoe, (c) minimum cleat diameter of 1/2 inch, and (d) maximum cleat length of 3/8 inch.

As a related factor, it has been postulated that the condition of the playing field contributes to the increased risk of lower extremity injury. In 1974 Mueller and Blyth (61) demonstrated in an experimental study that well-maintained playing fields decreased the risk of knee and ankle injuries with a 42.2% reduction in the number of injuries being observed when soccer-style shoes were used on the resurfaced fields.

The type of playing surface also may be a potential predisposing factor for lower extremity injury. In an effort to decrease foot fixation, artificial turf was developed, but a review of the literature shows a number of studies indicating this type of surface increases the number of time-loss lower extremity injuries by 30% to 50% (4, 20, 41, 88).

It is important to note that several studies have disputed the findings of increased injury risk from artificial turf. Based on football injury data obtained from 41 college teams during the 1975 season, it was found that "artificial turf did not constitute an imminent hazard" to football teams (24). In support of these findings, Henschen et al. (41) revealed that grass and artificial surfaces produced similar injury rates, but the most serious injuries occurred on artificial turf. Further evidence is provided by Culpepper et al. (29), who found that the probability of sustaining a knee or ankle injury at the high school level was the same for all types of fields.

An interesting finding in the literature revealed that the incidence of injury appears higher in the beginning of the season as well as early in the game for high school teams (10, 28, 38, 43). However, at the collegiate level Zemper (104, 105) reported that the highest rate of game injuries in his study occurred in the third quarter.

### 5.2.4 Equipment

In recent years there have been two pieces of football protective equipment that have been the focus of research. The helmet has received occasional attention in the literature, and more recently the preventive knee brace has been the subject of a number of articles.

Although a number of articles over the past 25 years have reported the incidence of cerebral concussions, only a few have actually looked at the football helmet. During the 1969 high school football season, Robey et al. (78) found essentially no difference in the incidence of second- or third-degree concussions among brands of padded helmets or brands of suspension helmets. However, the players wearing suspension helmets had lower rates of concussion overall. Data reported by Clarke and Powell (25) from a sample of high school and college teams during the 1975 to 1977 seasons indicated no difference in cerebral concussion rates in 13 brands of helmets. Most recently, Zemper (109) reported on a 5-year study of a national sample of college teams, which indicated that, out of 10 models of helmets studied, one had a statistically significant concussion rate higher than expected and one model had a significantly lower rate of concussions. He concluded that the laboratory testing currently done on football helmets is not sufficient to tell the whole story about the protective capability of helmets, and ongoing epidemiological studies to monitor field performance of helmets and other critical pieces of protective equipment are needed.

In an attempt to prevent the large numbers and severe nature of knee injuries in high school and college football, it is evident from the literature that the most significant trend has been toward the use of preventive (prophylactic) knee braces. A comparison of several studies of the efficacy of the knee brace is shown in Table 4.10.

A review of this table suggests that despite the wide use of these braces on high school and college football teams, there is little agreement among researchers about their effectiveness in preventing knee injury. Much of the skepticism and inconsistent results stems from the different study designs and methodologies implemented by each researcher. Studies by Hansen et al. (39), Hewson et al. (42), Rovere et al. (80), and Shaw and Brubaker (86) were longitudinal in design with distinct brace and nonbrace periods, but each had different criteria for brace use and compliance.

In an attempt to control for potentially confounding variables, Grace et al. (37) matched braced and unbraced players of similar position and size. In a similar vein, Teitz et al. (93) controlled factors such as skill level and position by analyzing different subgroups separately. Most of these studies are limited to one team or a small number of teams, which provides a very small sample size, and these studies provide conflicting results. The only national-scale studies using large

**Table 4.10   A Comparison of Epidemiologic Knee Brace Studies**

| Study | Design/injury criteria | Subjects/duration/brace use | Results |
|---|---|---|---|
| Grace et al., 1988 | Matched pairs<br>Injury based on time loss from practice<br>Injuries graded from mild to severe | 580 high school players over a period of two seasons<br>247 wore single-hinged braces<br>83 wore double-hinged braces<br>250 wore no braces | Significantly more knee injuries in the single-hinged braces group than in double-hinged and nonbraced groups<br>Foot and ankle injuries more common in braced players<br>More severe injuries to lower extremity in braced groups<br>More injuries to the knee than other lower extremity areas; MCL tears were most significant knee injury |
| Hansen et al., 1985 | Longitudinal<br>Number and type of knee surgeries were analyzed<br>Team medical records were used | University of Southern California (1980-1984) | 11% injury rate in nonbraced group; 5% injury rate in braced group<br>< 2% of braced players required surgery; 5% of nonbraced players required surgery<br>Braced players had one-quarter as many meniscectomies<br>1 braced player had severe knee injury; 6 nonbraced players had severe knee injuries<br>4% of braced linebackers were injured; 25% of nonbraced linebackers were injured<br>4% of braced offensive linemen were injured; 18% of nonbraced offensive linemen were injured<br>7% of braced defensive linemen were injured; 23% of nonbraced defensive linemen were injured |
| Hewson et al., 1986 | Longitudinal<br>Team rosters, treatment logs, NAIRS, medical records were analyzed<br>Injury rates based on number of exposures in games and practices | University of Arizona<br>1977-1980 no brace use<br>1981-1985 braces used | Number, type, and severity of knee injuries similar in both groups<br>Braced and nonbraced players had similar chances of being injured<br>Knee injury prevention not improved by brace use |
| Rovere et al., 1987 | Longitudinal<br>Injury records at University Sports Medicine Unit were analyzed<br>Injury rates based on incidence per 100 players | Wake Forest University<br>1981-1985 fall seasons and spring practices | More knee injuries, particularly Grade I MCL sprains, during the braced period<br>More knee operations performed during the braced period<br>Regardless of brace use, offensive team suffered more injuries<br>Knee injuries caused by body contact were fewer during braced period<br>More injuries occurred during games, with higher rates seen in the braced period |
| Schriner, 1985 | Survey<br>Based on rates per 100 players<br>Time-loss parameters used<br>Injuries classified by injury mechanism involved | 1,246 players from Michigan high schools<br>1984 season<br>197 players wore braces | Knee braces reduce injuries to the medial structures of the knee<br>No MCL, medial meniscus, and ACL injuries from lateral forces seen in braced players<br>Braced players did incur hyperextension knee injuries |
| Shaw and Brubaker, 1987 | Longitudinal<br>Criteria for bracing and injury definition not defined | Texas City High School varsity and junior<br>1983-1986 seasons<br>1983 no braces used<br>1984 all varsity players wore braces<br>1985-86 all players fitted with braces, but not required to wear them | In 1983, 19 knee injuries with 143 days of time loss<br>1984—17 injuries, 5 days time loss for braced players, 90 days for nonbraced<br>1985—9 injuries, 30 days time loss for braced players, 22 days for nonbraced<br>No associated structural damage to players wearing braces |

*(continued)*

**Table 4.10**    *(continued)*

| Study | Design/ injury criteria | Subjects/ duration/brace use | Results |
|---|---|---|---|
| Teitz et al., 1987 | Survey<br>Criteria for bracing, exposure while braced, and injury definition not stated | 71 NCAA Division I teams in 1984<br>61 NCAA Division I teams in 1985<br>7,010 players braced<br>4,584 players not braced | Braced players had higher injury rates, particularly running backs and defensive backs<br>MCL injuries were most common<br>Braced players missed as much or more playing time than nonbraced players<br>No difference in injury severity between braced and nonbraced players |
| Zemper, 1990 | 2-year prospective cohort study<br>Injury rates based on athlete-exposures<br>Brace use criteria determined by each school<br>One day or more time loss needed for injury to be reported | 1986 season: 32 NCAA and NAIA teams; 3,431 players<br>1987 season: 27 NCAA and NAIA teams; 2,798 players<br>28% of players wore braces | Braces do not reduce MCL injury rate<br>More time loss for those wearing braces<br>Approximately half of reported knee injuries occurred in games<br>No significant difference in knee surgery rate for braced and nonbraced players<br>No difference between the different brands of braces used<br>No relationship between brace use and ankle injuries<br>More MCL injuries among braced players who played on artificial turf<br>No significant effect of braces in reducing the severity of knee injuries |

numbers of teams were those of Teitz et al. (93) and Zemper (107). Both of these studies indicated preventive knee braces did not reduce the number or severity of MCL injuries, which these braces are specifically designed to prevent.

It is clear that until a sound epidemiologic model for future knee brace studies can be developed, the controversy over knee brace use as a preventive tool in minimizing the risk for lower extremity injury will continue.

# 6. Suggestions for Injury Prevention

As a preventive measure, the early detection, rehabilitation, and reevaluation of lower extremity strength imbalances and deficiencies must be stressed. This involves a rigorous strength program to develop the muscles in both limbs, as well as an effective strength testing and rehabilitative program (30, 51). A retrospective study conducted by Heiser et al. (40) demonstrated that early detection of muscle imbalances through isokinetic testing followed by a muscle imbalance rehabilitative program decreased the incidence of primary and recurrent hamstring strains in intercollegiate football players.

Prevention of facial injuries may be accomplished through the use of properly fitting helmets and padded chin straps, which will eliminate helmet rotation. Further decreases in injury may occur by padding the rim of the helmet. To reduce the injuries incurred by object penetration through the face mask, players should wear full-cage face masks. The stricter enforcement of rules, the proper use of protective equipment, and the elimination of illegal blocking and tackling techniques all will go a long way toward prevention and elimination of facial injuries (103).

A review of the literature indicates that oral injuries can be prevented through the use of mouth guards/protectors (49, 56, 85). There are several mechanisms contributing to the decreased incidence of oral trauma with mouth protector use: (a) mouth protectors separate the teeth from the soft tissues, thereby preventing lacerations and bruising during impact; (b) mouth protectors cushion opposing teeth and structures; and (c) mouth protectors cushion and distribute the impact and prevent superior and posterior displacement of the condyles. This helps in the prevention of concussions, cerebral hemorrhage, neck injuries, and possible death.

There appears to be consensus that mouth-guards offer some type and degree of protection, but there does not seem to be a consensus on which is the best type. Further research is needed to identify the factors associated with oral injuries and mouth protector use and to identify any other factors being influenced by their use. Research also needs to be directed at identifying which players are most susceptible to oral injury so that sound preventive and protective measures can be employed. Furthermore, research is needed to clarify and identify the most effective type of mouth protector for use in high school and college football.

With regard to other types of injuries, many studies in the literature identify and describe the causes, trends, patterns, and factors that contribute to the incidence of injury in football. A summary of preventive recommendations and measures, with discussion and support for each, is presented in tabular form in Table 4.11 to assist coaches, athletes, physicians, athletic trainers, sports administrators, and others to make informed decisions regarding the reduction and elimination of injuries from the game of football. Through careful implementation of and adherence to these preventive measures, football will become a safer and more enjoyable game for all.

# 7. Suggestions for Further Research

In an effort to continue the improvements being made in the area of high school and college football injury prevention, we present several recommendations for future epidemiologic injury research in this sport. These recommendations are provided to help researchers develop and improve a detailed and extensive body of knowledge relating to football injury at the high school and college levels, in an effort to make the game a safer sport for all involved.

1. An injury surveillance system combined with an accurate data collection system needs to be implemented and utilized at all institutions offering organized, competitive football. These programs should have the full cooperation of local physicians, team doctors, coaches, players, administrators, and any other parties involved with the football participants. Data also need to be collected for youth football, for which there currently is little information available.

2. A universally accepted definition of injury in conjunction with universally accepted injury rates, types, and severity measures needs to be developed. This would allow for injury data to be consistently reported and compared across studies. The most commonly used injury definition of "any football-related injury requiring medical attention and causing a player to limit or miss participation for one or more practices or games" is recommended, along with the use of an injury rate involving amount of exposure, such as injuries per 1,000 athlete-exposures or injuries per 1,000 minutes of exposure.

3. Attention should be directed at conducting studies with large sample sizes, equal groups, and an adequate length of study time to ensure the data are reliable and valid. Inconsistencies across studies along these parameters make comparisons difficult. Further attention also is needed to ensure that accurate and detailed methodologies and statistical analyses are provided across studies.

4. In addition to information on individual injury incidents, mechanism, and severity of injury, information concerning the exposure time for all participants (denominator data for calculating injury rates) must be reported and documented in as much detail as possible to make analysis and comparison across studies more effective. This may be accomplished through a universally accepted questionnaire and injury profile to be filled out in the event of an injury.

5. All injuries, regardless of their mechanisms, types, and/or severity levels, need to be reported by trained and experienced personnel (team physicians, athletic trainers, emergency room personnel) if a clear and accurate picture of the injury situation in football is to be established. Additionally, all injuries should be reported and recorded as soon as they occur to eliminate missing or inaccurate data.

6. All players on the football team, in addition to their amount of exposure to injury, need to be accounted for in the analysis of injuries. This would eliminate the problem of some players incurring a higher rate of injury because of their greater exposure times. Additionally, the population at risk and an adequate comparison (control) group needs to be identified in all studies.

7. There needs to be a greater awareness of and control for potential confounding variables and factors contributing to injury. These include age, size, weight, maturity level, skill level, intensity of competition, styles of play, playing conditions, equipment type, prior injury, and coaching experience and philosophy.

8. A qualified sports medicine team needs to be an integral part of all football programs. This should eliminate any bias that may occur in determining the occurrence of an injury.

**Table 4.11   Suggestions for Injury Prevention**

| Preventive recommendation | Discussion and Support |
| --- | --- |
| Preparticipation examination (Abdenour and Weir, 1986; Blackwell and McCullagh, 1990; Boynton, 1988; Brooks et al., 1976; Caine and Broekhoff, 1987; Coddington and Troxell, 1980; Lysens et al., 1989; Riley, 1978; Robey et al., 1971; Taylor and Luckstead, 1987) | A comprehensive medical history, physical and mental examination prior to athletic participation should be obtained and administered to all players. Abdenour and Weir (1986) demonstrated that historical information about the athlete was a significant predictor of physical well-being. The examination will then serve as a screening device to detect any preexisting medical abnormalities (cardiovascular, neurological, musculoskeletal, respiratory, etc.) and/or physical weaknesses. It will provide baseline information about the health and injury status of the player and will also aid in the detection of prior injury, which has been shown to increase the chance of further injury.<br>The psychological status of the athlete should also be examined and monitored because such factors as life stress, risk-taking behavior, and competitive anxiety have been shown to increase the likelihood of injury. |
| Maturity assessment (Caine and Broekhoff, 1987; Robey et al., 1971; Whieldon, 1978) | It appears that the risk of injury is not only related to age, but also to the size, physical, and sexual development of the athlete. Caine and Broekhoff (1987) recommend that players be matched according to their level of maturation (size, strength, power, skill level, fitness, experience) to prevent mismatching unequally developed players, thereby preventing unsafe and unfair play. |
| Year-round injury and health evaluation | This would provide the athletic program with an effective tracking system to constantly evaluate and identify any predisposing conditions that may make the players more susceptible to further more serious injury. |
| Adequate conditioning (physical and mental) and training of athletes (Boynton, 1988; Brooks et al., 1976; Lysens et al., 1989; Riley, 1978) | A year-round (preseason, inseason, and postseason) mandatory football-specific conditioning and training program should be aimed at improving muscular and ligament imbalances and weaknesses; coordination and timing; flexibility, mobility, and agility; and cardiovascular and endurance capacities. Cahill (1977) reported that players on a weight training program had a decreased incidence of knee injuries because of increased strength of the surrounding ligaments, muscles, and tendons.<br>The conditioning and training program should be a well-monitored gradual progression program with care taken not to overstress the athletes too soon. Physical contact should not be introduced until a general level of fitness has been established.<br>Boynton (1988) states that conditioning has an added quality in that improvement in physical conditioning will lead to subsequent improvements in the mental attitude of the players and of the team as a whole (e.g., confidence and controlled aggression).<br>An adequate and effective treatment and rehabilitation program should also be an integral part of the overall conditioning program of the athlete. |
| Limited contact activity (Blyth and Mueller, 1974; Cahill and Griffith, 1979; Robey et al., 1971) | Live contact between players can be limited by providing field equipment to teach and practice certain activities. However, safe techniques need to be established when using this equipment as several studies have shown a relationship between field equipment and the incidence of injury. When comparing injury incidence between limited and regular contact programs, Blyth and Mueller (1974) reported there were fewer injuries in the limited contact program (13.3%) than the regular contact program (86.5%). |
| Adequate provision of medical attention and treatment for the athletes (Blyth and Mueller, 1974; Boynton, 1988; Lackland et al., 1982; Truxal et al., 1981) | The early and effective diagnosis, evaluation, treatment, monitoring, and subsequent prevention of injuries may be accomplished by adequate on-field medical coverage (physicians, sports medicine personnel, and athletics trainers) at all games and practices. Blyth and Mueller (1974) reported that 2.4% of the injuries were the result of inadequate medical care and extreme heat, with only half of the coaches providing liquid to their players during activity. Lackland et al. (1982) demonstrated the value of athletic trainer/team physician services in their high school football injury study.<br>Proper medical supervision during football participation will ensure that activities are performed under safe playing conditions (e.g., avoiding extreme heat, humidity, and cold). |

| Preventive recommendation | Discussion and Support |
|---|---|
| Education, training, and certification of coaches (Caine and Broekhoff, 1987; Blyth and Mueller, 1974; Boynton, 1988) | All coaches should have adequate coaching and playing experience and be trained and evaluated in the fundamentals of the game. The use and coaching of illegal, unsafe techniques should not be tolerated. Coaches should be required to take educational and certification sport and exercise-related courses/clinics to improve, maintain, and refresh their knowledge of the game.<br>A capable, well-trained assistant coaching staff should be a part of all football programs. Schools with several assistant coaches were shown to have a lower incidence rate than those schools without assistant coaches (Blyth and Mueller, 1974). |
| Rules enforcement (Arnold and Coker, 1977; Blyth and Mueller, 1974; Boynton, 1988) | Coaches and athletes need to abide by the rules of the game, with referees and officials playing an active role in their enforcement. The 3.8% of injuries caused by illegal acts such as clipping, spearing, hitting while down and out-of-bounds, and personal fouls reported in the study by Blyth and Mueller (1974) may have been eliminated with proper rule awareness and enforcement. |
| Equipment (Blyth and Mueller, 1974; Boynton, 1988; Garrick et al., 1978; Johnson and Ritter, 1975; Schwank and Ryan, 1975; Slagle, 1983). | The use of proven protective equipment needs to be an integral part of all football programs. Additional padding and/or taping for the ribs, thighs, arms, hands, and ankles may help prevent some injuries. Additionally, the management of properly fitting and well-maintained equipment needs to be stressed. In the study directed by Blyth and Mueller (1974) 1.7% of all injuries were caused by ill-fitting, defective, or broken equipment.<br>The fields and playing surfaces need to be inspected and well-maintained. Garrick et al. (1978) recommends that a buffer zone be placed around the periphery of the playing field to prevent injuries occurring as the result of contact with people or objects out-of-bounds. Coaches and players should be prohibited from encouraging the use of protective equipment as offensive weapons.<br>Further research needs to be directed at improving the protective equipment being used by football players. |

# References

1. Abdenour, T.; Weir, N. Medical assessment of the prospective student athlete. Athletic Training. 21:122-123; 1986.
2. Albright, J.; Moses, M.; Harley, G.; Feldick, G.; Dolan, K.; Burmeister, L. Nonfatal cervical spine injuries in interscholastic football. JAMA. 236(11): 1243-1245; 1976.
3. Albright, J.; McAuley, E.; Martin, R.; Crowley, E.; Foster, D. Head and neck injuries in college football: An eight-year analysis. Am. J. Sp. Med. 13(3): 147-152;1985.
4. Alles, W.; Powell, J.; Buckley, W.; Hunt, E. The National Athletic Injury/Illness Reporting System 3-year findings of high school and college football injuries. J. Orthop. Sp. Phys. Ther. 1(2):103-108; 1979.
5. Alves, W.; Rimel, R.; Nelson, W. University of Virginia prospective study of football-induced minor head injury: Status report. Clin. Sp. Med. 6(1):211-218; 1987.
6. Arnold, J.; Coker, T. New football rules and athletic injuries. J. Ark. Med. Soc. 74(4):163-165; 1977.
7. Bailey, R. Head, neck and shoulder injuries. Texas Coach. 26-29; 1979.
8. Bandy, W.; McLaughlin, T.; McKitrick, B. A case study: The importance of dynamic evaluation in the assessment of posterior knee pain. J. Orthop. Sp. Phys. Ther. 5:132-133; 1983.
9. Blackwell, B.; McCullagh, P. The relationship of athletic injury to life stress, competitive anxiety and coping resources. Athletic Training. 25(1):23-27; 1990.
10. Blyth, C.; Mueller, F. When and where players get hurt. Physician Sp. Med. 2(9):45-52; 1974.
11. Boynton, D. A model for the prevention of football related injuries: A report to the Ontario Amateur Football Association. Audible. 14:20-23; 1988.
12. Brooks, W.; Young, B. High school football injuries: Prevention of injury to the central nervous system. Southern Med. J. 69(10):1258-1260; 1976.
13. Buckley, W. Concussion injury in college football: An eight-year overview. Athletic Training. 21(3): 207-211; 1986.

14. Buckley, W. Concussions in college football: A multivariate analysis. Am. J. Sp. Med. 16(1):51-56; 1988.

15. Buckley, W.; Powell, J. NAIRS: An epidemiological overview of the severity of injury in college football 1975-1980 seasons. Athletic Training. 17:279-282; 1982.

16. Cahill, B.; Griffith, E. Effect of preseason conditioning on the incidence and severity of high school football knee injuries. Am. J. Sp. Med. 6(4):180-184; 1978.

17. Cahill, B.; Griffith, E. Exposure to injury in major college football. Am. J. Sp. Med. 7(3):183-185; 1979.

18. Cahill, B.; Griffith, E.; Sunderlin, J.; Madden, T.; Weltman, A. High school football knee injuries. Ill. Med. J. 166(5):356-358; 1984.

19. Caine, D.; Broekhoff, J. Maturity assessment: A viable preventive measure against physical and psychological insult to the young athlete. Physician Sp. Med. 15(3):67-80; 1987.

20. Cameron, B.; Davis, O. The swivel football shoe: A controlled study. Am. J. Sp. Med. 16-27; 1973.

21. Canale, S.; Cantler, E.; Sisk, D.; Freeman, B. A chronicle of injuries of an American intercollegiate football team. Am. J. Sp. Med. 9(6):384-389; 1981.

22. Cantu, R. Cerebral concussion in sports. Sports Med. 14(1):65-74; 1992.

23. Carter, D.; Frankel, V. Biomechanics of hyperextension injuries to the cervical spine in football. Am. J. Sp. Med. 8(5):302-307; 1980.

24. Clarke, K.; Miller, S. Turf related injuries in college football and soccer. Athletic Training. 12(1):28-32; 1977.

25. Clarke, K.; Powell, J. Football helmets and neurotrauma—An epidemiological overview of three seasons. Med. Sci. Sp. 11(2):138-145; 1979.

26. Coddington, R.; Troxell, J. The effect of emotional factors on football injury rates: A pilot study. J. Human Stress. 6(4):3-5; 1980.

27. Culpepper, M.; Niemann, K. High school football injuries in Birmingham, Alabama. Southern Med. J. 76(7):873-878; 1983.

28. Culpepper, M.; Niemann, K. A comparison of game and practice injuries in high school football. Physician Sp. Med. 11(10):117-122; 1983.

29. Culpepper, M.; Morrison, T. High school football game injuries from four Birmingham municipal fields. Ala. J. Med. Sci. 24(4):378-382; 1987.

30. Darden, E. Prevention of the knee injury. Audible. 4(1):30-32; 1978.

31. Derscheid, G.; Garrick, J. Medial collateral ligament injuries in football. Am. J. Sp. Med. 9(6):365-368; 1981.

32. Dolan, K.; Feldick, H.; Albright, J.; Moses, J. Neck injuries in football players. AFP. 12(6):86-91; 1975.

33. Funk, F.; Wells, R. Injuries of the cervical spine in football. Clin. Orthop. 109:50-58; 1975.

34. Garrick, J.; Requa, R. Injuries in high school sports. Pediatrics. 60(3):465-469; 1978.

35. Gerberich, S.; Priest, J.; Boen, J.; Staub, C.; Maxwell, R. Concussion incidences and severity in secondary school varsity football players. Am. J. Publ. Health. 73(12):1370-1375; 1983.

36. Grace, T.; Sweetser, E.; Nelson, M.; Ydens, L.; Skipper, B. Isokinetic muscle imbalance and knee-joint injuries. J. Bone Joint Surg. 66-A(5):734-740; 1984.

37. Grace, T.; Skipper, B.; Newberry, J.; Nelson, M.; Sweetser, E.; Rothman, M. Prophylactic knee braces and injury to the lower extremity. J. Bone Joint Surg. 70-A(3):422-427; 1988.

38. Hale, R.; Mitchell, W. Football injuries in Hawaii 1979. Hawaii Med. J. 40(7):180-182; 1981.

39. Hansen, B.; Ward, J.; Diehl, R. The preventive use of the Anderson Knee Stabler in football. Physician Sp. Med. 13(9):75-77; 1985.

40. Heiser, T.; Weber, J.; Sullivan, G.; Clare, P.; Jacobs, R. Prophylaxis and management of hamstring muscle injuries in intercollegiate football players. Am. J. Sp. Med. 12(5):368-370; 1984.

41. Henschen, K.; Heil, J.; Bean, B.; Crain, S. Football injuries: Is grass or astroturf the culprit? Utah J. HPERD. 21:5-6; 1989.

42. Hewson, G.; Mendini, R.; Wang, J. Prophylactic knee bracing in college football. Am. J. Sp. Med. 14(4):262-266; 1986.

43. Hoffman, M.; Lyman, K. Medical needs at high school football games in Milwaukee. J. Orthop. Sp. Phys. Ther. 10(5):167-171; 1988.

44. Howe, D. Serious neck injuries. Coaching Review. 1979.

45. Johnson, D. Post-season knee injuries. Journal Clinics. 4:8; 1974.

46. Johnson, J.; Ritter, M. A computer analysis of football injuries. Sp. Med. 3(4):168-171; 1975.

47. Jones, R.; Henley, M.; Francis, P. Nonoperative management of isolated grade III collateral ligament injury in high school football players. Clin. Orthop. 213:137-140; 1986.

48. Kalenak, A.; Morehouse, C. Knee stability and knee ligament injuries. JAMA. 234(11):1143-1145; 1975.

49. Kaufman, R.; Kaufman, A. An experimental study on the effects of the MORA on football players. Basal Facts. 6(4):119-126; 1984.

50. Kelly, J.; Nichols, J.; Filley, C.; Lillehei, K.; Rubenstein, D.; Kleinschmidt-DeMasters, B. Concussion in sports. JAMA. 266(20):2867-2869; 1991.

51. Knight, K. Strength imbalance and knee injury. Physician Sp. Med. 8(1):140; 1980.

52. Lackland, D.; Akers, P.; Hirata, I. High school football injuries in South Carolina: A computerized survey. J. So. Carol. Med. Assoc. 78(2):75-78; 1982.

53. Lysens, R.; Ostyn, M.; Auweele, Y.; Lefevre, J.; Vuylsteke, M.; Renson, L. The accident-prone and overuse-prone profiles of the young athlete. Am. J. Sp. Med. 17(5):612-619; 1989.

54. Maroon, J.; Steele, P.; Berlin, R. Football head and neck injuries: An update. J. Clin. Neurosurg. 27:414-429; 1980.

55. Maroon, J. Catastrophic neck injuries from football in western Pennsylvania. Physician Sp. Med. 9(11):83-86; 1981.

56. McNutt, T.; Shannon, S.; Wright, J.; Feinstein, R. Oral trauma in adolescent athletes: A study of mouth protectors. Ped. Dent. 11(3):209-213; 1989.

57. Meeuwisse, W.; Fowler, P. Frequency and predictability of sports injuries in intercollegiate athletics. Can. J. Sp. Med. Sci. 13(1):35-42; 1988.

58. Moran, M.; Dvonch, V. Subtle Salter Type II distal femoral epiphyseal fracture. Orthopedics. 8(11): 1414-1416; 1985.

59. Moretz, J.; Walters, R.; Smith, L. Flexibility as a predictor of knee injuries in college football players. Physician Sp. Med. 10(7):93-97; 1982.

60. Moretz, J.; Harlan, S.; Goodrich, J.; Walters, J. Long-term followup of knee injuries in high school football players. Am. J. Sp. Med. 12(4):298-300; 1984.

61. Mueller, F.; Blyth, C. North Carolina high school football injury study: Equipment and prevention. J. Sp. Med. 2(1):1-10; 1974.

62. Mueller, F.; Schindler, R. Annual survey of football injury research 1931-1992. Orlando, FL: American Football Coaches Association; 1993.

63. Murray, P. Case study: Rehabilitation of a collegiate football placekicker with patellofemoral arthritis. J. Orthop. So. Phys. Ther. 10(6):224-227; 1988.

64. National Athletic Trainers Association. National high school injury registry report. Greenville, SC: NATA; 1987.

65. National Collegiate Athletic Association. Injury Surveillance System: Football. Overland Park, KS: NCAA; 1984.

66. National Collegiate Athletic Association. Injury Surveillance System: Football. Overland Park, KS: NCAA; 1985.

67. National Collegiate Athletic Association. Injury Surveillance System: Football. Overland Park, KS: NCAA; 1990.

68. National Collegiate Athletic Association. Annual Sports Sponsorship Survey. Overland Park, KS: NCAA; 1993.

69. National Federation of State High School Associations. Sports Participation Survey. Kansas City, MO: NFSHSA; 1993.

70. O'Donoghue, D. Diagnosis and treatment of injury to the anterior cruciate ligament. J. Orthop. Sp. Phys. Ther. 2(3):100-107; 1981.

71. Olson, O. The Spokane study: High school football injuries. Physician Sp. Med. 7(12):75-82; 1979.

72. Prager, B.; Fitton, W.; Cahill, B.; Olson, G. High school football injuries: A prospective study and pitfalls of data collection. Am. J. Sp. Med. 17(5):681-685; 1989.

73. Powell, J. Pattern of knee injuries associated with college football 1975-1982. Athletic Training. 20(2): 104-109; 1985.

74. Reid, S.; Reid, S., Jr. Advances in sports medicine: Prevention of head and neck injuries in football. Surg. Annual. 13:251-270; 1981.

75. Riley, C. The vital role the school plays in preventing athletic injuries. J. School Health. 1978.

76. Rishel, G.; Wilson, M.; Brodell, J. The management of severe recurrent ankle sprains in a starting high school running back. Athletic Training. 24(3):230-243; 1989.

77. Robertson, W.; Eichman, P.; Clancy, W. Upper trunk brachial plexopathy in football players. JAMA. 241(14):1480-1482; 1979.

78. Robey, J.; Blyth, C.; Mueller, F. Athletic injuries: Application of epidemiological methods. JAMA. 217(2):184-189; 1971.

79. Rogers, B. The mechanics of head and neck trauma to football players. Athletic Training. 16(2):132-135; 1981.

80. Rovere, G.; Haupt, H.; Yates, C. Prophylactic knee bracing in college football. Am. J. Sp. Med. 15(2): 111-116; 1987.

81. Saunders, R.; Harbaugh, R. The second impact in catastrophic contact-sports head trauma. JAMA. 252(4):538-539; 1984.

82. Schneider, R.; Reifel, E.; Crisler, H.; Oosterbahn, B. Serious and fatal football injuries involving the head and spinal cord. JAMA. 177(6):106-111; 1961.

83. Schriner, J.; Schriner, D. The effectiveness of knee bracing in preventing knee injury in high school athletes. Presented at the American College of Sports Medicine annual meeting, Nashville, TN, May 26-29, 1985.

84. Schwank, W.; Ryan, A. Stopping spear tackling. Physician Sp. Med. 3(9):72-78; 1975.

85. Seals, R.; Dorrough, B. Custom mouth protectors: A review of their applications. J. Prosth. Dent. 51(2):238-242; 1984.

86. Shaw, R.; Brubaker, D. The McDavid Guard (MKG) in preventing knee injuries. Texas Coach. 28-29; 1987.

87. Sherk, H.; Watters, W. Neck injuries in football players. J. Med. Soc. New Jersey. 78(9):579-583; 1981.

88. Skovron, M.; Levy, I.; Agel, J. Living with artificial grass: A knowledge update. Am. J. Sp. Med. 18(50):510-513; 1990.

89. Slagle, G. Prevention of neck injuries: The bar roll. Athletic Training. 18(2):63-66; 1983.

90. Slocum, D. The mechanics of common football injuries. JAMA. 170(14):1640-1646; 1959.

91. Tamberelli, A. Prevention and care of the knee injury. Athletic Journal. 58(6):103-105; 1978.

92. Taylor, S.; Luckstead, E. Medical concerns for the adolescent athlete. Iowa Medicine. 1987.

93. Teitz, C.; Hermanson, B.; Kronmal, R.; Diehr, P. Evaluation of the use of braces to prevent injury to the knee in collegiate football players. J. Bone Joint Surg. 69(9):1467-1470; 1987.

94. Torg, J.; Quedenfeld, T.; Landau, S. Football shoes and playing surfaces: From safe to unsafe. Physician Sp. Med. 1(3):51-54; 1973.

95. Torg, J.; Quedenfeld, T.; Moyer, R.; Truex, R.; Spealman, A.; Nichols, C. Severe and catastrophic neck

injuries resulting from tackle football. Delaware Med. J. 49(50):267-275; 1977.

96. Torg, J.; Vegso, J.; O'Neill, J.; Sennet, B. The epidemiologic, pathologic, biomechanical, and cinematographic analysis of football-induced cervical spine trauma. Am. J. Sp. Med. 18(1):50-57; 1990.

97. Truxal, B.; Shenker, I.; Nussbawn, M. On-field physician assessment of high school football injuries. Physician Sp. Med. 9(9):68-71; 1981.

98. Walsh, W.; Blackburn, T. Prevention of ankle sprains. Am. J. Sp. Med. 5(6):243-245; 1977.

99. Warren, R. Football knee injuries. Coaching Clinic. 20(4):16-21; 1982.

100. Weber, D. Prevention of toe, ankle and knee injuries in football. Athletic Purchasing and Facilities. 6(3):40-41; 1982.

101. Whieldon, D. Maturity sorting: New balance for young athletes. Physician Sp. Med. 6:127-132; 1978.

102. Whiteside, J.; Fleagle, S.; Kalanek, A.; Weber, H. Manpower loss in football: A 12-year study at the Pennsylvania State University. Physician Sp. Med. 13(1):103-114; 1985.

103. Wilson, K.; Rontal, E.; Rontal, M. Facial injuries in football. Am. Acad. Opthalm. Otolaryng. 77:434-437; 1973.

104. Zemper, E. Injury rates in a national sample of college football teams: A 2-year prospective study. Physician Sp. Med. 17(11):100-113; 1989a.

105. Zemper, E. A prospective study of injury rates in a national sample of American college football players. In: Proceedings of the First International Olympic Committee World Congress on Sport Sciences. Colorado Springs: USOC; 1989b:194-195.

106. Zemper, E. Cerebral concussion rates in various brands of football helmets. Athletic Training. 24(2):133-137; 1989c.

107. Zemper, E. A two-year prospective study of prophylactic knee braces in a national sample of college football players. Sports Training, Medicine and Rehabilitation. 1:287-296; 1990.

108. Zemper, E. Epidemiology of athletic injuries. In: McKeag, D.; Hough, D.; Zemper, E. Primary care sports medicine. Dubuque, IA: Brown & Benchmark;1993:63-73.

109. Zemper, E. Analysis of cerebral concussion frequency with the most commonly used models of football helmets. J. Athl. Training. 29(1):44-50; 1994.

# 5

# Baseball and Softball

*Stephan Walk, Michael A. Clark, and Vern Seefeldt*

## 1. Introduction

Today baseball is played professionally and recreationally in many countries, but nowhere with the attention and acclaim that it receives in the United States. Two professional leagues, the American and National, each with 14 teams, are provided with a steady stream of talented players by numerous levels of minor league baseball and by intercollegiate, interscholastic, and youth leagues. In the United States, the major leagues are supported by approximately 2,100 minor leaguers, 45,000 intercollegiate players, 433,684 who play at the interscholastic level, and approximately 2 million who play in the youth leagues (11, 122). Softball is a game derived from baseball, but played on a smaller diamond and playing surface and with a larger ball. The Amateur Softball Association of America (7) estimates that 40 million Americans play softball annually.

Two circumstances have influenced the incidence of injuries in baseball and softball in the last 2 decades. The popularity of baseball as an organized sport for young children and the propensity to extend the playing season by including competition at the intercity, state, regional, and national levels have influenced the number of baseball injuries among children and youth. The increasing popularity of softball as a sport for adults has increased the numbers who are potentially at risk of injury. In softball such extraneous factors as lack of skill, lack of proper physical conditioning, and—in leagues for adults—the consumption of alcohol in conjunction with play may contribute to injuries (78).

The purpose of this chapter is to interpret the published information on injuries in baseball and softball. Literature reviews included all available published reports in the English language since 1975; in addition, several studies involving large numbers of participants that paved the way for much of the subsequent research were also included in this review. Electronic searches included Medline (descriptors: baseball-softball injuries; search period 1983 to 1993); Sport Information Resource Center (descriptors: The Baseball File; articles retrieved from 1976 to the present); and references from printed articles and reports. Only those articles that focused on the incidence and causes of injuries in baseball and softball were included in this review. Articles that concentrated on the diagnosis, treatment, and rehabilitation of injuries in baseball and softball were excluded. The National Collegiate Athletic Association (NCAA) sponsors an ongoing effort to collect data on injuries, and this organization provided extensive information on both baseball and softball. Similarly, data from the National Federation of State High School Associations was available. However, national groups sponsoring baseball and softball and the national governing bodies of these sports do not routinely collect information relating to injuries; therefore, they were not able to provide useful data.

A review of the published literature on injuries in baseball and softball disclosed most of the methodological problems that were described by Walter and Hart (144). Nearly all of the reports of injuries were of the retrospective, case, or case series nature. Authors of only two studies used the cross-sectional method to obtain their data. None resorted to the prospective cohort method. The ages and levels of skill were frequently absent, as was the etiology of the injury. Estimating the rates of injury per athlete or per occasion for this chapter was complicated by the general lack of information about the population from which the athletes emerged. The data on injuries to young athletes, where overuse injuries are prevalent, no doubt suffer from under-reporting because many of the players with sore shoulders and elbows treat the injury by playing other positions that put less demand on the throwing arm or by withdrawing from baseball while the injury heals. Based on the methods reported in the literature that are commonly used to detect and record data, many of the injuries to youth and adults who play baseball or softball are probably not acknowledged.

# 2. Incidence of Injury

## 2.1 Injury Rates

### 2.1.1 Baseball

Reports of injury rates in baseball vary greatly, from the early study by Hale (60) in which he reviewed the number of injuries over a 5-year period from insurance claims filed by physicians, to the report by Martin et al. (96) of a 7-day competition during which a physician or a trainer was present to attend to athletes and file the injury report. Under such a diverse reporting system it is not surprising that the rates of injuries varied from 72 per 100 athletes over a 3-year period (126) to an injury–index factor of 0.14, whereby the index was calculated by factoring in the number of participant-hours and -weeks of exposure in the sport (20). At least part of this confusion is created by the manner in which injuries in baseball have been reported. In the example cited previously, Hale's (60) estimate that 2% of all youth baseball players were injured is likely to underestimate the actual injuries because only those who sought medical attention and whose forms were actually processed in the calculations are included in the determination. In the report of Martin et al. (96), it is likely that every detectable injury was reported.

A review of injury rate by level of competition does not provide any definitive answers. Although injuries are generally thought to occur in direct proportion to the intensity of the competition and the age of the athletes, the data in Table 5.1 do not permit such an interpretation. For example, Zaricznyj et al. (149) reported a rate of 9.5 injuries per 100 youth baseball players over the course of 1 year, while Grana (53) and Lowe et al. (92) reported rates of 0.015 and 1.22, respectively, in interscholastic baseball players over the same period of time. The data at the interscholastic level are equally unclear. For example, DuRant et al. (35) detected that 19.4 % of the athletes incurred an injury during the course of a season, while Splain and Rolnick (126) reported that 72% of their interscholastic

baseball players sustained an injury. Whether these vast differences are real or the result of variation in protocols for detecting and reporting injuries is impossible to determine on the basis of the information provided in the reports. Also note that the reports of injuries in Table 5.1 are approximately equally divided between prospective and retrospective studies.

### 2.1.2 Softball

The reports of injuries in softball present the same methodological dilemma that was reported for baseball, namely, that data were obtained in a variety of ways, without information that would permit the accurate calculation of rates. In addition, 4 of the 49 reports did not reveal whether the type of play was fast or slow pitch, and 5 additional reports provide no information regarding the gender of the players or the type of softball being played. Rates of injuries provided in Table 5.1 leave the general impression that there is no clear indication whether baseball or softball is safer at comparable levels of competition. For example, Grana (53) and McLain (97) reported fewer injuries in baseball than in softball, but Lowe et al. (92) and DuRant et al. (35) reported the reverse. Reports of injury rates in youth softball were not available, so no comparisons of injury rates were possible at an age where skill levels may have had less influence on injury rates than at the high school or interscholastic levels of play.

## 2.2 Practice Versus Competition

Only limited information compares injuries sustained during practices versus games. Of the 149 citations that addressed injuries in baseball and softball, only 3 presented data relative to this question. Whiteside (148) reported higher rates of injuries, both in reportable and significant injuries, during practices than in games when such variables as total number of games, total number of practices, and squad size were included in the calculations. Garrick and Requa's (48) data, at face value, seemed to support the data provided by Whiteside (148), while Duda (34) reported over twice as many injuries in baseball per 1,000 exposures during competition as during practices (5.80 vs 1.93). For a detailed description of the data available on injury rates during practice versus competition see Table 5.2.

The tendency to misinterpret the data regarding the occurrence of injuries in practices versus

**Table 5.1 Comparison of Injury Rates in Baseball and Softball**

| Study | Duration | Design* | Participants BB | Participants SB | # of teams BB | # of teams SB | # of injuries BB | # of injuries SB | Rate BB /100 aths | Rate BB /1,000 aths | Rate BB /1,000 ath exposures | Rate BB Other | Rate SB /100 aths | Rate SB /1,000 aths | Rate SB /1,000 ath exposures | Rate SB Other |
|---|---|---|---|---|---|---|---|---|---|---|---|---|---|---|---|---|
| **Youth** | | | | | | | | | | | | | | | | |
| Hale (60) | 5 years | Retro. | 771,810 | — | — | — | 15,444 | — | 2.0 | | | | | | | |
| Chambers (20) | 1 year | Prosp. | 740 | — | — | — | 2 | — | | | | 0.14[a] | | | | |
| Zaricznyj et al. (149) | 1 year | Retro. | 137 | — | — | — | 13 | — | 9.5 | | | | | | | |
| **High school** | | | | | | | | | | | | | | | | |
| Garrick & Requa (48) | 2 years | Prosp. | 249 | | 8 | | 46 | | | | 0.18 | | | | | |
| Garrick & Requa (47) | 2 years | Prosp. | | 16 | | 1 | | 7 | | | | | | | | 0.44[b] |
| Grana (53) | 1 academic year | Retro. | 1,969 | 715 | — | — | 29 | 9 | 0.015 | | | | 0.013 | | | |
| Lowe et al. (92) | 1 year | Retro. | 256 | 169 | — | — | 3 | 3 | 1.22 | | | | 1.78 | | | |
| McLain & Reynolds (97) | 1 year | Prosp. | 68 | 54 | — | — | 10 | 7 | 15.0 | | | | 13.0 | | | |
| DuRant et al. (35) | 1 academic year | Prosp. | 108 | 99 | — | — | 21 | 9 | 19.4 | | | | 9.1 | | | |
| **Intercollegiate** | | | | | | | | | | | | | | | | |
| Whiteside (148) | 2 years | Retro. | — | | — | | 133 | | | | 2.9 | | | | | |
| Haycock & Gillete (69) | 1 year | Retro. | — | — | | | | 230 | | | 1.3 | | | | 1.8 | |
| Clarke & Buckley (23) | 3 years | Prosp. | — | | 13 | 10 | | 11 | 9.2 | | | | 8.7 | | | |
| Ritter et al. (117) | 1 season | Prosp. | | 16 | — | 1 | | | | | 1.6[c] | | 68.0 | | 2.1[d] | |
| Powell (114) | 3 years | Prosp. | — | — | 40 | 29 | | | | | | | | | | |
| Splain & Rolnick (126) | 3 years | Retro. | 88 | 104 | 1 | 1 | 63 | 34 | 72.0 | | | | 33.0 | 3.37 | | |
| Duda (34) | 1 academic year | Retro. | — | — | — | | | | | | 3.37 | | | | | |
| NCAA (104) | 4 years | Prosp. | — | — | 694 | | 1,885 | | | | 2.86 | | | | | |
| NCAA (105) | 6 years | Prosp. | — | — | | 510 | | 704 | | | | | | | 2.57 | |
| **Amateur Event** | | | | | | | | | | | | | | | | |
| Lebrun et al. (87) | 2 weeks | Prosp. | — | — | — | — | 33 | 20 | | | | | | | | |
| Martin et al. (96) | 7 days | Prosp. | 148 | — | — | — | 8 | | 5.4 | | | | | | | |
| **Recreational adult** | | | | | | | | | | | | | | | | |
| Nadeau et al. (103) | 3 years | Retro. | — | | | | 150 | | | | | | | | | |
| **Professional** | | | | | | | | | | | | | | | | |
| Garfinkel et al. (46) | 2 seasons | Prosp. | — | | 1 | | 382 | | | | | | | | | |

*The distinction between retrospective and prospective studies was difficult to determine at times. "Retrospective" studies generally focused on interpreting previously collected injury data. Most of the studies listed as "prospective" established criteria, categories, and data collection protocols prior to starting the work. While strictly speaking this does not make a study "prospective," such a design is closer to the commonly accepted definition of such efforts.

[a]Injury index factor derived by formula: # of injuries $\times 10^4$ [(# of participants) $\times$ (avg. # of hrs. of part.) $\times$ (# wks. in sport)].

[b]Number of injuries per number of participants.

[c]Injuries per 1,000 athlete exposures averaged over 3 years (1975 = 1.1, 1976 = 2.1, 1977 = 1.6).

[d]Injuries per 1,000 athlete exposures averaged over 3 years (1975 = 2.1, 1976 = 1.9, 1977 = 2.3).

**Table 5.2    Comparison of Injury Rates in Practice Versus Competition**

| Study | Practice rates | | Competition rates | |
|---|---|---|---|---|
| | Injuries/1,000 athlete exposures | Other | Injuries/1,000 athlete exposures | Other |
| **Baseball** | | | | |
| Whiteside (148) | 4.1 (total injuries) | | 2.0 (total injuries) | |
| | 2.0 (serious injuries) | | 0.5 (serious injuries) | |
| Duda (34) | 1.93 | | 5.80 | |
| NCAA (104) | 2.30 (Division I) | | 6.38 (Division I) | |
| | 2.10 (Division II) | | 6.64 (Division II) | |
| | 1.79 (Division III) | | 4.87 (Division III) | |
| **Softball** | | | | |
| Garrick & Requa (47) | | 43%[a] | | 0.25[b] |
| Whiteside (148) | 8.6 (total injuries) | | 1.2 (total injuries) | |
| | 3.3 (serious injuries) | | 0.4 (serious injuries) | |
| NCAA (105) | 3.57 (Division I) | | 5.18 (Division I) | |
| | 3.14 (Division II) | | 5.54 (Division II) | |
| | 2.80 (Division III) | | 4.58 (Division III) | |

[a]Number of practice injuries as a percentage of total injuries.

[b]Number of injuries sustained during competitive events divided by number of participants.

games, even when numbers of games versus numbers of practices are included in the calculation of rate, was addressed by Garrick and Requa (48). Obscured by data that simply compare injuries by numbers of practices versus games is the fact that practices often place the entire squad at risk and games limit the numbers at risk at any given moment. Practices are often spent learning new skills and strategies in situations that often include all players in numerous repetitions of activities involving the risk of injury; however, competitions often place only the most skillful players at risk. Practices also receive an unfair portion of the attribution of injuries if the time per exposure is not included in the equation, because the time spent in actual player–ball and player–player contact during practices generally far exceeds these associations during games. Thus, although the data related to rates of injuries in practices versus games in baseball and softball are equivocal, the resultant values suggest that more injuries occur in games than in practices when the participant-hours are included in the calculation of rates. Therefore, the risk of injury is actually greater in games, but more injuries are likely to occur in practices if the exposure time is greater than in games.

# 3. Injury Characteristics

## 3.1 Injury Onset

The published literature on injuries in baseball and softball is overwhelmingly devoted to acute types of injuries. At all levels the types of injuries include such terms as *fractures*, *abrasions*, *lacerations*, *sprains*, and *contusions*. Injuries of a chronic nature, including stress fractures and overuse injuries of the elbow and shoulder joints, were seldom mentioned in the surveillance of injuries. The dramatic occurrence and ease of documentation has most likely influenced the imbalance of reporting many more acute-type rather than chronic injuries.

## 3.2 Injury Types

### 3.2.1 Baseball

The incidence of injuries, by type, provides a clear pattern of occurrences for participants at the youth, interscholastic, intercollegiate, and the professional levels. Although this discussion includes only the eight reports that provided interpretable information, the reports are consistent with regard to the pattern of occurrences (see Table 5.3). Abrasions were by far the most common type of injury in children and youth reported by Hale (60) and Heald (70), followed by fractures, sprains, and lacerations. At the interscholastic level, the only available report (92) divided the injuries evenly between fractures, lacerations, and sprains. Sprains were also the most common type of injury reported by Clarke and Buckley (23) and Whiteside (148) at the intercollegiate level, followed by strains. At the professional level, contusions, strains, and abrasions occurred most frequently (46).

The pattern of injury types presented in Table 5.3 suggests that at the youth level most injuries were caused by the inability of players to coordinate their bodies in relation to the playing field in the act of sliding, thus leading to abrasions and sprains. An inability to avoid contacts with other players or bases also was responsible for the high incidence of fractures. At the interscholastic level, the increased ability to produce force through increased muscularity may have contributed to the increase in sprains, while the still underdeveloped skill levels may have contributed to the higher percentage of lacerations and fractures. Intercollegiate baseball players incurred the vast majority of their injuries in sprains and strains, perhaps reflecting their ability to produce the force that is frequently associated with tearing of muscular and ligamentous tissue.

### 3.2.2 Softball

Only six reports provided evidence of injury types in softball (see Table 5.3), and there are no reports relating injuries to youth softball. The most interesting comparisons within this small group of reports was at the college level, where women's play could be contrasted to men's activity in baseball. Similarities at this level occurred in the percent of strains and sprains incurred by both genders. Differences in types of injuries were noted in fractures, where Clarke and Buckley (23) reported an occurrence rate of 27% for women and 10% for men. Concurring with the gender-based relationship, Whiteside (148) reported an incidence of 10.6% fractures for women and 3.4% for men.

Injuries at the adult recreational level also consisted primarily of sprains ($X = 33.9\%$) and strains ($X = 27\%$) as reported by Loosli et al. (90) and Nadeau et al. (103). Speculation about the causes for differences in the incidence of fractures between men and women appear to be unwarranted in light of the few studies that have addressed the issue and the lack of specific epidemiological data in the published reports. Although baseball and softball have many similarities, speculation about the causes for differences in occurrence of injuries in men and women should be replaced by well-designed studies that emphasize the epidemiology of injuries and the preventative measures that may be specific to each sport.

### 3.3 Injury Location

For baseball, the anatomical location of injuries that were described in 13 reports resulted in the emergence of a general pattern of injuries, by level of play (see Table 5.4). Note that the sources of data are generally from prospective studies, but several of the large databases—Hale (60), Splain and Rolnick (126), Whiteside et al. (147), and Whiteside (148)—use retrospective techniques. Conspicuous by their absence were reports that addressed the location of injuries to interscholastic players. At the youth level, injuries occurred most frequently to the upper extremity and head, each receiving approximately 35% of the injuries. The lower extremity received approximately 20% of the injuries, while the spine and trunk received 7% (56), 3% (113), and 4% (66), respectively.

For baseball at the intercollegiate level the location of injuries shifted to the upper and lower extremities (148, 149). While injuries to the lower extremity at the youth level were in the range of 19% to 22.5%, at the college level they ranged from 1.6 to to 60.3%. Although the distribution of injuries by general anatomical region is clearly displayed in Table 5.4, the footnotes (a–t) provide evidence that the literature did not reveal the locations of injuries in convenient categories. Despite the difficulty with classifications, the knee, ankle, and shoulder appear to have the greatest incidence of injuries at the intercollegiate level. This pattern of crediting the greatest incidence of injuries to the upper and lower extremities also prevailed at the amateur and professional levels, with relatively few injuries to the head and spine/trunk.

The anatomical location of injuries in softball is devoid of the pattern that appeared in baseball, primarily because only three studies addressed the issue of injuries in youth softball and none reported injuries at the interscholastic level (see Table 5.5). Data clearly indicate that the greatest percent of injuries occurred in the lower extremity, followed closely by the upper extremity, but the pattern within these general locations is not clear. For example, Whiteside (148) and Splain and Rolnick (126) reported that 15% of the injuries were located in the shoulder, but Zaricznyj et al. (149) reported only 2% at the shoulder. Whiteside reported that 24% of the injuries were at the pelvis and hip, but Zaricznyj et al. and Splain and Rolnick did not report any injuries at that location. However, data in all four reports implied that the head and spine/trunk received few injuries compared to the upper and lower extremities. The most common agreement regarding location of injuries in softball occurred at the adult recreational level, where Loosli et al. (90), Loosli et al. (91), and Wheeler (145) reported that 73%, 71%, and 71%, respectively, of the injuries occurred in the lower

**Table 5.3   Percent Comparison of Injury Types in Baseball and Softball**

| Level | # of subjects | # of injuries | Abrasions | Concussions | Dislocations | Fractures | Inflammations | Lacerations | Non-specific | Sprain | Strain | Other 1 | Other 2 | Other 3 |
|---|---|---|---|---|---|---|---|---|---|---|---|---|---|---|
| Baseball | | | | | | | | | | | | | | |
| Youth | | | | | | | | | | | | | | |
| Hale (60) | 771,810 | 15,444 | 52.0[a] | 3.0 | | 19.0 | | 10.0 | | 13.0 | | 3.0[b] | | |
| Heald (70) | ≈5,000,000 | ≈96,000 | 43.0[c] | 2.0 | | 19.0 | | 10.0 | | 18.0[d] | | 5.0[b] | 3.0[e] | |
| High school | | | | | | | | | | | | | | |
| Lowe et al. (92) | 256 | 3 | | | | 33.3 | | 33.3 | | 33.3 | | | | |
| College | | | | | | | | | | | | | | |
| Clarke & Buckley (23)‡ | — | — | | | | 10.0[f] | | | | 37.0 | 28.0 | 1.0[g] | 5.0[h] | |
| Whiteside (148)* | — | 133 | | | | 3.4 | | | | 34.5 | 26.1 | 6.7[g] | 29.4[i] | 19.0[e] |
| Amateur event | | | | | | | | | | | | | | |
| Martin et al. (96) | 148 | 8 | 25.0 | | | | | | 12.5 | 12.5 | 37.5 | 12.5[g] | | |
| Professional | | | | | | | | | | | | | | |
| Garfinkel et al. (46) | — | 382 | 16.7 | 0.5 | | 0.5 | 11.6[j] | 2.8 | 42.2[k] | 5.5 | 17.8 | 0.5[m] | 0.6[n] | 0.4[p] |
| Softball | | | | | | | | | | | | | | |
| High school | | | | | | | | | | | | | | |
| Lowe et al. (92) | 169 | 3 | | | | 33.3 | | | 33.3 | | 33.3 | | | |
| College | | | | | | | | | | | | | | |
| Clarke & Buckley (23)‡ | — | — | | | | 27.0[f] | | | | 40.0 | 12.0 | 4.0[g] | 4.0[h] | 13.0[e] |
| Whiteside (148)* | — | 76 | | | | 10.6[q] | | | | 32.0 | 25.3 | 12.0[g] | 20.0[i] | |
| Recreational adult | | | | | | | | | | | | | | |
| Loosli et al. (90)† | 81 | 66 | | | | 13.0 | | 8.0[a] | | 42.0 | 26.0 | 13.0[r] | | |
| Loosli et al. (90)§ | — | 285 | | | 5.01 | 6.0 | 10.0 | 7.0[a] | | 26.0 | 28.0 | 20.0[s] | | |
| Nadeau et al. (103)£ | — | 150 | 3.6 | | 0.9 | 14.5 | | | 14.5 | 33.6[d] | | 30.0[d] | 2.7[u] | |

[a]Includes contusions (no breakdown). [b]Dental injuries. [c]Includes contusions. [d]Includes sprains. [e]Other unspecified injuries. [f]Combines dental fractures with other types of fractures. [g]Neurotrauma. [h]Chronic orthopaedic. [i]General trauma (undefined). [j]Combines blisters (4.9), epicondylitis/tendinitis (4.1), rotator cuff tendinitis (1.6), bursitis (0.2), myositis (0.2), myositis ossificans (0.2), synovitis (0.2), and paronchia (0.2). [k]Combines contusions from hit by pitch (22.3) and other contusions (19.9). [m]Foreign body. [n]Combines effusion (0.2), fascial hernia (0.2), and thigh atrophy (0.2). [p]Combines nail avulsion and corns. [q]Includes subluxation. [r]Combines meniscus and other unknown injuries. [s]Combines overuse, meniscus, unknown, and degenerative injuries. [t]Includes digit sprains and contusions. [u]Knee injuries.

*Based on calculations of NAIRS data from 2 seasons. Combines practice and game-related frequencies.

‡Based on NAIRS data.

†Based on survey data. Percentages are estimates derived from histogram that does not list specific frequencies.

§Based on clinic data. Percentages are estimates derived from histogram that does not list specific frequencies.

£Based on 3 seasons of softball. Percentage figures calculated based on frequencies provided by authors.

**Table 5.4  A Comparison of Injury Location in Baseball by Percent of Occurrence**

| | Youth | Youth | Youth | Youth | Youth | College | College | College | College | College | Amateur event | Amateur event | Pro |
|---|---|---|---|---|---|---|---|---|---|---|---|---|---|
| | Chambers (20) | Hale (60) | Heald (70)[1] | Rutherford et al. (119)[2] | Zaricznyj et al. (149)[3] | Clarke & Buckley (23)[4] | Lowe et al. (92) | Whiteside (147) | Splain & Rolnick (126) | Whiteside (148)[5] | Lebrun et al. (87)[6] | Martin et al. (96)[7] | Garfinkel et al. (46)[8] |
| # of subjects | 740 | 771,810 | ≈5,000,000 | — | — | — | 256 | 708 | 88 | — | 18 | 148 | — |
| # of injuries | 2 | 15,444 | ≈96,000 | 86,500 | 146 | — | 3 | 5 | 63 | 133 | 33 | 8 | 382 |
| **Site of injury** | | | | | | | | | | | | | |
| Head | — | 33.0 | 38.0 | 39.5[o] | 40.4 | 2.0[a] | (67.0) | (40.0) | | (9.8) 8.8[a] | (3.0) | 25.0[m] | (4.9) |
| Skull | | | | | | | | | | 1.0 | | | |
| Face | | | | | | | 67.0 | 40.0 | | | | | 1.3 |
| Teeth | | | | | | | | | | | | | |
| Eyes | | | | | | | | | | | 3.0 | | 0.8 |
| Other | | | | | | | | | | | | | 2.8[n] |
| Spine/trunk | | 7.0 | 4.0 | 3.0[p] | | | | | (7.9) | 1.0[d] | (3.0) | | (6.8) |
| Neck | | | | | | | | | | | 3.0[j] | | |
| Upper back | | | | | | | | | 7.9[h] | | | | 4.2[h] |
| Lower back | | | | | | | | | | | | | |
| Ribs | | | | | | | | | | | | | 1.8 |
| Stomach | | | | | | | | | | | | | 0.8 |
| Upper extremity | (100.0) | 41.0 | 39.0 | (32.0) | (34.3) | | (33.0) | (20.0) | (31.7) | (49.5) | (60.1) | 12.5 | (42.9) |
| Shoulder | | | | | 0.7 | | | | 12.7 | 21.5[b] | | | 13.9 |
| Arm | | | | 32.0[q] | 0.7 | | | | 6.3 | | 60.1 | | 4.7 |
| Elbow | | | | | 5.5 | | 33.0 | | 6.3 | | | | 6.5 |
| Forearm | | | | | 3.4 | | | | | 28.0[c] | | | 3.7 |
| Wrist | | | | | 3.4 | | | | 4.8 | | | | 2.9 |
| Hand | 100.0 | | | | 4.8 | | | | | | | | 3.9 |
| Finger | | | | | 15.8 | | | 20.0 | 1.6 | | | | 7.3 |
| Lower extremity | | 19.0 | 19.0 | (22.5) | (24.7) | (44.0) | | (40.0) | (60.3)[i] | (39.8) | (15.2) | 62.5 | (42.2) |
| Pelvis, hip | | | | | 1.4 | 37.0 | | | 1.6 | 7.8[e] | | | 3.7 |
| Thigh | | | | | | | | | 14.3 | | | | 6.8 |
| Knee | | | | | 9.6 | 7.0 | | | 20.6 | 16.0 | 6.1 | | 12.0 |
| Leg | | | | 22.5[r] | 0.7[g] | | | | 3.2 | | 9.1[k] | | 6.8 |
| Ankle | | | | | 9.6 | | | | 14.2 | 16.0 | | | 2.4 |
| Heel/Achilles | | | | | | | | | | | | | 2.9 |
| Foot | | | | | 2.7 | | | 40.0 | 1.6 | | | | 3.9 |
| Toes | | | | | 0.7 | | | | | | | | 3.7 |

[a]Head, neck, and spine combined. [b]Shoulder and arm combined. [c]Forearm and hand combined. [d]Injuries classified under "torso". [e]Hip and leg combined. [f]Ankle and foot combined. [g]Tibia only. [h]Not specific as to location on back. [i]Neck and back combined. [j]Leg and ankle combined. [k]Head and back combined. [l]Refers to chest injuries. [m]Combines head, neck, and trunk injuries. [n]Unspecified head (1.0%), ear (1.0%), and throat (0.8%) injuries combined. [o]Head and face combined. [p]Upper and lower trunk injuries combined. [q]Arm and hand combined. [r]Leg and foot combined.

[1]Figures are from Little League, Inc. [2]Figures are averages of figures for organized and informal play. [3]Figures do not include a "not skeletal" injury, accounting for 0.7% of total. [4]Figures include "significant" injuries only, as defined by NAIRS. [5]Figures combine both "reportable" and "significant" injuries. [6]Figures refer to visits to physicians and other medical personnel and include treatment for illnesses that were not distinguished from injuries. Hence, not included in these figures were visits for ear, nose, and throat (6.1%), gastro-intestinal (3.0%), and skin (9.1%) conditions. [7]Figures include injuries and illnesses. Hence, not included in these figures were systemic injuries/illnesses (0.0%). [8]Percentage figures calculated from frequencies listed in article.

**Table 5.5　A Comparison of Injury Location in Softball by Percent of Occurrence**

| | Youth | | | College | | | Amateur event | Recreational adult | | |
|---|---|---|---|---|---|---|---|---|---|---|
| | Clarke & Buckley (23)[1] | Lowe et al. (92) | Zaricznyj et al. (149) | Splain & Rolnick (126) | Whiteside et al. (147)[2] | Whiteside et al. (148)[3] | Lebrun et al. (87)[4] | Loosli et al. (90)[5] | Loosli et al. (90)[6] | Wheeler (145)[7] |
| # of subjects | — | 169 | — | 104 | 250 | — | 20 | 81 | — | — |
| # of injuries | — | 3 | 49 | 34 | 2 | 76 | 21 | 66 | 285 | 93 |
| **Site of injury** | | | | | | | | | | |
| Head | 4.0[a] | | 32.7 | | | 5.6[a] | | | | |
| Skull | | | | | | | | | | (5.0) |
| Face | | | | | | 14.1 | | | | 5.0 |
| Teeth | | | | | | | | | | |
| Eyes | | | | | | | | | | |
| Spine/trunk | | | | | | | | | | |
| Neck | | | | 15.1[h] | | 6.9[d] | 5.0[i] | | | |
| Upper back | | | | | | | | | | |
| Lower back | | | | | | | | | | |
| Ribs | | | | | | | | | | |
| Stomach | | | | | | | | | | |
| Upper extremity | | | (55.0) | (27.3) | (100.0) | (31.4) | (30.0) | (27.0) | (26.0) | (13.1) |
| Shoulder | | | 2.0 | 15.1 | | 15.7[b] | | 3.0 | 17.0 | |
| Arm | | | | | | | 30.0 | | 2.0 | |
| Elbow | | | | | | | | 6.0 | 3.0 | |
| Forearm | | | 2.0 | | | 15.7[c] | | | | |
| Wrist | | | 4.1 | 6.1 | | | | 18.0[k] | 4.0[k] | |
| Hand | | | 38.8 | 6.1 | | | | | | |
| Finger | | | 8.1 | | 100.0 | | | | | 13.1 |
| Lower extremity | (59.0) | (100) | (12.2) | (60.5) | | (41.9) | (40.0) | (73.0) | (71.0) | (70.6) |
| Pelvis, hips | 40.0 | | | | | 24.2[e] | | | 3.0 | 3.3[l] |
| Thigh | 19.0 | 33.0 | 6.1 | 12.1 | | | | 26.0 | 10.0 | |
| Knee | | | 2.0[g] | 15.1 | | 5.2 | 25.0 | 26.0 | 44.0 | 23.9 |
| Leg | | | 4.1 | 21.2 | | | 15.0[j] | 4.0 | 4.0 | 9.7 |
| Ankle | | | | 9.1 | | 12.5[f] | | 17.0 | 7.0 | 33.7 |
| Heel/Achilles | | | | | | | | | | |
| Foot/toes | | 67.0 | | 3.0 | | | | 3.0 | 3.0 | |

[a]Head, neck, and spine combined. [b]Shoulder and arm combined. [c]Forearm and hand combined. [d]Injuries classified under "torso." [e]Hip and leg combined. [f]Ankle and foot combined. [g]Refers to tibia. [h]Does not specify location on back. [i]Neck and back combined. [j]Leg and ankle combined. [k]Hand, wrist, and finger combined. [l]Thigh and hip combined.

[1]Figures include "significant" injuries only, as defined by NAIRS.

[2]Figures refer to fractures only.

[3]Figures combine both "reportable" and "significant" injuries.

[4]Figures refer to visits to physicians and other medical personnel and include treatment for illnesses, which were not distinguished from injuries. Hence, not included in these figures were visits for ear, nose, and throat (15.0%), gastro-intestinal (5.0%), and skin (5.0%) conditions.

[5]Figures are from survey portion of study and are approximations based on histogram that does not specify exact percentages.

[6]Figures are from clinic portion of study and are approximations based on histogram that does not specify exact percentages. Injuries listed as "other/unknown" (approx. 6%) not included.

[7]Figures are of top 10 injuries only and are calculations based on frequencies.

extremity, while the remainder occurred in the upper extremity. Specific sites of greatest occurrence were the knees, ankles, and thighs.

### 3.3.1 Head/Spine/Trunk

Nearly all of the reports associated with injuries in baseball and softball discussed cases that involved either the shoulder, arm, elbow, or hand/fingers. The few studies that reported injuries to the head, spine, and trunk are listed in Table 5.6. Although significant by the nature of their severity, they represent a small proportion of the injuries involved in baseball or softball.

Perhaps no type of injury in baseball and softball features the frequency of occurrence, yet paucity of study, as those pertaining to the ocular region. The unprotected eye is particularly prone to penetration by fast-moving objects. Sport and play activities rank among the top contributors to all eye injuries (120,129), and balls of all varieties are the principle object by which such injuries occur (31). Interpretations of data collected by the Consumer Product Safety Commission have consistently shown that baseball ranks with basketball, hockey, football, and racquet sports as one of the leading causes of sports-related eye injuries (18, 139-143).

Eye injuries to children are predominantly sports-related (31), and it is not surprising that baseball injuries to the eye inordinately affect young players. Clearly, this is due to higher participation rates of children versus adults in baseball. Forty-five percent of eye injuries in a 6-year period were sustained by youth ages 5 to 14, with individuals in the 15 to 24 year age range sustaining another 26% of such injuries (141).

Reports indicate that when baseball has been identified as a source of eye injury, the injuries tend to be severe. As noted in the literature (85), sport-related eye injuries—of which baseball is a leading cause—have consistently been the leading source of hyphemas, a condition requiring hospitalization. Again, however, lack of specificity in the reporting of data makes such a conclusion speculative. Evidence shows a consistent pattern for the mechanism of eye injury in baseball and softball. Labelle et al. (83) reported that 92% of baseball injuries were caused by the ball, with the remainder being attributable to the bat. A similar pattern emerged in Fountain and Albert's (42) report of injuries in baseball and softball. The most frequent mechanism of severe eye injury in baseball involved blows to the eye by the ball. Yet, there are a number of other possible mechanisms of injury, including bats, fingers, and other foreign objects. What is evident, given the frequency of the occurrence of eye injury in baseball and softball, is that eye protection should be as standard a part of the baseball and softball uniform as the glove and helmet.

**Table 5.6  Case Reports, Case Studies, and Cross-Sectional Studies of Injuries Occurring in the Head/Spine/Trunk and Lower Extremities of Baseball Players**

| Study | Design | Subjects | Age | Level | Condition/diagnosis |
| --- | --- | --- | --- | --- | --- |
| Head | | | | | |
| Hart (67) | Case | 1 | 14 | — | Intracerebral hematoma |
| Trunk | | | | | |
| Strukel & Garrick (131) | Case | 4 | 16, 17, 20 | High school; college | Thoracic outlet compression |
| Gurtler et al. (59) | Case | 1 | 17 | — | Stress fracture of first rib on dominant side |
| Nuber et al. (109) | Case | 9 | 18-34 | Professional | Thoracic outlet compression |
| Abrunzo (1) | Case | 2 | 10, 11 | — | Commotio cordis, fatality |
| Glennon (51) | Case | 1 | 30 | Recreational | Lesion of branch of the infraspinatus of the suprascapular nerve |
| Lambert & Fligner (84) | Case | 1 | 15 | — | Large avulsion of the iliac crest with separation of fracture fragment |
| Thigh/leg | | | | | |
| Bowerman & McDonnell (12) | Case series | 29 | — | Professional | 14 cases of lower extremity abnormality |
| Monaco et al. (100) | Case | 2 | — | — | Partial tear of anterior cruciate ligament |
| Martin et al. (96) | Case | 1 | 22 | Professional | Stress fracture of the tibia and fibula |
| White (146) | Case | 1 | — | Professional | Open ankle sprain involving anterolateral capsule and torn lateral ligaments |

### 3.3.2 Upper Extremity

**3.3.2.1 Baseball.**   Fifty-four reports provided details of injuries to the upper extremity of baseball players. Of these, 7 addressed injuries to the shoulder, 26 were specific to the arm, 11 to the elbow, and 10 to the hand and fingers. Thirty-six of the reports were case studies, 15 were case series, and 3 were cross sectional in nature. Twenty-two of the 54 studies involved youth or teen-aged players, and 17 studies reported on professional players.

The attention directed to the upper extremity of baseball players indicates both the importance of the area (shoulder and elbow) to success in the sport and its vulnerability as an anatomical part of the body in relation to the skills demanded of baseball players. Table 5.7 provides both the general location and the specific condition/diagnosis of the injury in relation to the ages and playing levels of the subjects involved in the reports. Note that the six reports of injuries to the shoulder involved only adults, all at the college or professional levels, with the rotator cuff as the most frequent location of the problem.

Reports of injuries to the arms (see Table 5.7) of baseball players were so classified, in part, because the arm was designated in the title or in the general description by the authors. Scrutiny of the condition/diagnosis reveals that many of the reports could have been placed under the category of elbow (see Table 5.8); thus, the distinction between the reports within the categories of *arm* and *elbow* is not as precise as the subtitles suggest. Note that 11 of the 13 reports that involved injuries to youths appear under the subcategories of arm or elbow, frequently involving the epiphyses, apophyses, or spiral fractures of the humerus.

Ever since Dotter (33) identified the growth-related problems associated with the repetitive action of throwing a baseball, the shoulders and arms of youthful baseball players have been the source of considerable controversy and study (2, 3, 5, 14, 16, 25, 28, 39, 43, 55, 65, 81, 88, 111, 112, 124, 125, 136, 138). This extensive literature on the topic has resulted in changes in rules that limit the number of innings that young pitchers are allowed to pitch per week. However, the continuing reports in the medical literature since the modification of rules regarding pitching suggest that the problem persists.

The etiology of injuries to the pitcher's arm and shoulder is similar to that of other overuse syndromes. Repetitive throwing causes tissue breakdown, which may be in evidence as inflammation, fragmentation and avulsion of the apophysis, osteochondritis dissecans, and possibly osteoarthritis. Causes are attributed to excessive throwing, lack of flexibility, muscle imbalance, improper mechanics, and throwing pitches that involve a sidearm motion.

Reports of injuries to the hand and fingers were of two categories; namely, fractures of the hook of the hamate bone and circulatory disturbances involving functional constriction or obstruction of blood flow to the hand. None of the reports involved children or youth, and only 2 of 10 involved players of high-school age. Thus, baseball injuries to the hand/fingers that were reported in the literature pertained primarily to adults.

**3.2.2.2 Softball.**   The nine reports of injuries to the upper extremity of softball players also pertain primarily to adults. As noted earlier, the game of softball has not been the subject of study in any of the published literature in our reviews. Injuries to adults playing softball do not provide a pattern of injuries, probably because softball exists in varieties more numerous than baseball. The reader is referred to Table 5.9 for details of the condition/diagnosis of injuries reported for adult softball players.

### 3.3.3 Lower Extremity

Injuries to the lower extremities of baseball and softball players become more common as the level of competition and age of the competitors increase. Injuries to the lower extremity of youth baseball players (see Table 5.4) were in the range of 19% to 22.5% of total injuries. Data for interscholastic play were not available, but injuries to the lower extremities of intercollegiate and amateur baseball players were generally in the range of 40% to 60% of total injuries (see Table 5.4).

Reports of injuries to the lower extremity in youth and adult softball players (see Table 5.5) indicate that a high percentage of injuries involve the lower extremities at all levels. For example, Clarke and Buckley (23) reported 59% of injuries to youthful players were in the lower extremity. In collegiate play, Whiteside (148) reported 41.9% and Splain and Rolnick (126) reported that 60.5% of injuries involved the lower extremity. Injuries to the lower extremities of adults who played recreational softball were 73%, 71%, and 70.6%, respectively, as reported by Loosli et al. (90, 91) and Wheeler (145). Thus, the involvement of sliding by adult softball players markedly increases the incidence of injuries to the lower extremity (75-77).

**Table 5.7    Case Reports, Case Studies, and Cross-Sectional Studies of Injuries Occurring in the Shoulder and Arm of Baseball Players**

| Study | Design | Subjects | Age | Level | Condition/diagnosis |
|---|---|---|---|---|---|
| Shoulder | | | | | |
| DeBenedette (27) | Case series | 4 | — | Professional | Rotator cuff injuries |
| Fimrite (41) | Case | 2 | 31, 25 | Professional | Torn ligament/tear in rotator cuff |
| Gall (45) | Case | 1 | — | Professional | Torn rotator cuff |
| Haney (64) | Case | 1 | 20 | College | Elastofibroma under scapula of throwing arm |
| Lombardo et al. (89) | Case | 4 | 25, 22, 23, 24 | Professional | Lesions in the posterior capsule of the shoulder |
| Ringel et al. (116) | Case | 2 | 27, 34 | Professional | Suprascapular neuropathy |
| Arm | | | | | |
| Allen (6) | Case | 1 | 13 | — | Stress fracture of the humerus |
| Cahill (16) | Case series | 5 | 11-12 | — | Widening of the epiphyseal line with metaphyseal bone separation |
| Tullos & Fain (137) | Case | 1 | — | — | Osteochondrosis and possible stress fracture |
| Bowerman & McDonnell (12) | Case series | 29 | — | Professional | 22 cases of upper extremity and 14 cases of lower extremity abnormality |
| Ellman (37) | Case series | 4 | 10, 10, 12, 17 | — | Anterior angulation deformity of the radial head |
| Jackson (74) | Case series | 6 | 17-29 | Professional, college, high school | Impingement between the humeral head and the coracoacromial ligament |
| Gainor et al. (44) | Case series | 3 | 9, 18, 21 | — | Avulsion of medial epicondyle, spiral fracture of shaft of humerus, arterial clotting and pressure |
| Hang (65) | Case | 1 | 13 | — | Ulnar nerve compressed by fibrous tissue buildup |
| Moore (101) | Case | 2 | — | Professional | Decrease in range of motion in pitching arm |
| Hansen (66) | Case | 1 | 14 | — | Marked uniform widening of the proximal epiphysis of the humerus |
| Monaco et al. (100) | Case | 2 | — | — | Partial tear of anterior cruciate ligament |
| Barnett (10) | Case | 3 | 13 | — | Proximal humeral epiphysiolysis |
| Micheli (99) | Case | 1 | — | — | Injury to the growth plate of the medial epicondyle apophysis |
| Redler (115) | Case | 1 | 20 | — | Occlusion of the posterior humeral circumflex artery on full abduction |
| Garth et al. (49) | Case | 2 | — | — | Recurrent fractures of the humerus |
| Schemmel et al. (121) | Case | 1 | 18 | College | Tear in medial joint capsule and torn ulnar collateral ligament |
| Albert & Drvaric (4) | Case | 1 | 13 | — | Displaced spiral fracture of right midhumerus |
| Sterling et al. (127) | Case | 1 | 14 | — | Closed comminuted spiral fracture of the humerus |
| Branch et al. (13) | Case series | 12 | 36 | Recreational | 12 cases of spontaneous humeral shaft fractures |
| Nuber & Diment (107) | Case | 2 | 23, 21 | Professional, college | Olecranon stress fractures |
| DiCicco et al. (32) | Case | 1 | 30 | — | Displaced spiral fracture of the right humerus |
| Gross et al. (56) | Case | 1 | 12 | — | Stress fracture of the proximal humeral physis |

# 4. Injury Severity

## 4.1 Time Loss

Time lost from practice and competition in baseball and softball was the focus of only three reports. Garrick and Requa (48) reported that 27% of the baseball players missed 5 days of practice or competition due to injuries. Garfinkel (46) reported that 94% of professional athletes suffered injuries that prevented their participation for 8 days or less, 5% missed from 8 to 28 days of activity, and 1% did not participate in practices and games for 28 days or longer. Records of the NCAA indicate that for baseball and softball approximately 77% of the injuries permitted the player to return to practice or competition in less than 8 days (104, 105). Clearly, the time lost to injuries requires further

**Table 5.8　Case Reports, Case Studies, and Cross-Sectional Studies of Injuries Occurring in the Elbow and Hand/Fingers of Baseball Players**

| Study | Design | Subjects | Age | Level | Condition/diagnosis |
|---|---|---|---|---|---|
| Elbow | | | | | |
| Torg et al. (136) | Case | 1 | 16 | — | Nonunion of a stress fracture through the epiphyseal plate of the olecranon |
| Del Pizzo et al. (29) | Case | 19 | 17-31 | — | Ulnar nerve entrapment at the elbow |
| Indelicato et al. (72) | Case series | 25 | 19-28 | Professional | Elbow lesions |
| English et al. (38) | Case | 1 | — | Professional | Myofascial syndrome and acute recurrent somatic dysfunction |
| Selesnick et al. (123) | Case | 1 | 30 | — | Hyperextension and dislocation of elbow with large intra-articular displaced fracture of the coronoid process |
| Collins et al. (24) | Case | 1 | 27 | Professional | Posterior interosseous neuropathy of the elbow |
| Hand/fingers | | | | | |
| Carter et al. (17) | Case | 2 | 28, 31 | Professional | Un-united fractures of the hook of the hamate |
| Krishnan (82) | Case | 1 | 32 | — | Dislocation of distal and proximal joints of ring finger of dominant hand |
| Egawa & Asai (36) | Case series | 5 | 14, 14, 24, 24, 45 | — | Fracture of hook of hamate of the hand |
| Parker et al. (113) | Case | 6 | 29, 24, 24, 22, 24 | Professional | Fractured hook of hamate |
| Sugawara et al. (132) | Case | 8 | 16-26 | High school, college | Digital ischemia |
| Sugawara et al. (132) | Cross-sectional | 299 | — | High school | Digital ischemia (22.1%) |
| Sugawara et al. (132) | Cross-sectional | 72 | — | College | Digital ischemia (40.3%) |
| Itoh et al. (73) | Case | 3 | 24, 20, 21 | Professional, college | Circulatory disturbances of hand with ulcer formation |
| Nuber et al. (108) | Case | 11 | 23-47 | Professional | Ischemia of hand |
| Rotman & Pruitt (118) | Case | 1 | 24 | — | Avulsion fracture of nondominant wrist at base of long metacarpal |

study, especially in conjunction with the specific type of injury at specific levels of play.

## 4.2 Catastrophic Injury

Although there are numerous references in the literature to catastrophic nonfatal and fatal injuries related to baseball and softball in both children and adults, only 10 such events were described as case studies (see Table 5.10). All of the reports involved youth between the ages of 4 and 14 years, and 9 of the 10 involved children between 8 and 14 years. Seven of the 10 cases involved a pitched ball, and the remaining 3 involved a batted ball. Most of the catastrophic injuries occurred via a blow to the chest. Despite the infrequent occurrence of such incidences, it behooves administrators of programs and medical personnel to explore

ways, through protective equipment and modifications of rules, to determine if such devastating occurrences can be eliminated.

## 5. Injury Risk Factors

### 5.1 Intrinsic Factors

Considering the large number of studies reviewed, one is initially overwhelmed by the abundance of evidence about injuries in baseball, and to a more limited extent in softball, but is hard-pressed to find patterns emerging from the information. However, closer examination reveals that certain factors appeared to be associated with increased risk of injury and even with certain types of injuries. Generally, these factors could be separated into two categories: factors that are intrinsic to the

**Table 5.9   Case Reports, Case Studies, and Cross-Sectional Studies of Injuries Occurring in the Upper Extremity of Softball Players**

| Study | Design | Subjects | Age | Level | Condition/diagnosis |
|---|---|---|---|---|---|
| *Arm* | | | | | |
| Mutoh et al. (102) | Case | 1 | 19 | — | Stress fracture of ulna |
| Tanabe et al. (134) | Case | 3 | 20, 17, 16 | College; high school | Transverse fracture of middle of the ulna |
| *Hand/fingers* | | | | | |
| Kitagawa & Kashimoto (80) | Case | 1 | 36 | Recreational | Widening of the interphalangeal joint and small oval bone in the articular space of dominant hand |
| Parker et al. (113) | Case | 1 | 29 | Recreational | Hook of hamate fracture |
| Ferrier & Atkinson (40) | Case | 1 | 30 | Recreational | Intraarticular fracture of the base of the middle phalanx with dorsal subluxation of the PIP joint |
| *Spine/trunk* | | | | | |
| Haycock (69) | Case | 1 | 22 | Recreational | Disrupted kidney |
| *Thigh/leg* | | | | | |
| Monaco et al. (100) | Case | 2 | — | — | Partial tear of anterior cruciate ligament |
| Gross (57) | Case series | 5 | 14-35 | — | Dislocation of the patella |
| An et al. (8) | Case | 1 | 36 | Recreational | Acute anterior compartment syndrome of thigh |

**Table 5.10   Reports of Cases and Case Series of Catastrophic Injuries Occurring in Baseball and Softball**

| Study | Design | Subjects | Age | Level | Mechanism | Injury | Condition |
|---|---|---|---|---|---|---|---|
| Rutherford et al. (119)* | Case series | 1M | 14 | Youth | Pitched ball | Blow to chest | Fatal |
| | | 1M | 9 | Youth | Thrown ball | Blow to chest | Nonfatal |
| | | 1M | 14 | Youth | Pitched ball | Blow to chest | Fatal |
| | | 1M | 8 | Youth | Pitched ball | Blow to chest | Fatal |
| | | 1M | 11 | Youth | Batted ball | Blow to head | Fatal |
| | | 1F | 11 | Youth | Batted | Blow to head | Fatal |
| | | 1M | 4 | Youth | Batted | Blow to chest | Fatal |
| Abrunzo (1) | Case | 1M | 10 | Youth | Pitched ball | Blow to chest | Fatal |
| | | 1M | 11 | Youth | Thrown ball | Blow to chest | Nonfatal |
| Hart (67) | Case | 1M | 12 | Youth | Pitched ball | Blow to head | Nonfatal |

*Based on a listing of "selected cases" from among 51 reported baseball-related deaths and other cases.

athletes and those that are extrinsic to them. In the former group are the physical, functional, and psychological characteristics of the players. The latter includes items related to the level of exposure, coaching, and the playing environment. Many of these variables were revealed in quantitative studies, while others were hypothesized to be part of the mechanism that caused the injury; still others were revealed through analysis of how baseball and softball are played. Although Table 5.11 summarizes these conclusions, they merit more explanation than is possible here.

The most persuasive evidence regarding the association of injuries to intrinsic factors was related to the physical characteristics of the players.

Studies revealed that younger baseball players were more likely to suffer from injuries of the upper extremity and from being hit by pitched balls while batting (54, 55, 61). Older players were more likely to injure their knees, ankles, and other parts of the lower extremities. Not unexpectedly, pitchers of all ages reported arm injuries, but there were interesting differences in the nature of the complaints. Studies of younger pitchers reported elbow and shoulder pain, found to be associated with the epiphyseal areas (16, 137, for example). Older pitchers generally had injuries associated with repeated use that affected the rotator cuff (27, 50).

Because of the relative paucity of research done in softball, no clear patterns of injuries emerged.

**Table 5.11   Elements Affecting the Risk of Injuries Associated With Baseball and Softball**

| Intrinsic risks associated with . . . | Extrinsic risks associated with . . . |
| --- | --- |
| Physical characteristics of players<br>• Age/physical maturity<br>    Younger players<br>       More upper extremity injuries<br>    Older players<br>       More lower extremity injuries<br>    Young pitchers<br>       Epiphyseal problems<br>    Older pitchers<br>       Rotator cuff injuries<br><br>Functional characteristics of players<br>• Previous history of injury<br>• Poor pitching mechanics<br>• Poor sliding/base-running mechanics<br>• Imbalances in shoulder or upper leg musculature<br><br>Psychological characteristics of players<br>• Preparation for level of play | Level of exposure<br>• Level of competition<br>• Years in baseball/softball<br>• Position played<br>    Pitchers<br>       Number of pitches thrown<br>    Catchers<br>       Use of extra padding on glove hand<br>       Type of crouch used<br>       Time spent in crouch<br>• Number of practices/games per week<br>• Amount of sliding in practices/game<br>• Softball as opposed to baseball<br>    Softball pitchers<br>       Arm injuries uncommon<br>    Baseball pitchers<br>       Arm injuries relatively common<br><br>Coaching<br>• Instruction in correct pitching technique<br>• Instruction in throwing<br>• Instruction in proper sliding technique<br>• Instruction in avoiding pitched balls<br>• Instruction in proper use and maintenance of safety equipment<br><br>Environment<br>• Practice/playing conditions<br>• Type of base used<br>• Attention to safe field conditions<br>• Use of proper safety equipment |

However, there was some indication that injuries to the leg and foot were more common among older players (87, 91), and one of the studies suggested that softball pitchers might suffer the same consequences of overuse that are more commonly associated with baseball pitching (91).

A commonly suggested cause of arm injuries in young baseball pitchers was functional, namely, poor pitching mechanics. Specifically, dropping the elbow closer to horizontal was thought to increase the likelihood of injury (5). Among older pitchers, a suggested functional cause of injury was an imbalance in the musculature of the shoulder. For offensive players, poor mechanics were cited as a possible cause of injury when sliding (78). A history of previous injury indicated an increased risk of reinjury (49).

## 5.2 Extrinsic Factors

Numerous aspects of the games extrinsic to the athletes themselves might be related to an increase in the risk of injury. Generally, these were hypothesized as factors affecting the risk, but were more

related to the level of exposure. For example, the level of competition might be critical, because highly competitive athletes seemed to be injured more often (87). Similarly the number of years in the game could be expected to have an effect, and obviously the position played influences the risk. Clearly, pitchers suffer many injuries of the arm and shoulder, and it has been suggested that limiting their throwing would reduce this effect (21). Catchers were found to have circulatory and other problems with the glove hand (93, 108). The crouch traditionally used by catchers in both baseball and softball may influence the number of back and knee injuries with the rate of injury directly related to the amount of time spent in the crouched position.

Other elements related to the level of exposure to risk were the number of practices and games and the amount of sliding involved (78, 87, 103-105). Finally, although it has been suggested that pitching softball is easier on the arm than pitching baseball, Loosli et al. (91) and Tanabe et al. (134) documented arm injuries in the sport that raised concerns about this belief. Factors best described as related to the coaching of athletes were suggested as extrinsic risk elements. These ranged from improving the pitching and throwing mechanics of athletes (5) to instruction in proper sliding and fielding techniques (145). Instruction in avoiding pitched balls while batting (22) and the proper and expanded use of safety equipment were suggested (61). Finally, environmental factors were thought to have an influence on the risk of injury. Chief among these were the condition of the field and its surroundings (22) and the type of base used (78, 103).

### 5.2.1 Exposure Events

The events in baseball and softball that are most frequently associated with injuries at the youth level are being struck by a thrown or batted ball. Reports by Hale (60-62) and by Heald (70) place the incidences of being struck by a ball at 41.5% to 65%. Injuries that occurred while players were attempting to catch the ball and attempting to slide accounted for approximately 10% and 14% of the remaining injuries.

The events associated with injuries in baseball and softball at the adult level involved running— 36%, sliding—ranging from 27% to 71%, and collisions with other players—16% to 28% (60-62, 70, 76, 103, 117). More detailed discussion of the injuries associated with specific actions, such as throwing a baseball, catching, back and leg injuries, sliding, and playing particular positions follows.

*5.2.1.1 Throwing.* The results of 11 reports that pertain to injuries of the shoulder and elbow that have been attributed to the action of throwing are summarized here (9, 43, 52, 54, 58, 86, 95, 111, 130, 133, 135). Noteworthy in the major findings and conclusions is that injuries to the shoulders and elbows of baseball players have an early onset and are aggravated by the repetitive action of the overarm throwing motion.

*5.2.1.2 Catching.* Injuries to the hand in softball and baseball are closely associated with the act of catching, especially among catchers (26, 30, 68, 93). Among younger players and recreational softball players, the cause of injuries is frequently associated with an inability to accurately judge the flight of the ball and to intercept it within the gloved hand.

*5.2.1.3 The Back and Legs.* Two studies (71, 94) identified back and knee injuries associated with baseball. These injuries often are attributed to the

crouching position commonly used by catchers and in sliding.

*5.2.1.4 Sliding.* The special provision of progressive-release bases has added a dimension of safety to sliding that is absent when anchored bases are used (19, 106). Janda (78, 79) advocated that progressive-release bases that give way to the impact of a sliding player would substantially reduce the number of injuries sustained by adults in recreational softball.

*5.2.1.5 Position Play.* With respect to studying injuries that occur in players taking certain positions on the field, research on pitchers and pitching dominated the literature. From the early reports of Adams (2, 3) to the most recent work of Congeri (25) and Gross et al. (56), injuries affecting pitchers' arms have received most of the attention. The literature suggests that arm and shoulder injuries have an early onset, with younger pitchers often complaining of elbow and shoulder pain, and that these complaints are often associated with epiphyseal injuries; see Cahill (16) and Tullos and Fain (137). The common occurrence of pain and trauma to the elbow and shoulder joint of pitchers suggests that additional rule modifications, such as a limit to the number and kind of pitches thrown, in addition to the already present limit on the number of innings pitched, should be initiated. Adult pitchers generally had injuries associated with repeated use, especially in the rotator cuff—see, for example, DeBenedette (27) and Gates (50). These injuries are so common that some observers have suggested that every player who pitches will eventually suffer some sort of arm or shoulder injury.

As in the case of pitchers, repetitive actions are thought to be the chief mechanism of injury to catchers. Catchers were found to suffer from mallet fingers and injuries to the nerves and circulation of the glove hand (93, 108). Although not reported in the literature, an additional element potentially affecting injuries among catchers is the crouch position traditionally used in baseball and softball. Back and knee injuries as they relate to athletes playing in crouched position should receive additional study.

Other than the focus on pitchers and catchers, very little work has been reported on the occurrence of injury to players at various positions. Hale (61) reported data on the percentage of injuries occurring at each position in youth play. His findings were as follows: pitcher = 5%; catcher = 16%; first base = 5%; second base = 6%; third base = 5%; shortstop = 5%; outfielders = 14%; runners = 17%;

batter = 22%; on-deck batter = 2%; not categorized = 3%. This information from 1967 was presented only as percentages and *injury* was not defined. Nevertheless, several points emerge from Hale's report. Pitchers appear to be tremendously underrepresented in these data, as compared to subsequent reports of injuries. Injury rates among catchers and base runners seem to be consistent with the attention they have received in other reports. The relatively high rate of injuries to batters requires much closer attention than it has received to date. Garfinkel et al. (46) studied professional baseball players and discovered remarkably similar distribution: pitcher = 14.6%; catcher = 13.3%; first base = 1.8%; second base = 7.6%; third base = 3.4%; shortstop = 2.6%; outfielders = 9.8%; runners = 21.7%; batters = 23.8%; miscellaneous injuries = 1.1%. The issue of studying injuries in baseball and softball by position has received little attention and clearly is a topic that requires additional study.

## 6. Suggestions for Injury Prevention

Suggestions of the possible mechanisms that affect risk factors for injuries were many and varied, as noted in Table 5.12. Although the recommendations appear to be logical, most are based on experiential rather than experimental evidence. This does not discount the utility of the suggestions as a means of reducing injuries, but lack of scientific evidence in a sport such as baseball, where tradition is a major factor, is likely to be viewed as support for the status quo, rather than as a reason for change. Mechanisms included the personnel involved, the game, the environment in which the game is played, and the care of those who were injured.

Another important issue was the preparation of coaches—especially those in recreational and youth settings. It has been recognized and recommended that all coaches should receive formal preparation in a variety of areas, among them: the essential skills and mechanics of softball or baseball; certification in CPR and first aid; injuries and the mechanism of injuries commonly associated with baseball and softball; injury prevention techniques; and management skills relating to recording and reporting injuries and analyzing such data for patterns of injuries.

During actual baseball and softball games, several means of preventing or reducing injuries to athletes were suggested. Several of these recommendations involved improving techniques used

by players. Within this category were: throwing and pitching (15), sliding (63, 78, 103, 146), and avoiding pitched balls (34). A report by Clark and Seefeldt (22) also pointed out that injuries might be affected positively by modifying rules to emphasize elements of the game appropriate to the developmental level of the players involved. The issue of age-appropriate play prompted suggestions relating to rules changes, primarily involving the amount of time devoted to pitching baseball.

The equipment used in baseball and softball was the subject of numerous recommendations, and the playing environment was seen as an area in which more could be done to prevent injuries. Low-profile bases or ones easily dislodged by vigorous contact were proposed to reduce sliding injuries (61, 78, 90, 103). Other suggestions included: using a "double-wide" first base with the additional portion in foul territory for the use of the runner advancing from home plate; requiring hitters to wear individually fitted helmets that incorporate eye protection; having catchers wear extra padding on the hand in the mitt; using only NOCSAE approved balls in organized play for children under 13 (122); and not allowing shoes with metal cleats or spikes in any youth play (22, 61). Further, the size of the field should be proportional to the size of the athletes. A screened-in dugout or similar enclosures should protect all offensive team players (other than the batter) and the nonplaying members of the defensive team.

The general issue of health care could be seen as ultimately affecting the risk of injury. As previously mentioned, preparticipation physicals should be required of all players engaging in competitive baseball and softball. All agencies sponsoring baseball and softball games of any sort should establish injury reporting systems.

## 7. Suggestions for Further Research

Table 5.13 summarizes possible issues that should direct future research. First among the suggestions for further study is the basic problem of defining and accurately describing injuries. A number of the case studies described very specific injuries, but others simply categorized them by either type or location. This description lacks the precision needed, resulting in confusing and conflicting results when in reality such distinctions may not exist; rather, information on both type and location of injury is needed. Similarly, there should be more careful assessment of the injuries in terms of severity. This assessment should include the amount of

**Table 5.12  Injury Prevention Mechanisms in Baseball and Softball**

| Area of need | Suggestions from literature | Supporting evidence |
|---|---|---|
| **The personnel** | | |
| Education | Athletes should understand how the following elements affect injury: physical examination prior to play; appropriate level of physical fitness; warm-up/cool down; off-season and preseason training; need to report all injuries; caring for their own injuries; correct techniques; proper fitting and care of protective equipment; and environmental factors. | Congeri (25), Gross et al. (56), Kozar & Lord (81), Loosli et al. (90), O'Neill & Micheli (110) |
| | All coaches should receive formal education in the essentials of baseball/softball, CPR, and first aid; injuries and injury mechanisms; injury prevention techniques; recording, reporting, and analysis of patterns of injuries. | |
| Conditioning | Use appropriate conditioning to correct/avoid muscular imbalances, especially in pitchers. | Micheli (98) |
| **The game** | | |
| Techniques | Improve the throwing mechanics of young players, especially pitchers. | Brunet et al. (15) |
| | Teach correct sliding skills to all players. | Janda et al. (78), Nadeau et al. (103), Wheeler (145) |
| | Teach all players how to avoid pitched balls. | |
| Age-appropriate play | Emphasize elements of the game appropriate to the developmental level of the players. For example, do not expect young players to pitch to one another. | Clark & Seefeldt (22) |
| Rules | Limit the amount of pitching done by youth. | Clain & Hershman (21), Congeri (25), Sullivan (133) |
| | Count pitches rather than innings pitched. | Clark & Seefeldt (22) |
| Equipment | Bases that are easily dislodged by violent contact | Hale (61), Janda et al. (78), Loosli et al. (90), Nadeau et al. (103) |
| | "Double" first base | Clark & Seefeldt (22) |
| | Individually fitted helmets for eye protection | Stock & Cornell (128) |
| | Extra protection on glove hands of catchers | Itoh et al. (73), Haycock (68) |
| | Balls meeting NOCSAE recommendations for all organized play by children 12 years old and under | Clark & Seefeldt (22) |
| | No shoes with metal cleats or "spikes" in any youth play | Clark & Seefeldt (22) |
| **The environment** | | |
| Field | Proportional to the size of the players—not merely shortened distances for bases | Clark & Seefeldt (22) |
| Facilities | Offensive-team players stay behind a screened-in dugout or enclosure | Clark & Seefeldt (22) |
| | Fields free of debris and suitable for competition and practice, fences a reasonable distance from fair territory, in good repair, and no exposed edges | Clark & Seefeldt (22) |
| **Health care** | | |
| Medical exams | Require preparticipation examinations for all players. | |
| | Recommend medical exam for athletes suffering certain kinds of injuries, such as head injuries, sprains, dislocations, or ones remaining painful for more than a day. | |
| Injury recording and reporting | Sponsoring agencies should establish systems for recording, reporting, and tracking injuries that include kind and severity of injury, circumstances surrounding injuries, treatment required, and the outcome. | |

time lost from competition, regular activity, or both due to the injury.

In general, more complete information on both the athlete and the injury should be collected, such as the age and gender of the player; whether practice or play was involved; the type of game being played (baseball or softball, fast-pitch or slow-pitch softball, competitive or recreational); the

**Table 5.13  Suggestions for Further Research Into Baseball and Softball Injuries**

| Element to be studied | Suggestions |
|---|---|
| Injury definition | Injuries should be categorized on the basis of location and the type of injury. <br> Injuries should be assessed on the basis of competitive time lost and time away from regular activities (e.g., restriction of a day's activity, less than a week lost, more than a week lost). |
| Data collection | More complete data needed on both the athlete and the injury that includes age and gender of the player, the type of game being played, the specific activity involved, the ability level of the athletes, the position of the field, whether injuries occurred during practice or competition, in recreational or competitive settings, or simply involved equipment related to baseball or softball. <br> Distinguish injuries involving factors inherent to baseball and softball from those caused by faulty technique or poor skills. |
| Subjects | Injuries occurring in competitive, fast-pitch softball as it is played by females <br> The game of slow-pitch softball as it is played by adults <br> Injuries by the types of softball being played: competitive and recreational; fast-pitch and slow-pitch; games involving males or females or those including both genders <br> Injuries among males and females when they play the same game: youth baseball—including Little League, co-ed softball, recreational games |
| Research design | Studies need to include prospective and cross-sectional research. <br> Longitudinal research in areas where there is an indication of chronic injury, particularly in baseball and fast-pitch softball pitchers and catchers. |
| Researchers | More thorough and rigorous statistical analysis techniques. <br> Trained sport scientists, medical personnel, and experienced coaches and athletes. |

specific activity of the player at the moment of injury (hitting, bunting, running, sliding, fielding, throwing, pitching, catching); the ability level of the athletes; and the position assigned the injured player (hitter, runner, shortstop, outfielder). Such information would provide a much clearer picture of the mechanism of injury, a topic often neglected in the available reports. Such distinctions would also make it possible to distinguish injuries that are inherent to the games of baseball and softball from those resulting from faulty technique or poor skills. Additionally, such information would reveal whether certain acts common to the games (the catcher's crouch, for instance) present a serious injury risk. In addition, the relative risk to players in various positions could be assessed.

Due to the methodological weaknesses in the literature the studies mentioned in this chapter provided only a partial description of the injuries that occur in baseball and softball. Generally, the game of softball was not as thoroughly studied as baseball. Baseball was the focus of 98 studies, softball was the focus of 17, and another 34 either compared baseball and softball to one another or to other sports. Clearly, softball was underrepresented in the literature. Researchers also should attend to the differences and similarities in injuries occurring to males and females playing the same game. For example, youth baseball, including Little League, now commonly involves both genders being on the field at once; co-ed softball, which specifically requires five males and five females on each team, is a common variation of slow-pitch softball; women's professional baseball reappeared in 1994; and both genders commonly play together in recreational softball and baseball games. Clearly these settings provide interesting opportunities for study because of differences in perceived abilities to propel and receive baseballs and softballs.

Reports of injuries in baseball and softball underscore the fact that several research protocols have been neglected. The literature clearly is dominated by case studies and case series. Cross-sectional and especially prospective studies are required if researchers are to address the causes and mechanisms of injuries. Similarly, longitudinal research is indicated when other methodologies point to an indication of chronic injury. The issue of hand/circulatory injuries in catchers comes to mind as does the problem of arm/shoulder injuries to baseball and fast-pitch softball pitchers.

The topic of research teams also should be considered. Generally, the literature on baseball and softball injuries has been dominated by physicians, trainers, and other health care providers. These professionals have much to offer everyone concerned with the sports, but their efforts may be made even more meaningful if research teams were broadened to include trained sports scientists and experienced coaches and athletes. Such a diversified research team would probably expand the range of questions and draw different conclusions. Additionally, researchers generally should apply more thorough and rigorous statistical techniques to their data; far too many studies resulted in descriptive designs that included little more than counting the number of injuries per unit time.

# References

1. Abrunzo, T.J. Commotio cordis—the single, most common cause of traumatic death in youth baseball. American Journal of Diseases of Children. 145:1279-1282; 1991.
2. Adams, J.E. Injury to the throwing arm: A study of traumatic changes in the elbow joints of boy baseball players. California Medicine. 102(2):127-132; 1965.
3. Adams, J.E. Little league shoulder: osteochondrosis of the proximal humeral epiphysis in boy baseball pitchers. California Medicine. 105(1):22-25; 1966.
4. Albert, M.J.; Drvaric, D.M. Little league shoulder: case report. Pediatric Orthopedics. 13(7):779-781; 1990.
5. Albright, J.A.; Jokl, P.; Shaw, R.; Albright, J.P. Clinical study of baseball pitchers: correlation of injury to the throwing arm with the method of delivery. American Journal of Sports Medicine. 6(1):15-21; 1978.
6. Allen, M.E. Stress fracture of the humerus. American Journal of Sports Medicine. 12(3):244-245; 1974.
7. Amateur Softball Association. Personal communication. Oklahoma City, OK; 1994.
8. An, H.S.; Simpson, J.M.; Gale, S.; Jackson, W.T. Acute anterior compartment syndrome in the thigh: A case report and review of the literature. Journal of Orthopaedic Trauma. 1(2):180-182; 1987.
9. Andrews, J.R.; Carson, W.G.; McLeod, W.D. Glenoid labrum tears related to the long head of the biceps. American Journal of Sports Medicine. 13(5):337-341; 1985.
10. Barnett, L.S. Little league shoulder syndrome: proximal humeral epiphyseolysis in adolescent baseball pitchers. Journal of Bone and Joint Surgery. 67(3):495-496; 1985.
11. Benham, R.; DeJong, G.; Seefeldt, V. Sport opportunity: odds of competing at high school through professional levels. East Lansing, MI: Institute for the Study of Youth Sports; 1994. (Submitted for publication.)
12. Bowerman, J.W.; McDonnell, E.J. Radiology of athletic injuries: Baseball. Radiology. 116:611-615; 1975.
13. Branch, T.; Partin, C.; Chamberland, P.; Emeterio, E.; Sabetelle, M. Spontaneous fractures of the humerus during pitching. American Journal of Sports Medicine. 20(4):468-470; 1992.
14. Brogdon, B.G.; Crow, N.E. Little Leaguer's elbow. American Journal of Roentgenology. 83(4):671-675; 1960.
15. Brunet, M.E.; Haddad, R.J., Jr.; Porche, E.B. Rotator cuff impingement syndrome in sports. The Physician and Sportsmedicine. 10(12):86, 88-92, 94; 1982.
16. Cahill, B.R. Lesions of the proximal humeral epiphyseal plate. Journal of Sports Medicine. 2(3):150-152; 1974.
17. Carter, P.R.; Eaton, R.G.; Littler, J.W. Ununited fracture of the hook of the hamate. Journal of Bone and Joint Surgery. 59A(5):583-588; 1977.
18. Caveness, L.S. Ocular and facial injuries in baseball. International Ophthalmology Clinics. 28(3):238-241; 1988.
19. Centers for Disease Control and Prevention. Sliding-associated injuries in college and professional baseball—1990-1991. Journal of the American Medical Association. 269(15):1925; 1993.
20. Chambers, R.B. Orthopaedic injuries in athletes (ages 6 to 17). American Journal of Sports Medicine. 7(3):195-197; 1979.
21. Clain, M.; Hershman, E. Overuse injuries in children and adolescents. The Physician and Sportsmedicine. 17(9):111-112, 115-116, 119-120, 122-123; 1989.
22. Clark, M.A.; Seefeldt, V. Modifications that would improve skill development and safety in youth baseball. East Lansing, MI: Institute for the Study of Youth Sports; 1994.
23. Clarke, K.S.; Buckley, W.E. Women's injuries in collegiate sports. American Journal of Sports Medicine. 8(3):187-191; 1980.
24. Collins, K.; Storey, M.; Peterson, K.; Nutter, P. Nerve injuries in athletes. The Physician and Sportsmedicine. 16(1):92-96, 98-100; 1988.
25. Congeri, J. Treating—and preventing—little league elbow. The Physician and Sportsmedicine. 22(3):54-55, 59-60, 63-64; 1994.
26. Dawson, W.J.; Pullos, N. Baseball injuries to the hand. Annals of Emergency Medicine. 10(6):302-306; 1981.
27. DeBenedette, V. Rotator cuff problems among top athletes. The Physician and Sportsmedicine. 17(5):184-186; 1989.
28. DeHaven, K.; Evarts, C. Throwing injuries of the elbow in athletes. Orthopedic Clinics of North America. 4:801-808, 1973.
29. Del Pizzo, W.; Jobe, F.W.; Norwood, L. Ulnar nerve entrapment syndrome in baseball players. American Journal of Sports Medicine. 5(5):182-185; 1977.
30. DeGroot, H. III; Mass, D.P. Hand injury patterns in softball players using a 16 inch ball. American Journal of Sports Medicine. 16(3) 260-265; 1988.
31. DeRespinis, P.A.; Caputo, A.R.; Fiore, P.M.; Wagner, R.S. A survey of severe eye injuries in children. American Journal of Diseases of Children. 143:711-716; 1989.
32. DiCicco, J.D.; Mehlman, C.T.; Urse, J.S. Fracture of the shaft of the humerus secondary to muscular

violence. Journal of Orthopaedic Trauma. 7(1):90-93; 1993.

33. Dotter, W. Little Leaguer's shoulder: Fracture of the proximal epiphysial cartilage of the humerus due to baseball pitching. Guthrie Clinical Bulletin. 23:68-72; 1953.

34. Duda, M. News briefs: NCAA survey shows injury trends. The Physician and Sportsmedicine. 15(2):30; 1987.

35. DuRant, R.H.; Pendergrast, R.A.; Seymore, C.; Gaillard, G.; Donner, J. Findings from the preparticipation athletic examination and athletic injuries. American Journal of Diseases of Children. 146:85-91; 1992.

36. Egawa, M.; Asai, T. Fracture of the hook of the hamate: report of six cases and the suitability of computerized tomography. Journal of Hand Surgery. 8(4):393-398; 1984.

37. Ellman, H. Anterior angulation deformity of the radial head. Journal of Bone and Joint Surgery. 57(6):776-778; 1975.

38. English, W.R.; Young, D.R.; Moss, R.E.; Raven, P.B. Chronic muscle overuse syndrome in baseball. The Physician and Sportsmedicine. 12(3):111-115; 1984.

39. Ewing, J.D. Little league elbow. Nebraska Medical Journal. March:73-75; 1972.

40. Ferrier, J.A.; Atkinson, R.E. Acute flexor superficialis avulsion. Journal of Hand Surgery. 18A(3):514-515; 1993.

41. Fimrite, R. Stress, strain and pain. Sports Illustrated. 49(7):30-43; 1978.

42. Fountain, T.R.; Albert, D.M. The histopathology of sports-related ocular trauma. International Ophthalmology Clinics. 28:206-210; 1988.

43. Francis, R.; Bunch, T.; Chandler, B. Little league elbow: a decade later. The Physician and Sportsmedicine. 6(4):88-94; 1978.

44. Gainor, B.J.; Piotrowski, G.; Puhl, J.; Allen, W.C.; Hagen, R. The throw: biomechanics and acute injury. American Journal of Sports Medicine. 8(2):114-118; 1980.

45. Gall, S.L. News briefs: shoulder injury throws Hershiser a curve. The Physician and Sportsmedicine. 18(7):15-16; 1990.

46. Garfinkel, D.; Talbot, A.A.; Clarizio, M.; Young, R. Medical problems on a professional baseball team. The Physician and Sportsmedicine. 9(7):85-87, 90-91, 93; 1981.

47. Garrick, J.G.; Requa, R.K. Girls' sports injuries in high school athletics. Journal of the American Medical Association. 239(21):2245-2248; 1978a.

48. Garrick, J.G.; Requa, R.K. Injuries in high school sports. Pediatrics. 61(3):465-469; 1978b.

49. Garth, W.P.; Leberte, M.A.; Cool, T. A. Recurrent fractures of the humerus in a baseball pitcher. Journal of Bone and Joint Surgery. 70(2):305-306; 1988.

50. Gates, R.D. Ending the pitcher's nightmare: research in California on rotator cuff injuries may be putting a new lease on the life of athletes' shoulders. Coaching Review. 6:14-18; 1983.

51. Glennon, T.P. Isolated injury of the infraspinatus branch of the suprascapular nerve. Archives of Physical Medicine and Rehabilitation. 73:201-202; 1992.

52. Glousman, R.E.; Barron, J.; Jobe, F.W.; Perry, J.; Pink, M. An electromyographic analysis of the elbow in normal and injured pitchers with medial collateral ligament insufficiency. American Journal of Sports Medicine. 20(3):311-317; 1992.

53. Grana, W.A. Summary of 1978-79 injury registry for Oklahoma secondary schools. Journal of the Oklahoma State Medical Association. 72(10):369-372; 1979.

54. Grana, W.A. Little league elbow: Prevention and treatment. Sports Medicine Digest. 7(4):1-3; 1985.

55. Grana, W.A.; Rashkin, A. Pitcher's elbow in adolescents. American Journal of Sports Medicine. 8(5):333-336; 1980.

56. Gross, M.L.; Flynn, M.; Sonzogni, J.J. Overworked shoulders. The Physician and Sportsmedicine. 22(3):81-82, 85-86; 1994.

57. Gross, R.M. Acute dislocation of the patella: the Mudville mystery. Journal of Bone and Joint Surgery. 68A(5):780-781; 1986.

58. Gugenheim, J.J., Jr.; Stanley, R.F.; Woods, G.W.; Tullos, H.S. Little league survey: the Houston study. American Journal of Sports Medicine. 4(5):189-200; 1976.

59. Gurtler, R.; Pavlov, H.; Torg, J.S. Stress fracture of the ipsilateral first rib in a pitcher. American Journal of Sports Medicine. 13(4):277-279; 1985.

60. Hale, C.J. Injuries among 771,810 little league baseball players. Journal of Sports Medicine and Physical Fitness. 1(2):80-83; 1961.

61. Hale, C.J. Protective equipment for baseball. The Physician and Sportsmedicine. 7(7):58-63; 1979.

62. Hale, C.J. Vision in sports. Sports Vision. 8(2):26-27, 29; 1992.

63. Hall, R.E. The Rogers® break away base™: "State of the art." Transcript of testimony before a committee of the Michigan Senate. Elizabethtown, PA; 1991.

64. Haney, T.C. Subscapularelastofibroma in a young pitcher. American Journal of Sports Medicine. 18(6):642-644; 1990.

65. Hang, Y.S. Tardy ulnar neuritis in a little league baseball player. American Journal of Sports Medicine. 9(4):244-246; 1981.

66. Hansen, N.M. Epiphyseal changes in the proximal humerus of an adolescent baseball pitcher. American Journal of Sports Medicine. 10(6):380-384; 1982.

67. Hart, E.J. Little league baseball and head injury. Pediatrics. 8(3):520; 1992.

68. Haycock, C.E. Hand, wrist, and forearm injuries in baseball. The Physician and Sportsmedicine. 7(7):67-71; 1979.

69. Haycock, C.E.; Gillette, J.V. Susceptibility of women athletes to injury. Journal of the American Medical Association. 236(2):163-165; 1976.

70. Heald, J. Summary of baseball/softball injuries. Tullahoma, TN: Worth Sports Company; 1991.

71. Ichikawa, N.; Ohara, Y.; Morishita, T.; Taniguichi, Y.; Koshikawa, A.; Matsukura, N. An aetiological study of spondylolysis from a biomechanical aspect. British Journal of Sports Medicine. 16(3):135-141; 1982.

72. Indelicato, P.A.; Jobe, F.W.; Kerlan, R.K.; Carter, V.S.; Shields, C.L.; Lombardo, S.J. Correctable elbow lesions in professional baseball players: a review of 25 cases. American Journal of Sports Medicine. 7(1):72-75; 1979.

73. Itoh, Y.; Wakano, K.; Takeda, T.; Murakami, T. Circulatory disturbances in the throwing hand of baseball pitchers. American Journal of Sports Medicine. 15(3):264-269; 1987.

74. Jackson, D.W. Chronic rotator cuff impingement in the throwing athlete. American Journal of Sports Medicine. 4(6):231-240; 1976.

75. Janda, D.H. Prevention has everything to do with sports medicine. Clinical Journal of Sports Medicine. 2(3):159-160; 1992.

76. Janda, D.H.; Hankin, F.M.; Wojtys, E.M. Softball injuries: cost, cause and prevention. American Family Physician. 33(6):143-144; 1986.

77. Janda, D.H.; Wild, D.E.; Hensinger, R.N. Softball injuries. Sports Medicine. 13(4):285-291; 1992.

78. Janda, D.H.; Wojtys, E.M.; Hankin, F.M.; Benedict, M.E. Softball sliding injuries. Journal of the American Medical Association. 259(12):1848-1850; 1988.

79. Janda, D.H.; Wojtys, E.M.; Hankin, F.M.; Benedict, M.E.; Hensinger, R.N. A three-phase analysis of the prevention of recreational softball injuries. American Journal of Sports Medicine. 18(6):632-635; 1990.

80. Kitagawa, H.; Kashimoto, T. Locking of the thumb at the interphalangeal joint by one of the sesamoid bones. Journal of Bone and Joint Surgery. 66A(8): 1300-1301; 1984.

81. Kozar, B.; Lord, R.M. Overuse injury in the young athlete: reasons for concern. The Physician and Sportsmedicine. 11(7):116-122; 1983.

82. Krishnan, S.G. Double dislocation of a finger. American Journal of Sports Medicine. 7(3):204-205; 1979.

83. Labelle, P.; Mercier, M.; Podtetenev, M.; Trudeau, F. Eye injuries in sports: results of a five-year study. The Physician and Sportsmedicine. 16(5):126-129, 132, 135, 138; 1988.

84. Lambert, M.J.; Fligner, D.J. Avulsion of the iliac crest apophysis: a rare fracture in adolescent athletes. Annals of Emergency Medicine. 22(7):143-145; 1993.

85. Larrison, W.I.; Hersh, P.S.; Kunzweiler, T.; Shingleton, B.J. Sports-related ocular trauma. Ophthalmology. 97(10):1265-1269; 1990.

86. Larson, R.L.; Singer, K.M.; Bergstrom, R.; Thomas, S. Little league survey: the Eugene study. American Journal of Sports Medicine. 4(5):201-209; 1976.

87. Lebrun, C.M.; Morrell, R.; Sutherland, C. Organizing sports medicine coverage at the Canadian summer games. The Physician and Sportsmedicine. 14(11):118-120, 123-127; 1986.

88. Lipscomb. A.B. Baseball pitching injuries in growing athletes. Sports Medicine. 3(1):25-31; 1975.

89. Lombardo, S.J.; Jobe, F.W.; Kerlan, R.K.; Carter, V.S.; Shields, C.L., Jr. Posterior shoulder lesions in throwing athletes. American Journal of Sports Medicine. 5(3):106-110; 1977.

90. Loosli, A.R.; Requa, R.K.; Garrick, J.G.; Hanley, E. Injuries in slow pitch softball. The Physician and Sportsmedicine. 16(3):110-115, 118; 1988.

91. Loosli, A.R.; Requa, R.K.; Ross, W.; Garrick, J.G. Injuries to pitchers in women's collegiate fast-pitch softball. American Journal of Sports Medicine. 20(1):35-37; 1992.

92. Lowe, E.B.; Perkins, E.R.; Herndon, J.H. Rhode Island high school athletic injuries 1985-86. Rhode Island Medical Journal. 70(6):265-270; 1987.

93. Lowery, C.W.; Chadwick, R.O.; Waltman, E.N. Digital vessel trauma from repetitive impact in baseball catchers. Journal of Hand Surgery. 1(3):236-238; 1976.

94. Lucie, R.S.; Wiedel, J.D.; Messner, D.G. The acute pivot shift: clinical correlation. American Journal of Sports Medicine. 12(3): 189-191; 1984.

95. Magnusson, S.P.; Gleim, G.W.; Nicholas, J.A. Shoulder weakness in professional baseball pitchers. Medicine and Science in Sports and Exercise. 26(1):5-9; 1994.

96. Martin, R.K.; Yesalis, C.E.; Foster, D.; Albright, J.P. Sports injuries at the 1985 junior olympics. American Journal of Sports Medicine. 15(6):603-608; 1987.

97. McLain, L.G.; Reynolds, S. Sports injuries in a high school. Pediatrics. 4(3):446-450; 1989.

98. Micheli, L. Preventing youth sports injuries. Journal of Physical Education, Recreation and Dance. 56:52-54; 1985.

99. Micheli, L. Sports injuries commonly incurred by amateurs. Journal of Musculoskeletal Medicine. 3(2):13-30; 1986.

100. Monaco, B.R.; Noble, H.B.; Bachman, D.C. Incomplete tears of the anterior cruciate ligament and knee locking. Journal of the American Medical Association. 247(11):1582-1584; 1982.

101. Moore, M. Brief reports: arm range of motion decreased by pitching. The Physician and Sportsmedicine. 9(6):21; 1981.

102. Mutoh, Y.; Mori, T.; Suzuki, Y.; Sugiura, Y. Stress fractures of the ulna in athletes. American Journal of Sports Medicine. 10(6):365-367; 1982.

103. Nadeau, M.T.; Boatman, J.; Brown, T.; Houston, W.T. The prevention of softball injuries: the experience at Yokota. Military Medicine. 155:3-5; 1990.

104. National Collegiate Athletic Association. Injury surveillance system: 1992-93 baseball. Overland Park, KS: National Collegiate Athletic Association; 1993a.

105. National Collegiate Athletic Association. Injury surveillance system: 1992-93 softball. Overland Park, KS: National Collegiate Athletic Association; 1993b.

106. Newitt, P.A. The study of impact bases when compared to stationary bases. Unpublished thesis. Mt. Pleasant, MI: Central Michigan University; 1992.

107. Nuber, G.W.; Diment, M.T. Olecranon stress fractures in throwers. Clinical Orthopaedics and Related Research. 278:58-61; 1992.

108. Nuber, G.W.; McCarthy, W.J.; Yao, J.S.T.; Schafer, M.F.; Suker, J.R. Arterial abnormalities of the hand in athletes. American Journal of Sports Medicine. 18(5):520-523; 1990a.

109. Nuber, G.W.; McCarthy, W.J.; Yao, J.S.T.; Schafer, M.F.; Suker, J.R. Arterial abnormalities of the shoulder in athletes. American Journal of Sports Medicine. 18(5):514-519; 1990b.

110. O'Neill, D.; Micheli, L. Overuse injuries in the young athlete. Clinics in Sports Medicine. 7(3):591-610; 1988.

111. Pappas, A.M. Elbow problems associated with baseball during childhood and adolescence. Clinical Orthopedics. 164:30-41; 1982.

112. Pappas, A.M.; Zawacki, R. M. Baseball: too much on a young pitcher's shoulders? The Physician and Sportsmedicine. 19(3):107-110, 112-114, 117; 1991.

113. Parker, R.D.; Berkowitz, M.S.; Brahms, M.A.; Bohl, W.R. Hook of the hamate fractures in athletes. American Journal of Sports Medicine. 14(6):517-523; 1986.

114. Powell, J.W. Pros and cons of data-gathering mechanisms. In: Vinger, P.F.; Hoerner, E.F., eds. Sports injuries—an unthwarted epidemic. Littleton, MA: PSG Publishing Company, Inc.; 1981:31-35.

115. Redler, M.R. Quadrilateral space syndrome in a throwing athlete. American Journal of Sports Medicine. 14(6):511-513; 1986.

116. Ringel, S.P.; Treihart, M.; Carry, M.; Fisher, R.; Jacobs, P. Suprascapular neuropathy in pitchers. American Journal of Sports Medicine. 18(1):80-86; 1990.

117. Ritter, M.A.; Gioe, T.J.; Albohm, M. Sport-related injuries in women. JACHA. 28:267-268; 1980.

118. Rotman, M.B.; Pruitt, D.L. Avulsion fracture of the extensor carpi radialis brevis insertion. Journal of Hand Surgery. 18A(3):511-513; 1993.

119. Rutherford, G.W., Jr.; Kennedy, J.; McGhee, L. Baseball and softball related injuries to children 5-14 years of age. Washington, DC: U.S. Consumer Product Safety Commission; 1985.

120. Schein, O.D.; Hibberd, P.L.; Shingelton, B.J.; et al. The spectrum and burden of ocular injury. Ophthalmology. 95:300-305; 1988.

121. Schemmel, S.P.; Andrews, J.R.; Clancy, W.G. Acute ulnar collateral ligament injury in a baseball pitcher. The Physician and Sportsmedicine. 16(9):132-136, 138; 1988.

122. Seefeldt, V.; Ewing, M.; Walk, S. An overview of youth sports programs in the United States: report to the Carnegie council on adolescent development. East Lansing, MI: Institute for the Study of Youth Sports; 1992.

123. Selesnick, F.H.; Dolitsky, B.; Haskell, S.S. Fracture of the coronoid process requiring open reduction with internal fixation. Journal of Bone and Joint Surgery. 66A(8):1304-1305; 1984.

124. Slager, R.F. From little league to big league, the weak spot is the arm. The American Journal of Sports Medicine. 5(2):37-48, 1977.

125. Slocum, D.B. Classification of elbow injuries from baseball pitching. Texas Medicine. 64:48-53, 1968.

126. Splain, S.H.; Rolnick, A. Sports injuries at a non-scholarship university. The Physician and Sportsmedicine. 12(7):55-56, 58-60; 1984.

127. Sterling J.C.; Calvo, R.D.; Holden, S.C. An unusual stress fracture in a multiple sport athlete. Medicine and Science in Sports and Exercise. 23(3):298-303; 1991.

128. Stock, J.G.; Cornell, F.M. Prevention of sports-related eye injury. AFP. 44(2):515-520; 1991.

129. Strahlman, E.; Sommer, A. The epidemiology of sports-related ocular trauma. International Ophthalmology Clinics. 28:199-202; 1988.

130. Strauss, M.B.; Wrobel, L.J.; Neff, R.S.; Cady, G.W. The shrugged-off shoulder: a comparison of patients with recurrent shoulder subluxations and dislocations. The Physician and Sportsmedicine. 11(3):85-88, 93-94, 96-97; 1983.

131. Strukel, R.J.; Garrick, J.G. Thoracic outlet compression in athletes. American Journal of Sports Medicine. 6(2):35-39; 1978.

132. Sugawara, M.; Ogino, T.; Minami, A.; Ishi, S. Digital ischemia in baseball players. American Journal of Sports Medicine. 14(4):329-334; 1986.

133. Sullivan, J.A. Recurring pain in the pediatric athlete. Pediatrics Clinics of North America. 31(5):1097-1112; 1984.

134. Tanabe, S.; Nakahira, J.; Bando, E.; Yamaguchi, H.; Miyamoto, H.; Yamamoto, A. Fatigue fracture of the ulna occurring in pitchers of fast-pitch softball. American Journal of Sports Medicine. 19(3):317-321; 1991.

135. Torg, J.S.; Moyer, R.A. Non-union of a stress fracture through the olecranon epiphyseal plate observed in an adolescent baseball pitcher. Journal of Bone and Joint Surgery. 59A(2):264-265; 1977.

136. Torg, J.S.; Pollack, H.; Sweterlitsch, P. The effect of competitive pitching on the shoulders and elbows of preadolescent baseball players. Pediatrics. 49(2):267-272; 1972.

137. Tullos, H.S.; Fain, R.H. Rotational stress fracture of proximal humeral epiphysis. Journal of Sports Medicine. 2(3):152-153; 1974.

138. Tullos, H.S.; King, J.W. Lesions of the pitching arm in adolescence. Journal of the American Medical Association. 220(2):264-271; 1972.

139. Vinger, P.F. A sporting chance with protective eyewear. The Sightsaving Review. Spring:3-9; 1979.

140. Vinger, P.F. Sports-related eye injury: a preventable problem. Survey of Ophthalmology. 25(1):47-51; 1980.

141. Vinger, P.F. The incidence of eye injuries in sports. International ophthalmology Clinics. 21(4):21-46; 1981.

142. Vinger, P.F. The eye and sports medicine. In: Duane, T.D.; Jaeger, E.A., eds. Clinical Ophthalmology. Philadelphia: J.B. Lippincott Co; 1988.

143. Vinger, P.F.; Hoerner, E.F., eds. Sports injuries. Littleton, MA: PGS Publishing Company, Inc.; 1981.

144. Walter, S.; Hart, L. Application of epidemiological methodology to sports and exercise science research. In: Pandolf, K.; Holloszy, J. eds. Exercise and sports sciences reviews. Baltimore: Williams and Wilkens; 1990:417-448.

145. Wheeler, B.R. Slow-pitch softball injuries. American Journal of Sports Medicine. 12(3):237-240; 1984.

146. White, J. News briefs: Rare open ankle sprain sidelines Weiss. The Physician and Sportsmedicine. 19(9):47; 1991.

147. Whiteside, J.A.; Fleagle, S.B.; Kalenak, A. Fractures and refractures in intercollegiate athletes. American Journal of Sports Medicine. 9(6):369-377; 1981.

148. Whiteside, P.A. Men's and women's injuries in comparable sports. The Physician and Sportsmedicine. 8(3):130-135, 138, 140; 1980.

149. Zaricznjy, B.; Shattuck, L.J.M.; Mast, T.A.; Robertson, R.V.; D'Elia, G. Sports-related injuries in school-aged children. American Journal of Sports Medicine. 8(5):318-323; 1980.

# 6

# Basketball

*John Zvijac and William Thompson*

## 1. Introduction

Basketball has long been considered a noncontact sport. However, as the game has evolved, contact has become a significant factor. Basketball continues to increase in popularity as a participation sport at all levels of play, from recreational to professional. While the number and severity of injuries do not compare to football, a significant number of injuries do occur. As the sport grows in number of participants and in intensity, so do the number of injuries.

Specific studies comparing injury types and rates are relatively underrepresented in the literature when basketball is compared to football. Much of the data related to basketball are found in studies comparing various sports. This chapter attempts to provide a comprehensive review of research directed specifically at basketball as well as studies comparing basketball injuries to other sports. The rationale for this review is to clarify relative injury rates and to demonstrate the variability in the literature with regard to basketball.

Employing the terms basketball and injuries, the Medline database from 1970 to 1994 was explored. Textbook references were reviewed as dictated by journal bibliographies. Additional data were obtained from the National Collegiate Athletic Association Injury Surveillance System for Divisions I, II, and III men's basketball from 1988-1993. Literature containing any epidemiologic data with respect to basketball was included in this chapter. This chapter is designed to provide exposure to the limited epidemiologic data available for basketball and to provide an impetus for further and more standardized research into basketball injuries.

Much of the published literature on basketball-related injuries has been in the form of case reports or case series studies. While this gives us insight

to the possible causes of injuries and the possible risk-related factors attributable to these injuries, these types of studies limit our ability to obtain statistics that represent the morbidity of the general population of basketball players. Therefore, they cannot be used to calculate risks of injuries or identify either athletes that may be prone to injury or factors that increase the risk of injury. This is made evident throughout this chapter as we attempt to correlate data. The few prospective and retrospective studies that are available do provide insight to the nature and rate of injuries in basketball. The main difficulties with these studies in terms of interpretation of data include the relatively short periods of time in which the data were collected and the diversity of study populations, especially in regard to the level of competition. There is also notable variability in study design, data collection methods, and injury definitions. It is apparent that there is limited epidemiologic data regarding basketball. Nevertheless, the data that is available gives us impetus for further and more standardized research into basketball injuries.

## 2. Incidence of Injury

### 2.1 Injury Rates

The true rate of injury for the sport of basketball is difficult to ascertain. The available retrospective and prospective studies deal with unlike groups of age and athletic abilities. Furthermore, variability in the mathematical representation of the injury rates exists. Most of the literature includes basketball among many other sports rather than devoting a specific epidemiologic study exclusively to basketball. Raw data are not available, making it difficult to accurately determine even the most basic parameters. The exact number of males, females, and basketball players within a population of athletes is missing in most studies.

Table 6.1 provides a comparison of injury rates in women's basketball. The variability in the data prevents meaningful calculations. Of note is the relative increase in frequency, at all levels of play, of injury in women's basketball compared to other sports. Injury rates for women are among the highest in a number of studies (5, 6, 11, 17).

However, wide variability exists even when injury rates are expressed with the same parameters (5, 13). In any given group of injured athletes, a high percentage of injuries are accounted for by female basketball players (11, 66).

Similar data exist for men's basketball. Variability is common and precludes a collective injury rate for men participating in basketball. The National Collegiate Athletic Association (NCAA) maintains a yearly Injury Surveillance System (ISS) for reporting injuries in men's basketball divisions I, II, and III. It is the most consistent report in terms of update, time, completeness, and standardization of data. It is readily available to participating NCAA institutions and reports injuries per 1,000 exposures.

Table 6.2 represents injury rates in men's basketball. The similarity is evident in a number of studies that break injuries down per 1,000 hours of play or practice time (15, 71). However, wide variability exists in other well-designed studies comparing rates per 1,000 exposures (73).

Review articles have suggested that men have lower injury rates in basketball than women (18, 56). This has been demonstrated in large cross-sectional studies and in a study of professionals, but definite relative risks are not clear.

## 2.2 Rates During Practice Versus Competition

A significant difference in injuries sustained in practice versus competition has been demonstrated when comparing professional, intercollegiate, and interscholastic athletes (5, 21, 38, 71). The majority of injuries at the high school and recreational levels are sustained during practice. However, college and professional basketball players are injured

**Table 6.1  A Comparison of Injury Rates in Women's Basketball**

| Study | Duration | Injuries | Participants | Rate[a] |
|---|---|---|---|---|
| **Recreational** | | | | |
| Chan et al., 1984 (11) | 1 year | ? | 1,714[c] | ? (17.4% injuries accounted for by basketball)[b] |
| DeHaven et al., 1986 (16) | 7 years | 29 | ? | ? |
| Gutgesell, 1991 (21) | 1 year | 14 | 104 | 13.5% |
| Shambaugh et al., 1991 (54) | 1 year | 1 | 45 | 2% |
| **Club** | | | | |
| Yde et al., 1990 (71) | 1 year | 29[b] | 29 | 46%, 3/1,000 playing hours[b] |
| **High school** | | | | |
| DuRant et al., 1992 (17) | 1 year | 32 | 96 | 33.3% (highest among all female sports) |
| Backx et al., 1989 (6) | ? | ? | 105 | 1.99 risk ratio[d] (highest among all sports) |
| Backx et al., 1991 (5) | 7 months | ? | 19 | 998/1,000 athletes |
| Chandy et al., 1985 (13) | 3 years | 498 | 6,426[c] | 77.5/1,000 athletes |
| Emerson, 1993 (18) | 1 year | 76,624 | 333,149[c] | 23% |
| McClain et al., 1989 (41) | 1 year | 14 | 45 | 31% |
| Watson, 1984 (66) | 1 year | 9 | 6,799[c] | ? (7.8% injuries accounted for by basketball) |
| **College** | | | | |
| Barrett et al., 1993 (8) | 2 months | 1 | 47 | 2% |
| Young et al., 1981 (72) | 2 years | 22 | 188 | 12% |
| **Professional** | | | | |
| Colliander et al., 1986 (15) | 1 year | 73 | 118 | 2.85/1,000 hours |
| Klein et al., 1993 (33) | ? | 62 | 73 | 85% |
| Zelisko et al., 1982 (73) | 2 years | 134 | 13, 15 | 51.2/1,000 exposures |

[a]% of total players unless specified otherwise.

[b]Male and female data not separated.

[c]# of basketball players not specified.

[d]Risk ratio represents observed vs. expected injuries.

**Table 6.2   A Comparison of Injury Rates in Men's Basketball**

| Study | Duration | Injuries | Participants | Rate[a] |
|---|---|---|---|---|
| Recreational | | | | |
| Chan et al., 1984 (11) | 1 year | — | 1,714[c] | ? (17.8% injuries accounted for by basketball)[b] |
| Gutgesell, 1991 (21) | 1 year | 25 | 406 | 6.2% |
| Shambaugh et al., 1991 (54) | 1 year | 1 | 45 | 2% |
| Club | | | | |
| Sane, 1988 (53) | 6 years | 2,773 | 47,950[c] | 5.8% |
| Yde et al., 1990 (71) | 1 year | 29* | 27 | 46% (3/1,000 playing hours)[e] |
| High school | | | | |
| Backx et al., 1991 (5) | 7 months | — | 8 | 56/1,000 athletes |
| Backx et al., 1989 (6) | — | 105 | — | 1.99 risk ratio[b] |
| Chandy et al., 1985 (13) | 3 years | 404 | 7,209[c] | 6% |
| DuRant et al., 1992 (17) | 1 year | 20 | 132 | 15% |
| Emerson, 1993 (18) | 1 year | 83,772[c] | 380,783[c] | 22% |
| McClain et al., 1989 (41) | 1 year | 21 | 57 | 37% |
| Watson, 1984 (66) | 1 year | 9 | @ | ? (7.8% injuries from basketball) |
| College | | | | |
| Barrett et al., 1993 (8) | 2 months | 14 | 522 | 3% |
| NCAA ISS 1993 (28) Division I | 5 years | 1,600 | 26-44 teams | 5.66/1,000 exposures |
| Professional | | | | |
| Colliander et al., 1986 (15) | 1 year | 86 | 132 | 2.5/1,000 hours |
| Henry et al., 1982 (24) | 7 years | 576 | 71 | 69% |
| Klein et al., 1993 (33) | 1 year | 98 | 106 | 92% sustained ankle injuries |
| Zelisko et al., 1982 (73) | 2 years | 138 | 15, 15 | 32/1,000 exposures |

[a]% of total players unless otherwise specified.

[b]Male and female data not separated.

[c]# of basketball players not specified.

[d]Risk ratio represents observed vs. expected injuries.

[e]No male/female difference in injuries/10,000 playing hours.

@Unknown number reported.

more frequently during competition (5, 24). Henry et al. reported on 576 injuries in 76 professionals over a 7-year period and attributed 45% of the injuries to competition versus 23% attributed to practice (24). The trend toward increased injury during competition in elite athletes is clearly demonstrated by the NCAA ISS as well as studies on professionals (5, 24). Table 6.3 shows the rate is greater in competition. This may be due to the fact that practices are much more frequent than games. On the basis of Table 6.3, one would assume that games are more intense than practice. The intensity level may cause an increased risk of injury.

# 3. Injury Characteristics

## 3.1 Injury Onset

As noted in Table 6.4, the majority of injuries occurring in basketball at various levels are most often sudden-onset injuries. It is difficult to ascertain the percentage or extent of injury because the definition for injury onset is inconsistent across the studies. In addition, the acute injury that may have been superimposed on a chronic mechanism has not been separated.

## 3.2 Injury Types

Table 6.4 compares the occurrence of injury types in recreational, club, high school, college, and professional basketball. Where possible, the data are separated for males and females. However, many of the cross-sectional studies do not report separate injury types between males and females. Of note, Zelisko et al. (73) specifically compared male and female players and found similar injury-type distribution. In global terms, minor sprains and strains account for the majority of injuries; more significant sprains are less common.

**Table 6.3  A Comparison of Injury Rate in Practice vs. Competition in Basketball**

| Study | Practice | Competition |
|---|---|---|
| **Recreational** | | |
| Gutgesell, 1991 (21) | 10% | 90% |
| **Club** | | |
| Yde et al., 1990 (71) | 2.4/1,000 hours | 5.7/1,000 hours |
| **High school** | | |
| McCarthy et al., 1991 (38) | 60% | 40% |
| Backx et al., 1991 (5) | 1/1,000 hours[a] | 23/1,000 hours [a] |
| **College** | | |
| NCAA ISS, 1993[b] (28) | | |
| Division I | 4.41/1,000 exposures | 10.52/1,000 exposures |
| Division II | 4.98/1,000 exposures | 11.14/1,000 exposures |
| Division III | 4.15/1,000 exposures | 8.13/1,000 exposures |
| **Professional** | | |
| Henry et al., 1982[b] (24) | 23% | 45% |

[a]Male and female data not given.

[b]Males only.

## 3.3 Injury Location

The anatomic location of injuries occurring in school-aged, collegiate, and professional basketball players has been well documented. Injuries are classified as upper and lower extremity, spine and trunk, and oral and maxillofacial. Tables 6.5 and 6.6 give the percent comparison of injury location at the various athletic levels for women's and men's basketball. A review of Tables 6.5 and 6.6 suggests that injuries to the ankle are the most prevalent followed by injuries to the knee/hamstring area. Apart from the lower extremities, occurrence rates for injuries were next highest to the lower back and then the hand and wrist. Again, male and female differences are indicated when possible. Some studies concentrate on a specific anatomic site of injury and tend to report higher percentages for that given injury when compared to other, more general studies (35, 37, 65). Klein et al. (33) reported 98 ankle injuries among 106 professional players over one year.

### 3.3.1 Head/Spine/Trunk

As indicated in Tables 6.5 through 6.7, spine injuries in basketball are rare and infrequently reported in the literature. In a study of 263 club-level basketball players, no serious neck or spine injuries were reported (71). In the studies of professionals, no significant spine injuries were reported (15, 24, 73). Tables 6.5 and 6.6 demonstrate the relative occurrence of spine injuries. Table 6.7 shows the

**Table 6.4  A Percent Comparison of Injury Types in Men's and Women's Basketball**

| Level | Abrasion | Concussion | Contusion | Dislocation | Fracture | Inflammation | Laceration | Nonspecific | Sprain | Strain |
|---|---|---|---|---|---|---|---|---|---|---|
| **Recreational** | | | | | | | | | | |
| Gutgesell, 1991[a] (21) | — | — | 35.9 | — | 2.6 | — | 5.1 | 15.4 | 28.2 | 28.2 |
| Chan et al., 1984[a] (11) | 43 | — | 28 | — | — | — | — | — | 135 | 8 |
| **High school** | | | | | | | | | | |
| McClain et al., 1989[a] (41) | — | 3 | 13 | — | 10 | 7 | — | 6 | 34 | 23 |
| **College**[c] | | | | | | | | | | |
| NCAA ISS, 1993 (28) | .06 | .19 | .67 | .19 | .38 | .39 | .16 | .13 | 2.06 | .88 |
| **Professional** | | | | | | | | | | |
| Zelisko et al., 1982 (73) | 1.4 | — | 24.6 | 1.4 | 3.6 | 16.7 | 5.1 | — | 8.7 | 24.6 |

[a]Male to female data not given.

[c]Males only.

**Table 6.5   A Percent Comparison of Injury Location in Women's Basketball**

| | High school | | | College | | Professional | | Club | |
|---|---|---|---|---|---|---|---|---|---|
| | Maestrello (37)[a] 1989 | DuRant (17)[a] 1992 | Smith (16) 1986 | Whiteside (65)[b] 1981 | Lee-Knight (35) 1992 | Colliander (15) 1986 | Zelisko (73) 1982 | Chan (11) 1984 | Yde (71) 1990 |
| Head | 30.9 | 1.3 | | 0.0 | 2.5 | 0 | 10.4 | — | 0.0 |
| Skull | | | | | | | | | |
| Face | | | | | | | | | |
| Teeth | | | 2.5 | | | | | | |
| Spine/trunk | — | — | — | 0.0 | | 1 | | | 0.0 |
| Neck | | | | | | | | .02 | |
| Upper back | | | | | | | | | |
| Lower back | | | | | | | 8.2 | | |
| Ribs | | | | | | | | | |
| Stomach | | | | | | | | | |
| Upper extremity | | | | | | | | | |
| Shoulder | | 0.9 | | | | | 0.7 | .02 | |
| Arm | | 3.9 | | | | | 0.7 | | |
| Elbow | | | | | | | 5.2 | .07 | |
| Forearm | | | | 50 | | 3 | 0.7 | | |
| Wrist | | | | | | | 0.7 | | |
| Hand/fingers | | | | | | | 9.0 | .03 | 43 |
| Lower extremity | | | | | | | | | |
| Pelvis | | 8.3 | | | | 4 | 0.7 | | |
| Thigh | | | | | | 3 | 14.1 | | |
| Knee | | | | | | 17 | 19.3 | .18 | 5 |
| Leg | | | | | | 8 | 3.7 | | 5 |
| Ankle | | | | | | 56 | 17.9 | .1 | 33 |
| Heel | | | | | | — | | | |
| Foot | | | | 50 | | 8 | 6.0 | .3 | 0.0 |

[a]Male vs. female data not given separately.

[b]Fractures only.

various case reports, series, and unusual injuries occurring in the spine in basketball players as reported in the literature.

Eye and facial injuries have been documented in numerous injury surveillance system reports (37, 73). Ocular and maxillofacial injuries have generally been considered separately in the literature. These studies have compared basketball injuries with other sports injuries to ascertain relative risks.

In the 1989-1990 NCAA injury surveillance, ocular injuries comprised 2% of the total injuries (28). This represented 0.1 injuries per 1,000 sessions in practice or competition. A much higher percentage of ocular injuries was reported by the Consumer Product Safety Commission in 1982. In this report the eye accounted for close to 18% of all injuries, and basketball rated second only to baseball in ocular injury rates. Jones studied eye injuries in various sports and concluded that baseball accounted for 25% of all sports-related ocular injuries (73).

The majority of these injuries are conjunctival, corneal, and lid abrasions. The more serious injuries, which include retinal detachment or tear, vitreous hemorrhage, acute hyphema, and orbit fractures are less common. The preponderance of ocular injuries sustained in basketball are due to blunt trauma from fingers and elbows of other players. It is apparent that most eye injuries are preventable by the use of eye-protection devices. In a study of registered Finnish athletes over a 7-year period, maxillofacial injuries were compared for the sports of American football, bandy, handball, and basketball. In basketball, orofacial injuries represented 6.7 % of all injuries compared to 1.4% in football (53). Tables 6.5 and 6.6 give relative head and neck injuries.

### 3.3.2 Upper Extremity

Tables 6.5 and 6.6 give the percent comparison of upper extremity injury location. Upper extremity

**Table 6.6  A Percent Comparison of Injury Location in Men's Basketball**

| | High school | | | | College | | Professional | | | Recreation |
|---|---|---|---|---|---|---|---|---|---|---|
| | Maestrello 1989 (37) | DuRant 1992 (17) | West 1979 | Smith 1986 | Whiteside 1981 (65) | NCAA[a] 1993 (28) | Zelisko 1982 (73) | Colliander 1986 (15) | Henry 1982 (24) | Chan 1984 (11) |
| Head | 30.9 | 1.3 | — | — | 10 | .23 | 10.1 | 2 | 12 | — |
| Skull | | | | | | | | | | |
| Face | | | | | | | | | | |
| Teeth | | | | 0.8 | | | | | | |
| Spine/trunk | — | — | — | — | | .56 | | | 1 | .02 |
| Neck | | | | | | | | | | |
| Upper back | | | | | | | 13.0 | | | |
| Lower back | | | | | 5.0 | | 13.0 | | | |
| Ribs | | | | | | | 2.9 | 2 | 0.7 | |
| Stomach | | | | | | | | | 0.2 | |
| Upper extremity | | — | — | — | | .50 | 20.1 | | 7.0 | .38 |
| Shoulder | | 0.9 | | | | .18 | 2.9 | | 3.0 | .02 |
| Arm | | 3.9 | | | | 0.0 | 1.4 | | 2.0 | .07 |
| Elbow | | | | | | .09 | 2.9 | | | |
| Forearm | | | | | | .07 | 0.7 | 7.0 | | |
| Wrist | | | | | | .07 | 4.3 | | 2 | .03 |
| Hand | | | | | 20 | .09 | 7.9 | | 13 | .26 |
| Lower extremity | — | | | | | 3.42 | 35.7 | 78 | 39 | .58 |
| Pelvis | | | | | | .25 | 2.8 | 2 | 1 | |
| Thigh | | | | | | .27 | 6.5 | 2 | | |
| Knee | 8.3 | | | | 5 | .81 | 18 | 19 | 14 | .18 |
| Leg | | | | | | .17 | 3.6 | 2 | | |
| Ankle | 11 | | 47 | 70 | 50 | 1.59 | 20.3 | 48 | 18 | .10 |
| Foot | | | | | 45 | .33 | 0.7 | 5 | 6 | .30 |

[a]Injury/1,000 exposures.

**Table 6.7  Case Reports and Cross-Sectional Studies of Injuries Occurring in the Spine/Trunk of Male Basketball Players**

| Study | Design | Subjects | Age | Level | Condition/diagnosis |
|---|---|---|---|---|---|
| Head | | | | | |
| Chow, 1984 (10) | Case | 1 | 16 | High school | Optic nerve evulsion |
| Thun et al., 1982 (60) | Case | 26 | | High school | Keratoconjunctivitis; malfunctioning mercury vapor lamp |
| Sane, 1983 (53) | Case | 187 | 11-50 | Club | 187/47,950 with max/facial injury |
| Spine | | | | | |
| Clark, 1991 (14) | Case | 1 | 12 | High school | Lumbar apophyseal fracture |
| Garth et al., 1989 (19) | Case | 1 | 22 | College | Lumbar lamina fracture |
| Ribs/chest | | | | | |
| Woo, 1988 (70) | Case | 2 | | High school | Traumatic manubriosternal subluxation |
| Stiene, 1992 (58) | Case | 1 | 18 | College | Chest pain; syncope |
| Stomach | | | | | |
| Mucciolo et al., 1988 (47) | Case | 1 | 23 | Recreational | Traumatic incarcerated scrotal hernia |

injuries in basketball are common at all skill levels. As noted in Table 6.8, the hand and wrist are the most commonly injured upper extremity structures (11, 73).

The proximal interphalangeal joint is the most frequently sprained and dislocated joint in the hand, with dorsal P.I.P. joint dislocations being the most common subtype (62, 67). These result from

**Table 6.8   Case Reports and Cross-Sectional Studies of Injuries Occurring in the Upper Extremity of Male Basketball Players**

| Study | Design | Subjects | Age | Level | Condition/diagnosis |
|---|---|---|---|---|---|
| Shoulder/arm | | | | | |
| Hjelkrem et al., 1988 (27) | Case | 1 | 20 | Recreational | Synovial chondrometaplasia |
| Jobe et al., 1988 (   ) | Case | 25 | 15-26 | All | One basketball player in group of overhead athletes with shoulder instability treated with anterior capsulolabral repair |
| Wrist | | | | | |
| McClelland et al., 1988 (40) | Case | 1 | 23 | Recreational | Carpal, metacarpal, ankle fracture |
| Tehranzadeh et al., 1984 (59) | Case | 1 | 23 | Recreational | Osteochondral fracture detected with wrist arthroscopy in basketball player |
| Amadio et al., 1990 (3) | Cross-sectional | — | — | All | Basketball injuries accounted for 19% hand injuries |
| Hand | | | | | |
| Kirk et al., 1979 (32) | Case | 2 | | High school | Dunk lacerations |
| Rettig et al., 1989 (50) | Case | 53 | | All | Metacarpal fractures |
| Vicar, 1988 (62) | Case | 1 | 28 | Recreational | Volar PIP dislocation without fracture |

hyperextension and are usually associated with volar plate rupture and sparing of the collateral ligaments (62, 67). Thumb metacarpal-phalangeal joint injuries are next in frequency. More common injuries to this joint include trapezial-metacarpal joint fractures and ulnar collateral ligament sprains. The relative frequency of these injuries specifically in basketball players is not reported.

It is important to emphasize that Henry et al. (24) demonstrated that injuries to the wrist and hand accounted for only 4% of the total number of injuries. Furthermore, combined wrist and hand injuries accounted for only one missed game.

Table 6.8 represents the various upper extremity case reports, case series, cross-sectional studies and unusual injuries reported for basketball players in the literature.

### 3.3.3 Lower Extremity

The vast majority of injuries incurred during basketball are to the lower extremity (11, 15, 24, 28, 35, 37, 71, 73). A report of high school injury rates by the National Athletic Trainers' Association estimated 42% of all injuries to involve the ankle and foot and 10% to involve the knee in a survey of 380,783 participants (18).

Ankle sprains are the most common injury in basketball (11, 15, 24, 28, 35, 37, 71, 73). In the 7-year experience of professionals, ankle injuries accounted for 18.2% of all injuries (24). However, 18% of games were missed due to these ankle injuries as opposed to 66% missed due to knee injuries. In another study, ankle injuries accounted

for 17.9% and 20.3% in the females and males, respectively (73). This was twice the percentage of the second most common site, the head and neck. The frequency of ankle injuries is repeatedly demonstrated to be the most common injury in basketball at all levels.

Although less common than ankle injuries, knee injuries may account for greater loss of playing time (24). In Henry's study of professionals, knee injuries accounted for 18.2% of all injuries, but 66% of loss of playing time. As demonstrated in Tables 6.5 and 6.6 similar knee injury rates are reported. Klein et al. (33) reported 98 ankle injuries among 106 professional players over a 1-year period.

Specific knee injuries are variably reported in the literature. Baker and co-workers reviewed meniscal injuries in various sports (7). They found that basketball accounted for 18% of all meniscal tears sustained during sports. Of further note, the right knee was involved 80% of the time with 25% involving the lateral meniscus and 75% involving the medial meniscus. In contrast, a 7-year review of the National Basketball Association demonstrated a total of 38 meniscal tears in 36 players with 58% involving the lateral meniscus and 42% involving the medial meniscus (20).

Table 6.9 gives the rate of anterior cruciate ligament injury. Of particular recent interest is the comparison of male and female anterior cruciate ligament injury rates. Where possible, this is demonstrated in Table 6.11. Numerous anecdotal reports have suggested that women have a higher rate of anterior cruciate ligament tears than their male counterparts. As is shown in Table 6.11, scant literature exists but does suggest that females are at increased risk at all levels (16, 20, 48, 68).

Tables 6.10 and 6.11 report the various case reports in the literature specifically involving basketball players at all levels. Unusual injuries are also included, as well as separation between males and females where possible.

## 4. Injury Severity

### 4.1 Time Loss

Time loss has generally been reported as the number of games or days missed from practice,

competition, or both. Time frames are not standardized nor are percentages of total time missed uniform. Henry et al. (24) reported that for a given injury, a professional basketball player had a 7.6% chance of missing a game. The average time loss for given injuries in high school varies from 11.8 days in boys to 28.6 days in girls (41). Again the NCAA ISS report of time loss is the clearest and most standardized long-term report. The data are summarized in Table 6.12. It is notable that most injuries at the collegiate level are relatively minor with the time loss of 6 days or less in 76% of injuries.

### 4.2 Catastrophic Injury

Table 6.13 summarizes the literature of catastrophic injuries in case reports or series. As is apparent, these injuries are either rare or underreported.

## 5. Injury Risk Factors

Predictors of injury, specifically for basketball, are difficult to assess and are not well represented in the literature. A study by Shambaugh and co-workers attempted to correlate structural measures as predictors of injury in basketball players (54). In the study various structural measurements were taken from a small group of recreational athletes and correlated to injuries sustained during the league season. A formula was calculated and used to predict injury in an intercollegiate basketball team. The investigators state that the one player injured during the season had the highest

**Table 6.9 Anterior Cruciate Ligament Injury Rates in Basketball**

| Study | Duration | Participants | Male | Female |
|-------|----------|--------------|------|--------|
| High school | | | | |
| McClain et al., 1989 (41) | 1 year | 102 | 0/57 | 1/45 |
| Wirtz, 1982 (68) | 1 year | 22 teams | 1 | 16 |
| College | | | | |
| Gray et al., 1985 (20) | 30 months | 137 | 4/151 | 19/76 |
| NCAA 1992-93 (28) | 1 year | 102 schools | 13 | — |
| Professional | | | | |
| Emerson, 1993 (18) | 7 years | — | 3 | — |
| NBTA 1991 | 7 years | — | 22 | — |
| Henry et al., 1982 (24) | 7 years | 71 | 0 | — |
| Mixed | | | | |
| Noye et al., 1989 (48) | 7 years | 32 all sports | 5 | 0 |
| DeHaven et al., 1986 (16) | 7 years | — | 12 | 6 |

**Table 6.10 Case Reports of Injuries Occurring in the Lower Extremity of Female Basketball Players**

| Study | Design | Subjects | Age | Level | Condition/diagnosis |
|-------|--------|----------|-----|-------|---------------------|
| Knee | | | | | |
| Wirtz, 1982 (68) | Case | 16 | — | High school | Report of ACL ruptures in one season of B-varsity basketball players in Iowa public schools |
| Baker et al., 1985 (7) | Case | 31 | — | All | Comparison of medial and lateral meniscal tears in basketball players |
| Gray et al., 1985 (20) | Case | 19 | — | All | Survey of knee injuries in which ACL injuries accounted for 25% of injuries |
| Ankle | | | | | |
| Klein et al., 1993 (33) | Case | 73 | — | Professional | Series of fibular ankle sprains in professionals |
| Foot | | | | | |
| Alfred et al., 1992 (1) | Case | 1 | 17 | High school | Tarsal navicular stress fracture |

**Table 6.11    Case Reports of Injuries Occurring in the Lower Extremity of Male Basketball Players**

| Study | Design | Subjects | Age | Level | Condition/diagnosis |
|---|---|---|---|---|---|
| Knee | | | | | |
| Hanel et al., 1981 (23) | Case | 1 | 16 | High school | Patella fractures, consecutive |
| Hensal et al., 1983 (25) | Case | 1 | 17 | High school | Bilateral patella fractures |
| Maar et al., 1988 (36) | Case | 1 | 16 | High school | Bilateral tibial tubercle avulsion |
| Pape et al., 1993 (49) | Case | 1 | 15 | High school | Compartment syndrome complicating a tibial tubercle avulsion |
| Sacchetti et al., 1983 (52) | Case | 2 | | High school | Stress induced 1st rib fracture |
| Tibone et al., 1981 (61) | Case | 1 | 16 | College | Bilateral inferior patella pole fractures |
| Gray et al., 1985 (20) | Case | 4 | — | All | 4 ACL ruptures/30-month period in 76 females treated for basketball related injuries in a sports clinic |
| Baker et al., 1985 (7) | Case | 62 | — | All | Comparison of medial and lateral meniscal tears in basketball players |
| Krinsky et al., 1992 (34) | Case | 36 | — | Professional | Review of 38 meniscal tears in professionals with lateral > medial in frequency |
| Noyes et al., 1989 (48) | Case | 32 | 14-25 | All | Series of incomplete ACL tears treated in a group of athletes including 5 basketball players |
| Leg | | | | | |
| Rettig et al., 1988 (51) | Case | 8 | 14-23 | High school/ college | Delayed union tibia stress fractures |
| Ankle | | | | | |
| Shelbourne et al., 1988 (55) | Case | 4 | 18-23 | High school/ college | Medial malleolus stress fractures |
| Smith et al., 1986 | Case | 84 | — | High school | Of varsity basketball players studied, 70% reported ankle sprains during season |
| Klein et al., 1993 (33) | Case | 106 | — | Professional | Reports series of ankle sprains and recommended rehabilitation program |
| Foot | | | | | |
| Boitano et al., 1992 (9) | Case | 6 | — | College | Series of subtalar dislocations |
| Wolfe et al., 1989 (69) | Case | 1 | 22 | ? | Irreducible great toe IP joint dislocation |

**Table 6.12    Time Loss Injury Summary**

| | Time loss | Injuries | % of injuries |
|---|---|---|---|
| 1992-1993 | 1-2 days | 346 | 48.5 |
| | 3-6 days | 188 | 26.3 |
| | 7-9 days | 51 | 7.1 |
| | > 10 days | 129 | 18.1 |
| | Catastrophic | 0 | 0 |
| | Fatal | 0 | 0 |
| | | 714 | 100.0 |
| All years | 1-2 days | 1,972 | 48.1 |
| | 3-6 days | 1,148 | 28.0 |
| | 7-9 days | 267 | 6.5 |
| | > 10 days | 713 | 17.4 |
| | Catastrophic | 0 | 0 |
| | Fatal | 0 | 0 |
| | | 4,100 | 100.0 |

*Source.* 1992-93 Men's Basketball NCAA Injury Surveillance System.

calculated risk for injury determined by their formula. Based on the aforementioned study and the relative lack of data, proneness to injury in basketball is poorly understood and requires further research.

Studies relating structure or biomechanics to injury have been more successful in predicting injury than those focusing on strength, flexibility, or training. We believe that the most prudent method at present would be a prospective long-term study with preseason measurements of biomechanical parameters such as quadriceps girth, calf girth, Q angle of the knee, dorsiflexion of the ankle, forefoot varus, rearfoot valgus, and true apparent leg lengths. It is well documented that abnormalities in these parameters lead to overuse injuries. For example, excessive pronation or rear foot valgus can cause overuse injuries of the foot; a leg length discrepancy or internal tibial torsion may lead to Achilles tendinitis; combined increased Q angle and medial knee stress may be a risk factor for anterior knee pain due to patellofemoral misalignment.

**Table 6.13 Case Reports and Case Series of Catastrophic Injuries Occurring in Men's and Women's Basketball**

| Study | Design | Subjects | Age | Level | Condition/diagnosis |
|---|---|---|---|---|---|
| Chow et al., 1984 (10) | Case | 1 | 16 | High school | Optic nerve evulsion |
| NCAA Injury 1993 (28) | Case series | 0 | — | College | No catastrophic, fatal, or nonfatal injuries reported by participating institutions in Divisions I, II, III in 738,155 exposures in 5 years |

Identifying risk factors in basketball is an extremely complicated problem requiring a large data bank. While there are small studies that give us some insight as to the specific predictors of injury, it is obvious that there is insufficient data at present to give us substantial evidence that any particular parameter is a clear predictor of injury.

## 6. Suggestions for Injury Prevention

As with any sport, a preseason conditioning program for both cardiovascular and strengthening is indicated. Intuitively, one would believe that preseason conditioning would decrease the possibility of injuries. In addition, a continued maintenance program throughout the season would also help prevent injuries. During the season as minor injuries occur, the athlete who fatigues more readily will be creating abnormal stresses on all the joints of the lower extremity. This accumulating microtrauma could lead to overuse syndromes and injuries.

In terms of protective wear, the use of protective eye goggles would help prevent ocular injury. The use of braces, expecially on the lower extremity, is controversial at present and is not well tolerated by the basketball athlete. This is an area that requires further research.

## 7. Suggestions for Further Research

Aside from the injury surveillance systems of the National Athletic Trainers Association, National Collegiate Athletic Association, and the National Basketball Association, few prospective or retrospective studies exist related specifically to basketball. A far greater number of basketball players participate at the interscholastic level versus the intercollegiate and professional levels. It seems logical that the greatest database exists in this population. Further prospective study in this group with standardized data collection would lead to a clear understanding of specific injury types and rates in the sport of basketball.

Studies concerning reinjury rates are underrepresented. Those that do mention reinjury are unclear (15, 24, 44, 45). Further research into this area is needed. Useful data would include the patient's status prior to injury in terms of clinical examination and subjective complaints. In addition, a standardized collection process to separate players with prior injury would be most beneficial. The necessity for an objective clinical examination, as well as a subjective history, would be of great benefit in determining if a prior injury increases the risk for reinjury to the same location.

In addition to an injury surveillance system, it would be of benefit to have a prospective study, with a large database at the professional as well as the collegiate and scholastic levels, that deals with the structural parameters previously discussed. With a large database, potential predictors of injury relating to body structure and biomechanics may become clear. Knowing which players are at risk makes it possible to manipulate the parameters with rehabilitation, strengthening, and training. Mechanical devices such as braces or orthotics may reduce the structural imbalances and subsequent risk of injury. These studies must be long term and prospective for the greatest benefit and would require a large surveillance system. With these parameters, including a larger, more organized database, it is hoped that we may gain a clearer understanding of the risk and prevention of injury in the sport of basketball.

## References

1. Alfred, R.H.; Belhobek, G.; Bergfeld, J.A. Stress fractures of the tarsal navicular. A case report. Am. J. Sports Med. 20(6):766-768; 1992.
3. Amadio, P.C. Epidemiology of hand and wrist injuries in sports. Hand. Clin. 6:379; 1990.
4. Axe, M.J.; Newcomb, W.A.; Warner, D. Sports injuries and adolescent athletes. Del. Med. J. 63(6):359-363; 1991.

5. Backx, F.J.; et al. Injuries in high-risk persons and high-risk sports: A longitudinal study of 1818 school children. Am. J. Sports Med. 19:124; 1991.

6. Backx, F.J.; et al. Sports injuries in school-aged children: An epidemiologic study. Am. J. Sports Med. 17(2):234-240; 1989.

7. Baker, B.E.; Peckham, A.C.; Pupparo, F.; Sanborn, J.C. Review of meniscal injury and associated sports. Am. J. Sports Med. 13(1):1-4; 1985.

8. Barrett, Jr.; et al. High versus low top shoes for the prevention of ankle sprains in basketball players: A prospective randomized study. Am. J. Sports Med. 21(4):582-585; 1993.

9. Boitano, M.C. Subtalar dislocations in basketball players: Possible contributing factors. The Physician in Sports Medicine. 20(11):59-67; 1992.

10. Chow, A.Y.; Goldberg, M.F.; Frenkel, M. Evulsion of the optic nerve in association with basketball injuries. Ann. Ophthalmol. 16(1):35-37; 1984.

11. Chan, K.M.; Fu, F.; Leung, L. Sports injuries survey on university students in Hong Kong. Br. J. Sports Med. 18(3):195-202; 1984.

13. Chandy, T.A.; et al. Secondary school athletic injury in boys and girls: A three year comparison. Phys. Sports Med. 13:106-111; 1985.

14. Clark, J.E. Apophyseal fracture of the lumbar spine in adolescence. Orthop. Rev. 20(6):512-516; 1991.

15. Colliander, E.; et al. Injuries in elite Swedish basketball. Orthopedis. 9(2):225-227; 1986.

16. Dehaven, K.E.; et al. Athletic injuries: Comparison by age, sport and gender. Am. J. Sports Med. 14:218; 1986.

17. DuRant, R.H.; Pendergrast, R.A.; Seymore, C.; Gaillard, G.; Donner, J. Findings from the pre-participation athletic examination and athletic injuries. Am. J. Dis. Child. 146(1):85-91; 1992.

18. Emerson, R.J. Basketball knee injuries and the anterior cruciate ligament. Clin. Sports Med. 12(2):317-328; 1993.

19. Garth, W.P.; et al. Fractures of the lumbar lamina with epidural hematoma simulating herniation of a disc. JBJS. 71-A(5):771-772; 1989

20. Gray, J.; et al. A survey of injuries to the anterior cruciate ligament of the knee in female basketball players. Int. J. Sports Med. 6:314-316; 1985.

21. Gutgesell, M.E. Safety of a preadolescent basketball program. Am. J. Dis. Child. 145(9):1023-1025; 1991.

22. Guyette, R.F. Facial injuries in basketball players. Clin. Sports Med. 12(2):247-264; 1993.

23. Hanel, D.P.; Burdge, R.E. Consecutive indirect patella fractures in an adolescent basketball player. A case report. Am. J. Sports Med. 9(5):327-329; 1981.

24. Henry, J.H.; et al. The injury rate in professional basketball. Am. J. Sports Med. 1:16-18; 1982.

25. Hensal, F.; Nelson, T.; Pavlov, H.; Torg, J.S. Bilateral patellar fractures from indirect trauma. A case report. Clin. Orthop. (178):207-209; 1983.

26. Herskowitz, A.; Selesnick, H. Back injuries in basketball players. Clin. Sports Med. 12(2):293-306; 1993.

27. Hjelkrem, M.; Stanish, W.D. Synovial chondrometaplasia of the shoulder. A case report of a young athlete presenting with shoulder pain. Am. J. Sports Med. 16(1):84-86; 1988.

28. Injury Surveillance System. NCAA Men's Basketball. 1992-93.

29. Johnson, K.A.; Teasdall, R.D. Sprained ankles as they relate to the basketball player. Clin. Sports Med. 12(2):363-371; 1993.

30. Kelly, J.P.; Nichols, J.S.; Filley, C.M.; Lillehei, K.O.; Rubinstein, D.; Kleinschmidt-DeMasters. B.K. Concussion in sports. Guidelines for the prevention of catastrophic outcome. JAMA. 266(20):2867-2869; 1991.

32. Kirk, A.A.; et al. Dunk lacerations—Unusual injuries to the hands of basketball players. JAMA. 242(5):415; 1979.

33. Klein, J.; Hoher, J.; Tiling, T. Comparative study of therapies for fibular ligament rupture of the lateral ankle joint in competitive basketball players. Foot Ankle. 14(6):320-324; 1993.

34. Krinsky, M.B.; et al. Incidence of lateral meniscus injury in professional basketball players. Am. J. Sports Med. 20(1):17-19; 1992.

35. Lee-Knight, C.T.; Harrison, E.L.; Price, C.J. Dental injuries at the 1989 Canada games: An epidemiological study. J. Can. Dent. Assoc. 58(10):810-815; 1992.

36. Maar, D.C.; Kernek, C.B.; Pierce, R.O. Simultaneous bilateral tibial tubercle avulsion fracture. Orthopedics. 11(11):1599-1601; 1988.

37. Maestrello-deMayo, M.; et al. Orofacial trauma and mouth wear among high school varsity basketball players. J. Dentistry for Children. 36-39; 1989.

38. McCarthy, M.R.; Hiller, W.D.; Yates-McCarthy, J.L. Sports medicine in Hawaii: Care of the high school athlete in Oahu's public schools. Hawaii Med. J. 50(11):395-396; 1991.

39. McDermott, E.P. Basketball injuries of the foot and ankle. Clin. Sports Med. 12(2):373-393; 1993.

40. McClelland, S.J.; et al. Ipsilateral carpal, metacarpal and ankle fractures resulting from an attempted slam dunk. Am. J. Sports Med; 16(5):544-546; 1988.

41. McClain, L.G.; et al. Sports injuries in a high school. Pediatrics. 84(3):446-450; 1989.

42. Meyer, S.A.; Saltzman. C.L.; Albright, J.P. Stress fractures of the foot and leg. Clin. Sports Med. 12(2):395-413; 1993.

43. Micheli, L.J. Pediatric and adolescent sports injuries: Recent trends. Exerc. Sports Sci. Rev. 14:359; 1986.

44. Molnar, T.J.; Fox, J.M. Overuse injuries of the knee in basketball. Clin. Sports Med. 12(2):349-362; 1993.

45. Moretz, J.A.; et al. High school basketball injuries. Phys. Sports Med. 6:92-95; 1978.

46. Moyer, R.A.; Marchetto, P.A. Injuries of the posterior cruciate ligament. Clin. Sports Med. 12(2):307-315; 1993.

47. Mucciolo, R.L.; et al. Traumatic acute incarcerated scrotal hernia. J. Trauma. 28(5); 1988.

48. Noye, F.R.; et al. Partial tears of the anterior cruciate ligament: Progression to complete ligament deficiency. JBJS. 71-B(5):825-833; 1989.

49. Pape, J.M.; Goulet, J.A.; Hensinger, R.N. Compartment syndrome complicating tibial tubercle avulsion. Clin. Orthop. 295:201-204; 1993.
50. Rettig, A.C.; et al. Metacarpal fractures in the athlete. Am. J. Sports Med. 17(4):567-572; 1989.
51. Rettig, A.C.; et al. The natural history of delayed union stress fractures of the anterior cortex of the tibia. Am. J. Sports Med. 16(3):250-255; 1988.
52. Sacchetti, A.D.; Beswick, D.R.; Morse, S.D. Rebound rib: Stress-induced first rib fracture. Ann. Emerg. Med. 12(3):177-179; 1983.
53. Sane, J.; et al. Comparison of maxillofacial and dental injuries in four contact team sports: American football, bandy, basketball and handball. Am. J. Sports Med. 16(6):647-653; 1988.
54. Shambaugh, J.P.; et al. Structural measures as predictors of injury in basketball players. Med. Sci. Sports Exerc. 522-527; 1991.
55. Shelbourne, K.D.; et al. Stress fractures of the medial malleolus. Am. J. Sports Med. 16(1):60-63; 1988.
56. Sickles, R.T.; Lombardo, J.A. The adolescent basketball player. Clin. Sports Med.12(2):207-219; 1993.
57. Sonzogni, J.J., Jr.; Gross, M.L. Assessment and treatment of basketball injuries. Clin. Sports Med. 12(2):221-237; 1993.
58. Stiene, H.A. Chest pain and shortness of breath in a collegiate basketball player: Case report and literature review. Med. Sci. Sports Exerc. 24(5):504-509; 1992.
59. Tehranzadeh, J.; et al. Detection of loose intaarticular loose osteochondral fragments by double contrasts wrist arthrography. Am. J. Sports Med. 12(1):77-79; 1984.
60. Thun, M.J.; Altman, R.; Ellingson, O.; Mills, L.F.; Talansky, M.L. Ocular complications of malfunctioning mercury vapor lamps. Ann. Ophthalmol. 14(11):1017-1020; 1982.
61. Tibone, J.E.; Lombardo, S.J. Bilateral fractures of the inferior poles of the patellae in a basketball player. Am. J. Sports Med. 9(4):215-216; 1981.
62. Vicar, A.J. Proximal interphalangeal joint dislocations without fractures. Hand. Clinics. 4(1):5-13; 1988.
63. Vinger, P.F. Sports eye injuries a preventable disease. Ophthalmology. 88(2):108-113; 1981.
64. Weil, L.S.; et al. A biomechanical study of ankle sprains in basketball. J. Am. Podiatry Assn. 69(11):687-690; 1979.
65. Whiteside, J.A.; Fleagle, S.B.; Kalenak, A. Fractures and refractures in intercollegiate athletes. An eleven-year experience. Am. J. Sports Med. 9(6):369-377; 1981.
66. Watson, A.W. Sports injuries during one academic year in 6799 Irish school children. Am. J. Sports Med. 12(1):65-71; 1984.
67. Wilson, R.L.; McGinty, L.D. Common hand and wrist injuries in basketball players. Clin. Sports Med. 12(2):265-291; 1993.
68. Wirtz, P.D. High school basketball knee ligament injuries. J. Iowa Med. Soc. 105-106; 1982.
69. Wolfe, J.; et al. Irreducible dislocation of the great toe following a sports injury. Am. J. Sports Med. 17(5):695-696; 1989.
70. Woo, C.C. Traumatic manubriosternal joint subluxations in two basketball players. J. Manipulative Physiol. Ther. 11(5):433-437; 1988.
71. Yde, J.; et al. Sports injuries in adolescents' ball games: Soccer, handball and basketball. Br. J. Sp. Med. 24:51-54; 1990.
72. Young, M.L.; et al. Self concept and injuries among female college tournament basketball players. Am. Corr. Ther. J. 139-154; 1979.
73. Zelisko, J.A.; et al. A comparison of men's and women's professional basketball injuries. Am. J. Sports Med. 10:297-299; 1982.

# 7

# Bicycling

*Diane C. Thompson, Andrew L. Dannenberg,*
*Robert S. Thompson, and Frederick P. Rivara*

## 1. Introduction

The goal of this chapter is to present a comprehensive picture of all bicycle injuries using national or regional surveillance data, population based studies, and cohort or case control studies. Case series data are included only when more representative studies are not available. We have chosen to address bicycle injuries at all levels of the sport with specific references made to competitive injuries. There are 67 million bicyclists in the United States who ride approximately 15 billion hours per year (65). Bicycling is unlike many other sports in that the vast majority of bicyclists ride for recreation, transportation, or both, and only a small minority will ever ride in even a single competitive event. Approximately 94,000 cyclists are registered competitors with the United States Cycling Federation (USCF), National Off Road Bicycle Association (NORBA), or the Triathlon Federation (54, 82, 83). An unknown number belong to local or national cycling clubs and participate in bicycle tours ranging from short (15-20 mile) rides to centuries (100-mile tours) to multiday or multiweek trips. The 1990 toll of bicycle injuries is 900 deaths, 23,000 hospital admissions, 580,000 emergency department (ER) visits, and approximately 1.2 million visits to physicians' offices and clinics for treatment (65, 70).

The literature search covered publications available in Medline and SPORT Discus from 1975 to the present, published in English or with English abstracts. Key words with truncation were: bicycling, injuries, facial injuries, sports, helmets, statistics, morbidity, mortality, population-based studies, cost-effectiveness analysis, education, and legislation. The search strategy included identification of national, regional, and local databases at all levels of medical care.

The statistical profile for bicycle trauma can be described by using mortality data, hospitalization data, emergency department visits, and visits to physicians' offices or athletic trainers. As is true for all types of injuries, mortality data are the most universally available and completely reported. As injuries become less severe, the data are more difficult and expensive to obtain and the reporting is less complete. Injury rates are typically calculated using the entire population as the denominator since exposure data are often not available. A more accurate picture of the injury burden is obtained when exposure (cyclists' miles or trips) is used as the denominator. Comprehensive data on cyclists treated at hospital emergency departments, hospitalized for injuries, or killed are available for the entire population of cyclists, but the reason that the injured were cycling (competition/training/recreation) is not identified. The majority of the competitive and "serious" cyclists train on roadways and may commute to work as part of their weekly training program. Information on injuries resulting from competition are not available in organized format from any of the racing groups (54, 82, 83). Chronic or overuse injuries treated by athletic trainers and personal physicians are presented in the literature as case series.

This chapter will summarize the current literature on bicycle injuries and will include incidence data, descriptive epidemiology of bicycle injuries, injury risk factors, and injury prevention strategies.

## 2. Incidence of Injury

### 2.1 Injury Rates

Injury rates are calculated using both population and bicycling exposure as denominators. These rates vary by age and sex as illustrated in Tables 7.1 and 7.2. Females 5 to 9 years of age and males 10 to 14 years old have the highest injury rates per 100,000 population. Males have higher injury rates than females in all age categories.

Children age 5 to 15 and people over 50 have the highest injury rates per million trips: 430.7 injuries for children and 296.2 injuries for older adults (Table 7.2). Using cycling trips rather than population as the denominator suggests that the higher rates of injury in children and older adults are not explained by the amount of cycling exposure, but are due to a variety of personal characteristics.

Population-based studies in the United States that included data on bicycle injuries are summarized in Table 7.3. These data present an overall picture of bicycle injuries with bicycle-related head injuries emphasized because of their high importance. Depending on the study, injury rates are available for three different levels of medical care: outpatient, emergency department, and hospital. These are regional studies from Ohio (2), Massachusetts (24, 25), California (38, 39), and Washington (42, 63, 64, 78), as well as national data (1, 70).

The injury data from these different population based studies indicate that 5- to 14-year-old children are at highest risk for bicycle injuries (1, 24,

**Table 7.1   Bicycle-Related Injuries Treated in Emergency Departments 1987, 1989, 1990[1] by Age and Sex**

| Age in years | Male | | | Female | | | Total | | |
|---|---|---|---|---|---|---|---|---|---|
| | N | % | Rate[2] | N | % | Rate[2] | N | % | Rate[2] |
| 1-4 | 94,845 | 8.2 | 420 | 48,001 | 9.5 | 220 | 142,846 | 8.6 | 320 |
| 5-9 | 320,659 | 27.8 | 1,170 | 190,997 | 38.0 | 730 | 511,656 | 30.9 | 950 |
| 10-14 | 337,282 | 29.3 | 1,311 | 124,468 | 24.7 | 510 | 461,750 | 27.9 | 920 |
| 15-19 | 134,618 | 11.7 | 480 | 31,324 | 6.2 | 120 | 165,942 | 10.0 | 310 |
| 20-24 | 81,450 | 7.1 | 260 | 27,635 | 5.5 | 100 | 109,085 | 6.6 | 180 |
| 25-54 | 163,609 | 14.2 | 97 | 65,703 | 13.1 | 43 | 229,312 | 13.8 | 67 |
| 55-64 | 10,512 | 0.9 | 30 | 8,426 | 1.7 | 20 | 18,943 | 1.1 | 30 |
| 65+ | 9,892 | 0.9 | 30 | 6,382 | 1.3 | 10 | 16,274 | 1.0 | 20 |
| Total | 1,152,872 | – | 320 | 502,936 | — | 130 | 1,655,808 | — | 220 |

[1]National Electronic Injury Surveillance System (NEISS) average of 1987, 1989, and 1990 data.

[2]Rate per 100,000 population

**Table 7.2   Bicyclist Injuries and Deaths per Million Trips by Age[1]**

| Age | Annual average number of deaths (1987-1988)[2] | Annual average number of injuries (1987, 1989, 1990)[3] | Number of bicycle trips in millions (1990)[4] | Deaths/million bicycle trips | Injuries/million bicycle trips (hospital and ED)[5] |
|---|---|---|---|---|---|
| 5-15 | 401 | 342,407 | 795 | 0.50 | 430.7 |
| 16-19 | 105 | 37,520 | 145 | 0.72 | 258.8 |
| 20-29 | 167 | 61,441 | 407 | 0.41 | 151.0 |
| 30-39 | 110 | 33,136 | 232 | 0.47 | 142.8 |
| 40-49 | 61 | 14,551 | 72 | 0.85 | 202.1 |
| 50-64 | 60 | 10,015 | 34 | 1.76 | 296.2 |
| Total | 904 | 499,070 | 1,685 | 0.54 | 296.2 |

[1]Baker et al. *Injuries to bicyclists: a national perspective*, 1993.

[2]National Center for Health Statistics (NCHS).

[3]National Electronic Injury Surveillance System (NEISS).

[4]Nationwide Personal Transportation Survey (NPTS).

[5]Emergency Department.

**Table 7.3   Population-Based Studies in the United States 1980-1992: Bicycle Injuries and Deaths**

| Study | Level of medical care | Age | Head injury per 100,000 | Total injuries per 100,000 |
|---|---|---|---|---|
| San Diego 1978, 1981, Brain Injuries (38, 39) | Hospitalizations and deaths | 5-14 | 28 | |
| Statewide Childhood Injury Prevention Program (SCIPP) 1980-81 (25) | ED visits, hospitalizations, and deaths | 0-19 | 91 | 878 |
| National Electronic Injury Surveillance System (NEISS) 1987-89 (70) | ED and hospital | All | | 220 |
| | | 5-9 | 436 | 950 |
| | | 10-14 | 224 | 920 |
| Group Health Co-op of Puget Sound (GHC) 1987 (63, 76) | Outpatient, ED, hospitalizations | 5-9 | 566 | |
| | | 10-14 | 377 | |
| Group Health Co-op of Puget Sound (GHC) 1987 (76) | ED, hospital | All | 42 | 163 |
| | | 5-9 | 283 | 671 |
| | | 10-14 | 188 | 809 |
| Washington State Comprehensive Hospital Abstract Reporting (CHARS) 1989-91 (42) | Hospital | All | | 11.1 |
| | | 5-9 | | 29.8 |
| Group Health Co-op of Puget Sound (GHC) 1992 (64) | ED, hospital | 5-9 | 94.6 | |
| | | 10-14 | 60.9 | |
| National Electronic Injury Surveillance System (NEISS) 1984-88 (70) | Deaths from head injury | All | .25 | |
| | | 5-9 | .51 | |
| | | 10-14 | .86 | |
| National Center for Health Statistics (NCHS) 1987-88 (70) | Deaths | All | 0.41 | |
| | | 5-9 | 0.84 | |
| | | 10-14 | 1.26 | |
| Washington 1989-91 (42) | Deaths | All | | 0.2 |
| | | 5-9 | | 0.4 |
| | | 10-14 | | 0.7 |

42, 78). These children have three fourths of all bicycle head injuries. The scant data on competitive bicycling injuries indicates a 2% to 3% incidence rate for criteriums, track, and road races (7, 49). There is some evidence that mountain biking events have higher injuries rates (14).

## 3. Injury Characteristics

### 3.1 Injury Onset

Sudden onset injuries result from a bicycle crash (accident). Explanations or reasons for bicycle crashes in order of occurrence are falls (losing control or losing balance, swerving to avoid hazard); hitting a stationary object (road hazard, curb, parked vehicle, tree); hitting or being hit by a motor vehicle; hitting another bicycle, pedestrian, or animal; and malfunction of the bicycle (24, 75, 79). Motor vehicles are involved in bicycle crashes only 10% to 35% of the time (24, 48, 65, 67, 75, 79), but are responsible for approximately 90% of all fatalities. Falls are the major cause of head injuries, facial fractures, lacerations, and other types of injuries.

Gradual onset injuries include all nontraumatic injuries. These include neck pain, low back strain, ulnar nerve pain, ischial pain, pudendal nerve palsy, anterior and lateral knee pain, skin problems, hypothermia, heat illnesses, and dehydration (23, 30, 32, 49-51, 56, 62, 88). There are no prevalence or incidence data available for gradual onset injuries for a defined population of riders. One might speculate that there is a higher incidence of overuse injuries among competitive distance riders.

### 3.2 Injury Type

Abrasions and lacerations are the most frequent injuries in cyclists, while brain injuries are the most severe. Figure 7.1 shows the distribution of injury types treated in emergency departments (1). Abrasions or lacerations comprise 63% of injuries; other

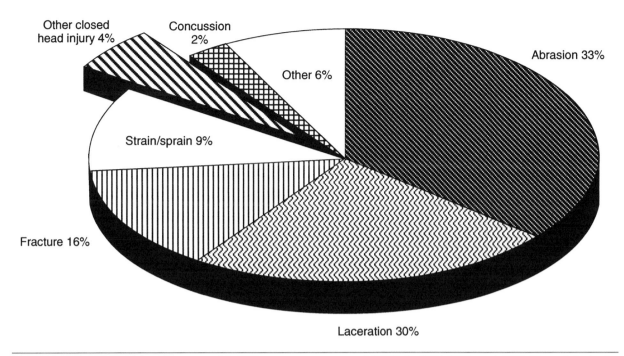

Other closed
head injury 4%

Concussion
2%

Other 6%

Abrasion 33%

Strain/sprain 9%

Fracture 16%

Laceration 30%

**Figure 7.1**    Injuries to bicyclists treated in U.S. emergency rooms, NEISS, in 1987, 1989, and 1990. From *Injuries to Bicyclists: A National Perspective* by S.P. Baker et al. (1).

injury types are fractures (16%), sprains/strains (9%), concussions (2%), and other closed head injuries (4%). Similar injury patterns have been found by other researchers with access to outpatient and emergency department data (75, 79).

Data from Washington State Comprehensive Hospital Abstract Reporting System (CHARS) database (1989-1990) are typical of a group of hospitalized cyclists (42). As expected, cyclists who were hospitalized for injuries had a higher proportion of head/brain injuries and fractures; 34% of the cyclists had head injuries, 27% lower limb fractures, and 26% upper limb fractures. Injuries suffered by 303 of 2,069 cyclists riding the Trans-America Bicycle Trail in 1976 were distributed as follows: 69% had abrasions, bruises, or lacerations; 3.3% fractures; 5% sprains; 3.3% concussions; and 10.9% miscellaneous or multiple injuries, including 0.7% deaths (1).

### 3.3 Injury Location

The body part distribution of bicycle injuries varies according to the age of the rider as described in Table 7.4. Head and facial injuries versus all injuries are higher in children, while injuries to the trunk are more prevalent in older cyclists.

#### 3.3.1 Head/Spine/Trunk

Head injuries comprise about one third of emergency-department treated bicycle injuries,

two thirds of all hospitalizations, and three fourths of all bicycle deaths (1, 6, 24, 70, 71, 79). The actual proportion of cyclists with head injury depends on helmet use in the cycling population. Until recently helmet use was quite low throughout the country. Helmet use has dramatically increased in some areas due to community-wide helmet campaigns and legislation (3, 15, 18, 20, 85). Helmets have been required for competition in the United States since 1986. As a result head injuries from racing have declined (14, 49, 69).

Bicycle crashes are a major cause of maxillofacial and dental injuries. Facial injuries resulting from bicycle crashes occur at almost the same rate as bicycle head injuries (43/100,000 vs. 45/100,000; 78). National Electronic Injury Surveillance Systems (NEISS) data from 1987-1990 indicate 20% of cyclists treated in hospitals and emergency departments in the United States suffered facial injuries (1). Head and facial injuries are usually grouped together so the precise number of facial injuries is unknown. Table 7.4 classifies forehead injuries as part of the face. The sex and age distribution of cyclists with facial and dental injuries reflects the demographics of the cycling population, predominately young (under 15) and male (6, 78). The pattern of facial fractures, predominantly mandibular fractures (65%) with a substantial portion located in the mandibular condyle, is unique to bicycle injuries (41, 44, 53, 74).

**Table 7.4   Area of Body Injured (by Age)**
**Bicyclists Treated in U.S. Emergency Departments[2]**

| Body area | Age in years | | | | | | | | | | | | | | | |
|---|---|---|---|---|---|---|---|---|---|---|---|---|---|---|---|---|
| | 1-4 | | 5-9 | | 10-14 | | 15-19 | | 20-24 | | 25-54 | | 55-64 | | 65+ | |
| | N | % | N | % | N | % | N | % | N | % | N | % | N | % | N | % |
| Head | 26,659 | 18.7 | 72,832 | 14.2 | 46,899 | 10.2 | 16,163 | 9.7 | 10,806 | 9.9 | 18,743 | 8.2 | 1,739 | 9.2 | 1,469 | 9.0 |
| Face[3] | 52,114 | 36.5 | 146,310 | 28.6 | 58,007 | 12.6 | 21,246 | 12.8 | 15,693 | 14.4 | 33,208 | 14.5 | 2,433 | 12.8 | 2,621 | 16.1 |
| Trunk | 3,834 | 2.7 | 38,033 | 7.4 | 28,547 | 6.2 | 12,003 | 7.2 | 8,161 | 7.5 | 27,358 | 11.9 | 3,264 | 17.2 | 3,363 | 20.7 |
| Upper extremity | 22,786 | 15.9 | 117,798 | 23.0 | 170,767 | 37.0 | 58,344 | 35.2 | 34,765 | 31.9 | 77,747 | 33.9 | 5,662 | 29.9 | 4,064 | 25.0 |
| Lower extremity | 34,448 | 24.1 | 113,620 | 22.2 | 130,348 | 28.2 | 40,577 | 24.5 | 25,901 | 23.7 | 47,297 | 20.6 | 4,477 | 23.6 | 3,034 | 18.6 |
| Multiple | 1,900 | 1.3 | 18,096 | 3.5 | 23,205 | 5.0 | 16,149 | 9.7 | 11,956 | 11.0 | 22,038 | 9.6 | 1,034 | 5.5 | 1,571 | 9.7 |
| Other unknown | 1,174 | 0.8 | 5,162 | 1.0 | 4,234 | 0.9 | 1,460 | 0.9 | 1,803 | 1.7 | 3,008 | 1.3 | 344 | 1.8 | 152 | 0.9 |
| Total | 142,915 | — | 511,831 | — | 462,004 | — | 165,942 | — | 109,085 | — | 229,399 | — | 18,943 | — | 16,274 | — |
| Grand total all injuries | 1,656,396 | | | | | | | | | | | | | | | |

[1]National Electronic Injury Surveillance System (NEISS), average visits 1987, 1989, and 1990.

[2]Baker et al. *Injuries to bicyclists: a national perspective.* 1993.

[3]Forehead injuries classified as facial injuries.

Ear and neck injuries are uncommon, comprising 0.3% and 0.6% of injuries respectively (1). Neck pain, low back strain, pudendal nerve palsy, and ischial pain are common overuse injuries in serious bicyclists (18b, 51, 88, 89). One of the concerns raised about bicycle helmets was that they would increase neck injuries (31). At the present time there is no evidence that bicycle helmets contribute to neck injury (73, 75, 79). Furthermore, this has not been found to be the case with motorcycle helmets (68).

### 3.3.2 Upper Extremity

Shoulder (clavicle) injuries are the most common upper extremity injury for cyclists over 15 years of age (1) and are a common injury in competitive cycling (7). Ulnar nerve pain and less frequently median nerve pain are common compression syndromes (62).

### 3.3.3 Lower Extremity

Knee injuries are the most common lower extremity injury beginning at age 10 (1). Anterior and lateral knee pain are common overuse injuries (32). "Spoke injuries," trapping the foot between the spoke and frame, happens to child passengers and can be prevented by using an approved mounted child seat (74, 81).

## 4. Injury Severity

Two commonly used injury scales are the Abbreviated Injury Scale (AIS) and the Injury Severity Score (ISS; 13). The AIS is an anatomically based system that classifies individual injuries by body region on a 6-point ordinal severity scale ranging from AIS-1 (minor) to AIS-6 (unsurvivable). Overall ISS are calculated from the sum of the squares of the highest AIS code in each of the three most severely injured ISS body regions. The AIS–ISS severity system was developed to predict the probability of survival and does not distinguish severity of injuries in terms of length of treatment and rehabilitation, cosmetic surgery, residual scarring, or psychological sequelae. The scale is not designed to measure injuries that restrict athletic practice or competition. For example, muscle sprains and strains serious enough to hinder performance are AIS-1 while muscle lacerations, ruptures, and tears are only AIS-2. The majority of bicycle injuries are not serious. Only 3.6% of over 3,200 cyclists treated in seven Seattle-area hospitals had ISS scores of 10 or higher. This group included 12 deaths (76). This distribution of injuries is typical of series that include emergency-department attended injuries.

### 4.1 Catastrophic Injury

The most common cause of death and serious disability from bicycle crashes is head injury. Head injury, or more specifically brain injury, is the primary or contributing cause of death in 62% to 90% of all bicycling fatalities (1, 22, 24, 38-40, 58, 70, 75, 91). Motor vehicle involvement is responsible for approximately one third of all bicycle related brain injuries and 90% of bicycle fatalities. The best evidence for this is the data from a population-based study in San Diego, California (38, 39). There are 700 to 900 deaths per year (34, 70). Table 7.5 indicates males have higher death and injury rates than females in all age categories. The death rate is highest for 10- to 14-year-olds of both sexes.

It is important to point out that when number of trips is used in the denominator the death rate is highest in 16- to 19-year-olds and cyclists over 50 years. The majority (56-62%) of bicyclist deaths occur in cyclists 16 and older (Tables 7.2 and 7.5).

## 4.2 Clinical Outcomes and Residual Symptoms

A cohort study evaluating the neurobehavioral outcomes of pediatric traumatic brain injury (TBI) suggested that mild TBI produces virtually no clinically significant long-term deficits in intellectual, neuropsychological, academic, or "real world" functioning and that moderately and severely brain injured children are at risk for problems in this area (35, 36).

Efforts to quantify costs of bicycle injuries have been mainly concerned with the costs of acute care and rehabilitation for head injured cyclists. The Consumer Product Safety Commission (CPSC) estimates the societal costs of medically attended bicycle-related injuries and fatalities to be about $8 billion annually, or $120 per rider per year (65). The cost effectiveness of bicycle helmet programs has been evaluated on local and national bases (28, 52, 80). A helmet subsidy of $10 was found to be cost effective for a health maintenance organization if helmet usage rates for members increased to 50% as a result (80). Nationwide it is estimated that each dollar spent on bicycle helmets saves $2 in medical care costs (52).

## 5. Injury Risk Factors

### 5.1 Intrinsic Factors

#### 5.1.1 Physical Characteristics

The incidence data for injuries and fatalities indicate that children ages 5 to 14 are at highest risk. The risk of death varies with age and severity of injury. Case fatality rate (CFR) is 18 deaths per 10,000 injuries and varies with cyclist age. Bicyclists 65 years of age and older have a CFR of 127 deaths per 10,000 injuries. Injured cyclists ages 15 to 19 are 3 times more likely to die than injured children ages 5 to 9. The higher mortality rate in 15- to 24-year-olds suggests that this group is subject to more severe injuries. Indeed this group rides at higher speeds and has the highest involvement with motor vehicles (1).

Males are injured far more frequently than females. As was noted earlier, up to 75% of injured cyclists are male. Males do ride more often, but when exposure is adjusted for, there is not much difference in the injury rate by sex (279 injuries per million trips for males and 303 for females) (1). Once a cyclist has crashed the risk of head injury does not vary by sex (79). Males are more likely to have more severe injuries (0.66 deaths/ million trips and 23.7 deaths/10,000 injuries vs.

**Table 7.5   Deaths From Bicycle-Related Injuries 1987-1988[1] by Age and Sex**

| Age in years | Male | | | Female | | | Total | | |
|---|---|---|---|---|---|---|---|---|---|
| | N | % | Rate[2] | N | % | Rate[2] | N | % | Rate[2] |
| 1-4 | 29 | 1.7 | 0.20 | 10 | 3.6 | 0.07 | 39 | 2.0 | 0.13 |
| 5-9 | 243 | 14.3 | 1.34 | 55 | 19.4 | 0.32 | 298 | 15.1 | 0.84 |
| 10-14 | 348 | 2.05 | 2.06 | 66 | 23.3 | 0.41 | 414 | 20.9 | 1.26 |
| 15-19 | 270 | 15.9 | 1.43 | 29 | 10.2 | 0.16 | 299 | 15.1 | 0.81 |
| 20-24 | 160 | 9.4 | 0.81 | 25 | 8.8 | 0.13 | 185 | 9.3 | 0.47 |
| 25-54 | 453 | 26.7 | 0.46 | 75 | 26.5 | 0.08 | 528 | 26.7 | 0.27 |
| 55-64 | 68 | 4.0 | 0.33 | 13 | 4.6 | 0.06 | 81 | 4.1 | 0.18 |
| 65+ | 127 | 7.5 | 0.59 | 10 | 3.5 | 0.04 | 137 | 6.9 | 0.24 |
| Total | 1,698 | — | 0.73 | 283 | — | 0.12 | 1,981 | — | 0.41 |

[1]National Center for Health Statistics, average of 1987 and 1988 data.

[2]Rate per 100,000 population.

0.27 and 9.0 for females) resulting in a population-based death rate that is 6 times the female rate (1). Bicyclists age 16 to 20 years had the highest crash rates of all cyclists traveling the TransAmerican Bicycle Trail in 1976. This group exhibited increased risk-taking behavior (such as high speeds on downhills) that may have contributed to its high crash rate (1, 9).

## 5.2 Extrinsic Factors

### 5.2.1 Exposure

Injury rates based on exposure by trips or miles ridden are discussed in Sections 2.1 and 4.1 and Table 7.2.

### 5.2.2 Training Methods or Conditions

Proper fit of the bicycle is essential to maximize rider performance and prevent overuse injuries. Once an injury occurs, medical treatment should be accompanied by evaluation of bicycle-fit to the rider and subsequent mechanical adjustment (10, 51, 56). Anterior and lateral knee pain, pudendal nerve palsy, ischial pain, ulnar nerve pain, neck pain, and low back strain all need to be treated with a combination of technique changes and modification of the bicycle components.

### 5.2.3 Environment

Population-based injury rates are the highest during periods when the largest numbers of cyclists are riding: months with good weather, daylight hours, and weekends (24, 34, 79). Using the Fatal Accident Reporting System (FARS) and the Nationwide Personal Transportation Survey (NPTS) data to adjust for exposure indicates that the highest risk period is from 10 p.m. to 6 a.m. when 5% of trips and 26% of all deaths occur (1, 33). During this period poor visibility of the cyclist, fatigue, and alcohol use both on part of motorist and cyclist are likely contributing factors.

The CPSC conducted a telephone survey of cyclists to determine bicycle use patterns (65). Riding patterns were distributed as follows: 44% on neighborhood streets, 20% on sidewalks and streets, 12% on bike paths, 12% on unpaved roads, 5% on highways, 8% on unpaved trails. Using FARS database Baker et al. (1) found over half of the fatal collisions occur in urban areas, but less than one third occurred at intersections. Approximately one third of cyclists of all ages were killed on roads with speed limits of 55 or greater. A recent survey of bicycle–motor vehicle collisions in Oregon found

that 48% of injuries occurred at intersections; however, 23% occurred as midblock dart outs (67). There is considerable debate about the safety of bike trails compared to roads and bike lanes (23, 45, 65, 72, 84, 86). Most competitive cyclists' high training mileage and speeds require road travel. Certainly the riding environment is one important area for further evaluation.

Bikecentennial data from 1976 (Table 7.6) provide information on injury rates and factors associated with bicycle crashes in a defined population that cycled more than 10 million miles on a defined route (1, 9).

Injury rates were higher for bicycles carrying full camping gear ( 83.4 injuries/million miles traveled vs. 22.2 injuries/million miles traveled for bicycles without gear). Factors contributing to bicycle-to-bicycle crashes (20% of total) included drafting and low responsiveness of heavily loaded bicycles in abrupt movements to avoid potholes and debris. Environmental factors such as potholes, broken pavement, rider fatigue, and excessive speed on downhill portions of the route contributed to 10.7% of all crashes. Motor vehicles were responsible for 17.5% of all crashes. Crashes were generally due to multiple causes, such as overloaded bicycles, excess speed, fatigue, motor vehicle traffic, and poor road conditions. Any of these combinations increase the bicyclists' crash risk.

There have been several reports in the literature about the role of alcohol in bicycle crashes. Fife's autopsy series reported 29% of cyclists tested had blood alcohol concentrations (BAC) from 0.18% to 0.30% (22). In Kraus' population-based study of brain-injured cyclists, more than half of all cyclists over 15 years of age who were tested were legally intoxicated (39). A case control study from Finland found that cyclists with BAC of 0.10% or more had 10 times the risk of injury compared to sober cyclists (57). Li and Baker recently reported the first nationwide study of alcohol use in fatally injured cyclists. They found 23% of the cyclists over 15 years of age who were tested had BAC $\geq$ 0.1% These cyclists were more likely to be male and to be killed at night. Ascertainment of alcohol use is incomplete for both injuries and deaths; blood alcohol levels are more likely to be obtained for deaths and in cases where there is a high index of suspicion. These authors suggest that the degree of overestimation due to selection bias was 10% (43).

### 5.2.4 Equipment: Bicycle Helmets

The biggest preventable risk factor for bicycle head injury is failure to wear a bicycle helmet. A number

**Table 7.6  Bicyclists Reporting at Least One Crash Versus Those Reporting No Crashes (p < .01): TransAmerica Bicycle Trail Cyclists, Summer 1976[1,2]**

|  | Reporting at least one crash[3]<br>(n = 308) | Reporting no crashes<br>(n = 1,761) |
|---|---|---|
| Age (years) | 16-20 | 31-35 and 46-55 |
| Education | High school diploma | Postgraduate work |
| Marital status | Single | Married |
| Occupation | Student |  |
| Failure of bicycle components | Pedals, brakes, rim, chain, packs, carrier |  |
| Number of flat tires | 5 or more | None |
| Bicycle packs | Used | Not used |
| Stop signs | Sometimes obey | Always obey |
| Rode 3 abreast | Often |  |
| Normal speed | 14-20 mph |  |
| Check bicycle mechanical condition |  | 1 time/day |
| Rode at night | Yes (sometimes without lights) | No |
| Illness | Rode while feeling ill | Did not ride while feeling ill |

[1]Characteristics for which no significant differences (p < .01) were identified included use of helmet, sex, height, weight, handedness, size of home community, automobile miles driven in past year, years of bicycling experience, length of time bicycle owned, bicycle frame style, frame size, wheel size, number of gears, type of brakes, type of handlebars, use of toe clips, type of tires, obeying traffic lights, use of brakes when going down hills, use of bright clothing, behavior near approaching animal, bicycling in bad weather, and riding alone.

[2]Baker et al. *Injuries to bicyclists: a national perspective.* 1993.

[3]Crash was defined as any injury requiring first aid treatment or greater care or more than $25.00 damage to the bicycle.

of studies have looked at the protective effect of helmets. These are summarized in Table 7.7. Each study indicates that bicycle helmets prevent serious head injury. The most compelling evidence was provided by a 1986-1987 case control study that evaluated the protective effect of helmets in a group of bicyclists who crashed, thus having the opportunity to sustain a head injury. Helmets were found to be 85% protective against head injury and 88% protective against brain injury (79). These results were corroborated by three recent case control studies (47, 48, 75). In Victoria, Australia, an increase in helmet wearing from 31% to 75% resulted in a 70% decrease in bicycle-related head-injury hospital admissions (12, 85). A recently published study from Queensland, Australia, (61) reported a decrease in hospital and emergency department treated bicycle-related head injuries after bicycle helmet use increased from 2.5% to 57%. Other bicycle-related injuries were unchanged (61). Medically treated head injuries declined 66% in a Seattle, Washington, HMO population following an increase in helmet use from 4.2% to 54% (64). The majority of helmets worn in the Seattle and Australian studies meet the stringent performance standards of ANSI, The Snell Memorial Foundation, or Australian National Standard (4, 5).

The independent effect of helmet use on facial injury is difficult to isolate due to the association of head and facial injuries and due to the imprecision of the ICD9-CM classification system that is available in automated databases. The prevalence of facial injuries in any series of bicycle injuries will vary depending on whether forehead is classified as part of the head or part of the face (1, 48, 77, 85). Evidence from a case control study indicates bicycle helmets offer protection against serious upper facial injuries (lacerations and fractures of eye/orbit, zygoma, nose), but do not protect against serious injuries to the lower face (maxillary, mandibular and dental fractures, and lacerations of chin and lips) (77). Full-face motorcycle helmets provide protection against injuries to the jaw, mouth, and teeth (68). Two helmet manufacturers, Giro and Bell, are developing full-face bicycle helmets following requests from mountain bike racers for additional injury protection.

## 6. Suggestions for Injury Prevention

A successful approach to bicyclist injury prevention should combine helmet use (the most important measure) with a variety of other measures designed to reduce the incidence of crashes, injuries, and deaths. Table 7.8, adapted from Brown

**Table 7.7   Studies of Bicycle Helmet Effectiveness**

| Investigators | Location | Data-year(s) | Design | Results | Comment |
|---|---|---|---|---|---|
| Lane, 1986 (40) | Victoria, Australia | 1983-1985 | Observational | Helmet campaign 1983-1986 | Helmet use observed |
| Wood and Milne, 1988 (91) | Same data set | | Time series | Helmet use ... 1983 1985 / Primary school 5% 58% / Secondary school 2% 18% / Adults 26% 44% / N = 180  N = 135 | Injuries (hospital attended); head injuries 25% down; other cycle injuries, stable |
| Dorsch et al., 1987 (21) | Adelaide, Australia | 1987 | Retrospective cohort; survey of bicycle club members; ascertained crashes in prior 5 years; helmet use at crash | 68% response rate (N = 197) 62% helmet use; helmets protective | Recall bias likely; multiple linear regression adjusted for age, sex, crash severity |
| Simpson et al., 1988 (72) | Oxford, England | 1983-1985 | Case series of road accidents (bicycle and motorcycle) | HI 33% of bicycle injuries; HI 15% of motorcycle injuries; compulsory helmet law for motorcycle helmets | Suggests bicycle HI decrease if helmet use was increased |
| Worrell, 1987 (92) | Portsmouth, England | 1985 | 100 consecutive cases of head injuries in bicyclists admitted to hospital | Plotted locations of injuries on standard diagram of head | Suggested that most could be prevented by helmet, based on location of injuries |
| Kiburz et al., 1986 (37) | Kansas City | 1985 | Survey of 492 adult cyclists asked if ever had bicycle crash | 61% response rate, 8.8% reported concussion; more severe HI and longer hospitalization in non-helmeted | Long recall period, may produce bias; suggests helmets protective |
| Wasserman et al., 1988 (87) | Vermont | 1984 | Survey that interviewed cyclists (N = 516) | 76% response rate; crude OR = 19.6; 95% CI (1.2-331) for HI in non-helmeted | Low power only 7 HI; 3 concussions, 4 lacerations |
| Cambridge et al., 1991 (11) | Christ Church, New Zealand | 1989 | Survey of injured cyclists from hospital surveillance (N = 86) | Crude OR = 0.35 for helmeted cyclists | Low and nonquantified response rate; suggests helmets protect |
| Thompson et al., 1989 (79) | Seattle, WA | 1986-1987 | Case control conducted in 5 area hospitals; ER control (433); population-based control group (588); HI cases (235); survey of cases and controls | 86% response rate; adjusted OR HI = 0.15; 95% CI (0.07, 0.29); OR brain injury = 0.12 95% CI (0.04, 0.40) | Used logistic regression analysis to adjust for age, sex, income, education, amount of cycling, severity of accident; suggests 85% reduction in HI and 88% in brain injury from helmets |
| Williams, 1991 (90) | Melbourne, Australia | 1987 | 1,892 bicycle injuries treated in ER; 432 riders helmeted, 64 damaged helmets tested | Examined helmets, recreated impacts, compared to standards. Of 5 persons with HI > AIS3, 4 helmets came off and one collapsed | Suggests helmet retention very important factor in protection; recommended changes in helmet construction and standards |

| Study | Location | Years | Population | Results | Comments |
|---|---|---|---|---|---|
| Bjornstig et al., 1992 (6) | Northern Sweden | 1985-1986 | 843 injured cyclists surveyed at time of ER visit | 321 HI; 105 deaths; 67 deaths from HI; estimated 48% reduction in HI if helmets had been worn based on location and clinical assessment | Recommended helmet legislation; 62% riders helmeted |
| Spaite et al., 1991 (73) | Arizona | 1986-1989 | Case series of bicyclist admitted to level I trauma center (N = 298); all involved in collision with motor vehicle | 5% of helmet wearers (6/116) and 47% with no helmets (79/168) had ISS scores > 15; suggests helmet users are careful riders | Biased case selection; no adjustment for age or sex; can derive estimate of protectiveness for helmets in those involved in MV crashes; crude OR = 0.03 |
| McDermott et al., 1993 (48) | Melbourne, Australia | 1987-1989 | Case-control study of 1,605 hospital-treated bicycle injuries; population based | Can estimate crude OR for helmet protection; OR = 0.6 (95% CI 0.47-0.80) helmets protective for head and facial injuries | Legislation beneficial; should use logistic regression to adjust for age and crash severity |
| Vulcan et al., 1992 (85) | Victoria, Australia | 1989-1991 | Population-based hospital admissions or deaths pre- and post-helmet law (7/1/91) | Helmet use 31% 1989-90; helmet use 75% 1990-91; HI admission or deaths 51% decrease; other bike injuries 24% decrease | Legislation increased helmet use, decreased HI; some reduction in cycling; before and after evaluation; no control city |
| Pitt et al., 1994 (61) | Queensland, Australia | 1985-1991 | Population-based helmet-use study; hospital and ER injuries of child cyclists | Helmet use 59% in 1991 vs. 2.5% in 1986; HI injury decreased to 18 per $10^5$ 1991 from 47 per $10^5$ 1986; other bicycle injuries no change | Some decrease in HI noncycling head injuries; evidence helmets are protective |
| Thomas et al., 1994 (75) | Queensland, Australia | 1991-1992 | Case-control HI cases (102); hospital controls (278) | Helmet use decreased HI by 63% (95% CI 34-80%) and brain injuries by 86% (95% CI 62-95%) | Logistic regression analysis adjusted for age, sex, hospital, parent education, object, crash severity; consider legislation |

HI = head injury.

OR = odds ratio. For case control studies the odds ratio approximates the relative risk of head injury in helmeted cyclists.

CI = confidence interval.

AIS = Abbreviated Injury Scale. Severity code 1, minor; 2, moderate; 3, serious; 4, severe; 5, critical; 6, fatal.

ISS = injury severity score. ISS is the sum of the squares of the highest AIS scores in three different body regions.

**Table 7.8  Interventions and Modifiable Risk Factors for Bicycle Injuries[1]**

| Phase | Human factors | Vehicle factors | Environmental factors |
|---|---|---|---|
| Preimpact | Cyclist education<br>Helmet laws<br>Alcohol laws | Brakes<br>Bicycle design | Road/path design<br>Modification of sewer grates, bridge deck gates<br>Road hazards |
| During impact | Bicycle helmets<br>Protective clothes | Redesign of injurious bicycle parts | Guardrail design<br>Less injurious car design |
| Postimpact | Age of cyclist<br>Physical condition | | Emergency services<br>Rehabilitation |

[1]Haddon Matrix: Adapted from Brown and Farley, 1989. In Baker et al. *Injuries to bicyclists: a national perspective.* 1993.

and Farley (8), gives examples of a broad selection of multidisciplinary strategies. It is based on a model developed by Haddon (26) that emphasizes the contributions of preventive measures that reduce the likelihood of an impact, the chance of injury when an impact occurs, and the consequences of injury. The model demonstrates that injury prevention is multifactorial; this discussion will cover a few selected interventions, cyclists' behavior, helmet use, alcohol laws, and environmental modifications.

## 6.1 Riders

Prevention of overuse injuries requires modification of equipment to ensure that the bicycle fits the rider properly. Stretching and strengthening exercises, the use of padded gloves and handlebars, and well-fitted and padded bicycle pants all contribute to increasing rider performance (62). Weather-related injuries can be prevented by the use of appropriate protective clothing for cold, wet, or hot weather and by sufficient replacement of fluids (30). Bicycle safety equipment, particularly lights and reflectors, should be required on all bicycles used for training, recreation, and transportation.

## 6.2 Sport

### 6.2.1 Promoting Bicycle Helmet Use With Campaigns

The first multifaceted community-based campaign to increase bicycle helmet use was established in 1986 by the Harborview Injury Prevention and Research Center (HIPRC), Seattle, Washington. The HIPRC campaign was based on research data, focused on a carefully selected target age group

(5-9 years old), had a very effective injury intervention device (the helmet), and had a built-in evaluation component (19, 20). These four elements combined with the multifaceted community-wide nature of the campaign were responsible for its success (3, 66). Between 1987 and 1993 child helmet use in Seattle increased from 5.5% to 58% (64). Adult helmet use increased from 56% to 70% between 1991 and 1993 (27). The HIPRC campaign design and strategy provided the basis for state, local, and nationwide campaigns. Narrowly focused campaigns (providing helmets in emergency departments, schools, and from pediatric offices) have not been particularly successful (16, 59, 60).

### 6.2.2 Promoting Bicycle Helmet Use With Administrative Rules and Legislation

Helmet use has been mandatory for bicycle races in the United States since 1986 (69b). Numerous cycling organizations require helmets for club rides. It is clear that legislation is quite effective in increasing helmet use and that the effect is not heavily dependent on enforcement (15, 18). It is our opinion that mandatory helmet legislation should be part of a comprehensive prevention program and should apply to cyclists of all ages (17, 64, 79). Legislation appears to be most effective when it is preceded by a well-coordinated helmet promotion campaign (46). The first major bicycle helmet law went into effect in Victoria, Australia, in 1990 after 8 years of public campaigns. Helmet wearing rates rose from 31% to 75% overall and approach 90% in some age groups (12, 85). Laws requiring helmets have been passed at state and local levels in the United States, Australia, Canada, and several European countries (4, 5, 75, 85).

These are our recommendations for preventing bicycle injuries:

- Helmet use by cyclists of all ages should be promoted using community-wide campaigns *and* mandatory legislation. Helmet effectiveness has been established by case control and cohort studies and preinjury and postinjury surveillance studies that document the reduction in head injuries in helmeted populations (Table 7.7). Both community campaigns and legislative approaches to increasing helmet use have been evaluated with presurveillance and postsurveillance studies and found effective.
- Alcohol laws similar to those for motor vehicle drivers should be applied consistently to bicyclists. Alcohol has been established as a risk factor for bike crashes in case series, case control studies, and nationwide injury surveillance (FARS). Legislation (DWI) has contributed to reductions in motor vehicle injuries as documented by time-series analysis.
- Bicycle-friendly riding environments should be established to encourage cycling and reduce crashes. This includes environmental modification and engineering solutions to construct safer roads with wide shoulders and minimal hazards. Well-engineered bicycle lanes should provide separate space for bicycles on roadways and connect with bicycle trails. Improvements in road design, bicycle design, and bicyclist behavior would all contribute to safety. Research in this area is mainly descriptive. Available studies are weakly designed, inadequately analyzed, or both; as a consequence, results are contradictory.

## 7. Suggestions for Further Research

### 7.1 Establish Sports Competition Databases

In this review we have described the relative lack of systematically collected information on injuries experienced by competitive cyclists during both training and competition events. In order to address these deficiencies, databases should be developed and maintained by the various bicycle racing organizations, specifically the United States Cycling Federation, National Off Road Bicycling Association, and the Triathlon Federation. The database should contain a description of the injury and how it occurred, including a description of the event and identification of the rider. These databases would provide the basis for developing the descriptive epidemiology of bicycle injuries in each competitive cycling event. Epidemiological studies utilizing case control or cohort design are needed to evaluate risk factors for injuries to competitive cyclists during competition and training.

### 7.2 Environmental Intervention

The effectiveness of different environmental designs for separating bicycles and motor vehicle traffic needs to be evaluated in a systematic manner. This evaluation should include a wide variety of bicycle lanes, paths, and changes in road design. Racing officials should consider environmental factors (physical terrain and traffic controls) when selecting courses for road races, criteriums, and mountain bike downhill races.

### 7.3 Education

It is widely believed in the bicycling community that cycling education for children and adults will improve bicycle safety by reducing crashes. There are no evaluations of bicycle safety programs. Evaluations of motor vehicle driver education programs for 16- to 18-year-old drivers have not shown that crash rates decline. It is important to determine whether bicycling skill courses or safety education courses effectively reduce bicycle crashes.

### 7.4 Bicycle Helmets

Our review of current bicycle helmet research suggests two further areas of investigation. To optimize helmet protection additional studies should evaluate helmet effectiveness in different age groups of cyclists and evaluate the role of fit and helmet retention in overall protection. Bicycle-related facial injuries are common, and current helmet design offers no protection for the lower face, jaw, mouth, and teeth. Helmets with a facial bar or similar protective piece may greatly reduce these injuries. The feasibility, acceptability, and effectiveness of these enhanced safety designs would be a valuable addition to bicycle safety.

## References

1. Baker, S.P.; Li, G.; Fowler, C.; Dannenberg, A.L. Injuries to bicyclists: a national perspective. Baltimore, MD: The Johns Hopkins University Injury Prevention Center; 1993.

2. Barancik, J.I.; Chatterjee, B.F.; Greene, Y.C.; et al. Northeastern Ohio Trauma Study: I. Magnitude of the problem. Am. J. Public Health 73:746-751; 1983.

3. Bergman, A.B.; Rivara, F.P.; Richards, D.D.; Rogers, L.W. The Seattle children's bicycle helmet campaign. Am. J. Dis. Child. 144:727-731; 1990.

4. Bicycle Helmet Safety Institute. A comparison of bicycle helmet standards. Bicycle Helmet Safety Institute. Arlington, VA. (BHSIDOC #185), September, 1994.

5. Bicycle Helmet Safety Institute. Helmet legislation update. Bicycle Helmet Safety Institute. Arlington, VA, 1994.

6. Bjornstig, U.; Ostrom, M.; Eriksson, A.; Sonntag-Ostrom, E. Head and face injuries in bicyclists—with special reference to possible effects of helmet use. J. Trauma 33:887-893; 1992.

7. Bohlmann, J.T. Injuries in competitive cycling. Physician Sportsmed. 9(5):117-124; 1981.

8. Brown, B.; Farley, C. The pertinence of promoting the use of bicycle helmets for 8 to 12 year old children. Chronic Diseases in Canada 10:92-94; 1989.

9. Burgess, B.; Burden D. Bicycle safety highway users information report. Report prepared by Bikecentennial in response to National Highway Traffic Safety Administration order number NHTSA-7-3200, July, 1977.

10. Burke, E.R. Proper fit of the bicycle. In: Mellion, M.B. & Burke, E.R., eds. Clinics in sports medicine. Philadelphia: W.B. Saunders; 1994: 1-15.

11. Cambridge, S. ed. Christchurch Cycle Safety Committee. Cycle use and collisions in Christchurch. Transit New Zealand Research Report. no. 7, 1989.

12. Cameron, M.H.; Vulcan, P.A.; Finch, C.F.; Newstad, S.V. Bicycle helmet use following a decade of helmet promotion in Victoria, Australia—An evaluation. Accid. Anal. & Prev. 26(3):325-337; 1994.

13. Champion, H.R.; Sacco, W.J.; Copes, W.S. Trauma Scoring. In: Moore E.E. et al., eds. Trauma. Norwalk: Appleton & Lang; 1991:47-65.

14. Chow, T.K.; Bracker, M.D.; Patrick, K. Acute injuries from mountain biking. West J. Med. 159:145-148; 1993.

15. Cote, T.R.; Sacks, J.J.; Lambert-Huber, D.A.; Dannenberg, A.L.; Kresnow, M.; Lipitz, A.L. Bicycle helmet use among Maryland children: effect of legislation and education. Pediatrics 89:1216-1220; 1992.

16. Cushman, R.; Down, J.; MacMillan, N.; Waclawik, H. Helmet protection in the emergency room following a bicycle injury: a randomized trial. Pediatrics 88:43-47; 1991.

17. Dannenberg, A.L.; Cote, T.R.; Kresnow, M.J.; Sacks, J.J.; et al. Bicycle helmet use by adults: the impact of companionship. Public Health Reports 108(2):212-217; 1993a.

18. Dannenberg, A.L.; Gielen, A.C.; Beilenson, P.L.; Wilson, M.H.; Joffe, A. Bicycle helmet laws and educational campaigns: an evaluation of strategies to increase children's helmet use. Am. J. Public Health 83:667-674; 1993.

18b. Desai, K.M.; Gingel, J.C. Hazards of long distance cycling. Br. Med. J. 298:1072-73; 1989.

19. DiGuiseppi, C.G.; Rivara, F.P.; Koepsell, T.D. Attitudes toward bicycle helmet ownership and use by school-age children. Am. J. Dis. Child. 144:83-86; 1990.

20. DiGuiseppi, C.G.; Rivara, F.P.; Koepsell, T.D.; Polissar, L. Bicycle helmet use by children. JAMA 262:2256-2261; 1989.

21. Dorsch, M.M.; Woodward, A.J.; Somers, R.L. Do bicycle safety helmets reduce severity of head injury in real crashes? Accid. Anal. Prev. 19:183-190; 1987.

22. Fife, D.; Davis, J.; Tate, L.; Wells, J.K.; Mohan, D.; Williams, A. Fatal injuries to bicyclists: the experience of Dade County, Florida. J. Trauma 23:745-755; 1983.

23. Forester, J. Effective cycling. Cambridge: MIT Press, 6th ed; 1993.

24. Friede, A.M.; Azzara, C.V.; Gallagher, S.S.; Guyer, B. The epidemiology of injuries to bicycle riders. Pediatr. Clin. North Am. 32:141-151; 1985.

25. Gallagher, S.S.; Finison, K.; Guyer, B.; Goodenough, S. The incidence of injuries among 87,000 Massachusetts children and adolescents: results of the 1980-81 Statewide Childhood Injury Prevention Program Surveillance System. Am. J. Public Health 74(12):1340-1347; 1984.

26. Haddon, W. Energy damage and the ten countermeasure strategies. J. Trauma 13(4):321-331; 1973.

27. Harborview Injury Prevention and Research Center (HIPRC). The 1991 Washington children's bicycle helmet campaign. (press releases 1991, 1993.)

28. Hatziandreu, E.J.; Brown, R.E.; Frank, S.R. Cost-effectiveness of three programs to increase use of bicycle helmets. Washington, DC: Battelle Medical Technology Assessment and Policy Research Center; 1993.

29. Hazinski, M.F.; Francescutti, L.H.; Lapidus, G.D.; Micik, S.; Rivara, R.P. Pediatric injury prevention. Ann. Emerg. Med. 22:456-467; 1993.

30. Helzer-Julin, M. Sun, heat, and cold injuries in cyclists. In: Mellion, M.B. & Burke, E.R., eds. Clinics in sports medicine. Philadelphia: W.B. Saunders; 1994: 219-235.

31. Hodgson, V. Impact, skid, and retention tests on a representative group of bicycle helmets to determine their head-neck protective characteristics. Detroit, Michigan, 1990. Report prepared in cooperation with the Michigan Bicycle Helmet Advisory Committee and the Michigan Department of Public Health.

32. Holmes, J.C.; Pruitt, A.L.; Whalen, N.J. Lower extremity overuse in bicycling. In: Mellion, M.B. & Burke, E.R., eds. Clinics in sports medicine. Philadelphia: W.B. Saunders; 1994:187-206.

33. Hoque, M. An analysis of fatal bicycle accidents in Victoria (Australia) with a special reference to nighttime accidents. Accid. Anal. Prev. 22:1-11; 1990.

34. Insurance Institute for Highway Safety. Flemming A., ed. Bicycles. Arlington, VA: IIHS. Fatality Facts, July 1994.

35. Jaffe, K.M.; Fay, G.C.; Polissar, N.L.; Martin, K.M.; Shurtleff, H.; Rivara, J.M.; Winn, H.R. Severity of pediatric traumatic brain injury and early neurobehavioral outcome: a cohort study. Arch. Phys. Med. Rehabil. 73:540-547; 1992.

36. Jaffe, K.M.; Fay, G.C.; Polissar, N.L.; Martin, K.M.; Shurtleff, H.; Rivara, J.M.; Winn, H.R. Severity of pediatric traumatic brain injury and neurobehavioral recovery at one year: a cohort study. Arch. Phys. Med. Rehabil.74:587-595; 1993a.

37. Kiburz, D.; Jacobs, R.; Reckling, F.; Mason, J. Bicycle accidents and injuries among adult cyclists. Am. J. Sports Med. 14:416-419; 1986.

38. Kraus, J.F.; Fife, D.; Conroy, C. Incidence, severity, and outcomes of brain injuries involving bicycles. Am. J. Public Health 77:76-78; 1987.

39. Kraus, J.F.; Rock, A.; Hemyari, P. Brain injuries among infants, children, adolescents and young adults. Am. J. Dis. Child. 144:684-691; 1990.

40. Lane, J.C. Helmets for child bicyclists, some biomedical considerations. Canberra City, Australia: Australia Federal Department of Transport. Federal Office of Road Safety. CR 47; 1986.

41. Le-Bescond, Y.; Lebeau, J.; Delgove, L.; Sadek, H.; Raphael, B. Mountain sports: their role in 2200 facial injuries occurring over 4 years at the University Hospital Center in Grenoble. Rev-Stomatol-Chir-Maxillofac. 93(3):185188; 1992.

42. LeMier, M. Strategies for prevention: bicycle injuries in Washington State. November 1992. Washington State Department of Health

43. Li, G.; Baker, S.P. Alcohol in fatally injured bicyclists. Accid. Anal. and Prev. 26(4)543-548; 1994.

44. Lindqvist, C.; Sorsa, S.; Hyrkas, T.; Santavirta, S. Maxillofacial fractures sustained in bicycle accidents. Intl. J. Oral Maxillofac. Surg. 15:12-18; 1986.

45. Lott, D.F.; Lott, D.Y. Effect of bike lanes on ten classes of bicycle-automobile accidents in Davis, California. J. Safety Res. 8:171-179; 1976.

46. Macknin, M.L.; Medendorp, S.V. Association between bicycle helmet legislation, bicycle safety education, and use of bicycle helmets in children. Arch. Pediat. Adolesc. Med. 148:255-259; 1994.

47. Maimaris, C.; Summers, C.L.; Browning, C.; Palmer, C.R. Injury patterns in cyclists attending an accident and emergency department: a comparison of helmet wearers and non-wearers. BMJ 308:1537-1540; 1994.

48. McDermott, F.T.; Lane, J.C.; Brazenor, G.A.; Debney, E.A. The effectiveness of bicyclist helmets: a study of 1710 casualties. J. Trauma 34:834-845; 1993.

49. McLennan, J.G.; McLennan, J.C; Ungersma, J. Accident prevention in competitive cycling. Am. J. Sports Med. 16(3):266-268; 1988.

50. Mellion, M.B. Common cycling injuries: Management and prevention. Sports Medicine 11(1):52-70; 1991.

51. Mellion, M.B. Neck and back pain in cycling. In: Mellion, M.B. & Burke, E.R., eds. Clinics in sports medicine. Philadelphia: W.B. Saunders; 1994:137-164.

52. Miller, T.R.; Pindus, N.M.; Douglass, J.B.; Rossman, S.B. Nonfatal injury incidence, costs, and consequences: a data book. Washington, DC: The Urban Institute; 1993.

53. Myral, R.T. Condylar injuries in children: what is different about them? In: Worthington, P. & Evans, J.R., eds. Controversies in oral and maxillofacial surgery. Philadelphia: W.B. Saunders; 1994.

54. National Off-Road Bicycle Association (NORBA). 1750 E. Boulder St., Colorado Springs, CO 80909. (personal communication), 1994.

55. Nationwide Personal Transportation Survey. 1990 NPTS Databook. U.S. Department of Transportation; Federal Highway Administration. 1990.

56. Nichols, C.E. Injuries in cycling in clinical practice of sports injury prevention and care: volume V. Encyclopaedia of sports medicine. Renstrom, P.A.F.H., ed; Oxford: Blackwell Scientific Publications; 1994.

57. Olkkonen, S.; Honkanen, R. The role of alcohol in nonfatal bicycle injuries. Accid. Anal. Prev. 22:89-96; 1990.

58. Ostrom, M.; Bjornstig, U.; Naslund, K.; Eriksson, R. Pedal cycling fatalities in northern Sweden. Inj. J. Epidemiol. 22(3):483-488; 1993.

59. Parkin, P.C.; Spence, L.J.; Hu, X.; Kranz, K.E.; Shortt, L.G.; Wesson, D.E. Evaluation of a promotional strategy to increase bicycle helmet use by children. Pediatrics 91:772-777; 1993.

60. Pendergrast, R.A.; Ashworth, C.S.; Durant, R.H.; Litaker, M. Correlates of children's bicycle helmet use and short-term failure of school-level interventions. Pediatrics 90:354-358; 1992.

61. Pitt, W.R.; Thomas, S.; Nixon, J.; Clark, R.; Battisutta, D.; Acton, C. Trends in head injuries among child bicyclists. BMJ 308:177; 1994.

62. Richmond, D.R. Handlebar problems in bicycling. In: Mellion, M.B. & Burke, E.R., eds. Clinics in sports medicine. Philadelphia: W.B. Saunders; 1994:165-174.

63. Rivara, F.P.; Calonge, N.; Thompson, R.S. Population-based study of unintentional injury incidence and impact during childhood. Am. J. Public Health 79(8):990-994; 1989.

64. Rivara, F.P.; Thompson, D.C.; Thompson, R.S.; Rogers, L.W.; Alexander, B.; Felix, D.; Bergman, A.B. The Seattle children's bicycle helmet campaign: changes in helmet use and head injury admissions. Pediatrics 93(4):567-569; 1994.

65. Rodgers, G.B., ed. Bicycle use and hazard patterns in the United States. Washington, DC: U.S. Consumer Product Safety Commission; 1994.

66. Rogers, L.W.; Bergman, A.B.; Rivara, F.P. Promoting bicycle helmets to children: a campaign that worked. J. Musculoskeletal Medicine 8:64-77; 1991.

67. Ronkin, M.; McAllister, W. Bicycle/motor vehicle accident summary. Oregon Department of Transportation; 1992

68. Rowland, J.; Rivara, F.P.; Salzberg, P.; Soderberg, R.; Maier, R.; Koepsell, T. Motorcycle helmet use, injury outcome and hospitalization costs: a statewide study

using linked motor-vehicle crash, hospital discharge and death certificate data. (in press); 1994.

69. Runyan, C.W.; Earp, J.L.; Reese, R.P. Helmet use among competitive cyclists. Am. J. Prev. Med. 7:232-236; 1991.

69b. Runyan, C.W. Traumatic injuries among North Carolinians. N.C. Med. J. 47:14-16; 1986.

70. Sacks, J.J.; Holmgreen, P.; Smith, S.M.; Sosin, D.M. Bicycle-associated head injuries and deaths in the United States from 1984 through 1988. How many are preventable? JAMA 266:3016-3018 and 3032-3033; 1991.

71. Selbst, S.M.; Alexander, D.; Ruddy R. Bicycle-related injuries. Am. J. Dis. Child. 141:140-144; 1987.

72. Simpson, A.H.R.W.; Unwin, P.S.; Nelson ,I.W. Head injuries, helmets, cycle lanes, and cyclists. Br. Med. J. 296: 1988.

73. Spaite, D.W.; Murphy, M.; Criss, E.A.; Valenzuela, T.D.; Meislin, H.W. A prospective analysis of injury severity among helmeted and nonhelmeted bicyclists involved in collisions with motor vehicles. J. Trauma 31:1510-1516; 1991.

74. Tanz, R.R.; Christoffel, K.K. Tykes on bikes: injuries associated with bicycle-mounted child seats. Pediatr. Emerg. Care 7:297-301; 1992.

75. Thomas, S.; Acton, C.; Nixon, J.; Battisutta, D.; Pitt, W.R.; Clark, R. Effectiveness of bicycle helmets in preventing head injury in children: case control study. BMJ 308:173-176; 1994.

76. Thompson, D.C.; Thompson, R.S.; Rivara, F.P. Bicycle helmet effectiveness and use in four age groups of cyclists. Abstract. Arch. Pediatrics Adolescent Med. 148:81; 1994.

77. Thompson, D.C.; Thompson, R.S.; Rivara, F.P. Incidence of bicycle-related injuries in a defined population. Am. J. Public Health 80:1388-1390; 1990.

78. Thompson, D.C; Thompson, R.S.; Rivara, F.P.; Wolf, M.E. A case-control study of the effectiveness of bicycle safety helmets in preventing facial injury. Am. J. Public Health 80:1471-1474; 1990a.

79. Thompson, R.S.; Rivara, F.P.; Thompson, D.C. A case-control study of the effectiveness of bicycle safety helmets. N. Engl. J. Med. 320:1361-1367; 1989.

80. Thompson, R.S.; Thompson, D.C.; Rivara, F.P.; Salazar, A.A. Cost-effectiveness analysis of bicycle helmet subsidies in a defined population. Pediatrics 91:902-907; 1993.

81. Timms, R.; Rivara, F. Bicycle child carriers: safety and convenience. Bicycle USA 9-12; 1990.

82. Triathlon Federation. 3595 East Fountain Blvd. Colorado Springs, CO 80910; Miller, T.K. (personal communication), 1994.

83. United States Cycling Federation (USCF). 1 Olympia Plaza, Colorado Springs, CO 80910; (personal communication), 1994.

84. U.S. Department of Transportation. National bicycling and walking study: transportation choices for a changing America. U.S. Department of Transportation: Federal Highway Administration, no. FHWA-PD-94-023, 1994.

85. Vulcan, P.A.; Cameron, M.H.; Watson, W.L. Mandatory bicycle helmet use: experience in Victoria, Australia. World J. Surgery 16:389-397; 1992.

86. Wachtel, A.; Lewiston, D. Risk factors for bicycle-motor vehicle collisions at intersections. ITE Journal 64:30-32; 1994.

87. Wasserman, R.C.; Waller, J.A.; Monty, M.J.; Emery, A.B.; Robinson, D.R. Bicyclists, helmets, and head injuries: a rider-based study of helmet use and effectiveness. Am. J. Public Health 78:1220-1221; 1988.

88. Weiss, B.D. Clinical syndromes associated with bicycle seats. In: Mellion, M.B. & Burke, E.R., eds. Clinics in sports medicine. Philadelphia: W.B. Saunders; 1994:175-186.

89. Weiss, B.D. Nontraumatic injuries in amateur long distance bicyclists. Am. J. Sports Med. 13:187-192; 1985.

90. Williams, M. The protective performance of bicyclists' helmets in accidents. Accid. Anal. Prev. 23:119-131; 1991.

91. Wood, T.; Milne, P. Head injuries to pedal cyclists and the promotion of helmet use in Victoria, Australia. Accid. Anal. Prev. 20:177-185; 1988.

92. Worrell, J. Head injuries in pedal cyclists: how much will protection help? Injury 18:5-6; 1987.

# 8

# Boxing

## Barry D. Jordan

## 1. Introduction

Unlike any other sport, boxing is associated with the intentional affliction of traumatic brain injury (i.e., a concussion or knockout). This proclivity of irreversible and/or permanent neurological injury in boxing introduces ethical, moral, medical, and social concerns. Although abolition of the sport has been advocated (21), its continued existence in society necessitates reforms to minimize injury and promote safety (9, 15). Accordingly, epidemiology will play a crucial role in documenting and establishing putative risk factors for injury in boxing and developing strategies for injury prevention. This comprehensive critical literature review of the epidemiological aspects of injury in boxing was undertaken to outline our current understanding of the subject matter and identify areas that need research and development.

Epidemiologic investigations of boxing injuries have been limited both in quantity and quality. The majority of investigations have been on anecdotal case reports or small clinical series that are often influenced by the "subjective" opinions of the proponents or opponents of boxing. There are only a limited number of epidemiological investigations in boxing that accurately present the descriptive characteristics (i.e., morbidity and mortality) or delineate the potential risk for injury.

## 2. Incidence of Injury

### 2.1 Injury Rates

Only a few epidemiological investigations of well-defined amateur or professional boxing populations present reliable incidence rates (Table 8.1).

Unfortunately, due to differences in data collection, study design, and population sample, comparisons between investigations yield minimum utility. Incidence rates are expressed as injuries per number of boxers, injuries per number of personal exposures, and injuries per time exposure (i.e., hours or rounds fought). Despite variations among the investigations, it is quite apparent that professional boxing is associated with a higher injury rate than amateur boxing.

### 2.2 Practice vs. Competition

Welch et al. (27) conducted a survey of boxing injuries that occurred during an instructional boxing program at the United States Military Academy (USMA) at West Point, New York, over 2 academic years (1983-1984 and 1984-1985). Injury rates were calculated by determining the number of hours spent boxing. During the 2-year period, there were 559 boxing injuries yielding an overall injury rate of less than 4%. The overall injury rate for instruction (practice) compared to competition was 9 and 43 injuries, respectively, per 1,000 hours. This higher injury rate during competition most likely reflects the increased intensity of boxing associated with competition.

## 3. Injury Characteristics

### 3.1 Injury Onset

Investigations involving the nature of injury onset in boxing have focused primarily on brain injury. The proper assignment of brain injury in boxing necessitates that sudden onset or acute brain injury (ABI) be differentiated from gradual onset or chronic brain injury (CBI). There are several aspects that distinguishes ABI from CBI (Table 8.2).

**Table 8.1    A Comparison of Injury Rates in Boxing**

| Study | Study design/ data collection methods | Population | Duration of injury surveillance | Number of participants | Exposure | Number of injuries | Injury rates | Comments |
|---|---|---|---|---|---|---|---|---|
| Estwanik et al. 1989 | Prospective monitoring of acute boxing injuries | Amateur boxers competing in the 1981 and 1982 USA national championships | 2 tournaments each lasting 5 days | — | 547 bouts 1,094 personal exposures | 100 | 9.1 injuries per 100 personal exposures | Injuries include 52 notable injuries and 48 injuries secondary to head blows |
| Welch et al. 1986 | Prospective monitoring of acute boxing injuries | Cadets at the U.S. Military Academy in West Point | 2 years | 2,100 | 25,305 boxing hours | 294 | 1) 14.0 injuries per 100 boxers 2) 11.6 injuries per 1,000 hours | Only include moderate injuries |
| Jordan et al. 1988 | Retrospective review of injury reports | Professional boxers licensed in New York | 2 years | 906 | 3,110 rounds fought | 376 | 1) 41.5 injuries per 100 boxers 2) 1.2 injuries per 10 rounds fought | |
| McCown, 1959 | Retrospective review of injury records | Professional boxers licensed in New York State | 7 years | 11,173 | — | 2,351 | 21.0 injuries per 100 boxers | |

**Table 8.2    A Comparison Between Acute and Chronic Brain Injury in Boxing**

| | Acute brain injury (ABI) | Chronic Brain injury (CBI) |
|---|---|---|
| Onset of symptoms | Immediate | Typically delayed, usually occurring years after exposure and/or cessation of boxing career. |
| Symptoms | 1) Concussion (i.e. transient impairment of neurologic dysfunction) 2) Focal neurological deficits if associated with intracranial hemorrhage | 1) Dementia/personality changes 2) Cerebellar dysfunction 3) Parkinsonism 4) Pyramidal tract dysfunction 5) Intellectual impairment |
| Pathophysiology | Acceleration of the brain (usually rotational) | Unknown: Perhaps multiple petechial hemorrhage that are replaced by gliosis or progressive neuronal dropout |
| Pathology | 1) Usually none 2) Diffuse axonal injury 3) Intracranial hemorrhage | 1) Neurofibrillary changes 2) Cerebellar atrophy 3) Degeneration of substantia nigra 4) Diffuse cerebral atrophy 5) "Diffuse" amyloid placques |
| Treatment | 1) Usually none required except for neurological observation 2) Hospitalization and neurosurgical intervention | Anti-Parkinsons medications such as L-Dopa and Selegiline as well as anti-cholinergic agents |

Acute brain injury attributable to boxing is usually of immediate onset and associated with transient neurological impairment such as loss of consciousness, amnesia, or loss of motor tone. On occasion, severe ABI may be associated with both intracranial hemorrhage and focal neurologic deficits. In contrast, CBI typically has a delayed onset after the initiation of a boxing career and may progress for years after retirement from boxing. Chronic brain injury has been recognized by a variety of names including dementia pugilistica, chronic traumatic encephalopathy, and the punch syndrome. Chronic brain injury associated with boxing has been classically described as a variable constellation of symptoms including dementia, personality changes, cerebellar dysfunction, pyramidal tract dysfunction, and extrapyramidal disease (17).

The diagnosis of ABI is usually nonproblematic because it is typically associated with obvious neurological symptoms (e.g., loss of consciousness, loss of motor control) that are immediately observed in response to a boxer's punch. However, if a boxer experiences neurologic symptoms that are not obvious (e.g., amnesia, headache), the diagnosis of ABI may go unacknowledged, unless the boxer is examined at the termination of the bout by the ringside physician.

Unlike ABI, CBI is not temporally related to the immediate effects of a boxer's punch and is, therefore, more difficult to diagnose. For example, if a boxer develops neurological symptoms in later life, such as dementia or motor impairment, the establishment of a causal association between the neurologic symptoms and the boxing career is problematic. First, it is unknown whether an individual would have developed neurologic symptoms without exposure to boxing. Second, it would be difficult to control for confounding variables that may be present with neurologic dysfunction, such as alcohol and drug abuse, head trauma outside of the ring, and other environmental and occupational exposures.

## 3.2 Injury Type

Epidemiological investigations of boxing injuries typically classify specific injuries according to anatomic site. The documentation of injury type (e.g., strain, sprain, laceration, contusion) without specification of location is uninformative and potentially misleading because of the predilection for head injury in boxing. Accordingly, injury characteristics are more appropriately classified by location.

## 3.3 Injury Location

Specific injuries will be broadly classified as head/spine/trunk, upper extremity, lower extremity, and other. Further specification of injury type according to anatomic site will be addressed in subsequent sections of this chapter. The percent distribution of boxing injuries according to location is presented in Table 8.3.

### 3.3.1 Head/Spine/Trunk

Depending upon the investigation cited, 27% to 93% of boxing injuries involve the head (Table 8.3). However, the interpretation of comparison percent distributions of head injuries in boxing is limited by the relatively flexible definition of head injury. Head injury that is associated with brain injury should be distinguished from injury to the face, eyes, ears, nose, and oral cavity that is not associated with neurological injury (Table 8.4). Accordingly, this discussion of head injury attempts to distinguish ABI from nonneurological head injury.

Brain injury represents the most devastating type of injury encountered in boxing and is the primary public health concern. The cerebral concussion is the most frequently encountered brain injury and is the essence of the knockout. Rarely, acute catastrophic brain injury, such as diffuse axonal injury or intracranial hemorrhage, is encountered.

Larsson et al. (19) reported acute head injuries among amateur boxers at the 1950 and 1951 Swedish Junior Championships and the 1951 Swedish Championships. Seventy-five boxers were examined in connection with 102 matches. Among the 75 boxers, 35 had been knocked down and 14 of these were knockouts. Blonstein and Clarke (1) assessed acute boxing injuries among 3,000 boxing contests that included almost 5,000 boxers who were licensed by the London Amateur Boxing Association. During a 7-month period, 23 boxers were knocked out twice and 6 had been severely concussed on one occasion. These 29 boxers represented 0.58 percent of boxers active during that year.

Estwanik et al. (7) reported on acute boxing injuries that occurred during the 1981 and 1982 U.S.A. National Amateur Boxing Championships. During the two tournaments there were 547 bouts with 1,094 personal exposures. Forty-eight matches (8.7 percent) were terminated because of severe blows to the head. This yielded a rate of 4.38 head injuries per 100 personal exposures. The majority of these head injuries were not associated with loss of consciousness. This study established

**Table 8.3   A Comparison of Percent Distribution of Boxing Injuries by Location**

| Study | Head %(#) | Upper/extremity %(#) | Lower/extremity %(#) | Spine/trunk %(#) | Other %(#) | Comments |
|---|---|---|---|---|---|---|
| Estwanik et al. 1984 | 73(73) | 23(23) | 2(2) | 2(2) | 0(0) | Total 100 injuries excluded minor injuries such as episaxis and unsutured lacerations. Amateur boxers. |
| Welch et al. 1986 | 48(142) | 46(134) | 4(12) | 2(6) | 0(0) | Total 294 injuries. Cadets at the U.S. Military Academy West Point. |
| Jordan and Campbell 1988 | 93(351) | 2(9) | 0(0) | 3(11) | 1(5) | Total 376 injuries. Professional boxers. |
| Enzenauer et al. 1989 | 68(272) | 17(67) | 5(25) | 7(29) | 2(8) | Total of 401 injuries among U.S. Army personnel. |
| Jordan et al. 1990 | 27(121) | 33(147) | 24(107) | 16(72) | 0(0) | Total of 447 injuries. Survey of injuries among amateur boxers at the U.S.O.T.C. |

**Table 8.4   Head Injury**

I. Neurological
  1) Concussion
  2) Diffuse axonal injury
  3) Focal brain injury
    a) Subdural hematoma
    b) Epidural hematoma
    c) Intracerebral hemorrhage
    d) Cerebral contusion
II. Non-neurological
  1) Facial
  2) Ocular
  3) Nasal
  4) Auricular
  5) Oral/mandibular
  6) Other

a head injury rate for a selected sample of highly skilled amateur boxers in the United States.

Jordan et al. (12) reviewed all boxing injuries sustained by amateur boxers at the United States Olympic Training Center (USOTC) from January 1, 1977, through August 30, 1987. During this 10-year period, there were a total of 447 injuries. There were only 29 acute brain injuries, which comprised 6.5% of the total injuries. Twenty-eight of these injuries were concussions, and one boxer was diagnosed as experiencing a posttraumatic headache (i.e., postconcussion syndrome). The neurologic manifestations of these concussions could not be

determined from the method of data collection employed by these investigators.

Enzenauer et al. (6) retrospectively reviewed all hospitalizations for boxing-related injuries in the U.S. Army hospitals worldwide from January 1980 through December 1985. Head injuries were broadly classified and included neurological and nonneurological injuries such as fracture of facial bones, ocular injuries, and head/neck contusion. During the 6-year period of observation, there were 401 admissions for boxing-related injuries, which yielded an average of 67 hospitalizations annually. Head injuries accounted for 68% of all injuries.

Among professional boxers in New York State from 1952 through 1958, McCown (22) observed 325 knockouts and 789 technical knockouts among 11,173 participants. Among the 325 knockouts, which were defined as those boxers who were counted out (i.e., took the 10-second count), all except 10 were able to arise from the floor and walk to their respective corners unaided, without need of further medical assistance. However, 10 boxers were more severely concussed and required hospitalization lasting from 24 hours to 10 days.

Jordan and Campbell (9) conducted a 2-year survey of medical injuries among active professional boxers, licensed in New York State during a 2-year period. Data were extracted from medical injury report forms at the New York State Athletic Commission (NYSAC) from August 1, 1982, through

July 31, 1984. Injury report forms are routinely completed by the ringside physician on any professional boxer who sustains an injury in the ring during competitive boxing. Injuries were divided into craniocerebral and noncraniocerebral injuries. Craniocerebral injuries were defined as any technical knockout or knockout from head blows. A technical knockout or knockout in which the nature of the injury was not specified was assumed to be craniocerebral injury. All other injuries were classified as noncraniocerebral injuries. During the 2-year observation period 3,110 rounds were fought with 376 craniocerebral injuries. This yielded a frequency of 0.8 craniocerebral injuries per 10 rounds fought. Rarely did craniocerebral injuries result in neurologic dysfunction. Four boxers required immediate neurologic evaluation after their fights. One of these four boxers died as a result of bilateral subdural hematomas. During the 2 years of study, there was a mean of 453 boxers licensed to box in New York State. On the basis of these findings, it was concluded that severe, acute catastrophic neurological injuries are rare in professional boxing when strict medical supervision is present.

Approximately 20% to 40% of all boxing injuries involve the face, eye, ear, nose, mandible, and oral cavity (Table 8.5). The most common non-neurological head injuries are nasal injuries and facial lacerations. Eye injuries are relatively uncommon and do not exceed 5 percent of all boxing injuries.

Injury to the spine/trunk are relatively infrequent in boxing and comprises 2% to 16% of all boxing injuries (Table 8.3). Trunk injuries typically include rib contusions/fractures and abdominal contusions. Testicular trauma and kidney contusions are rarely encountered because these areas are illegal targets. The majority of spinal injuries are soft tissue injuries (e.g., strain, sprain, muscle spasm).

### 3.3.2 Upper Extremity

Injuries to the upper extremity in boxing represent 2% to 46% of all boxing injuries (Table 8.3). The majority of upper extremity injuries involve the hand and wrist (see Table 8.6). The second most common site of upper extremity injury involves the shoulders. As expected, the repetitive and forceful delivery of punches is responsible for the relatively high frequency of upper extremity injury.

### 3.3.3 Lower Extremity

Injuries to the lower extremity are relatively uncommon in boxing. With the exception of the data reported from the USOTC over a 10-year period (12), the majority of epidemiologic investigations of boxing injuries (Table 8.3) indicate that lower extremity injuries in boxing represent 6% or less of all boxing injuries. The relatively high percentage of lower extremity injuries (24%) among amateur boxers at the USOTC probably reflects the distribution of acute as well as chronic injuries sustained during sparring, training, and competitions (1). Lower extremity injuries that occur during training are more likely to include overuse injuries associated with jogging and jumping rope (12).

## 4. Injury Severity

### 4.1 Time Loss

Injury statistics regarding time loss from sports participation, work, or school are largely unavailable. However, Enzenauer et al. (6) retrospectively

**Table 8.5    A Comparison of Percent Distributions of Non-Neurological Head Injury**

| | Estwanik et al. 1984 n=1094[a] | Welch et al. 1986 n=2100 | Jordan et al. 1988 n=906[b] | Jordan et al. 1990 n=447[c] | Total |
|---|---|---|---|---|---|
| Injury | %(#) | %(#) | %(#) | %(#) | |
| Facial Laceration | 14(14) | 0(0) | 18(66) | 2(8) | 88 |
| Eye | 3(3) | 0(0) | 3(13) | 5(23) | 39 |
| Ear | 3(3) | 0(0) | 0(1) | 1(5) | 9 |
| Nose | 3(3) | 39(114) | 1(5) | 8(34) | 156 |
| Oral | 2(2) | 0(0) | 0(0) | 3(13) | 15 |
| Mandibular | 0(0) | 2(6) | 1(4) | 2(7) | 17 |
| Other | | | | 0(2) | 2 |
| Total | 25(25) | 41(120) | 24(89) | 21(92) | 326 |

[a]Personal exposures.

[b]Number of participants over a two year period that were licensed annually (some may be counted twice).

[c]Total number of injuries. Actual number of participants is unknown.

**Table 8.6   A Comparison of Percent Distributions of Upper Extremity Injuries**

| Study | Estwanik et al. 1984<br>n=1094[a]<br>%(#) | Welch et al. 1986<br>n=2100<br>%(#) | Jordan et al. 1988<br>n=906[b]<br>%(#) | Jordan et al. 1990<br>n=447[c]<br>%(#) | Total |
|---|---|---|---|---|---|
| Hand/wrist | 22(22) | 18(54) | 2(8) | 21(92) | 176 |
| Shoulder | 1(1) | 22(66) | 0(1) | 7(32) | 100 |
| Elbow | — | 5(14) | — | 4(16) | 30 |
| Upper arm | — | — | — | 1(4) | 4 |
| Forearm | — | — | — | 1(3) | 3 |
| Total | 23(23) | 46(134) | 2(9) | 33(147) | 313 |

[a]Personal exposures.

[b]Number of participants over a two year period that were licensed annually (some boxers may be counted twice).

[c]Total number of injuries. Actual number of participants is unknown.

reviewed all hospitalizations for boxing-related injuries in the U.S. Army hospitals worldwide from January 1980 through December 1985. During the 6-year period of observation, there were 401 admissions for boxing-related injuries, which yielded an average of 67 hospitalizations annually. The morbidity associated with all types of boxing injuries included an average of 5.1 days in bed and 8.9 days disabled or unfit for duty.

## 4.2 Catastrophic Injury

Acute catastrophic injury (i.e., death or permanent disability) is a relatively uncommon occurrence in modern-day boxing. This is a reflection of increasing medical and safety reforms. The vast majority of boxing deaths are attributable to severe neurological injury, in particular the subdural hematoma (10). Enzenauer et al. (6) reported one fatality from a serious head injury during a 6-year period. McCown (22) reported that among professional boxers in New York State only two experienced what was classified as severe cerebral injury. There were no fatalities recorded during this 7-year period. Another survey of acute boxing injuries in New York State noted one boxing death over a 2-year period (9). In addition to acute neurologic injury, ocular injuries represent the other major type of visual impairment and represent another permanent disability. Although uncommon, retinal detachments are the most serious vision-threatening injuries in boxing. Serious vision-threatening ocular injuries are frequently associated with withdrawal from boxing participation.

## 4.3 Clinical Outcome/Residual Symptoms

The long-term cumulative effects of repetitive head trauma encountered in boxing can result in chronic brain injury (CBI) and significant neurological disability. CBI represents a spectrum of progressive neurological dysfunction that typically occurs after the cessation of a boxing career (17).

Two epidemiological investigations of CBI among retired boxers have been performed (24, 26). Thomassen et al. (26) conducted a case control study comparing 53 former champion amateur boxers with 53 former soccer players and found no significant differences in neurological and electroencephalogram (EEG) evaluations. Nonetheless, neuropsychological testing demonstrated that the boxers exhibited significantly more dysfunction than the controls on several subtests. However, these findings were inconclusive because the boxers differed from the soccer players in important background variables such as age and education.

Roberts (24) conducted a prevalence study of CBI among retired professional boxers. This investigator randomly sampled 250 of 16,781 ex-professional boxers who were licensed by the British Board of Control for at least 4 years from 1929 through 1955. Among the 250 boxers, 224 were examined. Thirty-seven boxers, or 17%, had clinical evidence of central nervous system (CNS) lesions attributable to boxing. Clinically, these findings were stereotyped with predominantly cerebellar and extrapyramidal signs with relatively less clearly defined impairment of intellectual function. Among the 224 boxers examined, 11 had evidence of CNS lesions not attributed to boxing. Of major importance, Roberts demonstrated that the prevalence of CBI attributable to boxing increased with increasing age and exposure. This was evidenced by an increased prevalence of CBI among boxers who had longer boxing careers (10 years or more), greater number of professional fights (150 fights or more), later age at retirement (28 years or older), and age at the time of examination (50 years or older). The significance of this investigation is that it provided risk factors for the development of CBI attributable to boxing. Theoretically, this could provide guidelines for criteria to recommend retirement of boxers with high boxing exposure and increased risk of CBI.

Although CBI has been primarily described among retired boxers, several investigations have attempted to document subtle clinical evidence of chronic neurological dysfunction among active amateur and professional boxers (see Table 8.7). These studies have relied primarily on the case control method and have utilized various neurodiagnostic tests.

# 5. Injury Risk Factors

Intrinsic and extrinsic risk factors for injury in boxing are not well delineated, often speculative, and require further epidemiological confirmation.

## 5.1 Intrinsic Factors

### 5.1.1 Age

Age of retirement from professional boxing is a risk factor for CBI. According to Roberts (24), British boxers that retired after the age of 28 years exhibited an increased risk of chronic traumatic encephalopathy attributable to boxing. This older age at retirement, more than likely, represents a longer exposure to a boxing career and potential traumatic brain injury. McLatchie et al. (23) observed that decreasing age was a risk factor for exhibiting an abnormal EEG. In contrast, increasing age was observed to be a risk factor for exhibiting an abnormal EEG among active professional boxers (2).

Age does not appear to be a risk factor for ABI associated with boxing. There is no existing epidemiological evidence that older boxers are more likely to experience a cerebral concussion or knockout (KO). However, among 143 boxers that experienced a technical knockout (TKO)/KO, boxers with abnormal or borderline computerized tomography (CT) scans were older than those with normal CT scans (13).

The age at examination of retired boxers will influence the examiner's ability to detect neurological dysfunction. Boxers that are examined after 50 years of age have a higher likelihood of exhibiting neurological deficits compared to those who are younger (24). Theoretically, this may be attributable to a longer period of neuronal dropout associated with the normal aging process superimposed on preexisting neuronal loss, secondary to the neurotrauma associated with boxing. Thus far, there is no evidence that the age of initiation of a boxing career or the age of retirement from amateur boxing influences the risk of ABI or CBI attributable to boxing.

### 5.1.2 Weight

There is relatively little epidemiological data to indicate whether heavier weight increases the risk of neurologic injury in boxing. One might suspect that the heavier boxers are capable of generating more forceful punches compared to lighter weight boxers. Blonstein and Clarke (1) noted that more prolonged knockouts were more common in the heavier weight classes. In a clinical survey, Critchley (4) reported that lighter weight boxers who fight heavier weight boxers may be at increased risk of CBI.

### 5.1.3. Boxing Skills/Performance

Intuitively, one would expect that less skilled boxers who lack the proper defensive techniques would be at increased risk of neurotrauma associated with boxing. Larsson et al. (19) observed that the more experienced boxers displayed better defensive skills and were able to protect themselves against hard blows more efficiently than less experienced boxers who exposed themselves more. Drew et al. (5) noted that the number of professional losses plus draws correlated inversely with performance on neuropsychological testing. In a CT scan survey of 338 professional boxers in New York State, boxing records were not associated with an increased risk of abnormal CT scans. However, a self-reported history of a TKO or KO was associated with increased risk of exhibiting brain atrophy on CT scan (13). Progressive changes on serial CT scanning may be associated with having more than 10 losses (14).

## 5.2 Extrinsic Factors

### 5.2.1 Sparring

Training for a bout involves considerable sparring (i.e., noncompetitive boxing) during which brain injury can occur. Large scale epidemiological studies have not confirmed the hypothesis that an increased exposure to head blows during sparring increases the risk of brain injury (25). A preliminary investigation suggests that increased sparring

**Table 8.7  A Comparison of Studies Assessing Chronic Brain Injury Among Active Boxers**

| Study | Study Design | Population | Neurodiagnostic Testing | Findings |
|---|---|---|---|---|
| Drew et al. (1986) | Case Control | Professional boxers (N = 19) | Neuropsychological Testing | Boxers demonstrated decreased performance on certain neuropsychological tests that correlated with total # of professional bouts and # of professional losses plus draws |
| McLatchie et al. (1987) | Case Control | Amateur boxers (N = 20) | Neurological examination, EEG, CT, Neuropsychological Testing | Abnormal clinical examination correlated with increasing numbers of fights. Abnormal EEG correlated with decreasing age. |
| Brooks et al. (1987) | Case Control | Amateur boxers (N = 29) | Neuropsychological Testing | Boxers exhibited lower scores on immediate and delayed recall and intelligence. No correlation with boxing exposure. |
| Levin et al. (1987) | Prospective Case-Control | Amateur and Professional (N = 13) | Neuropsychological Testing, MRI | No significant differences noted at six months follow-up evaluation. |
| Jordan et al. (1992) | Cross-Sectional | Professional boxers (N = 338) | CT | Brain atrophy was associated with cavum septum pellucidum. History of abnormal CT scan associated with history of TKO/KO. |
| Stewart et al. (1994) | Prospective Cohort | Amateur boxers (N = 484) | Neuropsychological Testing, EEG, BAER, Atoxea | Increasing numbers of bouts at baseline correlated with impaired performance in memory, visuoconstruction, and perceptual/motor ability. |

exposure is related inversely to performance on neuropsychological testing of memory and concentration (18). A clinical observation in the boxing community is that the majority of injuries occur during sparring. This finding probably reflects the longer duration of time spent sparring compared to active competition. According to data from the USMA (27), the absolute number of boxing injuries is higher during sparring, but the injury rate per unit time of exposure is higher for competitive boxing.

### 5.2.2 Exposure

According to Roberts (24), boxers who boxed longer than 10 years or had more than 150 fights had an increased risk of CBI attributable to boxing compared to those who boxed fewer years. According to Stewart et al. (25), the total number of amateur boxing contests was associated with impaired neuropsychological test performance. McLatchie et al. (23) noted that abnormal neurological examinations correlated with increasing number of fights.

## 6. Suggestions for Injury Prevention

### 6.1 Players

Boxers should avoid excessive sparring and prolonged exposure to boxing as evidenced by duration of career, age at retirement, and number of fights. Accordingly, medical research needs to be conducted in order to recommend or estimate a "relatively" safe level of boxing exposure that minimizes injury. Boxers who continue to box should be proficient at their craft. Poor performance increases the risk of brain injury, and therefore, boxers with consistently poor performances should undergo a comprehensive medical and neurological evaluation with possible consideration for suspension.

### 6.2 Sport

Regulatory agencies or governing organizations in professional boxing should collectively enforce uniform medical standards nationwide. Currently, the regulation of professional boxing varies from state to state. Accordingly, enforcement of medical suspensions and surveillance of serious medical injuries that prohibit competitive boxing are less than optimal. A national registry of professional boxers would allow the tracking of boxers as they travel among the various boxing jurisdictions and help identify boxers who are medically suspended.

### 6.3 External Environment

In modern-era boxing, the condition of the boxing venue or arena is rarely a source of significant injury risk. However, it is paramount that an ambulance be present at boxing matches or that an alternate, preplanned mechanism for rapid evacuation of an injured boxer be implemented. This evacuation procedure should include the designation of a hospital that offers neurosurgical and neuroradiological services for medical evaluation and treatment. The ring floor should be padded with ensolite. Ring ropes should be attached securely to the ring or corner posts to prevent the boxer from being propelled out of the ring. The corner posts should also be adequately padded.

### 6.4 Health Support System

The ringside physician and health support system are extremely important for injury prevention. Physicians who provide medical services to boxers should be trained in the diagnosis, management, and prevention of boxing-related injuries. Duties of the ringside physician should include prefight medical and neurological examinations, injury surveillance during boxing competitions, and postfight evaluations of suspected injuries.

## 7. Suggestions for Further Research

Brain injury represents the major health concern of modern-day boxing. The continuation of boxing in our society depends on maximizing safety and minimizing severe permanent irreversible traumatic brain injury. The focus of future medical research will be preventing neurological injury. Epidemiological investigation will be essential in expanding our current knowledge. Unfortunately, our current understanding is poorly delineated and is limited by too few good-quality epidemiological studies.

The scarcity of good-quality epidemiological investigations is largely attributed to methodological limitation in study design that adversely influences the validity and precision of the data and information collected. Failure to recognize and address methodological issues can limit the interpretation of the study. Several factors may influence the efficacy of an epidemiological investigation of boxing injuries and potentially introduce bias. These factors include injury definition, study population, study design, data-collection methods, and the members of the research team.

## 7.1 Injury Definition

Epidemiological investigations will need to distinguish neurological from nonneurological injuries. In addition, ABI will need to be differentiated from CBI. Prospective investigations of large, well-defined boxing populations with adequate controls exemplify the prototypic epidemiological investigation. Furthermore, detailed and sophisticated diagnostic procedures will be necessary to more accurately define injury.

## 7.2 Study Population

The ascertainment of an adequate study population along with appropriate controls is an important methodological consideration in the epidemiologic investigation of boxing injuries (16). The cases should be clearly identified as being representative of a particular boxing population (e.g., active vs. retired or amateur vs. professional; 16). The control groups should share similar socioeconomic and educational levels to prevent introduction of unintentional brain injury (16).

## 7.3 Study Design

There are essentially three epidemiological approaches to the investigation of boxing-related injury. These include cross-sectional, case control, and cohort studies (16). The ideal epidemiological investigation would include a cohort of boxers and controls matched according to age, race, education, and socioeconomic level that were evaluated before participation in boxing and followed prospectively through life with periodic medical evaluations.

## 7.4 Data Collection Methods

Prospective data collection is unequivocally superior to retrospective data collection that may be influenced by selective recall. In boxing, the documentation of and measurement of boxing exposure is crucial in the establishment of a causal relationship via applicable dose-response curves. Accordingly, the documentation of boxing exposure

during competition and sparring/training is a paramount epidemiological consideration (16).

## 7.5 Research Team

The ideal research team for the epidemiological investigation of boxing-related injuries should include a knowledgeable clinical epidemiologist and strong biostatistical support. In addition, the team should have clinical and practical experience related to boxing and sports medicine as it pertains to various organ systems (e.g., nervous system, visual system, musculoskeletal system).

# References

1. Blonstein, J.L.; Clarke, E. Further observations on the medical aspects of amateur boxing. Br. Med. J. 1:362-364; 1957.
2. Brookler, K.H.; Itil, T.; Jordan B.D. Electrophysiologic testing in boxers. In: Medical aspects of boxing. Ed. B.D. Jordan. CRC Press, Boca Raton, 1993: 207-214.
3. Brooks, N.; Kupshik, G.; Wilson, L.; et al. A neuropsychological study of active amateur boxers. J. Neurol. Neurosurg. Psych. 50:997-1000; 1987.
4. Critchley, M. Medical aspects of boxing, particularly from a neurological standpoint. Br. Med. J. 1:357-362; 1957.
5. Drew, R.H.; Templer, D.I.; Schuyler, B.A.; et al. Neuropsychological deficits in active licensed professional boxers. J. Clin. Psych. 42:520-525; 1986.
6. Enzenauer, R.W.; Montrey, J.S.; Enzenauer, R.J.; et al. Boxing-related injuries in the U.S. Army, 1980 through 1985. JAMA 261:1463-1466; 1989.
7. Estwanik, J.J.; Boitano, M.; Ari, N. Amateur boxing injuries at the 1981 and 1982 USA/ABF national championships. Phys. Sportsmed. 12:123-128; 1984.
8. Jordan, B.D. Medical and safety reforms in boxing. JNMA 80:407-412; 1988.
9. Jordan, B.D.; Campbell, E. Acute boxing injuries among professional boxers in New York State: a two-year survey. Phys. Sportsmed. 16(1):87-91; 1988.
10. Jordan, B.D. Neurologic injuries in boxing. In: Sports neurology. Ed. B.D. Jordan, P. Tsairis, R.F. Warren. Aspen Press, Maryland, 1989:219-228.
11. Jordan, B.D.; Zimmerman, R.D. Computerized tomography (CT) and magnetic resonance imaging (MRI) comparisons in boxers. JAMA 163:1670-1674; 1990.
12. Jordan, B.D.; Voy, R.O.; Stone, J. Amateur boxing injuries at the United States Olympic training center. Phys. Sportsmed. 18(2):80-90; 1990.
13. Jordan, B.D.; Jahre, C.; Hauser, W.A.; et al. CT of 338 active professional boxers. Radiology 185:509-512; 1992a.

14. Jordan, B.D.; Jahre, C.; Hauser, W.A.; et al. Serial computed tomography in professional boxers. J. Neuromag. 2:181-185; 1992b.

15. Jordan, B.D. Increasing medical safety in boxing. In: Medical aspects of boxing. Ed. B.D. Jordan. CRC Press, Boca Raton, 1993a:17-21.

16. Jordan, B.D. Epidemiology of brain injury in boxing. In: Medical aspects of boxing. Ed. B.D. Jordan. CRC Press, Boca Raton, 1993b:147-168.

17. Jordan, B.D. Chronic neurologic injuries in boxing. In: Medical aspects of boxing. Ed. B.D. Jordan. CRC Press, Boca Raton, 1993c:178-185.

18. Jordan, B.D..; Matser, E.; Zimmerman, R.D.; et al. Sparring and neuropsychological test performance among professional boxers (in preparation).

19. Larsson, L.W.; Melin, K.A.; Nortstrom-Ohrberg, G.; et al. Acute head injuries in boxers. Acta. Physhiat. Neurol. Scand. (Suppl.) 95:1-42; 1954.

20. Levin, H.S.; Lippold, C.S.; Goldman, A.; et al. Neurobehavioral functioning and magnetic resonance imaging findings in young boxers. J. Neurosurg. 67:657-667; 1987.

21. Lundberg, G.D. Medical arguments for non participation in boxing. In: Medical aspects of boxing. Ed. B.D. Jordan. CRC Press, Boca Raton, 1993c:11-15.

22. McCown, I.A. Boxing injuries. Am. J. Surg. 98:509-616; 1958.

23. McLatchie, G.; Brooks, N.; Galraith, S.; et al. Clinical neurological examination, neuropsychology, electroencephalography, and computed tomographic head scanning in active amateur boxers. J. Neurol. Neurosurg. Psych. 50:96-99; 1987.

24. Roberts, A.H. Brain damage in boxers. London: Pitman Medical Scientific Publishing Co.; 1969.

25. Stewart, W.F.; Gordon, B.; Selves, O.; et al. Prospective study of central nervous system function in amateur boxers in the United States. AJE 139:573-588;1994.

26. Thomassen, A.; Juul-Jensen, P.; Olivarius, B.; et al. Neurological electroencephalographic, and neuropsychological examination of 53 former amateur boxers. Acta Neurol. Scand. 60:352-362; 1979.

27. Welch, M.J.; Sitler, M.; Kroeten, H. Boxing injuries from an instructional program. Phys. Sportsmed. 14(9):81-89; 1986.

# 9

# Dance

*Caroline G. Caine and James G. Garrick*

## 1. Introduction

The art and science of dance has long been a part of the study of human motor performance. Dancers are not only artists; they are also athletes in that they train like athletes, possess the same high degree of fitness and endurance attributes (22, 127), and sustain many of the same injuries as other athletes (8). Physical activity whether for artistic, fitness, social, or purely kinesthetic purposes has become an integral aspect of our culture (187), thus involving ever-increasing numbers of participants at all levels of commitment. Dance is no exception. With theatrical, fitness, and recreational options available to anyone who wishes to participate, dance plays a significant role in the way we live our daily lives as casual participants in dance and the way we fulfill dreams as devotees of a selected dance idiom.

Regardless of the level of participation, injuries are inevitable. The purpose of this chapter is to provide an integrated perspective of the current dance injury information, based on the research literature, as it relates to theatrical dance idioms (e.g., ballet, modern dance, jazz dance, "show biz" dance) and aerobic dance, or dance for fitness. It is not within the scope of this chapter to address those dance forms that exist predominantly as a sociocultural manifestation (e.g., break dancing, folk dancing, ballroom and current social dance forms, Morris dancing, Flamenco, or other dance forms that reflect a particular cultural heritage).

The literature search for this chapter was limited to published, English-language, peer-reviewed reports since 1975 and involved the ancestral approach as well as searches in the following databases: Medline, January 1975 through December 1993 (descriptors: injury/ies, injured in combination with dance, danced, dance-like, dancer,

dancers, dances, dancing, dancing injuries, dancing physiology, dancing psychology, dancing trends), and SPORT Discus, January 1975 through June 1993 (descriptors: dance, dance injuries). Those reports that seemed to be written for the popular audience rather than from a research perspective were eliminated as were those that seemed to duplicate an author's previously reported data and those that reported data incompletely, thus making it impossible to assess them.

The kinds of questions this chapter has set out to illuminate are the following: Which dance idioms seem to contribute to the most injuries and to the most injuries of a serious nature? Which participants, and in which dance idioms, are at highest risk of injury? To what extent are dance injuries avoidable, whether in one of the theatrical dance idioms or aerobic dance? There are clues throughout the literature, but there are yet few definitive answers; the research literature is replete with limitations, originating in the characteristic case report and case series design that makes up most of the dance injury literature. Unfortunately, much of what is espoused in the dance community concerning injuries, their causes, and their cures is based seemingly on an unrestrained enthusiasm about information that these data cannot support because of inherent biases in their research designs. Therefore, it is essential that undeserved credence not be given to the data extracted from the research reports that are reviewed in this chapter without first realizing that all investigations are not equally valid. Limitations in the dance literature that impede our making comparisons between and among studies and progressing toward bottom-line answers include *lack of* the following:

- Uniform injury definition, particularly in terms of injury rate

- Uniform definition of specific injury types, such as "shin splints"
- Distinction between injury types (e.g., sprains, strains, fractures), and injury locations (e.g., shoulder pain)
- Standard nomenclature for injury types and injury locations, which are well-established in the medical literature
- Uniform terms by which to report injury severity
- Adequate sample sizes
- Information about the population from which the injured dancers came (denominator)
- Controlled data collection

To correct these limitations, we need to conduct randomized control studies that will substantiate the implications found in case and case series studies. In spite of the limitations, it is the intent of this chapter to find the best answers possible at this point in time by presenting the various properties and findings of the studies in as integrative a way as possible so as to approach a global picture of theatrical dance and aerobic dance injuries.

## 2. Incidence of Injury

### 2.1 Injury Rates

How injuries occur in dance, and at what rate, depends largely on the prevailing conditions at the time of injury: Was the injury incurred by a ballet dancer or an aerobics dancer, by a child or an adult, by a student or a professional? We present injury-rate data, first in terms of the different dance forms and then in terms of participant-specific data, in order to answer these kinds of questions.

#### 2.1.1 Injury Rates in Theatrical Dance Forms

Only three prospective studies from which injury rates can be deduced or calculated have been conducted in theatrical dance idioms. Table 9.1 presents data from those studies. All of these data should be interpreted with caution, as the range of study results is too diverse to support an integrative analysis. Obviously, the differences in study designs, populations, methodologies, and definitions contribute to this variability. Nonetheless, the following points can be made:

- Injury rates among the studies reflect the differences in the studies themselves. Although all three studies are prospective in design, Reid's study (141) of ballet students, aged 10.4

to 18.8 years who danced between 2 and 25 hours per week, reflects a different injury picture from the study conducted by Clanin et al. (24), who followed advanced and professional college-age dancers through a typical multi-disciplinary college dance curriculum. By the same token, a typical college dancer will experience dance differently from a typical pre-professional dancer who is training at a performing arts center, as reflected in the prospective study conducted by Rovere and colleagues (151).

- Medical diagnosis was employed in the data collection for all three studies, but injury definition was lacking in all of them. Furthermore, it seems that only those injuries that were reported by the dancers were recognized. No information regarding unreported injuries or complaints was provided.
- While no injury rates per 1,000 hours of exposure could be calculated, a rate based on 100 hours of exposure could be estimated from the information provided in the reports. A further calculation of the number of hours of activity required for a complaint to occur has also been provided in Table 9.1.

What the data in Table 9.1 do not indicate is the relationship of injury rate to skill level. As dancers advance, they spend more time in the studio and on stage performing increasingly challenging steps. Clearly, there is a need for well-designed studies in all age and proficiency groups before accurate injury rates can be ascertained.

#### 2.1.2 Injury Rates in Fitness Dance Forms

The eight epidemiologic studies concerning aerobic dance injuries from which injury rates can be deduced or calculated are presented in Table 9.2. The magnitude of the aerobic dance population, at one time estimated at 39 million participants (108), suggests a greater medical and public health problem than that presented by all other dance forms in aggregate, thereby spawning more research and producing more epidemiologic data in aerobics than in theatrical dance idioms. Thus, the rates in Table 9.2 may be considered with slightly more confidence than those in Table 9.1. Yet again, the rates must be interpreted with caution because of differences in injury definition, study design and conduct, and study population. Nonetheless, a general injury picture can be drawn, as follows:

- Among the retrospective studies in which a comparison can be made, the injury rate per

**Table 9.1    A Comparison of Injury Rates in Theatrical Dance**

| Study | Design | Methods | Duration | Injuries (number) | Sample size | Age | Rate: # injuries/100 participant seasons | Rate: # injuries/100 hours of exposure | Hours of activity/injury |
|---|---|---|---|---|---|---|---|---|---|
| Ballet: | | | | | | | | | |
| Reid (1987) (students) | Prospective | Questionnaire interview physical exam medical records | 6.4 yr[a] | 252 | 75 | mean 13.5 yr | 336.0 | 0.09 | 1,159.2 |
| Mixed idioms: | | | | | | | | | |
| Clanin et al. (1986) (collegiate) | Prospective | Physical exam Medical diagnosis | 2 academic yr (approx. 39 wk/yr) | 335 (in 159 dancers) | 268 | mean 26 yr | 125.0 | 0.11 | 936.0 |
| Rovere et al. (1983) (advanced students) | Prospective | Medical diagnosis | 9 mo | 352 (in 185 dancers) | 218 | 15-22 yr | 161.5 | 0.28 | 357.1 |

[a]All subjects had danced at least 1 yr at 3 hr/wk minimum; average number of weeks off season was 10.6 wk/yr.

**Table 9.2   A Comparison of Injury Rates in Aerobic Dance**

| Study | Method (% responce rate) | Duration | Proficiency level | Injuries (number) | Sample size | Age | Rate: # injuries/100 participant seasons | Rate: # injuries/100 hours of exposure | Hours of activity/injury |
|---|---|---|---|---|---|---|---|---|---|
| **Prospective** | | | | | | | | | |
| Allen et al. (1986) | Questionnaire (baseline) | 6 mo | Moderate-to-intense | 38 | 229 | —a | 16.6 | 3.5 | 289.3 |
| students | | | | | | | | | |
| judo surface | Goniometer | | | 20 | 146 | | 13.7 | 2.9 | 350.4 |
| gym surface | Med. exam | | | 18 | 83 | | 21.7 | 4.5 | 221.3 |
| | Squat test | | | | | | | | |
| Garrick et al. (1986) | Questionnaire (baseline) | 16 wk^b | — | 327 | 411 | | 79.6 | 1.09 | 91.7 |
| students | Interview (weekly) | | | 244 | 351 | 32.54 yr | 69.5 | 1.16^c | 86.2 |
| instructors | | | | 83 | 60 | 31.73 yr | 138.3 | 0.93^c | 107.5 |
| **Retrospective** | | | | | | | | | |
| Francis et al. (1985) instructors | Questionnaire (67.5) | —d | — | 220 | 135 | 15-50+ yr (77% of them were 20-35 yr old) | 163.0 | 0.22 | 454.5 |
| Hayes (1985) students | Questionnaire (51.3) | — | — | 615 | 410 | 27.2 yr | 150.0 | — | — |
| Janis (1990)^e students/ instructors | Questionnaire (—) | —f | 20% low impact 30% intermediate 40% advanced 10% extended advanced | 206 | 375 | 15-60 yr | 27.5 | — | — |
| high impact | | | | | 309 | | | | |
| low impact | | | | | 66 | | | | |
| Mutoh et al. (1988) | Questionnaire (—) | 5 yr | Mixed | | | | | | |
| students | | | | 250 | 800 | 19-41 yr | 15.6 | —g | |
| instructors | | | | 196 | 161 | 24.7 ± 3.21 | 40.4 | —g | |
| Richie et al. (1985) | Questionnaire (> 50%) | — | Mixed | | | | | | |
| students | | | | 1180 | 1291 | — | 91.4 | | |
| instructors | | | | 1075 | 1233 | 11-71 yr | 87.2 | 1.01 | 99.0 |
| | | | | 105 | 58 | 20-60 yr | 72.4 | 0.29 | 344.8 |
| Rothenberger et al. (1988) students | Questionaire (99.8) | — | Mixed | 1228 | 726 | 13-70 yr mean 31.5 yr | 84.6 | 0.50 | — |

a Broad cross-section of university students, staff, and faculty.
b Students completed an average of 12.26 weeks; instructors 12.73 weeks.
c These rates include Grade I through Grade IV complaints. If Grade I is dropped, the number of time-loss injuries becomes 84 and the injury rates become 0.29 per 100 hours of activity for students and 0.26 for instructors.
d Average duration of teaching was 2 years; therefore, amassed hours = approx. 100,246.
e Included 2 low impact, 3 intermediate, 4 advanced, and 1 extended advanced classes.
f Average length of participation was 129 weeks for females and 75 weeks for males; instructors had been teaching at least 2 years.
g Mutoh reports an injury rate in this category as low as 0.17 for instructors and 0.15 for students, but that rate represents only 1 of 13 fitness facilities.

100 participant seasons seems higher in instructors (range = 40.4-163.0) (50, 126, 145) than in students (range = 15.6-150.0) (74, 126, 145, 149); yet, when based on exposure (number of injuries per 100 hours of activity), students seem to experience more injuries (range = 0.15-1.01) than instructors (range = 0.17-0.29). The stronger evidence from the prospective reports seems to support these comparisons (3, 57).

- Injury rates may be characterized by frequency of classes per week (50, 57, 74, 85, 145, 149, 163). On average, retrospective data indicate that taking three classes per week is safer than taking four or more classes per week (85, 145, 149, 163), if for no other reason than the difference in exposure (time at risk). Yet, when the injury rate was calculated per class or per hour in a prospective study by Garrick et al. (57), the injury rate (per hour) steadily decreased as the number of classes per week increased from one class per week to four classes per week and from one class per week to nine classes per week. It is not known whether a selection process was taking place here.

- Retrospective data suggest that the longer someone participates in this activity, the more likely an injury will occur (50, 145, 149, 163). Although they provided no injury rates, Stephens and Ransom (163) confirmed that the proportion of injured versus uninjured dancers in their retrospective study increased after participating 12 months or more. They also found that more dancers get injured in the 1st month of activity than in the ensuing 11 months, hypothesizing that a generally poor fitness condition prior to participation may predispose the relatively new participants to injuries. Unfortunately, none of the studies reported these findings in terms of rates (e.g., number of injuries per 100 hours of activity), nor did they mention drop-out subjects.

- Age may correlate to injury rate (85, 149, 163). Rothenberger et al. (149) and Janis (85) found higher injury frequencies in middle-age participants, whereas Stephens and Ransom (163) reported higher injury frequencies in the 21 to 25 and 31 to 35 age groups. On the other hand, Richie et al. (145) and Mutoh et al. (126) found no correlation between age and injury. Again, none of the studies reported their findings in terms of rates or drop-out subjects.

## 2.2 Reinjury Rates

The lack of information regarding reinjury rates in dancers is alarming, given both the anecdotal knowledge and the empirical evidence that reinjury occurs in athletic endeavors. The definition of reinjury is also unclear in the dance literature wherein such terms as old, repeated, or recurrent injuries may be found. Reinjury implies that a previous injury has healed prior to its recurrence and that its recurrence is characterized by the same type, location, and onset as the original injury. Without this clarification, there is no assurance that reinjuries, and not chronic injuries, are being reported.

The few studies that report reinjury rates in theatrical dancers employ a variety of implied definitions for "rate." Expressed as a percentage of all injuries, Clanin et al. (24) and Rovere et al. (151) reported reinjury rates as 16.1% and 4.5%, respectively. It was also possible to convert Clanin's data into rates expressed as number of reinjuries per 100 participant seasons (20.2), as well as per 100 hours of exposure (0.02). Clanin et al. identified strains as the most frequent type of recurring injury, and Rovere et al. located most recurring injuries in the spine. On a different note, Reid et al. (141) expressed reinjury rate in terms of injured dancers, which made it impossible to compare his data with others.

Among aerobic dance studies, Francis et al. (50) reported a reinjury rate of 35.9%, expressed as a percentage of all injuries in their study. Garrick et al. (57) examined both the frequency and location of reinjuries. Among students, 57.5% of those with a history of prior injuries were reinjured whereas only 39.8% of those previously uninjured became casualties. Among instructors, the proportions were 70.6% and 76.7%, respectively. In aggregate, 31% of the injuries were reinjuries. While the severity of the reinjuries appeared to be no greater than the original injuries, anatomic sites appeared to be linked to likelihood of reinjury. For example, students with a history of foot, ankle, leg/shin, or knee injuries were twice as likely to be reinjured as were those without previous problems.

## 2.3 Injury Rates in Class Practice vs Rehearsal vs Performance

There are virtually no epidemiologic data available that address this aspect of injury rates. In theatrical dancers, only Bowling (12) provides us with data, as follows: 15.5% of injuries occur in class, 27.6%

in rehearsal, 32.8% during performance, and 24.1% of injuries could not be attributed specifically to any of the situations. Unfortunately, there is no denominator information allowing the calculation of rates, so these percentages are somewhat meaningless. Nonetheless, it is interesting to note the potential dangers of performance in light of the fact that more time is spent in class and rehearsal than in performance.

# 3. Injury Characteristics

## 3.1 Injury Onset

It is generally understood that most injuries to theatrical and aerobic dancers are characterized by gradual onset or overuse. Unfortunately, specific figures go largely unreported, for only one epidemiologic study was found that reported such data in theatrical dance idioms and only two in aerobic dance.

- Of their 335 reported injuries, Clanin et al. (24) identified the etiologies of 109 injuries in their prospective study. Of these, 41.6% were attributed to overuse, although overuse injury was not defined in their study. They also reported that ballet class was responsible for two times and five times as many overuse injuries as modern dance and jazz classes, respectively.
- Among aerobic dance studies, Garrick et al. (57) and Mutoh et al. (126) found that approximately 80% of injuries are overuse whereas Allen et al. (3) reported 16.6%. This astonishing difference in results may be attributed to the populations studied—dancers from aerobic fitness facilities (in the two former studies) versus dancers from a university recreation program (in the latter study). Furthermore, Allen et al. sought different data than the other two studies, which may have affected the results.

## 3.2 Injury Types

The current shortage of prospective and retrospective dance injury studies prevents assessment of injury type from an integrative perspective. As shown in Table 9.3, inconsistent categorization and, in some cases, vague diagnoses of injury types among the studies preclude comparisons.

To enable comparison by providing a larger pool of data, case series data are shown in Table 9.4. While data in prospective and retrospective studies are considered the more cogent in that they can show the incidence of specific injury types within a population of both injured and uninjured dancers, series data are capable of showing how prevalent specific injury types are only within the injured population of dancers. In spite of this sample bias, series data can be valuable.

### 3.2.1 Injury Types in Theatrical Dance Forms

There are 464 injuries to 627 theatrical dancers represented in the prospective and retrospective studies shown in Table 9.3, and most of these are strains and sprains. Similarly, most of the injuries presented in Table 9.4 were strains although there is some confusion with the data in two of the case series. Solomon and Micheli (161) report a relatively large proportion of ligamentous injuries; Washington (179) reports relatively large proportions of both ligamentous injuries and back pain, yet he shows no sprains or strains. It is speculated that some of these injuries may have been strains or sprains.

According to Solomon and Micheli (161), Reid (141), and Schaflé et al. (157), the back seems to be most vulnerable to strains. Rovere et al. (151) goes further in his prospective study to report that cervical and upper back strains occurred roughly twice as often in modern dancers as in ballet dancers, and strains of the lower back and hamstrings, as well as shin splints, occurred roughly twice as often in ballet dancers as in modern dancers. These results are not comparable among the studies, however, because the data vary widely in terms of definition of some types of injuries, which subsequently affects how the data were recorded in each study.

Although fractures do not appear to be prevalent among dancers as represented in Tables 9.3 and 9.4, increasing evidence is emerging that shows a strong correlation between bone injuries and irregular or absent menses. The strongest evidence comes from the randomized control trial conducted by Benson et al. (10), although there were only 49 subjects. They found that dancers with abnormal menstrual function had more bone injuries than normally menstruating dancers ($p < .05$). Kadel and associates (88) corroborate this finding in their retrospective investigation of stress fractures in 54 dancers whose heavy (> 5 hours/day) training schedules and prolonged amenorrheic intervals contribute independently to the risk of fracture ($p < .025$ and $p < .001$, respectively). Similar findings were reported by Warren et al. (178) in their retrospective and cross-sectional

**Table 9.3   A Percent Comparison of Injury Types in Prospective and Retrospective Dance Studies**

| Injury type | N/Level: | Theatrical idioms: Bowling (1989) Retrospective 141/professional | Clanin et al. (1986) Prospective 268/college | Rovere et al. (1983) Prospective 218/advanced | Aerobic Dance: Rothenberger et al. (1988) Retrospective 726/students |
|---|---|---|---|---|---|
| Abrasion | | 0.0 | 0.0 | 0.0 | 0.0 |
| Back Pain | | —[a] | 3.7 | — | 0.0 |
| Chondromalacia patella | | 0.0 | 1.8 | 3.4 | 0.0 |
| Contusion | | 12.1[b] | 3.7 | 4.3 | 0.0 |
| Dislocation | | 15.5[a] | 1.8 | 0.0 | 0.0 |
| Fracture | | 10.3 | 0.0 | 0.0 | 1.8 |
| Hip pain | | 0.0 | 0.0 | 14.2 | 0.0 |
| Impingement | | 0.0 | 0.0 | 0.3 | 0.0 |
| Inflammation | | 0.0 | 7.4 | 1.7 | 2.9 |
| Knee pain | | 0.0 | 0.0 | 1.1 | 0.0 |
| Ligamentous injury | | —[c] | 0.0 | 3.4 | 5.9 |
| Muscle spasm | | 0.0 | 11.1 | 0.0 | 0.0 |
| Nonspecific pain | | 0.0 | 0.0 | 0.0 | 0.0 |
| Sprain | | 60.3[c] | 18.5 | 15.6 | 6.5 |
| Strain | | —[c] | 20.4 | 17.6[d] | 14.8 |
| Stress fracture | | 0.0 | 1.8 | 0.8 | 5.3 |
| Stress lesion (shin splint) | | 1.7 | 0.0 | 5.4 | 10.7 |
| Tendinitis | | 0.0 | 13.0 | 13.9 | 12.4 |
| Torn/pulled muscle | | —[c] | 0.0 | 0.0 | 0.0 |
| Other | | 0.0 | 16.7 | 13.4 | 40.2[e] |
| Total Injuries | | 58 | 54 | 352 | 1228 |
| Total % | | 99.9 | 99.9 | 99.9 | 100.0 |

[a]Includes problems with the back (including vertebrae) and injuries to cartilage.

[b]Includes bruising, swelling, or inflammation of muscles or tissues.

[c]Includes sprains, strains, tears, or pulls of muscles or ligaments.

[d]Mostly strains to the upper and lower back.

[e]Includes 385 injuries not diagnosed by a physician.

study on bone mineral content and menstrual function. While the correlation between stress fractures and delayed menarche was not statistically significant, secondary amenorrhea ($p < .01$) and its duration ($p < .05$) were statistically significant. They also found a high incidence of fracture (61%) in the 75 dancers studied, and 69% of these were medically confirmed stress fractures. In a 1989 cross-sectional study, Hamilton et al. (66) also found a positive relationship between amenorrhea and stress fractures ($p < .05$), and correlated stress fractures in both male and female dancers to age upon entering their companies ($p < .05$). Warren et al. (177) also report the only epidemiologic evidence to date that addresses scoliosis in dancers—a prevalence of 24%, and the frequency rose with increased age at menarche ($p < .03$).

### 3.2.2 Injury Types in Fitness Dance Forms

The retrospective data in Table 9.3 reveal that, out of 1,228 injuries to 726 students, most aerobic students incur strains, tendinitis, and shin splints. By comparison, case series data reveal that mixed populations of injured aerobics instructors and students incur mostly shin splints and inflammation injuries. These figures are not comparable, however, because the data vary widely in terms of definition of some types of injuries, which subsequently affects how the data were recorded in each study.

## 3.3 Injury Location

Some interesting trends concerning injury location appear in Tables 9.5-9.8 that signal the kind of activity indigenous to each dance form. For instance, the implication from prospective and retrospective data (see Tables 9.5 and 9.7) is that the knee (range = 12.1-20.1) is the most frequently injured site in theatrical dancers and the leg/shin

**Table 9.4  A Percent Comparison of Injury Types Among Dancers in Case Series**

| Injury type | Theatrical idioms: | | | | | Aerobic Dance: | |
| | Garrick (1985) Ballet | Garrick (1985) Modern | Solomon & Micheli (1986) Mixed* | Washington (1978) Mixed | Garrick (1985)** | Hayes (1985)** | Vetter et al. (1985)* |
| N = | 1055 | 354 | 164 | — | 681 | 100 | 61 |
| Abrasion | — | — | 0.5 | 0.0 | — | 0.0 | 0.0 |
| Back pain | — | — | 0.0 | 16.7 | — | 7.5 | 6.2 |
| Chondromalacia patella | — | — | 6.1 | 2.2[a] | — | 17.7 | 15.4 |
| Contusion | 3.7 | 2.5 | 0.5 | 0.0 | 5.9 | 0.0 | 0.0 |
| Dislocation | 2.7 | 2.0 | 8.2 | 3.9[a] | 1.5 | 0.0 | 0.0 |
| Fracture | 8.2[b] | 8.5[b] | 5.6 | 10.4 | 13.7 | 0.0 | 0.0 |
| Hip pain | — | — | 0.0 | 6.3 | — | 4.7 | 0.0 |
| Impingement | — | — | 0.0 | 0.0 | — | 0.0 | 0.0 |
| Inflammation | 14.4 | 20.1 | 0.0 | 1.2 | 24.5 | 0.0 | 23.1 |
| Knee pain | 16.0[c] | 20.9[c] | 3.1 | 2.2 | 15.0[c] | 0.0 | 4.6 |
| Ligamentous injury | — | — | 20.9 | 17.6 | — | 0.0 | 0.0 |
| Muscle spasm | — | — | 2.0 | 0.0 | — | 0.0 | 0.0 |
| Nonspecific pain | — | — | 0.0 | 13.3 | — | 1.9 | 0.0 |
| Sprain | 10.7 | 12.4 | 4.1 | 0.0 | 6.0 | 0.0 | 0.0 |
| Strain | 23.6 | 22.3 | 14.3 | 0.0 | 24.8 | 12.1 | 3.1 |
| Stress fracture | —[b] | —[b] | 2.6 | 0.0 | — | 0.0 | 7.7 |
| Stress lesion (shin splint) | — | — | 5.1 | 15.0 | — | 39.3 | 21.5 |
| Tendinitis | — | — | 11.7 | 0.7 | — | 2.8 | 3.1 |
| Torn/pulled muscle | — | — | 6.6 | 1.7 | — | 0.0 | 0.0 |
| Other | 7.7[d] | 8.2[d] | 8.7 | 8.9 | 6.6 | 12.1 | 15.4 |
| Total injuries | — | — | 196 | 414 | — | 107 | 65 |
| Total % | 87.0 | 96.9 | 100.0 | 100.1 | 98.0 | 99.9 | 100.1 |

*Categorized as a mixed-idiom study; no control for injuries associated with either dance idiom.

**Includes both students and instructors.

[a]Includes dislocations of the knee and chondromalacia patella.

[b]Includes both acute and stress fractures.

[c]Includes patellofemoral disease and Osgood Schlatter syndrome.

[d]Includes degeneration and impingement injuries.

**Table 9.5   A Percent Comparison of Injury Location in Prospective and Retrospective Dance Studies: Theatrical Idioms**

| Anatomical site | Ballet: Reid (1987) (student) N = 75 prospective | Mixed Idioms: Bowling (1989) (professional) N = 141 retrospective | Mixed Idioms: Clanin et al. (1986) (collegiate) N = 268 prospective | Mixed Idioms: Rovere et al. (1983) (advanced) N = 185 prospective |
|---|---|---|---|---|
| Head/spine/trunk | (16.7) | (—) | (21.8) | (17.6) |
| Neck | 4.8[a] | 25.9[b] | 1.5 | 1.7 |
| Back | 10.7 | —[b] | 19.4 | 12.2 |
| Torso/abdomen | 1.2 | —[c] | 0.9 | 3.7 |
| Upper extremity | (9.6) | (5.2) | (4.5) | (0.0) |
| Shoulder | 2.4 | — | 2.7 | — |
| Arm | 1.2 | — | 1.8[e] | — |
| Elbow | 1.2 | — | —[e] | — |
| Wrist/hand | 4.8 | — | —[e] | — |
| Lower extremity | (73.7) | (—) | (60.9) | (71.1) |
| Hip/groin | 7.2 | 12.1[c] | 7.8 | 14.2 |
| Thigh | 9.5 | 10.3[d] | — | — |
| Knee | 20.1 | 12.1 | 14.9 | 14.5 |
| Leg/shin | 8.4 | —[d] | 18.2 | 5.4 |
| Ankle | 15.4 | 18.9 | 9.3 | 22.2[g] |
| Heel/achilles | 0.0 | 0.0 | 0.0 | —[g] |
| Foot/toes | 13.1 | 15.5 | 10.7 | 14.8 |
| Other | 0.0 | 0.0 | 12.8[f] | 11.4 |
| Total injuries | 252 | 58 | 335 | 352 |
| Total % | 100.0 | 100.0 | 100.0 | 100.1 |

[a]Includes both head and neck injuries.

[b]Includes both back and neck injuries.

[c]Includes hip/groin/ribs injuries.

[d]Includes thigh and leg injuries.

[e]Includes all upper extremity injuries except shoulder injuries.

[f]Includes 9 "other" injuries and 34 injuries unaccounted for by the authors.

[g]Includes both ankle and Achilles injuries.

(range = 16.8-40.5) in aerobic dancers. How reliable are these conclusions?

Although the study populations and designs differ markedly, the prospective and retrospective data in Table 9.5 reveal that the knee may be the most vulnerable site in theatrical dancers, but it is difficult to ignore the high percentages of back injuries in the mixed idioms. The case series data in Table 9.6 seem to confirm the knee as the most frequently injured site in dancers overall, followed closely by foot and ankle injuries. Yet again, focusing on only the mixed-idiom studies, the back emerges as a vulnerable site, thus adding credence to the prospective and retrospective data.

Suspected injury mechanisms for knee injuries in dancers have traditionally been related to malalignment through the segments of the lower extremity from hip to ankle. Clippinger-Robertson et al. (28) demonstrated in their combined retrospective and cross-sectional study that both lack of perfect turnout and a shallow *demi-plié* can lead theatrical dancers toward knee injuries. Injuries to the knee and tibia have been prospectively correlated with malalignment through the lower extremity and subtalar pronation in aerobic dancers (3).

In aerobic dancers, it is not surprising that both students and instructors suffer from leg/shin pain (see Table 9.7). Like runners, aerobic dancers repetitively stress the structures of the lower leg, with little variation in rhythm.

In addition to the epidemiologic evidence presented in Table 9.7, data from case series are presented in Table 9.8. Injuries to the knee are

**Table 9.6   A Percent Comparison of Injury Location in Case Series*: Theatrical Idioms**

| | Ballet: | | | | Modern: | Mixed idioms: | |
|---|---|---|---|---|---|---|---|
| Anatomical site   N= | Garrick (1985) 1055 | Garrick (1988) — | Micheli (1983) — | Quirk (1983) 664 | Garrick (1985) 354 | Solomon & Micheli** (1986) 164 | Washington (1978) — |
| Head/spine/trunk | (9.0) | (8.0) | (13.3) | (8.5) | (10.5) | (27.8) | (24.1) |
| Neck | — | — | 0.0 | 0.0 | — | 4.4 | 5.5 |
| Back | 9.0 | 8.0 | 13.3 | 8.5 | 10.5 | 23.2 | 18.6 |
| Torso/abdomen | — | — | — | — | — | 0.2 | 0.0 |
| Upper extremity | (3.8) | — | (3.6) | (0.0) | (2.5) | (2.2) | (12.0) |
| Shoulder | 2.1 | — | 0.0 | 0.0 | 1.1 | 2.2 | 6.0 |
| Arm | 1.7[a] | — | 0.0 | 0.0 | 1.4[a] | — | 0.0 |
| Elbow | — | — | 0.0 | 0.0 | — | — | 1.9 |
| Wrist/hand | — | — | 0.0 | 0.0 | — | — | 4.1 |
| Lower extremity | (84.9) | (81.7) | (83.2) | (80.4) | (85.5) | (70.0) | (61.1) |
| Hip/groin | 9.7 | 10.0 | 20.5[b] | 8.6 | 7.6 | 11.4 | 7.5 |
| Thigh/hamstring | 2.7 | — | — | 4.3 | 3.9 | 4.8 | 0.0 |
| Knee | 22.9 | 20.6 | 38.6 | 17.3 | 34.7 | 20.1 | 14.7 |
| Leg/shin | 11.4 | 12.7 | 0.0 | 7.8 | 5.1 | 7.0 | 15.0 |
| Ankle | 16.6 | 15.8 | 24.1[c] | 22.3 | 11.0 | 19.7 | 13.3 |
| Heel/Achilles | — | — | —[c] | 0.0 | — | — | 0.0 |
| Foot/toes | 21.6 | 22.6 | —[c] | 20.1 | 23.2 | 7.0 | 10.6 |
| Other | — | — | 0.0 | 11.1 | — | — | 2.6 |
| Total injuries | — | 1243 | 83 | 2113 | — | 229 | 414 |
| Total % | 97.7 | 89.7 | 96.5 | 100.0 | 98.5 | 100 | 99.8 |

*Does not include case series that focused on selected injury types.

**Categorized as a mixed-idiom study because there was no control for injuries associated with either dance idiom.

[a]Includes all upper extremity injuries except shoulder injuries.

[b]Includes all lower extremity injuries except foot and ankle injuries.

[c]Includes all foot and ankle injuries.

**Table 9.7  A Percent Comparison of Injury Location in Prospective and Retrospective Dance Studies: Aerobic Dance**

| Anatomical site | Francis et al. (1985) instructor N = 135 Retrospective | Garrick et al. (1986) student/instructor N = 351/50 Prospective | Hayes (1985) student N = 410 Retrospective | Janis (1990) student N = 375 Retrospective | Mutoh et al. (1988) student/instructor N = 800/161 Retrospective | | Richie et al. (1985) student/instructor N = 1233/58 Retrospective | | Rothenberger et al. (1988) student N = 726 Retrospective |
|---|---|---|---|---|---|---|---|---|---|
| Head/spine/trunk | (13.2) | (14.3) | (15.6) | (18.0) | (12.1) | (15.8) | (13.9) | (14.3) | (21.5) |
| Head | 0.0 | 0.0 | 0.0 | 0.5 | 2.4 | 0.5 | 0.0 | 0.0 | 0.2 |
| Neck | 0.0 | 1.2 | 0.0 | 4.9 | 1.6 | 2.6 | 4.8 | 4.8 | 4.4 |
| Back | 13.2 | 11.9 | 15.6 | 12.6 | 6.4 | 11.7 | 9.1 | 9.5 | 15.4 |
| Torso/abdomen | 0.0 | 1.2 | 0.0 | 0.0 | 1.7 | 1.0 | 0.0 | 0.0 | 1.5 |
| Upper extremity | (0.0) | (2.8) | (13.0) | (5.9) | (4.0) | (2.5) | (3.9) | (5.7) | (9.0) |
| Shoulder | 0.0 | 1.6 | — | 3.9 | 2.8 | 2.0 | 3.9 | 5.7 | 5.5 |
| Arm | 0.0 | 1.2 | — | 1.0 | 0.4 | 0.5 | 0.0 | 0.0 | 0.9 |
| Elbow | 0.0 | 0.0 | — | 0.5 | 0.4 | 0.0 | 0.0 | 0.0 | 0.6 |
| Wrist/hand | 0.0 | 0.0 | — | 0.5 | 0.4 | 0.0 | 0.0 | 0.0 | 2.0 |
| Lower extremity | (80.5) | (81.5) | (71.3) | (76.2) | (84.4) | (80.7) | (74.4) | (63.7) | (63.1) |
| Hip/groin | 5.5 | 4.5 | 0.0 | 1.9 | 8.4 | 5.6 | 3.0 | 1.9 | 2.9 |
| Thigh | 0.0 | 0.0 | 0.0 | 1.0 | 7.6 | 2.6 | 3.0 | 0.9 | 2.4 |
| Knee | 11.8 | 14.7 | 15.1 | 16.5 | 15.2 | 12.8 | 8.9 | 8.6 | 9.2 |
| Leg/shin | 34.5 | 28.7 | 40.5[a] | 25.7 | 16.8 | 24.5 | 35.4 | 33.3 | 30.9 |
| Ankle | 10.9 | 10.7 | 0.0 | 13.6 | 8.8 | 8.7 | 7.3 | 5.7 | 12.2 |
| Heel/Achilles | 0.0 | 0.0 | 0.0 | 3.4 | 6.4 | 4.1 | 3.1 | 1.9 | 0.0 |
| Foot/toes | 17.7 | 22.9 | 15.7 | 14.1 | 21.2 | 22.4 | 13.7 | 11.4 | 5.5 |
| Other | 6.4 | 1.2 | 0.0 | 0.0 | 0.0 | 3.6 | 7.8 | 16.2 | 6.3 |
| Total injuries | 220 | 244 | 615 | 206 | 250 | 209 | 1075 | 105 | 1228 |
| Total % | 100.0 | 99.8 | 99.9 | 100.1 | 100.5 | 102.6 | 100.0 | 99.9 | 99.9 |

[a]Includes shin splints (26.7%) and muscle cramps (13.8%).

**Table 9.8    A Percent Comparison of Injury Location in Case Series: Aerobic Dance**

| Anatomical site | N = | Belt (1990) 48 | Garrick (1985) 681 | Hayes (1985) 100 | Vetter et al. (1985) 61 |
|---|---|---|---|---|---|
| Head/spine/trunk | | (1.9) | (11.0) | (7.5) | (7.7) |
| Neck | | 0.0 | 0.0 | 0.0 | 1.5 |
| Back | | 1.9 | 11.0 | 7.5 | 6.2 |
| Torso/abdomen | | 0.0 | 0.0 | 0.0 | 0.0 |
| Upper extremity | | (1.9) | (4.5) | (3.8) | (3.1) |
| Shoulder | | 1.9 | 3.2 | 1.9 | 3.1 |
| Arm | | 0.0 | 1.3[a] | 0.0 | 0.0 |
| Elbow | | 0.0 | — | 0.0 | 0.0 |
| Wrist/hand | | 0.0 | — | 1.9 | 0.0 |
| Lower extremity | | (94.1) | (83.3) | (76.6) | (84.6) |
| Hip/groin | | 3.8 | 8.7 | 6.5 | 6.2 |
| Thigh | | 1.9 | 4.8 | 1.9 | 0.0 |
| Knee | | 32.7 | 32.6 | 17.7 | 21.5 |
| Leg | | 19.2 | 16.4 | 39.3 | 27.7 |
| Ankle | | 17.3 | 6.9 | 4.7 | 6.2 |
| Heel/Achilles | | 3.8 | 0.0 | 2.8 | 1.5 |
| Foot/toes | | 15.4 | 13.9 | 3.7 | 21.5 |
| Other | | 1.9 | 0.0 | 12.1 | 4.6 |
| Total injuries | | 52 | — | 107 | 65 |
| Total % | | 99.8 | 98.8 | 100.0 | 100.0 |

[a]Includes all upper extremity injuries except shoulder injuries.

prominent in the series data. Garrick (55), in finding that the knee was the most frequently injured site across all nine sports in his series that included dancers from all idioms, cautions that the knee may not necessarily be the most frequently injured anatomic site. Rather, he suggests, the data may reflect the degree of concern about and interest in knee injuries by the patients because of the potential complications of such injuries.

One retrospective aerobics study reported injury location as a function of age. Rothenberger et al. (149) found that the shin was most vulnerable in aerobic dancers under age 40 and that the lower back sustained more injuries in dancers over age 40. One case series on ballet dancers presented a general analysis of injury location in relation to age group and concomitant performance demands. In that study, Garrick (56) found the following relationships:

- Back injuries were seen more commonly in dancers over age 40
- Hip injuries were seen more commonly in 13- to 38-year-old dancers as well as those over 40
- Knee injuries ravaged every age group and increased with age and dancing commitment
- Leg injuries are most prevalent during the ages 13-25 years

- Ankle injuries are highest in 6- to 12-year-old dancers, in spite of their lower skill and participation levels. By contrast, between ages 13 and 25 the dancer increases both skill and participation levels, yet shows lower proportions of ankle injuries
- Foot injuries are seen more in age groups where learning and perfecting of *pointe* technique takes place, usually between 10 and 18 years

In general, Garrick's series data support the reasoning that injury patterns parallel aging problems wherein symptomatic residuals of previous injuries, as well as accumulated microtraumas over the years, might account for the prevalence of injuries at specific anatomical sites at certain stages of life.

An examination of injury types and frequency in relation to anatomical site can be accomplished through a summary of case reports, case series, and cross-sectional studies, which characterize most of the dance injury literature. The data from these studies are of limited statistical value, but they may enhance an understanding of the dance injury situation and are presented by general anatomic region below.

### 3.3.1 Head/Spine/Trunk

As shown in Tables 9.5 and 9.7, head/spine/trunk injuries comprise 20.9% of injuries in theatrical dancers and 15.6% and 13.8% in aerobic students and instructors, respectively. The more numerous case series data (see Tables 9.6 and 9.8) suggest that 10.5% may be an equally realistic figure for theatrical dancers and 9.9% for aerobic dancers, based on the limitations among studies presented in both the epidemiologic tables (Tables 9.5 and 9.7) and case series tables (Tables 9.6 and 9.8).

Most of the injuries in this anatomic region are to the spine, characterized by low back strain or other soft tissue injuries (24, 117, 151, 161, 179). Also, spondylolysis and spondylolisthesis are thought to be more prevalent in dancers than in the general population, and six cases have been reported in the series literature (161, 179). Two cases are described in reports by Abel (1) and Ireland and Micheli (83). In both cases, bilateral fractures occurred in the pedicles, which are mechanically stronger than the par interarticularis where fractures ordinarily occur, and are thought to be so situated because of the movements peculiar to classical ballet (e.g., dancing on *pointe* and thereby shifting the axis of stress through the pedicles). Table 9.9 shows these and other injuries to the head/spine/trunk in theatrical dancers.

Warren et al. (177) also found a prevalence of scoliosis in ballet dancers who experience delayed menarche. Although the scoliotic dancers did not complain of back pain or injuries, their data suggested a high risk of injury in that their bone age was delayed by 2 to 4 years and 2 subjects still had no fusion of the iliac apophyseal plates at age 19, thus leaving them vulnerable to possible growth plate injury, stress fractures, or both. Low lumbar bone density values have also been reported by Horváth and Holló (79) in four Hungarian ballerinas and by Armann et al. (5) in their cross-sectional study.

There are no case studies in aerobic dance that describe injuries to this anatomic region. However, Vetter et al. (175) reported one neck strain and four cases of low back pain without radiation in their series of 65 injuries.

### 3.3.2 Upper Extremity

Previous epidemiologic tables in this chapter show very few upper extremity injuries in theatrical dancers (4.0%) and aerobic dancers (9.1% in students, 5.6% in instructors). From Tables 9.6 and 9.8, theatrical dancers suffered 2.3% injuries to this body region, and aerobic dancers 4.2%. Strains and dislocations are typical shoulder injuries (138, 161, 179).

No case reports, case series, or cross-sectional studies were found to illustrate upper extremity injuries in theatrical dancers. In aerobic dancers Vetter et al. (175) reported two cases of shoulder impingement syndrome in their series of 65 injuries.

### 3.3.3 Lower Extremity

Lower extremity injuries to theatrical dancers, as reported in the epidemiologic literature, range from 60.9% to 73.3% (see Table 9.5). This includes all levels and age groups. In case series, the range is slightly higher, 63.7% to 85.5% (see Table 9.6). The most frequently injured component of the lower extremity is the knee that accounts for 18.8% and 22.9% of all injuries in the epidemiologic and case series literature, respectively.

Aerobic dance students incur 63.1% to 84.4% of total injuries to the lower extremity, and instructors 63.7% to 88.0% (see Table 9.7). The leg/shin is the site most affected at 16.8% to 40.5% and 24.1% to 34.5% for students and instructors, respectively. Case series data, which do not distinguish students from instructors, show 76.6% to 94.1% of injuries to the lower extremity with the knee as the most frequently reported site of complaint (see Table 9.8). The two studies with the smaller sample populations ($N = 48$ and $N = 61$) demonstrated the higher percentages of lower extremity injuries; therefore, the case series data are somewhat fallible.

#### 3.3.3.1 Lower Extremity Injuries in Theatrical Dance Forms.
Several informative discussions of lower extremity injuries in theatrical dancers exist in the literature (8, 27, 28, 43, 48, 67-71, 73, 80, 81, 92, 93, 100, 113, 139, 142, 143, 154, 159, 167, 168, 171, 172, 182, 185), and these should be consulted for detailed descriptions of diagnoses and treatments associated with the various injuries suffered by dancers.

Table 9.10 summarizes specific injuries to the lower extremity that were identified in case series and cross-sectional studies. For brevity, case reports have not been included in Table 9.10 except where they were discussed in the literature as case series. Instead, cases will be cited where appropriate to support the discussion below. While the data in Table 9.10 are not representative of injuries to the dance population as described in the epidemiologic literature (refer to Table 9.5), they expand

**Table 9.9   Case Reports, Case Series and Cross-Sectional Studies of Injuries Occurring in the Head/Spine/Trunk of Theatrical Dancers**

| Study | Idiom | Design | Subjects | Age | Level | Condition/diagnosis |
|---|---|---|---|---|---|---|
| Head | | | | | | |
| Spine | | | | | | |
| Abel (1985) | Ballet | Case | 1 F | 17 | — | Bilateral "jogger's" fracture of the pedicle of L4 with surrounding sclerosis |
| Horváth & Holló (1986) | Ballet | Cross-sectional | 4 F | 21-30 | Professional | 3 of 4 dancers had decreased bone mineral content in the spine, perhaps due to delayed menarche |
| Ireland & Micheli (1987) | Ballet | Case | 1 F | 18 | Professional | Bilateral fracture of the pedicle of L2 with surrounding sclerosis |
| Miller et al. (1975) | Ballet | Case | 1 M | 37 | Professional | Degenerative changes in the right sacroiliac joint and in the upper thoracic spine |
| | | | 1 M | 36 | Professional | Translumbar low back pain without radiation |
| Warren et al. (1986) | Ballet | Cross-sectional | 75 F | 18-36 | Professional | 24% had scoliosis, which may be related to delayed menarche; 2 of these had no fusion of the iliac apophyseal plates at age 19 |
| Trunk | | | | | | |
| Collins (1981) | Tassel dancing | Case | 1 F | 33 | Professional | Dilated duct system of the breast, with some periductal fibrosis, due to pierced nipple |

knowledge about specific injuries to dancers. Within limitations, generalizations about those injuries can be made as follows:

*Hip/pelvis.* Injuries to the hip/pelvis area have been described in case reports. These include hypertrophic osteoarthritic changes, contusion to the greater trochanter, and traction-type fatigue fractures in the femoral neck (123); and "snapping hip" syndrome (156). In their cross-sectional study of 11 patients with snapping hip, Jacobs and Young (84) probed the phenomenon of the snapping hip and discovered that the dancers with a narrower bi-iliac width are predisposed to this condition. Obviously, a study of 11 patients does not provide conclusive information, yet it offers potential direction for investigation.

Another type of hip injury, an unusual case of femoral head collapse associated with anorexia nervosa, was reported by Warren et al. (178). Because dancers generally neglect their diets and are at high risk for anorexia nervosa and delayed menarche (18, 54, 63, 64), they are subject to skeletal aberrations that do not often appear in the nondancer population.

*Thigh.* Case reports of thigh injuries in dancers have described two cases of femoral nerve injury, both in advanced-to-professional-level modern dancers (122, 153).

*Knee.* Complaints of chondromalacia patella have not yet appeared in case reports and cross-sectional studies, although the incidence could be as high as 8.2% (151). The difficulty with tracking the incidence of chondromalacia patella is that the term is often used loosely in the literature, or it may be lumped with anterior knee pain (141). Clippinger-Robertson and colleagues (28) did not verify by X ray, MRI, or arthroscopy that the subjects in their retrospective survey had this condition; however, they did select subjects for their cross-sectional follow-up study who presented with three or more classic symptoms of chondromalacia patella in order to compare their performance of second position *plié* cinematographically and electromyographically with matched controls. Their results, although limited by the research design, suggest that activation patterns during the *plié* can be altered in order to prevent knee problems.

Other examples of knee injuries in case reports include "jumper's knee," or patellar tendon tendinitis (47), meniscal tears (123), osteochondral fracture of the tibial plateau (115), and a rare posterolateral subluxation of the proximal fibula at the

**Table 9.10   Case Series and Cross-Sectional Studies of Injuries Occurring in the Lower Extremity of Theatrical Dancers**

| Study | Idiom | Design | Subjects | Age | Level | Condition/diagnosis |
|---|---|---|---|---|---|---|
| **Hip/pelvis** | | | | | | |
| Jacobs (1978) | Modern dance | Cross-sectional | 11 F | Collegiate | Student | Compared cases with "snapping hip" to matched controls; dancers with narrower bi-iliac width may be predisposed to this condition |
| Schaberg et al. (1984) | Ballet | Cases[a] | 2 F | 19, 20 | — | Snapping hip syndrome; both were treated with steroid injections; 1 patient is still symptomatic |
| **Knee** | | | | | | |
| Ferretti et al. (1983) | Ballet | Case[a] | 1 F | 20 | — | "Jumper's knee," or patellar tendon tendinitis; 34 months after surgery, results considered poor |
| Clippinger-Robertson et al. (1986) | Mixed | Cross-sectional | 14 F | — | Intermediate to professional | Compared cases with clinical chondro-malacia patella to matched controls and found that injured dancers displayed greater anterior pelvic tilt, lumbar lordosis, and P angles; greater amplitude and dominance of quadriceps activity during the 2nd position grand plié |
| **Leg** | | | | | | |
| Daffner (1984) | Modern dance | Cases[a] | 2 F | — | Professional | Identified stress fractures (horizontal striations of the anterior cortex of the tibia); present only in athletes who leap and not in runners |
| Gans (1985) | Ballet | Case series | 16 F | 16-31 | Student | Compared jumping techniques of dancers with a history of "shin splints" and those without the condition; shin-splint victims demonstrated more double heel strikes upon landing ($p = .02$) than the other group |
| Holder & Michael (1985) | Ballet | Case[a] | 1 F | 30 | — | Clinically differentiated the diagnosis of "shin splints" from stress fractures using 3-phase bone scintigraphy |
| Nussbaum et al. (1988) | Ballet | Case series | 22 F, 1 M | 8-63 mean 21 | All | 19 of 23 dancers had stress fractures and stress reactions, confirmed by scintigraphic bones scans |
| | | | | | | Stress reaction was seen most often in tibiae (17 dancers exhibiting bilateral cases), followed by femora (11) |
| **Ankle/Achilles** | | | | | | |
| Brodsky & Khalil (1987) | Ballet | Cases[b] | 5 F, 1 M | 18-23 | Professional | Successfully treated 8 cases of talar compression syndrome in 6 dancers with surgical removal of the accessory ossicle; all have remained asymptomatic for 7 yr |
| Fernandez-Palazzi et al. (1990) | Ballet | Case series | 10 F, 3 M | — | Professional | Treated 19 cases of Achilles tendinitis in 13 dancers; 13 cases were located in the middle of the tendon, 4 at the insertion of the calcaneous, and 2 at the musculo-tendinous junction. |
| | | | | | | Incidence by clinical phase: 7 (36.8%) Phase I cases, pain only after dancing; 3 (15.8%) Phase II cases, pain on starting dancing that decreases once warmed up but reappears after dancing; 9 (47.4%) Phase III cases, pain during and after dancing |

| Study | Idiom | Design | Subjects | Age | Level | Condition/diagnosis |
|-------|-------|--------|----------|-----|-------|---------------------|
| Hamilton (1982) | Ballet | Case series | 100 | — | Professional | Out of 100 ankle injuries in 15 months, 17 were sprains, 16 were Grade I and II, 1 was a Grade III sprain |
| Marotta & Micheli (1992) | Ballet | Case series | 9 F, 3 M | 14-34 | Advanced & professional | Operated on 15 ankles (12 patients) with os trigonum impingement; all but one patient returned to dancing |
| Stoller et al. (1984) | Mixed | Cross-sectional | 26 F, 6 M | 18-40 mean 23 | Advanced & professional | Found 59.3% of the dancers had anterior talar exostoses compared to 4% of controls; significant because the dancers were younger than controls and development of these lesions is time related |
| Wredmark et al. (1991) | Ballet | Case series | 9 F, 4 M | 14-31 | Professional | 14 os trigonums or other prominent lateral posterior processes of the talus were surgically removed, together with division of the thickened flexor hallucis longus tendon sheath in at least half of the cases; all but 1 case returned to dancing |

Foot/Toes

| Study | Idiom | Design | Subjects | Age | Level | Condition/diagnosis |
|-------|-------|--------|----------|-----|-------|---------------------|
| Ambré & Nilsson (1978) | Ballet | Cross-sectional | 20 F | 28±7 | Professional | Range of dorsiflexion of the big toe was significantly decreased after a performance, compared to 34 controls |
| Grahame et al. (1979) | Ballet | Cases[b] | 8 F, 1 M | 14-61 | All | Identified 10 stress lesions (fractures) in 8 dancers by using scintigraphy in the diagnosis; assured 1 patient that he did not have stress lesions |
| Kliman et al. (1983) | Ballet | Case[a] | 1 F | 22 | — | Osteochondritis of right lateral hallux sesamoid, a "fracture" secondary to aseptic necrosis; bilateral bipartite medial sesamoids |
| | Modern dance | Case[a] | 1 F | 40 | Recreational | Bilateral bipartite medial sesamoids |
| Marshall & Hamilton (1992) | Ballet | Case series | — | — | Professional | Cuboid subluxations accounted for 17.5% of foot and ankle injuries incurred in a 3-week period and a later 3-week rehearsal period, compared to 4% among other athletes |
| Micheli et al. (1985) | Ballet | Cases[b] | 4 F | 16-35 | — | Stress fractures of the Lisfranc (2nd tarsometatarsal) joint |
| Nussbaum et al. (1988) | Ballet | Case series | 22 F, 1 M | 8-63 mean 21 | All | 19 of 23 dancers had stress fractures and stress reactions, confirmed by scintigraphic bones scans |
| | | | | | | Stress reaction seen most often in tibiae (17 dancers exhibiting bilateral cases) |
| | | | | | | Stress fracture most common in the feet (17 in 8 dancers); 10 dancers had stress reactions in feet |
| Torg et al. (1982) | Ballet | Case[a] | 1 F | 22 | Recreational | Complete, nondisplaced stress fracture of the tarsal navicular; failure to treat 7 of the fractures with nonweight-bearing resulted unsatisfactorily (some prolonged morbidity and disability) |
| Warren et al. (1986) | Ballet | Cross-sectional | 75 F | 18-36 | Professional | 26 of 27 stress fractures in the metatarsals |

[a]Obtained from case series data.

[b]Discussed as a series.

superior tibio-fibular joint (59). Usually this kind of dislocation injury occurs with a twisting fall and displaces antero-laterally, but the dancer in this case landed awkwardly on a minimally flexed knee that resulted in a surprising (because of the minor injury) peroneal nerve palsy.

*Leg.* Injuries to the lower leg are replete in dancers. It is not unusual for dancers to present with multiple stress (fatigue) fractures and stress reactions throughout the lower extremity (120, 123, 130, 131, 133, 150). Furthermore, a retrospective study of 54 professional ballet dancers found that the risk of stress fractures increased in dancers who danced more than 5 hours per day and in those whose amenorrheic intervals extended beyond 6 months (88).

In a series that included a variety of athletes, Daffner (38) scintigraphically analyzed the striations on the cortex of the tibia and determined that leaping athletes, such as dancers, will experience different stress fractures than running athletes. Holder and Michael (78) also studied a variety of athletes presenting with "shin splints" (also referred to as *soleus syndrome* and *medial tibial stress syndrome*), and believe that they have scintigraphically differentiated shin splints from stress fractures. Whereas Daffner identified most lesions on the anterior aspect of the tibia, Holder and Michael obtained anterior, posterior, lateral, and medial images to determine that shin splints do not originate in the tibialis posterior muscle as previously believed, but rather that the condition is related to the origin of the soleus muscle and causes abnormal activity along the posterior medial cortex of the lower middle third of the tibia. However, these findings should be applied with caution, for shin splints is a term too imprecise to be attributed to a single etiology.

*Ankle.* A prevalence of the following complaints in the ankle exists in the case, series, and cross-sectional literature that was not apparent from Tables 9.5 and 9.6: talar compression syndromes, usually with an os trigonum present, and caused by weight-bearing on *pointe* or *demi-pointe* (16, 112, 137, 186); flexor hallucis longus tendinitis, which can be easily misdiagnosed as Achilles tendinitis (48); Achilles tendinitis (46, 134), often located in the middle of the tendon but not always; ruptured peroneus brevis tendon (37); osteochondral fracture of the upper surface of the talus (123); sprains (69); and anterior impingement syndromes (123,

131, 132, 164). Dancers have been found to exhibit anterior talar exostoses at a frequency rate of 59.3% versus 4.0% in controls (164). The significance of this finding is that this kind of lesion is time related, usually appearing in older age groups than the 32 professional dancers involved in Stoller's (164) cross-sectional study. The average age of the dancers was 23 years versus 45.8 years for the controls.

*Foot/toes.* Injuries to the foot/toes consist mainly of damage to the flexor hallucis longus tendon[1] resulting in tendinitis and trigger toe (35, 58, 107, 152, 173); loose or dislocated metatarsophalangeal joints (123, 169); cuboid subluxations (114); sesamoiditis (97, 184); and stress fractures and reactions (60, 119, 130). It seems that stress fractures in dancers occur most often in the feet, and stress reactions most often in the tibiae (130). This is also borne out in the series conducted by Kadel and associates (88), who studied amenorrheic professional ballet dancers.

Two reports in the literature provided information on unusual overuse injuries to the feet. Lehman et al. (106) described Iselin's disease in a 12-year-old ballet student. This condition is caused by repetitive overstress to the forefoot and results in an enlarged apophysis of the proximal fifth metatarsal. Micheli et al. (119) reported four stress fractures of the Lisfranc's (second tarsometatarsal) joint in ballet dancers. This injury is found only in female dancers whose hyperflexed forefoot during *pointe* work concentrates all mechanical forces at the tarsometatarsal junction of Lisfranc's joint, thus rendering it vulnerable.

***3.3.3.2 Lower Extremity Injuries in Fitness Dance Forms.*** Very little evidence of aerobic dance injuries comes from case reports, but the few cases do bear out the epidemiologic evidence that most injuries in the lower extremities of aerobic dancers are undoubtedly stress-related, overuse injuries (see Table 9.11). No cross-sectional studies or case series were found that address lower extremity injuries in aerobic dancers.

# 4. Injury Severity

## 4.1 Time Loss

### 4.1.1 Time Loss in Theatrical Dance Idioms

In theatrical dancers, epidemiologic data concerning absence from training are not only scarce but

---

[1]Flexor hallucis longus injuries are usually categorized as ankle injuries; however, because the damage was experienced in the foot/toes by the dancer, these complaints have been categorized as foot/toe injuries.

**Table 9.11   Case Reports, Case Series, and Cross-Sectional Studies of Injuries Occurring in the Lower Extremity of Aerobic Dancers**

| Study | Design | Subjects | Age | Level | Condition/diagnosis |
|---|---|---|---|---|---|
| Hip/pelvis | | | | | |
| Thigh | | | | | |
| Knee | | | | | |
| Leg | | | | | |
| Read (1984) | Case | 1 F | 31 | Instructor | Runner's stress fracture; fibular, just proximal to the tibiofibular syndesmosis |
| Strudwick & Goodman (1992) | Case | 1 F | 32 | Student | Proximal fibular stress fracture |
| Ankle | | | | | |
| Green & Maltz (1992) | Case | 1 F | 32 | Student | Bilateral ankle pain related to sarcoidosis with Stage I lung involvement and secondary erythema nodosum; diagnosis confirmed that the patient had a musculoskeletal manifestation of sarcoid, not overuse injury |
| Foot/toes | | | | | |
| Cross et al. (1984) | Case | 1 F | 41 | Instructor | First reported case of elastofibroma in the plantar surface of the foot |
| Riddle & Freeman (1988) | Case | 1 F | 27 | Instructor | Bilateral plantar fasciitis and Achilles tendinitis were successfully managed with permanent orthoses |

also lacking in uniform definitions of time loss. Yet, the following inferences can be made from the one randomized control trial (10), one retrospective (12), and two prospective studies (141, 151) that include time-loss data.

- Approximately 28.8% (12) to 35.6% (141) of dancers incurred injuries that kept them out of training for more than a week.
- Dancers with a body mass index < 19.0 and who experienced irregular menstrual cycles spent more days injured than dancers with a body mass index > 19.0 and with regular menses (10).
- Tendinitis about the hip resulted in the longest period of absence from training (6.9 days), followed by low-back strain (4.7 days), chondromalacia patellae (4.1 days), Achilles tendinitis (2.5 days), and ankle sprain (2.1 days) (151).

### 4.1.2 Time Loss in Aerobics

There are two prospective (57, 74) and two retrospective (145, 149) studies on aerobic dance injuries that present time-loss data. Although the data were expressed as a percentage of participants in some of the studies and as a percentage of injuries in other studies, the following information could be extrapolated from the studies.

- Approximately 30.8% of students and 34.1% of instructors suffered a time-loss injury.
- Approximately 8.1% of students' injuries and 2.2% of instructors' injuries were diagnosed by a physician.
- Aerobic dancers seem to see a physician mostly for foot and shin/leg injuries. Back injuries are more common among students than instructors, and ankle injuries are more common among instructors than students.
- Strain and tendinitis are the most frequently mentioned diagnoses.

## 5. Injury Risk Factors

One of the realities of theatrical dance is that it takes years of intense, disciplined motoric patterning to achieve the necessary economy of movement and simplicity of line that are the hallmark of the dancing artist. Once achieved, it is expected that dancers will use that artistry for as long as their careers will allow. In aerobic dance, like other endurance activities, the goal is to achieve maximum fitness through cardiovascular improvement. However, in the quest for aerobic fitness the participant can suffer musculoskeletal injury that may discourage further participation. Identifying injury risk factors and preventing injury, thereby enabling the prolonged theatrical dance career or the prolonged pursuit of fitness, is the goal of all research into dance injuries.

## 5.1 Intrinsic Factors

### 5.1.1 Physical Characteristics

An impressive body of knowledge concerning the physical and physiological characteristics of the theatrical and aerobic dancer has emerged in the last 10 years. These studies are based on the premise that, before a problem can be addressed, we must first know about the individual who presents with the problem. Once that profile is established, it can then be investigated in relation to injury.

Studies that profile the physical and physiological characteristics of theatrical dancers can be categorized as follows:

- Body build and body composition (5, 10, 18, 26, 31, 40, 44, 76, 77, 91, 105, 118, 129, 148)
- Musculoskeletal characteristics, including flexibility, hypermobility, muscular strength, range of motion, and bone mass (4, 5, 7, 28, 46, 72, 84, 86, 90, 91, 94-96, 98, 101, 104, 117, 118, 125, 143, 160, 164, 168, 172)
- Neuromuscular adaptations (7, 98)
- Physiological characteristics, including cardiovascular fitness and muscular endurance (23, 26, 29, 30, 32, 33, 91, 105, 118, 125, 128, 129, 147, 158)
- Nutritional habits (5, 11, 13, 18, 26, 31, 45, 63, 64, 162)
- Anorectic and other psychosocial behaviors (10, 13, 19, 41, 45, 53, 54, 62-66, 87, 103, 109, 110, 116, 155, 166, 181)
- Training status (109)
- Hematologic status (31, 111)
- Menstrual function and hormonal status (2, 5, 10, 17, 18, 30, 39, 51, 63, 86, 88, 124, 176, 177).

The body of knowledge profiling aerobic dancers is less extensive. It provides information primarily on benefits of aerobic dance as they relate to

- body composition (42, 174),
- musculoskeletal characteristics (3, 144),
- physiological characteristics (21, 42, 49, 82, 99, 121, 135, 170, 174, 180), and
- psychological changes (42).

The aforementioned studies on theatrical and aerobic dancers are worth perusing, for they provide baseline data on dancers as a population.

Many of them correlate the characteristic(s) under investigation with injuries in dancers or with risk of injury. Those studies are discussed in the remainder of this section on injury risk factors.

*5.1.1.1 Physical Characteristics in Theatrical Dancers.* Table 9.12 presents only analytical studies that attempted to identify factors that may predispose theatrical dancers to injury or skeletal change. These results must be interpreted with caution, however, because some study designs and methodology, which are indicated in the table, compromise the results. Within the limitations of the analytical studies, the following information on risk factors is emerging in the literature:

- In spite of the interest in researching the body composition of dancers, only Benson et al. (11) have provided analytical data. They found that dancers with a lower percent body fat spent more days recovering from low-grade injuries than those with greater body mass index (BMI) ($p < .05$).
- Menarcheal history and menstrual function may predispose dancers to injury. Benson et al. (10) reported more injuries to the bone in dancers with irregular cycles than with regular cycles. Furthermore, a relationship clearly exists between stress fractures and amenorrhea (66, 88, 177). Research suggests a strong relationship between menstrual dysfunction and reduced bone mineral content in the lumbar spine and wrist of dancers, thus compromising skeletal integrity (39, 79, 86).

*5.1.1.2 Physical Characteristics in Aerobic Dancers.* Table 9.13 presents analytical evidence that identifies predisposing factors to injury in aerobic dancers. These results must be interpreted with caution, however, because some study designs and methodology, which are indicated in the table, compromise the results. The numerous analytical studies that support the physiological benefits of aerobic dancing were not included in Table 9.13 because they do not relate their findings to injuries. However, these have been referenced in Section 5.1.1 for perusal.

Regarding physical characteristics, only Garrick et al. (57) provide evidence of risk factors. They suggest that prior injury may predispose aerobic dancers to greater risk of injury than dancers who have not been previously injured. They point out, however, that the severity of the reinjury will likely be no greater than the primary complaint.

**Table 9.12  Analytical Evidence Regarding Potential Risk Factors for Theatrical Dance Injuries**

| Study | Duration | Design | Method | n | Purpose | Results |
|---|---|---|---|---|---|---|
| **Intrinsic factors** | | | | | | |
| **Physical characteristics** | | | | | | |
| Benson et al. (1989) | 6 mo | RCT | Injuries: questionnaire and monthly telephone interviews; menstrual function: self-reported; BMI; food frequency questionnaire, analyzed by Practocare software | 56 | To investigate the relationship between nutrient intake, body mass index (BMI), menstrual function, and injury | Dancers with BMI < 19.0 spent more days with a low-grade injury than those with BMI > 19.0 ($p < .05$); dancers with abnormal menses had more bone injuries than normally menstruating dancers ($p < .05$). |
| Jacobs & Young (1988) | — | Cross-sectional | Goniometric and cable-tensiometric measurements; anthropometry | 11 | To determine generic characteristics in dancers with snapping-hip problem | Dancers with narrower bi-iliac width are more predisposed to snapping-hip problems ($p < .10$). |
| Warren et al. (1986) | — | Retrospective & cross-sectional | Injury history; interviews; medical tests; orthopedic exam; longitudinal endocrine status evaluation (N = 10); blood tests; x-ray and bone scan; EAT-26 | 75 | To determine the prevalence of scoliosis and fractures among dancers in relation to menarcheal history | 18 (24%) dancers had scoliosis, and the prevalence rose as the age at menarche rose; delayed menarche ($p < 0.04$), secondary amenorrhea, duration of amenorrhea ($p < 0.05$), and anorectic behavior are significantly higher in dancers with scoliosis than without scoliosis; delayed menarche, secondary amenorrhea ($p < 0.01$) and its duration ($p < 0.05$), and prolonged hypoestrogenism are significantly correlated with incidence of fractures and stress fractures. |
| **Motor/functional characteristics** | | | | | | |
| Barrack et al. (1983) | — | Cross-sectional | Joint laxity criteria (Nicholas); custom-made Jobst air splints | 12 | To determine the relationship between joint laxity and joint position sense in the knee | Dancers did worse ($p < .03$) than controls on joint position sense and overestimated the angle to which knee joint had been passively moved ($p < .01$); may indicate below normal protective reflexes. |
| Gans (1985) | — | Cross-sectional | Cinematography | 16 | To correlate heel contact during jumps with shin splints | Dancers with a history of shin splints showed more double heel strikes than other group ($p = .02$). |
| Hamilton, W.G. et al. (1992) | — | Cross-sectional | Medical exam, Cybex, goniometer | 14 F, 14 M | To profile musculoskeletal characteristics and correlate them to injury | Certain flexibility patterns (ability to assume the lotus position and increased total turnout) may predispose male dancers to overuse injury ($p < .05$). Conversely, women with less turnout were predisposed to overuse injury ($p < .05$); also implicated were less bilateral plié ($p < .01$) and decreased left ankle dorsiflexion ($p < .05$) in women. |
| Klemp et al. (1984) | — | Cross-sectional | Beighton's modification of the Carter and Wilkinson method for measuring joint mobility | 377 | To determine the prevalence of hypermobility in a large ballet school and the rate of genetic and acquired factors; the risk of injury and mitral valve prolapse (MVP) in hypermobile dancers | 36 (9.5%) of the dancers showed hypermobility and had more injuries than nonhypermobile dancers ($p < .05$); forward flexion can be acquired through prolonged ballet training ($p < .0015$); none of the 36 hypermobile dancers showed evidence of MVP, but the sample was too small to add to that research question. |

(continued)

**Table 9.12**  (continued)

| Study | Duration | Design | Method | n | Purpose | Results |
|---|---|---|---|---|---|---|
| Klemp & Chalton (1989) | 4 yr | Cross-sectional & retrospective | Beighton's method, as above | 102 | To determine the influence of 4 years additional training on articular mobility | Forward flexion is usually acquired and develops after 4 or more years of training (p < .0001); the mobility score may assist in predicting who will continue dancing (p < .03), but hypermobility is not necessarily associated with excellence in dancing. |
| Koceja et al. (1991) | — | Cross-sectional | Laboratory tests for tendon-tap reflex | 7 | To examine force-time characteristics of the Achilles tendon-tap reflex and its resultant neuromuscular adaptations in relation to several years of dance training | Dancers exhibited less unilateral isometric force and longer half-relaxation times (p < 0.05) than the untrained subjects; also, a conditioning tap to the Achilles tendon produces a long-latency inhibition of the contralateral Achilles tendon-tap reflex force for trained subjects. These differences in reflexes may reflect differences in muscle stiffness, tissue compliance, or neural organization. |
| Kushner et al. (1990) | — | Cross-sectional | Goniometer and Leighton flexometer | 22 | To determine how much turnout is necessary for maximum hip abduction | The greater the position of external rotation, the more abduction achieved (p < .05); insufficient range of turnout or faulty technique may predispose the dancer to injury. |
| Reid et al. (1987) | 1 school year | Cross-sectional & retrospective | Observation, interview, goniometric measurements | 30 | To determine the prevalence of lateral hip and knee pain and snapping problems in the hip and knee of dancers | Dancers had significantly greater passive external hip rotation and significantly less passive hip adduction and internal rotation (p < .05); ranges of motion increased with longer training. Dancers with lateral symptoms had significantly reduced hip adduction versus dancers without symptoms (p < .001); no differences were found between dancers with or without anterior hip pain or snapping. 9 (30%) of dancers had experienced lateral hip or knee problems, and 7 of these required treatment; 5 (16.7%) of controls experienced problems, but none required treatment. Iliotibial band tightness may predispose dancers to lateral hip and knee pain or snapping (p < .05). |
| **Psychosocial characteristics** | | | | | | |
| Hamilton et al. (1989) | — | Cross-sectional | Self-report questionnaire (API); a manual for measures of occupational stress, strain, and coping | 14 F, 15 M | To explore personalities, stresses, and injury patterns of leading dancers | Stress fractures were higher in dancers who entered the company at a later (≥ 20 yr) age (p < .05). Relationship between stress fractures and amenorrhea exists (p < .05). Older dancers (≥ 30 yr) had more major injuries and were disabled longer (p < .05) than younger dancers. Personality factors suggestive of the over-achiever, combined with physical stress, correlated positively with dancers who were most injured over their careers (.001 < p < .05). Women may be psychologically better suited to the profession than men; women were more adjusted (p < .001), tough-minded (p < .001), and caring (p < .001). Male dancers experienced more stress related to erratic work schedules and personal isolation than females (p < .05). Male dancers scored lower on self-care (p < .05), suffered more strain due to disrupted personal relationships, and experienced more symptoms of poor health, fatigue, and overuse of alcohol than female dancers. |

| Study | Exposure/Duration | Design | Method | N | Purpose | Results |
|---|---|---|---|---|---|---|
| Liederbach et al. (1992) | 5 wk | Prospective | Observation, weekly urine specimens, weekly profile of mood states | 12 | To examine physiologic and psychological changes in relation to mood to see if staleness develops | Urinalysis reflected possible stress as the performance period continued (p < .001). Mood states also changed during week 4 (p < .001), then reversed in week 5 as vacation approached. |
| **Extrinsic factors** | | | | | | |
| *Exposure* | | | | | | |
| Kadel et al. (1992) | — | Retrospective | Questionnaires on 1-week diet history; stress fracture history; physical traits | 54 | To compare whether stress fractures in dancers were related to nutritional or menstrual abnormalities and rigorous training schedules | Risk of stress fractures in professional ballet dancers increases in dancers who dance > 5 hours per day (p < .025) and in those with amenorrheic intervals exceeding 6 months (p < .001). |
| **Training methods or conditions** | | | | | | |
| Ambré & Nilsson (1978) | — | Cross-sectional | Range of dorsiflexion of big toe joint measured by a square rule | 20 | To determine whether dancing on pointe produces any degenerative changes in the big toe joint | No significant change in ROM with age in either the dancers or controls; but there was a significant difference between groups (0.02 > p > 0.01); no difference in dancers before and immediately after performance; concluded that dancing on pointe may not be as harmful to the forefoot as has been proposed |
| Clippinger-Robertson et al. (1986) | — | Retrospective | Questionnaire | 362[a] | To ascertain the incidence of patellofemoral complaints in dancers | Difference in knee pain vs. no pain increases for modern dancers as they progress to higher levels (p < 0.01), but not in ballet dancers (p < 0.05). |
| Kravitz et al. (1986) | — | Cross-sectional | Electrodynogram | 16 | To examine the forces that may contribute to bunion formation in ballet dancers | High percentage of body weight shifts to the medial aspect of the 1st metatarsal head and medial aspect of the hallux interphalangeal joint when performing passé relevé; foot abducts (a pronatory component) so the weight can rest against the joint as described; because of small sample size and large number of outliers, no statistical analysis was completed |
| Teitz et al. (1985) | — | Cross-sectional | Kulite semi-conduction | 13[b] | To determine the relative pressures on the 1st and 2nd toes and 1st metatarsophalangeal joint while on pointe; and as a function of toe length and foot position | Ballet dancers may be predisposed to arthritis or hallux rigidus in the 1st MTP joint due to marked pressure when on pointe; 1st toe always took equal or greater pressure than the 2nd toe; pressures on the 2nd toe as well as pressure ratios between the 1st and 2nd toes differed between Groups 1 and 2 (p < .05 and p < .01, respectively). No significant difference between Group 3 and other groups was found. |
| **Equipment** | | | | | | |
| Skrinar et al. (1981) | — | Cross-sectional | Cinematography | 12 | To examine differences in pelvic tilt between 1st position flat and on pointe and relationship between brand of pointe shoe | Dancers who wear Capezio shoes showed increased pelvic tilt on pointe (p < .01); may be at risk of muscular imbalance in the foot and upward through the body |

BMI = body mass index.

EAT = Eating Attitudes Test (Garner & Garfinkel, 1979).

MTP = metatarsophalangeal joint.

[a] Includes 156 ballet and 206 modern dancers at the advanced and professional levels.

[b] Group 1 (N = 4): first 3 toes were of even length. Group 2 (N = 5): first 3 toes were of decreasing length. Group 3 (N = 4): 2nd toe was longer than 1st and 3rd.

**Table 9.13   Analytical Evidence Regarding Potential Risk Factors for Aerobic Dancers**

| Study | Duration | Design | Method | n | Purpose | Results |
|---|---|---|---|---|---|---|
| **Intrinsic factors** | | | | | | |
| **Physical characteristics** | | | | | | |
| Garrick et al. (1986) | 16 wk | Prospective | Questionnaire | 411 | To identify the nature of aerobic injuries and possible contributing factors | People with a history of prior injuries are at greater risk (p < 0.01) of being injured in aerobics, but average severity of the reinjury is no greater than primary complaints |
| **Motor/functional characteristics** | | | | | | |
| Allen et al. (1986) | 6 mo | Prospective | Goniometer; physical exam; squat test; interviews | 229 | To determine whether lower extremity malalignment or floor surface was responsible for aerobic dance injuries | High malalignment scores and abnormal squat tests were correlated with injuries (p < .05) |
| Richie et al. (1993) | — | Cross-sectional | Biomechanical exam of the foot for subtalar joint position; EMG | 12 | To determine the effect of 3 different floor surfaces on the medial shin musculature during stationary running | Participants who registered greater EMG values during eccentric muscle activity during the run-in-place test were more likely to incur shin pain (p < .05); they also had excessive pronation of the feet. |
| **Extrinsic factors** | | | | | | |
| **Exposure** | | | | | | |
| Garrick et al. (1986) | 16 wk | Prospective | Questionnaire | 411 | To identify the nature of aerobic injuries and possible contributing factors | Instructors are at greater risk of injury than students because of greater exposure time. Students who use aerobic dance as their only fitness activity are at greater risk of injury than students who participate in multiple fitness activities (p < 0.001). |
| Richie et al. (1985) | —[a] | Retrospective | Questionnaire | 1,291[b] | To identify factors related to causes and prevention of aerobics injuries | People who participate more times per week (e.g., instructors) are at greater risk of injury (p < 0.001). The longer someone participates in aerobics, the greater the chance of being injured (p < 0.001). |
| Rothenberger et al. (1988) | —[c] | Retrospective | Questionnaire | 726 | To document the nature of aerobic dance injuries and determine predisposing factors of injuries | Participating in 4 or more classes/week increases the risk of injury (p < 0.05) and number of injuries (p < 0.05). Participating sporadically in consecutive classes increases the risk of injury (p < 0.001) over always or never taking consecutive classes. |
| **Training methods or conditions** | | | | | | |
| Janis (1990) | 129 wk | Retrospective | Questionnaire | 375 | To determine injury rates in high-impact vs. low-impact aerobics | Students in high-impact aerobics are at greater risk of injury than students in low-impact aerobics. |
| **Environment** | | | | | | |
| Allen et al. (1986) | 6 mo | Prospective | Goniometer; physical exam; squat test; interviews | 229 | To determine whether lower extremity malalignment or floor surface was responsible for aerobic dance injuries | For participants with similar malalignment and squat test scores, there is no significant difference between number of injuries incurred on gym floor or on judo/wrestling mats. |
| Richie et al. (1993) | — | Cross-sectional | EMG | 12 | To determine the effect of 3 different floor surfaces on the medial shin musculature during stationary running | Dancing on nonresilient surfaces and on carpet can predispose the dancer to injury (p < 0.05). |

| Study | Duration | Design | Method | $n$ | Purpose | Results |
|---|---|---|---|---|---|---|
| Rothenberger et al. (1988) | —[c] | Retrospective | Questionnaire | 726 | To document the nature of aerobic dance injuries and determine predisposing factors of injuries | Resilient plywood surfaces may increase the risk of injury over exercising on padded and carpeted concrete ($p < 0.05$). Resilient plywood surfaces may increase the risk of lower extremity injuries over exercising on padded and carpeted concrete ($p < 0.08$). |
| **Equipment** Clark et al. (1989) | 15 wk | Prospective | Questionnaires at 5-wk intervals | 139 | To determine whether use of viscoelastic insoles decreases the frequency of musculoskeletal injury | The findings do not support the hypothesis that viscoelastic shoe inserts might decrease injuries, but they were "liked" better than the placebos ($p < 0.01$). |
| Rothenberger et al. (1988) | —[c] | Retrospective | Questionnaire | 726 | To document the nature of aerobic dance injuries and determine predisposing factors of injuries | Specially designed aerobic shoes may increase the risk of lower extremity injuries over other types of footwear or bare feet ($p < 0.001$). |

EMG = electromyography.

[a]Average length of participation for students was 6.08 months and for instructors, 30.5 months.

[b]Number of students = 1,233, and number of instructors = 58.

[c]28% of the subjects had been exercising for 1 to 2 years, and 26% had been exercising 2 years or longer.

### 5.1.2 Motor/Functional Characteristics

Research suggests that the following motor/functional characteristics may predispose the theatrical dancer to injury:

- Certain flexibility patterns (e.g., ability to assume the lotus position and increased total turnout in males) and general hypermobility as defined by Beighton's modification of the Carter and Wilkinson criteria may predispose the dancer to overuse injury (72, 94, 96). Conversely, lack of certain flexibility patterns (e.g., less turnout from the hip and less ankle dorsiflexion) also predispose female dancers to overuse injury (52, 72, 104, 143).
- Flaws in technique may predispose the dancer to injury. Gans (52) found a significant correlation between double heel strikes when landing jumps and shin splints.
- Below normal protective reflexes in dancers may develop over time (7, 98).

In aerobic dancers, some attention has been given to malalignments in the lower extremity as a possible injury risk factor. Specifically, pronation of the feet has been correlated with injuries (3, 144), as shown in Table 9.13. Richie and colleagues (144)

went so far as to demonstrate electromyographically that pronation produces greater eccentric muscular forces and, therefore, more shin pain.

### 5.1.3 Psychosocial Characteristics

Table 9.12 shows that two analytical studies have been conducted on theatrical dancers in relation to stress, personality, and demographic factors. They confirm that a hectic schedule (66, 109) and increasing age (66) can adversely influence injury patterns.

In addition to the studies presented in Table 9.12, numerous analytical studies address dietary behaviors that may predispose the dancer to injury, poor health, or death. While it is not the intent of this chapter to explore psychiatric epidemiology, that science, which identifies individuals at risk for developing life-threatening conditions such as anorexia nervosa, directly affects the world of dance. Salient findings of those studies indicate the following:

- Dancers are at risk for nutrient deficiency at a range of significance of $0.0001 > p < .05$ (13, 45, 64, 103, 111).
- Dancers are at risk for anorexia nervosa at a range of significance of $0.003 > p \le .05$ (13, 19, 45, 63, 87, 103, 116).

- Hamilton et al. (62) reported that white dancers are at higher risk of anorexia nervosa than black dancers ($p < .10$); black dancers had more positive body images ($p < .01$) and were less concerned about dieting ($p < .01$) than white dancers. With further reference to demographics, professional dancers are more likely to practice anorectic behavior ($p < .05$) than dancers in regional companies (62) or university dance students (54).

## 5.2 Extrinsic Factors

### 5.2.1 Exposure

Only one retrospective study has been found that addresses exposure as it relates to injury in theatrical dancers. Kadel et al. (88) found greater risk of stress fractures in dancers who dance more than 5 hours per day.

In aerobic dancers Rothenberger et al. (149) found that participating in four or more classes per week increased the risk of injury. More exposure time to aerobics at both the instructor and student levels increases the risk of injury (57, 145). Furthermore, if it is the student's only fitness activity, or if the student sporadically participates in consecutive aerobic classes, the risk of injury increases (57, 149).

### 5.2.2 Training Methods or Conditions

#### 5.2.2.1 In Theatrical Dancers. Three cross-sectional studies have addressed concerns to the forefoot as a result of dancing on *pointe*. Two studies confirmed that the first metatarsophalangeal (MTP) joint sustains marked pressure during ascending and suspending on *pointe*, thereby predisposing the ballerina to bunion deformity (102) or possibly arthritis in the first MTP joint (168). However, a third study (4) claims that dancing on *pointe* may not be as harmful as the literature suggests. The researchers looked for degenerative changes in the first MTP joint by measuring the range of motion in dancers before and after a performance and found no significant change. This study perhaps could have offered more convincing evidence had it been conducted longitudinally.

Relatively weak research into a specific style or idiom of dance reveals that modern dancers may experience increasing knee pain as they progress to higher levels of technique and performance, but ballet dancers do not (28). This may have some merit depending on the style of modern dance involved. For instance, Solomon and Micheli (161) in their case series identified Graham technique as contributing to more knee injuries than ballet and the other major modern dance techniques (i.e., Limon, Cunningham, Horton, and Humphrey-Weidman). Furthermore, Chmelar et al. (23) found in their cross-sectional study that professional ballet dancers had greater hamstring strength than professional modern dancers and university ballet and modern dancers. To date, no research has been conducted to correlate this finding with possible predisposition to knee injuries.

Another difference between ballet and modern dancers has been identified in their physiology. Chmelar et al. (23) found professional ballet dancers to be less aerobically fit than professional modern dancers and university ballet and modern dancers. Unfortunately, they did not follow the dancers prospectively in order to relate this information to injuries between the groups.

#### 5.2.2.2 In Aerobic Dancers. Only one study has addressed training methods or conditions in aerobics. Janis (85) found higher injury rates in high-impact aerobic students than in low-impact aerobics.

### 5.2.3 Environment

The dance floor itself is important to both theatrical and aerobic dancers. The only study that investigated floor surfaces in ballet is descriptive in nature, and it identifies hard surfaces as a possible contributing factor to 9 out of 19 cases of Achilles tendinitis (46).

In aerobics, the evidence in Table 9.13 is inconclusive. Given the different study designs, this is not surprising. Allen et al. (3) present prospective evidence that malalignment, not floor surface, contributes to injury. Richie et al. (144) and Rothenberger et al. (149) did not include leg/foot alignment in their studies, and they reported contradictory evidence concerning resilient versus nonresilient surfaces. The evidence provided in the cross-sectional study conducted by Richie and colleagues may be more convincing at this time because it included electromyographical (EMG) measurements while the subjects performed on three different floor surfaces. They determined that both a concrete and a carpet-over-concrete surface may place aerobic dancers at greater risk than a sprung hardwood floor.

### 5.2.4 Equipment

Shoes have been investigated in both ballet and aerobics. Skrinar et al. (160) studied the effect of three brands of *pointe* shoes on dancers' posture when standing in first position and when on *pointe*. They found a relationship between Capezio *pointe* shoes and increased pelvic tilt that may predispose the dancer to muscular imbalances in the foot and possibly upward through the body. In a descriptive study by Carlson et al. (20), molds of the feet while inside three selected brands of *pointe* shoes verified that the fit of the Capezio shoe is generally too short for the foot. This may contribute to the finding in Skrinar's study.

In aerobic studies, Rothenberger et al. (149) reported disturbing findings about the ineffectiveness of aerobic shoes in reducing injuries, and Clark et al. (25) prospectively determined the ineffectiveness of viscoelastic shoe inserts in reducing injuries.

# 6. Suggestions for Injury Prevention

While a variety of suggestions for injury prevention have been presented in the dance literature, few have actually been tested. What is needed is the assurance, acquired through valid research strategies, that what seems like logical advice is indeed helpful prescription for injury prevention. How long did dancers treat their injuries with a nice hot soak in the tub before researchers demonstrated that ice therapy was the most effective immediate treatment? Now, little more than a decade later, the number of preventive strategies has grown, but there is still much more work to be done to verify what we know today and to further delineate that knowledge in terms of the dancer, dancing, the environment and equipment, and the health support system.

Tables 9.14 and 9.15 present preventive measures that have been suggested in the literature, and those measures have been organized around the four categories delineated in the previous paragraph. What will not appear in Table 9.14 is the myriad of evidence that discloses physiological profile, menstrual dysfunction, and poor dietary practices among theatrical dancers. While research clearly supports the need for nutrition to sustain strength, both mentally and physically, its direct relationship to dancers' injuries has not yet been fully explored. Only those preventive measures that have been linked to injury are presented.

Similarly, Table 9.15 does not include the many reports on the physiological benefits of aerobic dancing. While it is known that aerobic capacity in individuals helps to define their fitness level, its relationship to injuries has not yet been fully explored.

# 7. Suggestions for Further Research

As stated early in this chapter, there is a dearth of truly valid research in dance injuries that identifies rates and causes of injury. The control data are simply too few. The state of the dance injury literature constitutes a basic theme in the recommendations for further research.

It is essential that, until more well-designed, prospective, cohort studies are conducted, the reader who delves into the literature distinguish between the levels of evidence presented in the many studies. Not all published data are equally robust, and not all published reports deserve the same credibility. Hopefully, the effort to identify information in this chapter by the type of research design will assist the reader in making this distinction. A future challenge will be to "weight" the studies by attaching some sort of value or index to them, based on their internal and external validities. This topic is currently being explored by epidemiologists and may result in such an index for future use in analyses such as this.

In addition to the need for better designed studies, succinct recommendations for further research based on the data presented in this chapter are outlined in Table 9.16. The recommendations are organized according to the section headings used throughout the chapter.

Having finished an analysis of the literature, dare we attempt to answer the questions posed at the beginning of this chapter? Although it is impossible to offer definitive responses based on the nonintegratability of the data available, we volunteer the following remarks.

- In spite of cases illustrative of negative consequences, dancing is not a dangerous activity. Furthermore, based on injury rates, neither theatrical nor aerobic dancing can be considered more risky than the other, although specific kinds of injuries and their anatomical sites can be attributed to specific dance idioms.
- Injuries are inevitable, and some risk factors have been identified. In theatrical dance idioms, the highest risk of injury may be to participants who have been previously injured and not yet fully recovered; have relatively low body mass index; have experienced menstrual dysfunction; display anorectic characteristics; possess either hypermobile or tight joints; dance more than 5 hours per day; wear *pointe* shoes that alter the anatomically sound functioning of the foot; dance on *pointe* without

**Table 9.14 Suggestions for Injury Prevention in Theatrical Dancers**

| Preventive measure | Examples/suggestions | Study/level of evidence |
| --- | --- | --- |
| **The dancer** | | |
| Nutritional education | • Dancers do not consume enough calories or specific nutrients to support normal growth and healing. | Armann et al., 1990/prospective and cross-sectional<br>Benson et al., 1985/cross-sectional<br>Benson et al., 1989/RCT<br>Braisted et al., 1985/cross-sectional<br>Calabrese et al., 1983/cross-sectional<br>Cohen et al., 1985/cross-sectional<br>Evers, 1987/cross-sectional<br>Hamilton, L.H. et al., 1986/cross-sectional<br>Kurtzman et al., 1990/cross-sectional<br>Mahlamäki & Mahlamäki, 1988/intervention<br>Sawyer-Morse et al., 1989/cross-sectional<br>Stensland & Sobal, 1992/retrospective |
| | • Relationship exists between incidence of bone injuries and body mass index ($p < .05$). | Benson et al., 1989/RCT |
| | • Sound nutrition may be helpful in preventing fractures and stress fractures in dancers. | Kadel et al., 1992/retrospective<br>Micheli & Solomon, 1990/case series<br>Warren et al., 1986/retrospective |
| | • Athletic amenorrhea and its resultant bone loss must be combated with evaluation of each dancer's vitamin and mineral deficiencies and with forced vacation leave. | Jonnavithula et al., 1993/prospective<br>Reid, 1987/cross-sectional<br>Warren, 1980/prospective |
| | • Implementation of the Body Profile Analysis System (BPAS) to estimate ideal body size and shape. | Katch, 1993/N.A. |
| | • Aspiring dancers should become aware of the detrimental effects of excess body fat on performance. | Evans et al., 1985/case series |
| Accommodation of anatomical flaws | • Structured ballet warm-up should include static iliotibial band stretches. | Reid et al., 1987/prospective |
| Stress reduction | • Dancers feel that pressure and overwork contribute to their injuries. | Bowling, 1989/retrospective |
| | • Pressure to be thin, augmented by high performance standards, contribute to anorectic behavior in dancers. | Garner & Garfinkel, 1980/cross-sectional |
| | • Personality factors suggestive of the overachiever, combined with physical stress, correlated positively with number of injuries. | Hamilton, L.H. et al., 1989/cross-sectional |
| | • Women may be psychologically better suited to the profession than men. | Hamilton, L.H. et al., 1989/cross-sectional |
| **Dancing** | | |
| Correction of flaws in technique | • To counteract dominance of quadriceps activity during pliés, which may aggravate the knee, dancers should be encouraged to co-contract the adductors and hamstrings during the plié. With cueing from the teacher, dancers are able to profoundly alter their pattern. | Clippinger-Robertson et al., 1986/cross-sectional |
| | • Dancers with chondromalacia patellae (CP) displayed greater anterior pelvic tilt during 2nd position grand plié than dancers without CP. | Clippinger-Robertson et al., 1986/cross-sectional |
| | • Teachers should emphasize femoral rotation from the hip rather than foot position. | Reid, 1987/prospective |
| | • Tendinitis of the ankle and stress fractures of the 2nd metatarsal involving Lisfranc's joint in ballet dancers can be prevented by watching that the dancer does not "knuckle over" or otherwise allow the foot to over-arch with full body weight stressing the metatarsals. | Braver, 1988/clinical report<br>Micheli et al., 1985/case series |
| | • Limiting excessive pronatory forces can decrease the tendency to develop first metatarsophalangeal joint deformity associated with the stresses produced from pronatory motions. | Kravitz et al., 1986/cross-sectional |
| Limiting of rigorous training schedules | • Dancers who dance > 5 hours per day may increase their risk of stress fractures. | Kadel et al., 1992/retrospective |
| | • The young dancer should be allowed at least a 6-week block of rest once a year. | Reid, 1987/prospective |

| Preventive measure | Examples/suggestions | Study/level of evidence |
|---|---|---|
| Slow, progressive training | • Prevention of stress fractures may lie in a slow, progressive approach to training with careful attention to avoiding rapid changes of style or technique; a reasoned attempt to match the anatomical characteristics of the individual dancer to the demands of the technique; and a general awareness of body mechanics, especially as they pertain to avoiding excessive fatigue. | Micheli & Solomon, 1990/case series |
| | • Dancing beyond the dancer's current technical capability can contribute to injuries. | Clanin et al., 1986/prospective<br>Solomon & Micheli, 1986/case series |
| **Environment and equipment** | | |
| Avoidance of slippery, sticky, or hard floors | • A sprung floor is best for absorbing shock. | Bowling, 1989/retrospective |
| | • A slippery floor for ballet dancers and a sticky floor for modern dancers have been attributed to injuries. | Reid, 1987/prospective<br>Clanin et al., 1986/prospective<br>Werter, 1985/case reports |
| | • Most of the cases of Achilles tendinitis developed while dancing on hard surfaces. | Fernández-Palazzi et al., 1990/case series<br>Klemp & Learmonth, 1984/cross-sectional |
| | • Shin splints were notably absent when dancers trained primarily on sprung floors, and they developed when the company was on tour and danced mostly on rigid floors. | |
| Appropriate shoe selection | • Pointe shoes have their own fitting characteristics; each dancer must be willing to try on every available brand of pointe shoe to find one which allows anatomically sound mechanics of rising and balancing on the pointes. | Carlson et al., 1981/cross-sectional |
| | • For instance, Capezio shoes are generally shorter than the dancer's foot and, consequently, force the dancer to perform on either flexed or hyperextended toes and with increased pelvic tilt. | Skrinar et al., 1981/cross-sectional |
| | • The best way to distribute the pressures on the forefoot while on pointe is to align the toes side by side so that as many toetips as anatomically possible can bear the weight. Pointe shoes, however, are not made wide enough in the vamp to accommodate an appropriate side-by-side alignment of the toes. Padding may assist the distribution of weight for shorter toes. | Teitz et al., 1985/cross-sectional<br>Tuckman et al., 1991/cross-sectional |
| | • Use alginate molding technique to evaluate chronic forefoot conditions and dynamic changes on pointe and help in the placement of paddings, toe spacers, toe extendors, and selection of proper pointe shoe style. | Tuckman et al., 1991/cross-sectional |
| **Health support system** | | |
| Awareness | • University health care centers need to be sensitive to dancers as a unique population with regard to eating disorders. | Kurtzman et al., 1990/cross-sectional |
| | • Unlike anorexia nervosa patients whose condition is motivated by a fear of failure, dancers adopt anorectic behavior because of an inner motive to achieve. | Weeda-Mannak & Drop, 1985/cross-sectional |
| | • As a rule, students in university dance programs do not receive the same medical attention as the competitive athletes. | Werner et al., 1991/retrospective |
| Availability | • Dancers are often unable to seek medical help for injuries when they should because it was not available to them while on tour, or it was difficult to obtain an appointment. | Bowling, 1989/retrospective |

*(continued)*

**Table 9.14**  *(continued)*

| Preventive measure | Examples/suggestions | Study/level of evidence |
|---|---|---|
| Screening techniques | • Preparticipation exams have resulted in fewer injuries in dancers. Students should be screened annually for overall conditioning and rehabilitation of prior injuries; detection of orthopedic abnormalities or limitations; and assessment of dietary habits and menstrual function. | Plastino, 1987/clinical report<br>Rovere et al., 1983/prospective<br>Weeda-Mannak & Drop, 1985/cross-sectional<br>Werner et al., 1991/retrospective |
| | • The bi-iliac width may be used as a screening device to isolate those dancers who require exercises to regain and retain muscular balance and keep the soft tissues from adaptively shortening. | Jacobs & Young, 1988/cross-sectional |
| | • Insufficient turnout, as determined by passive hip abduction, may predispose the dancer to injury. | Kushner et al., 1990/cross-sectional |
| | • National ballet dancers who have undergone a stringent selection process through the company school may be less susceptible to develop eating problems. 42% of dancers who were selected by general audition had an obese family member compared to dancers who came up through the company school. | Hamilton, L.H. et al., 1988/retrospective |
| | • Hypermobile dancers are at greater risk of injury (p < .05) and should not make dancing a career. | Hamilton, W.G. et al., 1992/cross-sectional<br>Klemp et al., 1984/retrospective |
| Use of orthotics | • The Braver ballet device is an orthotic that limits excessive pronation and supination as well as corrects for the mechanical disadvantages imposed by enlarged and extra bones in the forefoot. However, no statistical data describe its effectiveness. | Braver, 1989/clinical report |

**Table 9.15  Suggestions for Injury Prevention in Aerobic Dancers**

| Preventive measure | Examples/suggestions | Study/level of evidence |
|---|---|---|
| **The dancer** | | |
| Accommodation of anatomical flaws | • Pronation is correlated with incidence of injury. | Allen et al., 1986/prospective<br>Richie et al., 1993/cross-sectional<br>Stephens & Ransom, 1988/retrospective |
| | • Athletes who are susceptible to shin pain should be placed in a preconditioning program to strengthen the lower leg. | Richie et al., 1993/cross-sectional |
| **Dancing** | | |
| Appropriate exposure | • Limit the number of classes per week to 3 and no more than 4. | Hayes, 1985/retrospective<br>Janis, 1990/retrospective<br>Richie et al., 1985/retrospective<br>Rothenberger et al., 1988/retrospective |
| Effective stretches and warm-up | • The best type of stretch for a dancer's warm-up is the static stretch. | Rothenberger et al., 1988/retrospective<br>Stephens & Ransom, 1988/retrospective |
| Exercise prescription | • Aerobic dance routines should be modified to fit the aerobic capacity level of the class. | Francis et al., 1985/retrospective<br>Janis, 1990/retrospective<br>Thomsen & Ballor, 1991/prospective<br>Carroll et al., 1991/RCT |
| | • Individuals who must limit complete ROM in the shoulders should replace above shoulder level arm movements with below shoulder level arm movements with weights to maintain cardiovascular stimulus. | |
| | • Students with prior orthopedic complaints should receive precautionary instruction to prevent reinjury. | Garrick et al., 1986/prospective |

| Preventive measure | Examples/suggestions | Study/level of evidence |
|---|---|---|
| Slow, progressive training | • Prevention of stress fractures may lie in a slow, progressive approach to training with careful attention to avoiding rapid changes of style or technique; a reasoned attempt to match the anatomical characteristics of the individual dancer to the demands of the technique; and a general awareness of body mechanics, especially as they pertain to avoiding excessive fatigue. | Rothenberger et al., 1988/retrospective |
| | • For beginners, preconditioning exercises may be required, such as walking or other gradual approach to conditioning. | Stephens & Ransom, 1988/retrospective |
| Instructor certification | • It is believed that adequate training and certification can reduce the risk of injury. | Richie et al., 1985/retrospective<br>Stephens & Ransom, 1988/retrospective |
| **Environment and equipment** | | |
| Appropriate shoe selection | • Aerobic shoes do not necessarily prevent injuries, and in fact most injuries in some studies were found among dancers using aerobic shoes.<br>• Viscoelastic insoles may prevent injuries in aerobic dancing and may improve comfort and provide pain relief for some high-level aerobic dancers, if proper shoe fit is achieved. | Janis, 1990/retrospective<br>Richie et al., 1985/retrospective<br>Rothenberger et al., 1988/retrospective<br>Clark et al., 1989/prospective |
| Dancing surface | • Hardwood, sprung floors, which can absorb shock and produce the lowest amount of eccentric muscle activity of the lower leg musculature, have been demonstrated to best serve the dancer. | Richie et al., 1993/cross-sectional |
| | • The closest kind of floor to that ideal is the suspended wood floor, and its effectiveness is controversial. Allen et al. (1986) found no difference between a regular gym floor and a judo/wrestling mat in relation to injuries, rather malalignment was the causative factor leading to injury. Janis (1990) found it effective in injury prevention; Rothenberger et al. (1988) found the padded and carpeted concrete floor most effective. | Allen et al., 1986/prospective<br>Janis, 1990/retrospective<br>Rothenberger et al., 1988/retrospective |
| **Health support system** | | |
| Screening techniques | • A squat test, in conjunction with assessment of malalignments in the lower extremity, can help identify aerobics participants who may be predisposed to injury. | Allen et al., 1986/prospective<br>Stephens & Ransom, 1988/retrospective |
| | • A thorough evaluation of lower extremity alignments has been effective in identifying runners who may be predisposed to injury. | James et al., 1978/case series |
| Use of orthotics | • Orthotic devices have been effective in rehabilitating and/or preventing injuries in dancers and runners. | Allen et al., 1986/prospective<br>Baitch, 1987/clinical report<br>James et al., 1978/case series<br>Riddle & Freeman, 1988/case report<br>Vetter et al., 1985/case series |

ensuring an equal pressure ratio between the first two toes; experience stress in their personal lives; dance on nonresilient, sticky, or slippery floors; and dance inefficiently.

• In aerobic dancers, although the verdict is not yet in concerning all risk factors, participants may be at highest risk of injury who have experienced prior injuries; display malalignments in the lower extremities; participate more than 4 times per week; dance on non-resilient floors; wear specific brands of aerobic shoes; and are in a certain age group, although research results among the various studies are not yet adequately controlled to report which age group is the most likely to incur injuries.

• Finally, injuries can be avoided if one takes precautions. More intervention studies must be conducted to augment the few modalities which have resulted from studies on orthotics and iron supplementation.

**Table 9.16    Suggestions for Further Research**

| Research component | Research directions/questions |
|---|---|
| **Literature** | |
| Research design | Most data come from case series and cross-sectional studies, which provide information only on injured dancers. Without information about the population of dancers who are not injured, series and cross-sectional data cannot contribute information about injury rates or possible causative factors. |
| Injury definition | How is injury defined among studies and among dance forms? |
| Data collection | Data collection needs to be uniform among studies so that injury rates can be calculated in terms of exposure to risk of injury. |
| **Incidence of injury** | |
| Injury rates | More prospective cohort studies need to be conducted because of their stronger controls for bias. Determine injury rates among skill levels and age groups. |
| Reinjury rates | Define reinjury. Is it necessarily the same as a recurrent injury? More studies need to be conducted with reinjuries in mind. |
| Practice versus performance | Comparing a relative risk of practicing versus performing requires very precise denominator information (i.e., the amount of time actually spent dancing). If injuries occur during class, cross-tabulate them with reference to phase of dancing season (e.g., peak season, end of season). |
| **Injury characteristics** | |
| Injury onset | Determine onset of injury as it relates to age, skill level, idiom. Define sudden and gradual onset injuries more clearly and use uniform terminology among studies. |
| Injury type | Define ambiguous conditions, such as "shin splints," according to the current medical knowledge and use terminology consistently among dance forms. Cross-tabulate types with age, skill level, dance idiom. Design studies to address and test suspected mechanisms of injury. Which ones actually contribute to injuries, and specifically what kinds of injuries, where, etc.? |
| Injury location | Data collection needs to be more specific to anatomic sites, not to broader anatomical regions. Differentiate among the number of dancers who participate in each idiom and those who participate in an eclectic dance experience. How do the injury patterns differ? |
| **Injury severity** | |
| Time loss | Establish uniform measures of amount of time lost due to injury. Implement a uniform grading scale for severity of specific types of injuries. |
| Catastrophic injury | Make the definition of catastrophic injury uniform from study to study. Is every head and spine injury catastrophic? The definition should include specific criteria beyond death and paralysis. |
| Clinical outcome/ residual symptoms | Record data according to clinical outcome and medical costs. There is no central database for collecting costs associated with medical treatment of dancers; it should include information from physicians, surgeons, psychologists, dietitians, chiropractors, and physical therapists. |
| **Injury risk factors** | |
| Intrinsic factors | Explore further the comparison of injuries between dancers whose bodies are naturally suitable to ballet and those that are forced into the ideal image. In a few studies, age of participants was correlated to injury. More research should take this factor into account from the onset of designing the study. Investigate musculoskeletal, physiologic, and psychosocial characteristics of dancers other than professional ballerinas. |
| Extrinsic factors | Data collection should include exposure time to practice, rehearsal, and performance. (Aerobic dance studies have already begun addressing exposure.) Also, explore the differences between styles within idioms (e.g., Bournonville, Cecchetti, Russian in ballet; Graham, Limon, Cunningham in modern dance; high-impact versus low-impact aerobics; step aerobics versus power aerobics, etc.) in terms of uniquenesses, teaching approaches, etc. Environment and shoe studies need to be controlled for other variables such as age of participants, their injury history, exposure, etc. |
| Injury prevention | Conduct prospective studies to address and test injury prevention measures suggested by previous research. |

Clearly, what we know about dance injuries has mushroomed a hundredfold since 1975. As future dance research increasingly incorporates control data, the reliability of bottom-line answers obtained through stringent integrative analysis of the literature will ripen.

# References

1. Abel, M.S. Jogger's fracture and other stress fractures of the lumbo-sacral spine. Skeletal. Radiol. 13:221-227; 1985.

2. Abraham, S.F.; Beaumont, P.J.V.; Fraser, I.S.; Llewellyn-Jones, D. Body weight, exercise and menstrual status among ballet dancers in training. Brit. J. Obstet. Gynaecol. 89:507-510; 1982.

3. Allen, M; Webster, C.A.; Stortz, M.; Bruno, J.; Cove, L. Fitness class injuries: floor surface, malalignment, and a new "squat test." Ann. Sp. Med. 3(1):14-18; 1986.

4. Ambré, T.; Nilsson, B.E. Degenerative changes in the first metatarso-phalangeal joint of ballet dancers. Acta Orthop. Scand. 49:317-319; 1978.

5. Armann, S.A.; Wells, C.L.; Cheung, S.S.; Posner, S.L.; Fischer, R.J.; Pachtman, J.A.; Chick, R.P. Bone mass, menstrual abnormalities, dietary intake, and body composition in classical ballerinas. Kines. Med. Dance 13(1):1-15; 1990.

6. Baitch, S.P. Aerobic dance injuries: a biomechanical approach. JOHPERD May-June:57-58; 1987.

7. Barrack, R.L.; Skinner, H.B.; Brunet, M.E.; Cook, S.D. Joint laxity and proprioception in the knee. Phys. Sportsmed. 11(6):130-135; 1983.

8. Bejjani, F.J. Occupational biomechanics of athletes and dancers: a comparative approach. Clinics in Podiatric. Med. and Surg. 4(3):671-711; 1987.

9. Belt, C.R. Injuries associated with aerobic dance. Am. Fam. Physician 41(6):1769-1772; 1990.

10. Benson, J.E.; Geiger, C.J.; Eiserman, P.A.; Wardlaw, G.M. Relationship between nutrient intake, body mass index, menstrual function, and ballet injury. J. Am. Diet. Assoc. 89(1):58-63; 1989.

11. Benson J.; Gillien, D.M.; Bourdet, K.; Loosli, A.R. Inadequate nutrition and chronic calorie restriction in adolescent ballerinas. Phys. Sportsmed. 13(10):79-90; 1985.

12. Bowling, A. Injuries to dancers: prevalence, treatment, and perceptions of causes. Br. Med. J. 298:731-734; 1989.

13. Braisted, J.R.; Mellin, L.; Gong, E.J.; Irwin, C.E., Jr. The adolescent ballet dancer. Nutritional practices and characteristics associated with anorexia nervosa. J. Adolesc. Health Care 6(5):365-371; 1985.

14. Braver, R.T. Tendonitis rond de ankle, part 3: improper dance technique. Kines. for Dance 11(2):5-8; 1988.

15. Braver, R.T. Tendonitis rond de ankle, part 5: imbalance of muscle strength and elasticity. Kines. for Dance 11(4):5-8; 1989.

16. Brodsky, A.E.; Khalil, M.A. Talar compression syndrome. Foot Ankle 7(6):338-344; 1987.

17. Brooks-Gunn, J.; Warren, M.P.; Hamilton, L.H. The relationship of eating problems and amenorrhea in ballet dancers. Med. Sci. Sports Exerc. 19(1):41-44; 1987.

18. Calabrese, L.J.; Kirkendall, D.T.; Floyd, M.; Rapoport, S.; Williams, G.W.; Weiker, G.G.; Bergfeld, J.A. Menstrual abnormalities, nutritional patterns, and body composition in female ballet dancers. Phys. Sportsmed. 11(2):86-98; 1983.

19. Campbell, J. Anorexia nervosa: body dissatisfaction in a high risk population. CAHPER J. July/August:36-42; 1985.

20. Carlson, K.; Skrinar, M.; Jeglosky, L. Selected differences between foot configuration and shoe dimensions among three brands of pointe shoes (abstract). Int. J. Sports Med. 2:284; 1981.

21. Carroll, M.W.; Otto, R.M.; Wygand, J. The metabolic cost of two ranges of arm position height with and without hand weights during low impact aerobic dance. Res. Q. Exerc. Sport 62(4):420-423; 1991.

22. Chambers, B. Fitness of dancers and varsity athletes. JOPERD 52(5):46,49; 1981.

23. Chmelar, R.D.; Schultz, B.B.; Ruhling, R.O.; Shepherd, T.A.; Zupan, M.F.; Fitt, S.S. A physiologic profile comparing levels and styles of female dancers. Phys. Sportsmed. 16(7):87-96; 1988.

24. Clanin, D.R.; Davidson, D.M.; Plastino, J.G. Injury patterns in university dance students. In: Shell, C.G., ed. The dancer as athlete. Champaign, IL: Human Kinetics Publishers; 1986:195-199.

25. Clark, J.E.; Scott, S.J.; Mingle, M. Viscoelastic shoe insoles: their use in aerobic dancing. Arch. Phys. Med. Rehabil. 70:37-40; 1989.

26. Clarkson, P.M.; Freedson, P.S.; Keller, B.; Carney, D.; Skrinar, M. Maximal oxygen uptake, nutritional patterns and body composition of adolescent female ballet dancers. Res. Q. Exerc. Sport 56(2):180-184; 1985.

27. Clippinger-Robertson, K. A unique challenge; biomechanical considerations in turnout. JOHPERD May/June: 37-40; 1987.

28. Clippinger-Robertson, K.S.; Hutton, R.S.; Miller, D.I.; Nichols, T.R. Mechanical and anatomical factors relating to the incidence and etiology of patello-femoral pain in dancers. In: Shell, C.G., ed. The dancer as athlete. Champaign, IL: Human Kinetics Publishers; 1986:53-72.

29. Cohen, J.L.; Gupta, P.K.; Lichstein, E.; Chadda, K.D. The heart of a dancer: noninvasive cardiac evaluation of professional ballet dancers. Am. J. Cardio. 45:959-965; 1980.

30. Cohen, J.L.; Kim, C.S.; May, P.B., Jr.; Ertel, N.H. Exercise, body weight, and amenorrhea in professional ballet dancers. Phys. Sportsmed. 10(4):92-101; 1982.

31. Cohen, J.L.; Potosnak, L.; Frank, O.; Baker, H. A nutritional and hematologic assessment of elite ballet dancers. Phys. Sportsmed. 13(5):43-54; 1985.

32. Cohen, J.L.; Segal, K.R.; McArdle, W.D. Heart rate response to ballet stage performance. Phys. Sportsmed. 10(11):120-133; 1982.

33. Cohen, J.L.; Segal, K.R.; Witriol, I.; McArdle, W.D. Cardiorespiratory responses to ballet exercise and the VO$_2$max of elite ballet dancers. Med. Sci. Sports Exerc. 14(3):212-217; 1982.

34. Collins, R.E.C. Breast disease associated with tassel dancing. Br. Med. J. 283:1660; 1981.

35. Cowell, H.R.; Elener, V.; Lawhorn, S.M. Bilateral tendonitis of the flexor hallucis longus in a ballet dancer. J. Pediatric Orthop. 2:582-586; 1982.

36. Cross, D.L.; Mills, S.E.; Kulund, D.N. Elastofibroma arising in the foot. Southern Med. J. 77(9):1194-1196; 1984.

37. Cross, M.J.; Crichton, K.J.; Gordon, H; Mackie, I.G. Peroneus brevis rupture in the absence of the peroneus longus muscle and tendon in a classical ballet dancer. Am. J. Sports Med. 16(6):677-678; 1988.

38. Daffner, R.H. Anterior tibial striations. Am. J. Roentgenol. 143:651-653; 1984.

39. Dhuper, S.; Warren, M.P.; Brooks-Gunn, J.; Fox, R. Effects of hormonal status on bone density in adolescent girls. J. Clin. Endocrinol. Metab. 71(5): 1083-1089; 1990.

40. Dolgener, F.A.; Spasoff, T.C.; St. John, W.E. Body build and body composition of high ability female dancers. Res. Q. Exerc. Sport 51(4):599-607; 1980.

41. Druss, R.G.; Silverman, J.A. Body image and perfectionism of ballerinas. Gen. Hosp. Psychiatry 1(2):115-121; 1979.

42. Eickhoff, J.; Thorland, W.; Ansorge, C. Selected physiological and psychological effects of aerobic dancing among young adult women. J. Sports Med. 23:273-280; 1983.

43. Ende, L.S.; Wickstrom, J. Ballet injuries. Phys. Sportsmed. 10(7):101-118; 1982.

44. Evans, B.W.; Tiburzi, A.; Norton, C.J. Body composition and body type of female dance majors. Dance Res. J. 17(1):17-20; 1985.

45. Evers, C.L. Dietary intake and symptoms of anorexia nervosa in female university dancers. J. Am. Diet. Assoc. 87(1):66-68; 1987.

46. Fernández-Palazzi, F.; Rivas, S.; Mujica, P. Achilles tendinitis in ballet dancers. Clin. Orthop. Related Re. (257):257-261; 1990.

47. Ferretti, A.; Ippolito, E.; Mariani, P.; Puddu, G. Jumper's knee. Am. J. Sports Med. 11(2):58-62; 1983.

48. Fond, D. Flexor hallucis longus tendinitis—a case of mistaken identity and posterior impingement syndrome in dancers: evaluation and management. J. Orthop. Sports Phys. Ther. 5(4):204-206; 1984.

49. Foster, C. Physiological requirements of aerobic dancing. Res. Q. 46:120-122; 1975.

50. Francis, L.L.; Francis, P.R.; Welshons-Smith, K. Aerobic dance injuries; a survey of instructors. Phys. Sportsmed. 13(2):105-111; 1985.

51. Frisch, R.E.; Wyshak, G.; Vincent, L. Delayed menarche and amenorrhea in ballet dancers. N. Engl. J. Med. 303(1):17-19; 1980.

52. Gans, A. The relationship of heel contact in ascent and descent from jumps to the incidence of shin splints in ballet dancers. Phys. Ther. 65(8):1192-1196; 1985.

53. Garner, D.M. You are what you don't eat. Anorexia nervosa and the dancer. Dance in Canada (20):5-8; 1979.

54. Garner, D.M.; Garfinkel, P.E. Socio-cultural factors in the development of anorexia nervosa. Psychological Med. 10:647-656; 1980.

55. Garrick, J.G. Characterization of the patient population in a sports medicine facility. Phys. Sportsmed. 13(10):73-76; 1985.

56. Garrick, J. Age and injury in ballet. In: Grana, W.A., ed. Advances in sports medicine and fitness. Chicago: Year Book Medical Publishers; 1988.

57. Garrick, J.G.; Gillien, D.M.; Whiteside, P. The epidemiology of aerobic dance injuries. Am. J. Sports Med. 14(1):67-72; 1986.

58. Garth, W.P. Flexor hallucis tendinitis in a ballet dancer. J. Bone Joint Surg. 63A(9):1489; 1981.

59. Gillham, N.R.; Villar, R.N. Postero-lateral subluxation of the superior tibio-fibular joint. Brit. J. Sports Med. 23(3):195-196; 1989.

60. Grahame, R.; Saunders, A.S.; Maisey, N. The use of scintigraphy in the diagnosis and management of traumatic foot lesions in ballet dancers. Rheum. Rehab. 18: 235; 1979.

61. Green, G.A.; Maltz, B.A. Case report: bilateral ankle pain in an aerobic dancer. Med. Sci. Sports Exerc. 24(12): 1316-1320; 1992.

62. Hamilton, L.H.; Brooks-Gunn, J.; Warren, M.P. Sociocultural influences on eating disorders in professional female ballet dancers. Int. J. Eating Disorders 4(4): 465-477; 1985.

63. Hamilton, L.H.; Brooks-Gunn, J.; Warren, M.; Hamilton, W.G. The impact of thinness and dieting on the professional ballet dancer. CAHPER J. 52(4): 30-35; 1986.

64. Hamilton, L.H.; Brooks-Gunn, J.; Warren, M.P. Nutritional intake of female dancers: a reflection of eating problems. Int. J. Eating Disorders 5(5): 925-934; 1986.

65. Hamilton, L.H.; Brooks-Gunn, J.; Warren, M.P.; Hamilton, W.G. The role of selectivity in the pathogenesis of eating problems in ballet dancers. Med. Sci. Sports Exerc. 20(6): 560-565; 1988.

66. Hamilton, L.H.; Hamilton, W.G.; Meltzer, J.D.; Marshall, P.; Molnar, M. Personality, stress, and injuries in professional ballet dancers. Am. J. Sports Med. 17(2): 263-267; 1989.

67. Hamilton, W.G. Tendonitis about the ankle joint in classical ballet dancers. Am. J. Sports Med. 5: 84-88; 1977.

68. Hamilton, W.G. The dancer's ankle. Emergency Med. 14: 42-48; 1982.

69. Hamilton, W.G. Sprained ankles in ballet dancers. Foot Ankle 3(2): 99-102; 1982.

70. Hamilton, W.G. Stenosing tenosynovitis of the flexor hallucis longus tendon and posterior impingement upon the os trigonum in ballet dancers. Foot Ankle 3(2): 74-80; 1982.

71. Hamilton, W.G. Foot and ankle injuries in dancers. Clin. Sports Med. 7(1): 143-173; 1988.

72. Hamilton, W.G.; Hamilton, L.H.; Marshall, P.; Molnar, M. A profile of the musculoskeletal characteristics of elite professional ballet dancers. Am. J. Sports Med. 20(3): 267-273; 1992.

73. Hardaker, W.T., Jr. Foot and ankle injuries in classical ballet dancers. Orthop. Clin. No. Amer. 20(4): 621-627; 1989.

74. Hayes, G.W. Injuries arising from aerobic fitness classes. Can. Fam. Physician 31: 1517-1519; 1985.

75. Hergenroeder, A.C.; Brown, B.; Klish, W.J. Anthropometric measurements and estimating body composition in ballet dancers. Med. Sci. Sports Exerc. 25(1): 145-150; 1993.

76. Hergenroeder, A.C.; Fiorotto, M.L.; Klish, W.J. Body composition in ballet dancers measured by total body electrical conductivity. Med. Sci. Sports Exerc. 23(5): 528-533; 1991.

77. Hergenroeder, A.C.; Wong, W.W.; Fiorotto, M.L.; Smith, E.O.; Klish, W.J. Total body water and fat-free mass in ballet dancers: comparing isotope dilution and TOBEC. Med. Sci. Sports Exerc. 23(5):534-541; 1991.

78. Holder, L.E.; Michael, R.H. The specific scintigraphic pattern of "shin splints in the lower leg": concise communication. J. Nuclear Med. 25(8):865-869; 1984.

79. Horváth, Cs.; Holló, I. Scoliosis and fractures in young ballet dancers. N. Engl. J. Med. 315(22):1417-1418; 1986.

80. Howse, A.J.G. Posterior block of the ankle joint in dancers. Foot Ankle 3(2):81-84; 1982.

81. Howse, J. Disorders of the great toe in dancers. Clin. Sports Med. 2(2):499-505; 1983.

82. Igbanugo, V.; Gutin, B. The energy cost of aerobic dancing. Res. Q. 49(3):308-316; 1978.

83. Ireland, M.L.; Micheli, L.J. Bilateral stress fracture of the lumbar pedicles in a ballet dancer. J. Bone Joint Surg. 69A (1):140-142; 1987.

84. Jacobs, M.; Young, R. Snapping hip phenomenon among dancers. Am. Correct. Ther. J. 32(3):92-98; 1978.

85. Janis, L.R. Aerobic dance survey. A study of high-impact versus low-impact injuries. J. Am. Podiatr. Med. Assoc. 80(8):419-423; 1990.

86. Jonnavithula, S.; Warren, M.P.; Fox, R.P.; Lazaro, M.I. Bone density is compromised in amenorrheic women despite return of menses: a 2-year study. Obstet. Gynecol. 81(5, Part I):669-674; 1993.

87. Joseph, A.; Wood, I.K.; Goldberg, S.C. Determining populations at risk for developing anorexia nervosa based on selection of college major. Psychiatric Res. 7:53-58; 1982.

88. Kadel, N.J.; Teitz, C.C.; Kronmal, R.A. Stress fractures in ballet dancers. Am. J. Sports Med. 20(4):445-449; 1992.

89. Katch, F.I. The body profile analysis system (BPAS) to estimate ideal body size and shape: application to ballet dancers and gymnasts. World Rev. Nutr. Diet. 71:69-83; 1993.

90. Kirkendall, D.T.; Bergenfeld, J.A.; Calabrese, L.; Lombardo, J.A.; Street, G.; Weiker, G.G. Isokinetic characteristics of ballet dancers and the response to a season of ballet training. J. Orthop. Sports Phys. Ther. 5(4):207-211; 1984.

91. Kirkendall, D.T.; Calabrese, L.H. Physiological aspects of dance. Clin. Sports Med. 2(3):525-537; 1983.

92. Kleiger, B. Anterior tibiotalar impingement syndrome in dancers. Foot Ankle 3(2):69-73; 1982.

93. Kleiger, B. The posterior tibiotalar impingement syndrome in dancers. Bull. Hosp. Jt. Dis. Orthop. Instit. 47(2):203-210; 1987.

94. Klemp, P.; Chalton, D. Articular mobility in ballet dancers, a follow-up study after four years. Am. J. Sports Med. 17(1):72-75; 1989.

95. Klemp, P.; Learmonth, I.D. Hypermobility and injuries in a professional ballet company. Brit. J. Sports Med. 18(3):143-148; 1984.

96. Klemp, P.; Stevens, J.E.; Issacs, S. A hypermobility study in ballet dancers. J. Rheumatol. 11(5):692-696; 1984.

97. Kliman, M.E.; Gross, A.E.; Pritzker, K.P.H.; Greyson, N.D. Osteochondritis of the hallux sesamoid bones. Foot Ankle 3(4):220-223; 1983.

98. Koceja, D.M.; Burke, J.R.; Kamen, G. Organization of segmental reflexes in trained dancers. Int. J. Sports Med. 12:285-289; 1991.

99. Koltyn, K.F.; Morgan, W.P. Efficacy of perceptual versus heart rate monitoring in the development of endurance. Brit. J. Sports Med. 26(2):132-134; 1992.

100. Kravitz, S.R. The mechanics of dance and dance-related injuries. In: Subotnick, S.I., ed. Sports medicine of the lower extremity. New York: Churchill Livingstone; 1989:595-603.

101. Kravitz, S.R.; Fink, K.L.; Huber, S.; Bohanske, L.; Cicilioni, S. Osseous changes in the second ray of classical ballet dancers. J. Am. Podiatr. Med. Assoc. 75(7):346-348; 1985.

102. Kravitz, S.R.; Murgia, C.J.; Huber, S.; Fink, K.; Shaffer, M.; Varela, L. Bunion deformity and the forces generated around the great toe: a biomechanical approach to analysis of pointe dance, classical ballet. In: Shell, C.G., ed. The dancer as athlete. Champaign, IL: Human Kinetics Publishers; 1986:213-225.

103. Kurtzman, F.D.; Yager, J.; Landsverk, J.; Wiesmeier, E.; Bodurka, D.C. Eating disorders and associated symptoms among dancers and other student populations at UCLA. Kines. Med. Dance 13(1):16-32; 1990.

104. Kushner, S.; Saboe, L.; Reid, D.; Penrose, T.; Grace, M. Relationship of turnout to hip abduction in professional ballet dancers. Am. J. Sports Med. 18(3):286-291; 1990.

105. Lavoie, J.M.; Lèbe-Nèron, R.M. Physiological effects of training in professional and recreational jazz dancers. J. Sports Med. 22:231-236; 1982.

106. Lehman, R.C.; Gregg, J.R.; Torg, E. Iselin's disease. Am. J. Sports Med. 14(6):494-496; 1986.

107. Lereim, P. Trigger toe in classical ballet dancers. Arch. Orthop. Trauma Surg. 104:325-326; 1985.

108. Levine, A.; Wells, S.; Kopf, C. New rules of exercise. U.S. News & World Report 101:52; 1986.

109. Liederbach, M.; Gleim, G.W.; Nicholas, J.A. Monitoring training status in professional ballet dancers. J. Sports Med. Phys. Fitness 32(2):187-195; 1992.

110. Lowenkopf, E.L.; Vincent, S.M. The student ballet dancer and anorexia. Hillside J. Clin. Psychiatry 4:53-64; 1982.

111. Mahlamäki, E.; Mahlamäki, S. Iron deficiency in adolescent female dancers. Brit. J. Sports Med. 22(2):55-56; 1988.

112. Marotta, J.J.; Micheli, L.J. Os trigonum in dancers. Am. J. Sports Med. 20(5):533-536; 1992.

113. Marshall, P. The rehabilitation of overuse foot injuries in athletes and dancers. Clin. Podiatr. Med. Surg. 6(3):639-655; 1989.

114. Marshall, P.; Hamilton, W.G. Cuboid subluxation in ballet dancers. Am. J. Sports Med. 20(2):169-175; 1992.

115. McDonnell, M.F.; Butler, J.E. III. Osteochondral fracture of the tibial plateau in a ballerina. Am. J. Sports Med. 16(4):417-418; 1988.

116. Meermann, R. Experimental investigation of disturbances in body image estimation in anorexia nervosa patients, and ballet and gymnastic pupils. Int. J. Eating Disorders 2(4):91-100; 1983.

117. Micheli, L.J. Back injuries in dancers. Clin. Sports Med. 2(3):473-484; 1983.

118. Micheli, L.J.; Gillespie, W.J.; Walaszek, A. Physiologic profiles of female professional ballerinas. Clin. Sports Med. 3(1):199-209; 1984.

119. Micheli, L.J.; Sohn, R.S.; Solomon, R. Stress fractures of the second metatarsal involving Lisfranc's joint in ballet dancers. J. Bone Joint Surg. 67A(9):1372-1375; 1985.

120. Micheli, L.J.; Solomon, R. Stress fractures in dancers. In: Solomon, R.; Minton, S.C.; Solomon, J., eds. Preventing dance injuries: an interdisciplinary perspective. Reston, VA: AAHPERD; 1990: 133-153.

121. Milburn, S.; Butts, N.K. A comparison of the training responses to aerobic dance and jogging in college females. Med. Sci. Sports Exerc. 15(6):510-513; 1983.

122. Miller, E.H.; Benedict, F.E. Stretch of the femoral nerve in a dancer. J. Bone Joint Surg. 67(2):315-317; 1985.

123. Miller, E.H.; Schneider, H.J.; Bronson, J.L.; McLain, D. A new consideration in athletic injuries; the classical ballet dancer. Clin. Orthop. Rel. Res. 111:181-191; 1975.

124. Moisan, J.; Meyer, F.; Gingras, S. Leisure physical activity and age at menarche. Med. Sci. Sports Exerc. 23(10):1170-1175; 1991.

125. Mostardi, R.A.; Porterfield, J.A.; Greenberg, B.; Goldberg, D.; Lea, M. Musculoskeletal and cardiopulmonary characteristics of the professional ballet dancer. Phys. Sportsmen. 11(12): 53-61; 1983.

126. Mutoh, Y.; Sawai, S.; Takanashi, Y.; Skurko, L. Aerobic dance injuries among instructors and students. Phys. Sportsmen. 16(12):81-86; 1988.

127. Nicholas, J.A. Risk factors, sports medicine and the orthopedic system: an overview. J. Sp. Med. 3(5): 243-259; 1975.

128. Noble, R.M.; Howley, E.T. The energy requirement of selected tap dance routines. Res. Q. 50(3):438-442; 1979.

129. Novak, L.P.; Magill, L.A.; Schutte, J.E. Maximal oxygen intake and body composition of female dancers. Euro. J. Appl. Physiol. 39:277-282; 1978.

130. Nussbaum, A.R.; Treves, S.T.; Micheli, L. Bone stress lesions in ballet dancers: scintigraphic assessment. A.J.R. 150:851-855; 1988.

131. Oliver, W. Problems in technique: ankle block—a case study. Kines. for Dance 9(4):18-19; 1987.

132. Parkes, J.C.; Hamilton, W.G.; Patterson, A.H.; Rawles, J.G., Jr. The anterior impingement syndrome of the ankle. J. Trauma 20(10):895-898; 1980.

133. Passa, A.; Rampoldi, M. Fatigue fracture of the tibia in dancers (report of 3 cases). Ital. J. Orthop. Traumatol. 13(2):235-240; 1987.

134. Percy, E.C.; Telep, G.N. Anomalous muscle in the leg: soleus accessorium. Am. J. Sports Med. 12(6): 447-450; 1984.

135. Perry, A.C.; Shaw, M.H.; Hsia, L.; Nash, M.S.; Kaplan, T.; Signorile, J.F.; Appleyate, B. Plasma lipid levels in active and sedentary premenopausal females. Int. J. Sports Med. 13(3):210-215; 1992.

136. Plastino, J.G. The university dancer, physical screening. JOHPERD May/June:49-50; 1987.

137. Quirk, R. Talar compression syndrome in dancers. Foot Ankle 3(2):65-68; 1982.

138. Quirk, R. Ballet injuries, the Australian experience. Clin. Sports Med. 2(3):507-513; 1983.

139. Quirk, R. Stress fractures of the foot. Am. Fam. Phys. (Aust) 16(8):1101-1102; 1987.

140. Read, M.T.F. Runner's stress fracture produced by an aerobic dance routine. Brit. J. Sports Med. 18(1):40-41; 1984.

141. Reid, D.C. Preventing injuries to the young ballet dancer. Physiother. Canada 39(4):231-236; 1987.

142. Reid, D.C. Prevention of hip and knee injuries in ballet dancers. Sports Med. 6:295-307; 1988.

143. Reid, D.C.; Burnham, R.S.; Saboe, L.A.; Kushner, S.F. Lower extremity flexibility patterns in classical ballet dancers and their correlation to lateral hip and knee injuries. Am. J. Sports Med. 15(4):347-352; 1987.

144. Richie, D.H.; DeVries, H.A.; Endo, C.K. Shin muscle activity and sports surfaces. J. Am. Podiatr. Med. Assoc. 83(4): 181-190; 1993.

145. Richie, D.H.; Kelso, S.F.; Bellucci, P.A. Aerobic dance injuries: a retrospective study of instructors

and participants. Phys. Sportsmed. 13(2):130-140; 1985.

146. Riddle, D.L.; Freeman, D.B. Management of a patient with a diagnosis of bilateral plantar fasciitis and Achilles tendinitis—a case report. J. Phys. Ther. 68(12):1913-1916; 1988.

147. Rimmer, J.H.; Rosentswieg, J. The maximum $O_2$ consumption in dance majors. Dance Res. J. 14(1 & 2):29-31; 1981-82.

148. Rosentswieg, J.; Tate, J.; Fuller, P. Body composition specificity of female dancers (abstract). Med. Sci. Sports 11:102-103; 1979.

149. Rothenberger, L.A.; Chang, J.I.; Cable, T.A. Prevalence and types of injuries in aerobic dancers. Am. J. Sports Med. 16(4):403-407; 1988.

150. Round, M.J.; Rothschild, B.M. Shin pain in a ballet dancer. Illinois Med. J. 161(2):109-111; 1982.

151. Rovere, G.D.; Webb, L.Z.; Gristina, A.G.; Vogel, J.M. Musculoskeletal injuries in theatrical dance students. Am. J. Sports Med. 11:195-198; 1983.

152. Sammarco, G.J.; Miller, E.H. Partial rupture of the flexor hallucis longus tendon in classical ballet dancers. J. Bone Joint Surg. 61A:149-150; 1979.

153. Sammarco, G.J.; Stephens, M.M. Neurapraxia of the femoral nerve in a modern dancer. Am. J. Sports Med. 19(4):413-414; 1991.

154. Saunders, A.J.S.; El Sayed, T.F.; Hilson, A.J.W.; Maisey, M.N.; Grahame, R. Stress lesions of the lower leg and foot. Clin. Radiol. 30:649-651; 1979.

155. Sawyer-Morse, M.K.; Smolik, T.; Mobley, C.; Saegert, M. Nutrition beliefs, practices, and perceptions of young dancers. J. Adolesc. Health Care 10(3):200-202; 1989.

156. Schaberg, J.E.; Harper, M.C.; Allen, W.C. The snapping hip syndrome. Am. J. Sports Med. 12(5):361-365; 1984.

157. Schaflé, M.; Requa, R.K.; Garrick, J.G. A comparison of patterns of injury in ballet, modern, and aerobic dance. In: Solomon, R.; Minton, S.C.; Solomon, J., eds. Preventing dance injuries: an interdisciplinary perspective. Reston, VA: AAHPERD; 1990:1-4.

158. Schantz, P.G.; Åstrand, P.O. Physiological characteristics of classical ballet. Med. Sci. Sports Exerc. 16(5):472-476; 1984.

159. Scheller, A.D.; Kasser, J.R.; Quigley, T.B. Tendon injuries about the ankle. Clin. Sports Med. 2(3):631-641; 1983.

160. Skrinar, M.; Carlson, K.; Jeglosky, L. Effect of three brands of pointed[sic] shoe on pelvic tilt (abstract). Int. J. Sports Med. 2:283; 1981.

161. Solomon, R.; Micheli, L. Concepts in the prevention of dance injuries: a survey and analysis. In: Shell, C.G., ed. The dancer as athlete. Champaign, IL: Human Kinetics Publishers; 1986:201-212.

162. Stensland, S.H.; Sobal, J. Dietary practices of ballet, jazz, and modern dancers. J. Am. Diet. Assoc. 92(3):319-324; 1992.

163. Stephens, R.E.; Ransom, S.B. Epidemiology of aerobic dance injuries. J. Osteopathic Sports Med. 2(4):7-11; 1988.

164. Stoller, S.M.; Hekmat, F.; Kleiger, B. A comparative study of the frequency of anterior impingement exostoses of the ankle in dancers and nondancers. Foot Ankle 4(4):201-203; 1984.

165. Strudwick, W.J.; Goodman, S.B. Proximal fibular stress fracture in an aerobic dancer. Am. J. Sports Med. 20(4):481-482; 1992.

166. Szmukler, G.I.; Eisler, I.; Gillies, C.; Hayward, M.E. The implications of anorexia nervosa in a ballet school. J. Psychiat. Res. 19(2/3):177-181; 1985.

167. Teitz, C.C.; Harrington, R.M. Patellar stress fracture. Am. J. Sports Med. 20(6):761-765; 1992.

168. Teitz, C.C.; Harrington, R.M.; Wiley, H. Pressures on the foot in pointe shoes. Foot Ankle 5(5):216-221; 1985.

169. Thomasen, E. The loose metatarsophalangeal joint in dancers. In: Ryan, A.J.; Stephens, R.E., eds. Dance medicine: a comprehensive guide. Chicago: Pluribus Press; 1987:135-138.

170. Thomsen, D.; Ballor, D.L. Physiological responses during aerobic dance of individuals grouped by aerobic capacity and dance experience. Res. Q. Exerc. Sport 62(1):68-72; 1991.

171. Torg, J.S.; Pavlov, H.; Cooley, L.H.; Bryant, M.H.; Arnoczky, S.P.; Bergfeld, J.; Hunter, L.Y. Stress fractures of the tarsal navicular. J. Bone Joint Surg. 63A(5):700-712; 1982.

172. Tuckman, A.S.; Werner, F.W.; Bayley, J.C. Analysis of the forefoot on pointe in the ballet dancer. Foot Ankle 12(3):144-148; 1991.

173. Tudisco, C.; Puddu, G. Stenosing tenosynovitis of the flexor hallucis longus tendon in a classical ballet dancer. Am. J. Sports Med. 12(5):403-404; 1984.

174. Vaccaro, P.; Clinton, M. The effects of aerobic dance conditioning on the body composition and maximal oxygen uptake of college women. J. Sports Med. 21(3):291-294; 1981.

175. Vetter, W.L.; Helfet, D.L.; Spear, K.; Matthews, L.S. Aerobic dance injuries. Phys. Sportsmed. 13(2):114-120; 1985.

176. Warren, M.P. The effects of exercise on pubertal progression and reproductive function in girls. J. Clin. Endocrin. Metab. 51: 1150-1156; 1980.

177. Warren, M.P.; Brooks-Gunn, J.; Hamilton, L.H.; Warren, L.F.; Hamilton, W.G. Scoliosis and fractures in young ballet dancers: relation to delayed menarche and secondary amenorrhea. N. Engl. J. Med. 314(21):1348-1353; 1986.

178. Warren, M.P.; Shane, E.; Lee, M.J.; Lindsay, R.; Demptster, D.W.; Warren, L.F.; Hamilton, W.G. Femoral head collapse associated with anorexia nervosa in a 20-year-old ballet dancer. Clin. Orthop. Rel. Res. (251):171-176; 1990.

179. Washington, E.L. Musculoskeletal injuries in theatrical dancers: site, frequency and severity. Am. J. Sports Med. 6:75-98; 1978.

180. Watterson, V.V. The effects of aerobic dance on cardiovascular fitness. Phys. Sportsmed. 12(10):138-145; 1984.

181. Weeda-Mannak, W.L.; Drop, M.J. The discriminative value of psychological characteristics in anorexia nervosa. Clinical and psychometric comparison between anorexia nervosa patients, ballet dancers and controls. J. Psychiat. Res. 19(2/3):285-290; 1985.

182. Weiker, G.G. Dance injuries: the knee, ankle, and foot. In: Clarkson, P.M.; Skrinar, M., eds. Science of dance training. Champaign, IL: Human Kinetics Publishers; 1988:147-192.

183. Werner, M.J.; Rosenthal, S.L.; Biro, F.M. Medical needs of performing arts students. J. Adolesc. Health 12(4):294-300; 1991.

184. Werter, R. Dance floors—a causative factor in dance injuries. J. Am. Podiatr. Med. Assoc. 75(7):355-358; 1985.

185. Wittenbecker, N.L.; Dinitto, L.M. Successful treatment of patellofemoral dysfunction in a dancer. J. Orthop. Sp. Phys. Ther. 10(7):270-273; 1989.

186. Wredmark, T.; Carlstedt, C.A.; Bauer, H.; Saartok, T. Os trigonum syndrome: a clinical entity in ballet dancers. Foot Ankle 11(6):404-406; 1991.

187. Zeigler, E.F. Philosophical perspective. In: Krotee, M.L., ed. Cross-cultural dimensions of scientific inquiry. JOPERD 51(9):40; 1980.

# 10

# Disability Sports

*Peter A. Harmer*

## 1. Introduction

Although it has been almost 50 years since the first international sporting event for spinal cord injured (SCI) persons took place at Stoke Mandeville Hospital in England and more than 30 years since the Special Olympics first provided international sporting opportunities to persons with mental retardation, very little effort has been directed towards investigating injuries in disability sports (4, 13, 17, 20, 25, 31). However, increasing participation in athletic activities by persons with disabilities, because of legislative initiatives and changing social standards, has meant the possibility of more activity-related injuries, especially at the elite sporting level (7, 8, 19, 32, 44). Unfortunately, the dearth of published information makes it very difficult "to make definitive statements regarding sports-related injury patterns" in disability sports (6).

Identifying injury patterns in disability sports is important for a number of reasons.

- It allows participants or prospective participants to make informed choices about participating based on the risk of injury.
- It provides medical and health care professionals information to ensure appropriate and adequate care in disability sports.
- It directs researchers, coaches, and administrators to develop the safest possible circumstances for participation.

To ascertain the current state of data-based knowledge involving injury characteristics in disability sports and to make recommendations to promote the interests of athletes in disability sports, a literature search was undertaken.

As participants in disability sports have unique physical and physiological characteristics independent of those related to sporting activity, the search was conducted on both Medline and the SPORT Discus databases. Search terms were combined: (athletic injuries, sports injuries) and (handicapped, special populations, wheelchair, disabled). The search covered the period 1966 to 1994 and identified manuscripts published in English. In addition to the electronic database searches, the reference lists and bibliographies of cited works were examined for further sources of information.

A total of 28 studies containing some type of data related to injuries in disability sports was retrieved. The same data were the substance of three manuscripts (10-12) while progressive analysis of a longitudinal study produced three reports (14-16). However, one of the latter contained information not subsequently reanalyzed. Thus, a total of 25 studies (grouped into four categories: wheelchair, cross-disability, Special Olympics, and other) were retained for analysis and discussion. Several cross-disability studies included wheelchair athletes but did not differentiate injury information by disability type. Thus, the cross-disability grouping has some wheelchair data irretrievably embedded in it.

These papers represented approximately one half of the articles produced by the literature search. The remainder were reviews (9, 41), synthesis papers (30), or articles aimed at educating health care professionals and the general public about the medical needs of athletes in disability sports (5, 26-29, 34, 40). These articles tended to focus on prevention and treatment of injuries in very general terms.

The multiplicity of conditions and the range of activities that constitute disability sports present significant difficulties in conducting epidemiological research in this area. Simply defining the population of interest can be daunting. For example, Laskowski and Murtaugh (25), in their study of injuries sustained at instructional ski schools by skiers with disabilities, noted that 45 different disabilities were represented including "amputation, hemiplegia, vision and hearing impairments, spinal cord injuries, multiple sclerosis, and muscular dystrophy." Curtis (10) identified 32 different sports played by a sample of 127 wheelchair athletes; McCormack et al., (31) reported 90 wheelchair athletes representing at least seven types of disability participating in 19 different sports; and Paciorek & Jones (36) listed 53 sports and recreational activities supported by nine different disability sports organizations.

Additionally, levels of disability are accounted for differently within various governing bodies (e.g., Wheelchair Sports - USA [WS-USA], formerly the National Wheelchair Athletic Association [NWAA], has an eight-level classification system, whereas the National Wheelchair Basketball Association [NWBA] has a three-level system). Moreover, different organizations sponsor the same sports (e.g., track in Special Olympics [SO], WS-USA, United States Cerebral Palsy Athletic Association [USCPAA], United States Association for Blind Athletes [USABA], etc.), making meaningful comparisons between and across groups difficult.

Apart from the difficulties of dealing with the array of disability groupings and sports, fundamental methodological issues such as a standard operational definition of an injury are unresolved. Ferrara and associates (14-19) have consistently regarded an injury as "any trauma to the participant that occurred during any practice, training or competition session that caused the athlete to stop, limit, or modify participation for one day or more." This is the most useful definition found in the disability sports literature because it contains a means of estimating severity. Apart from the work of Ferrara, there is little consistency or commonality among the studies surveyed: "a reportable illness/ injury that was evaluated by the US medical staff during the duration of the 1988 Paralympics" (38); "trauma incurred while training, practicing or competing in wheelchair sports" (31); any complication of activity (grouped under the headings "pressure sores," "urinary tract infections," "strains and sprains," and "other"; 35); "a significant injury was defined as one which was severe enough to cause the athlete to take time off training and/or competition" (7); and injuries or preexisting conditions that can be exacerbated by activity (3). The variety of definitions makes it difficult to combine findings that deal with the same population, complicates comparisons across studies, and may distort the risk involved in participation (too

broad a definition may artificially inflate the risk and a too narrow definition may underestimate it).

The majority of the studies also suffer from one or more of the following: small sample sizes, short data collection periods, lack of exposure information, and data collection bias.

Finally, because of the limited numbers of participants and the great range of sports and disability types and levels, injury data can not be meaningfully related to specific types or levels of disability. Thus, most researchers have been required to sacrifice precision in data interpretation in favor of a global view. As research on risk factors and sports injury incidence "should be undertaken on groups that are homogeneous with regards to age, sex, level of competition and type of sport" (43) and in light of the methodological problems noted, the conclusions and recommendations based on these less sensitive data must be viewed with caution. Although the conclusions of prospective studies generally can be regarded with more confidence than retrospective research, few of the small number of prospective studies in disability sports are free of the flaws mentioned above. Therefore, the caveat on data interpretation applies to the literature as a whole.

## 2. Incidence of Injury

### 2.1 Injury Rates

Few studies calculated injury rates or recorded the exposure data necessary for these calculations. The majority presented raw data or computations such as the percentage of athletes injured, frequency of a particular type of injury, or the relative percentages of each type of injury to the total number of injuries. Some researchers did attempt to extend their analyses but overlooked important considerations in the process. Curtis (10), for example, presented an injury risk graph for various sports based on reported injuries per participant; but only sports in which at least 30 athletes indicated they participated were included, and no adjustment was made for athletes who participated in more than one sport. A summary of information from various studies pertaining to the relative risk of participation based on injury rates is contained in Table 10.1.

The following general observations are derived from the six studies that calculated exposure data.

- Complications from sports activity for SCI individuals in a rehabilitation setting are low (2.51/1,000 hours of exposure; 35).

- Skiing is a low risk undertaking for athletes with disabilities, whether competing (2 injuries/1,000 skier days; 32) or learning (3.5 injuries/1,000 skier days; 25).
- The risk of injury in competitive athletes of various disability groups is not high (9.45/1,000 athlete exposures [AE]; 14), but does vary according to sport (from 9.21 per 1,000 AE for track to 6.21/1,000 AE for weight lifting of four sports surveyed; 16).
- Special Olympians have an extremely low risk of injury while engaged in competition (0.4 injuries/1,000 hours of exposure; 33).

With due regard to the problems inherent in discussing risk in terms of the percentage of athletes injured or the number of injuries per 100 athletes, data from the remaining studies indicate that generally

- a majority of wheelchair athletes will sustain one or more injuries in training or competition with the risk related to the sports undertaken,
- athletes with cerebral palsy seem to have a smaller percentage of injuries compared to athletes with other disabilities,
- as a group, the percentage of Special Olympians needing treatment for illness or injury at competitions is the lowest of any disability group (approximately 10%), and
- a high percentage of amputee soccer players sustain injuries, but few are even of moderate severity.

## 2.2 Reinjury Rates

No work published to date has addressed the issue of reinjury rates in any disability sports population or activity. The most commonly discussed conditions in this regard are urinary tract/bladder infections and pressure sores in SCI individuals involved in wheelchair activities. Several authors (18, 21, 31, 35, 45) identified these problems and discussed the interaction of neurologic defect and requirements of activity (e.g., position in a wheelchair) that may contribute to them but did not provide any information on the rate of recurrence. However, in a study of 42 SCI athletes and nonathletes, Stotts (42) found athletes to be significantly more successful in avoiding these major complications than nonathletes. Sports activity as a possible mediator of conditions that have a significant impact on activity levels in SCI individuals, such as urinary tract infections (UTI) and pressure

sores, argues for the need for an expanded definition of athletic "injury" in disability sports.

## 2.3 Practice vs. Competition

Only one study (38) provided information on injury rates during practice versus competition. In the small sample of U.S. cerebral palsy athletes at the 1988 Paralympics ($n = 75$), 7 of 27 injuries (27%) occurred in competition with the remaining 20 (73%) sustained during practice (training and scrimmages). No exposure information (time involved in each condition) was provided.

# 3. Injury Characteristics

## 3.1 Injury Onset

Few authors have attempted to evaluate the nature of onset of injury. Table 10.2 outlines information contained in the literature on percent comparisons of injury onset in disability sports.

The limited information indicates that

- elite wheelchair athletes report more acute injuries,
- injuries reported in cross-disability groups, such as teams attending the Paralympics, are closely divided between acute and chronic in nature, but careful consideration should be given to the prevalence of chronic conditions, and
- cerebral palsy athletes in international competition record significantly more acute injuries than chronic ones.

Although the data sampling periods may explain some of the findings (e.g., in studies conducted during competitions it is not unusual to record more acute injuries than chronic ones), more data are necessary before the relationship between levels of activity, types of disability, and the nature of injury onset can be accurately identified and explained.

## 3.2 Injury Type

Most authors have noted that athletes with disabilities present injury profiles similar to those of the general athletic population. The significant difference between the two groups seems to be related to medical care for conditions secondary to a particular disability (e.g., pressure sores or carpal tunnel syndrome [CTS] in wheelchair athletes) rather

**Table 10.1   A Comparison of Injury Rates in Disability Sports**

| Study | Design | Data collection | Duration injury survey | # injuries (definition varies greatly) | # participants | Rate: injuries/100 participants | Rate: injuries/ 1,000 hours of exposure | Rate: injuries/1,000 athletic exposures |
|---|---|---|---|---|---|---|---|---|
| **Wheelchair** | | | | | | | | |
| Curtis, 1982 | R | Q | Any previous injury | 291 | 129 | 225.6 | — | — |
| Hoeberigs & Verstappen, 1984 | R | Q | 1980 Paralympics basketball (2 weeks) | —[a] | 89 | 6-41[*b] | — | — |
| Nilsen et al., 1985 | R | RR | 10 years | 30 | 61 | 49.18 | 2.51 | — |
| Ahsoh, 1987 | R | — | Any previous injury | — | — | 70.0* | — | — |
| Ferrara & Davis, 1990 | R | I | 1 year | 50 | 19 | 263.15 | — | — |
| Hoeberigs et al., 1990 | P | DM | 1986 International Flower Marathon (1 week) | 20 | 40 | 50 | — | — |
| McCormack et al., 1991 | R | Q | Any previous injury | 346 | 90 | 384.4 | — | — |
| Wilson & Washington, 1993 | R | Q | Any previous injury | — | 83 | Track: 97* Swim: 91* Field: 22* | — | — |
| Burnham et al., 1994 | R | Q | 1 year | 189 | 116 | 162.9 | — | — |
| **Cross-disability** | | | | | | | | |
| Jackson & Fredrickson, 1979 | R | DM | 1976 Paralympics (all participants) | 127 | > 1,500 | 8.46 | — | — |
| McCormick, 1985 | R | Q | Any previous injury (skiing) | 23 | 60 | 38.3 | 2.0[c] | — |
| Burnham et al., 1991 | R | RR | 1988 Paralympics (Canadian team) | 108 | 151 | 71.5 | — | — |
| Ferrara & Buckley, 1992 | P | — | 18 months | — | — | — | — | |
| Overall | | | | | | | | 9.30 |
| Track | | | | | | | | 9.21 |
| Basketball | | | | | | | | 8.16 |
| Swimming | | | | | | | | 7.34 |
| Weight lifting | | | | | | | | 6.21 |
| Ferrara et al., 1992a | R | Q | 6 months | | | | | |
| Overall | | | | 388 | 426 | 91.07 | — | — |
| NWAA[d] | | | | 100 | 87 | 114.9 | — | — |
| USABA[e] | | | | 144 | 122 | 118.0 | — | — |
| USCPAA[f] | | | | 144 | 217 | 66.4 | — | — |
| Ferrara et al., 1992b | R | Q | 6 months (skiing) | 100 | 68 | 147.05 | — | — |
| Laskowski & Murtaugh, 1992 | R | RR | 2-4 years (skiing) | 268 | — | — | 3.5[c] | — |
| Ferrara & Buckley, 1994 | P | — | 2 years | 128 | 319 | 40.12 | Range: 0.26-14 | 9.45 |

| Study | Design | Method | Event | Injuries | Athletes | Rate | *Percent | |
|---|---|---|---|---|---|---|---|---|
| **Special Olympics** | | | | | | | | |
| Bedo et al., 1976 | P | DM | 1975 international | 274 | 3,200 | 8.56 | — | — |
| Birrer, 1984 | P | DM | 2 years (state c'ships) | 43 | 2,056 | 2.09 | — | — |
| McCormick et al., 1990 | P | DM | 3 days (state c'ships) | 4 | 777 | 0.5 | 0.4[g]/70[h] | — |
| Robson, 1990 | P | DM | 1989 international (7 days) | 157 | 1,512 | 10.38 | — | — |
| Wekesa & Onsongo, 1992 | P | DM | 10 days (training camp) | 110 | 38 | 289.47 | — | — |
| **Other** | | | | | | | | |
| Richter, 1988 (cerebral palsy) | — | — | 1988 state games | 11 | 350 | 3.14 | — | — |
| Richter et al., 1991 (cerebral palsy) | P | DM | 1988 Paralympics (USA team) | 27 | 75 | 36 | — | — |
| Kegel & Malchow, 1994 (amputee soccer) | R | Q/I | Any previous injury | 61 | 75 | 81.3 | — | — |

*Percent injured.

*Note.* P denotes prospective; R denotes retrospective. DM denotes direct monitor; I denotes interview; RR denotes record review; Q denotes questionnaire.

[a] Investigated muscle soreness only.

[b] From beginning to end of tournament.

[c] 1,000 skier days.

[d] National Wheelchair Athletic Association (now Wheel Sport-USA).

[e] United States Association for Blind Athletes.

[f] United States Cerebral Palsy Athletic Association.

[g] Rate based on event time (duration of event).

[h] Rate based on measured activity time (actual time athlete was active).

**Table 10.2   A Percent Comparison
of Nature of Injury Onset in Disability Sports**

| Study | # injuries | # participants | Acute | Chronic |
|---|---|---|---|---|
| Wheelchair | | | | |
| Ferrara & Davis, 1990[a] | 50 | 19 | 65 | 23 |
| Cross-disability | | | | |
| Burnham et al., 1991 (Paralympics) | 108 | 151 | 49 | 51 |
| Ferrara et al., 1992a (3 disability groups) | 388 | 426 | 45 | 55 |
| Ferrara et al., 1992b (skiing) | 100 | 68 | 40 | 60 |
| Other | | | | |
| Richter et al., 1991 (cerebral palsy) | 27 | 75 | 73 | 27 |

[a]Excludes 12% of injuries not sports related.

than injuries related to a particular sport per se. A summary of injury types is shown in Table 10.3.

The information provided in the literature can be summarized as follows;

- The majority of injuries to wheelchair athletes are minor (abrasions, lacerations, sprains, and strains). Serious injuries such as concussions, dislocations, and fractures are few.
- Athletes represented in the cross-disability group also have a high percentage of sprains and strains but suffer more contusions. The percentage of lacerations, dislocations, and fractures reported in this group is higher than in other groups but is activity-related (skiing). Nonetheless, skiers with a disability suffered a statistically significant fewer number of fractures and lacerations than nondisabled skiers (25).
- Special Olympians suffer mostly abrasions and contusions of a minor nature.
- The small sample of cerebral palsy athletes suggests that strains are the primary injury type for this group.

## 3.3 Injury Location

As a general observation, the distribution of injury locations in disability sports is disability dependent. As might be expected, upper extremity injuries (both chronic and acute) are most common in wheelchair athletes (1, 17, 35). For ambulatory athletes, lower extremity injuries are more prevalent. However, the distribution of injuries in disability sports is also influenced by the sport played, as in the general athletic population (e.g., 8, 25). A summary of injury locations is shown in Table 10.4. Observations from these data are discussed in more detail below.

### 3.3.1 Head/Spine/Trunk

Head, spine, or trunk injuries account for approximately 10% of recorded injuries in wheelchair athletes (range = 7-18%), whereas in the few studies available on athletes with cerebral palsy these injuries range between 13% and 30%. From the single study on amputee soccer, a distribution of 20% of injuries in these regions it not surprising given the nature of the game (24). Injuries to the head, spine, or trunk do not seem to be a problem for Special Olympics athletes.

### 3.3.2 Upper Extremity

Because of the primary role the upper extremities play in both activities of daily living and sport in wheelchair athletes, it is not surprising to find the preponderance of injuries in this area. Data from the studies surveyed indicate that upper extremity injuries account for approximately 75% of the injuries reported by wheelchair athletes (range = 58-87%). Closer examination reveals the hands and fingers to be the most commonly injured site followed by the shoulder. These findings are in keeping with the unique characteristics of wheelchair use: The close proximity of the fingers to wheelchair spokes and the function of the hand as the point of force application to the wheel for propulsion means that hands and fingers are repeatedly subject to trauma. However, the majority of hand and finger injuries are minor (abrasions, blisters, lacerations) and account for only approximately 13% of time loss injuries (7). On the other hand, in addition to the considerable repetitive stress that accompanies its role as the primary force generator for wheelchair motion, the shoulder is subject to the normal acute and chronic stresses arising from sport-specific motion, for example, throwing and hitting. Despite the lower percentage of injuries occurring in the shoulder compared to the hands and fingers, shoulder injuries account for a significantly higher percentage of time loss injuries (85%, including elbow and wrist injuries [7]). Side dominance does not seem to be a factor in developing injury (19). This is not unexpected given the bilateral nature of wheelchair use.

**Table 10.3  A Percent Comparison of Injury Types in Disability Sports**

| Study | # participants | # injuries | Abrasion | Concussion | Contusion | Dislocation | Fracture | Inflammation | Laceration | Nonspecific | Sprain | Strain | Other/ unknown |
|---|---|---|---|---|---|---|---|---|---|---|---|---|---|
| **Wheelchair** | | | | | | | | | | | | | |
| Curtis, 1982* | 129 | 291 | 35[a] | 2 | 0 | 0 | 5 | 0 | — | 0 | 33[b] | — | 21 |
| Ferrara & Davis, 1990 | 19 | 50 | 22 | 0 | 10 | 0 | 6 | 0 | 2 | 0 | 4 | 48 | 8 |
| McCormack et al., 1991* | 90 | 346 | 22.5 | 2 | 7.8 | 0.6 | 2 | 17.1 | 3.8 | 0 | 0 | 16.3 | 29.6 |
| **Cross-disability** | | | | | | | | | | | | | |
| McCormick, 1985 (skiing) | 60 | 23 | 0 | 4.3 | 13.04 | 4.3 | 30.43 | 4.3 | 13.04 | 21.74 | 4.3 | 0 | 4.3 |
| Burnham et al., 1991 (Paralympics) | 151 | 108 | 5.5 | 0 | 0.9 | 0 | 0.9 | 15.7 | 0 | 34.3 | 3.7 | 22.2 | 16.7 |
| Laskowski & Murtaugh, 1992 (skiing) | — | 268 | 3.4 | 0 | 19.4 | 2.6 | 9.7 | 0 | 6.3 | 0 | 36.2 | 8.6 | 13.8 |
| **Special Olympics** | | | | | | | | | | | | | |
| Bedo et al., 1976 | 3,200 | 274 | 29.6 | 1.5 | 9.1 | 0 | 1.1 | 0.4 | 7.3 | 0 | 9.5 | 4 | 37.6 |
| Birrer, 1984 | 2,056 | 43 | 34.9[a] | 0 | 30.2 | 0 | 0 | 0 | 0 | 0 | 9.3 | 18.6 | 7 |
| Wekesa & Onsongo, 1992 | 38 | 110 | 2.7 | 0 | 59.1 | 0 | 0 | 2.7 | 0.9 | 34.6 | 0 | 0 | 0 |
| **Other** | | | | | | | | | | | | | |
| Richter et al., 1991 (cerebral palsy) | 75 | 27 | 3.7 | 0 | 3.7 | 7.4 | 0 | 3.7 | 0 | 3.7 | 7.4 | 66.7 | 3.7 |

*Data in manuscript did not total 100%.

[a]Includes lacerations.

[b]Includes strains.

**Table 10.4   A Percent Comparison of Injury Location in Disability Sports**

| Location | Wheelchair | | | Special Olympics | Other | |
|---|---|---|---|---|---|---|
| | Ferrara & Davis 1990 (*n* = 19) | McCormack et al. 1991 (*n* = 90) | Burnham et al. 1994 (*n* = 116) | Wekesa & Onsongo 1992 (*n* = 38) | Richter et al. 1991 (*n* = 75) | Kegel & Malchow 1994 (*n* = 75) |
| Head/spine/trunk | (18.0) | (10.7) | (6.9) | (0.0) | (18.5) | (19.6) |
| Skull | — | 5.3[a] | — | — | — | 4.9 |
| Face | — | — | — | — | — | 9.8 |
| Teeth | — | — | — | — | — | — |
| Neck | — | 0.9 | 3.2 | — | 7.4 | 4.9 |
| Back | — | 4.5 | 3.7 | — | 11.1 | — |
| Upper extremity | (58.0) | (78.9) | (86.8) | (23.5) | (40.7) | (34.5) |
| Shoulder | 16.0 | 16.2 | 16.9 | 7.2 | 25.9 | 9.8 |
| Arm | 2.0 | 11.6 | — | 0.9 | 11.1 | 6.6 |
| Elbow | 8.0 | 6.7 | 10.6 | 2.7 | — | 6.6 |
| Forearm | 2.0 | 2.1 | — | — | — | 3.3 |
| Wrist | 12.0 | 4.6 | 8.5 | 2.7 | — | 4.9 |
| Hand/fingers | 18.0 | 37.7 | 50.8 | 10.0 | 3.7 | 3.3 |
| Lower extremity | (22.0) | (6.7) | (6.4) | (38.2) | (29.6) | (42.6) |
| Pelvis/hips | — | — | — | — | — | — |
| Thigh | — | — | — | 12.7 | 11.1 | — |
| Knee | — | — | — | 18.2 | 7.4 | 18.0 |
| Leg | — | — | — | 1.8 | — | — |
| Ankle | — | — | — | 5.5 | 7.4 | 16.4 |
| Foot/toes | — | — | — | — | 3.7 | 8.2 |
| | excl. 2% illness | orig. < 100% | | excl. 38% unknown | | excl. 3.3% other |

| Location | Cross-disability | | | | | | | | |
|---|---|---|---|---|---|---|---|---|---|
| | McCormick, 1985 (*n* = 60) | Burnham et al., 1991 (*n* = 151) | Ferrara et al., 1992a | | | | Ferrara et al., 1992b (*n* = 68) | Laskowski & Murtaugh, 1992 | Ferrara & Buckley, 1994 (*n* = 319) |
| | | | Total (*n* = 426) | NWAA (*n* = 87) | USABA (*n* = 122) | USCPAA (*n* = 217) | | | |
| Head/spine/trunk | — | — | (14.0) | (10.0) | (17.0) | (13.0) | (12.1) | (20.0) | (22.7) |
| Skull | 4.3 | — | — | — | — | — | 1.0 | — | — |
| Face | — | — | — | — | — | — | — | — | — |
| Teeth | 4.3 | — | — | — | — | — | — | — | — |
| Neck | — | 3.7 | — | — | — | — | 11.1 | — | — |
| Back | 8.7 | 6.5 | — | — | — | — | — | — | — |
| Upper extremity | — | — | (44.0) | (65.0) | (30.0) | (43.0) | (51.0) | (20.0) | (35.9) |
| Shoulder | 8.7 | 29.6 | 22.0 | 40.0 | 15.0 | 17.0 | 28.0 | — | — |
| Arm | — | 0.9 | 7.0[b] | 17.0 | 1.0 | 5.0 | 14.0[b] | — | — |
| Elbow | — | 1.9 | — | — | — | — | — | — | — |
| Forearm | — | — | 5.0[c] | 4.0 | 3.0 | 7.0 | 6.0[c] | — | — |
| Wrist | — | 6.5 | — | — | — | — | — | — | — |
| Hand/fingers | 8.7 | 1.9 | 10.0 | 4.0 | 11.0 | 14.0 | 3.0 | — | — |
| Lower extremity | — | — | (42.0) | (25.0) | (53.0) | (44.0) | (36.0) | (57.4) | (21.1) |
| Pelvis/hips | — | 4.6 | 6.0[d] | 3.0 | 6.0 | 7.0 | 9.0 | — | — |
| Thigh | — | 9.3 | — | — | — | — | — | — | — |
| Knee | 26.1 | 1.9 | 15.0 | 12.0 | 10.0 | 21.0 | 26.0[d] | — | — |
| Leg | 8.7 | 4.6 | 17.0[e] | 6.0 | 26.0 | 15.0 | 1.0 | — | — |
| Ankle | 4.3 | 4.6 | — | — | — | — | — | — | — |
| Foot/toes | — | 1.9 | 4.0 | 4.0 | 11.0 | 1.0 | — | — | — |
| | 6 locations not specified | 24 locations not specified | | | | | | excl. 38 unknown 2.6% other | excl. 20% illness |

[a]Includes facial injuries.
[b]Includes elbow injuries.
[c]Includes wrist injuries.
[d]Includes thigh injuries.
[e]Includes ankle injuries.

Upper extremity injuries in other groups of disability-sports athletes also show disability and sport-related patterns. In two studies of athletes with cerebral palsy, upper extremity injuries accounted for approximately 40% of all injuries, with approximately half of these related to the shoulder (17, 38). However, it was reported that only 30% of injuries recorded in a group of blind athletes involved the upper extremity, although the shoulder was also the site of 50% of these injuries (17). In a small sample of amputee soccer players, 35% of injuries were found to be upper extremity, but in contrast to the other groups, no single site predominated (24). The high percentage of upper extremity injuries and the even distribution through the upper extremities in amputee soccer players may be attributed to use of crutches for ambulation by all players (except goal keepers). The need to support the running body through the upper extremities means that these athletes are more susceptible to upper extremity injuries than athletes who can run without crutches.

### 3.3.3 Lower Extremity

In general, ambulatory athletes in disability sports experience approximately the same percentage of lower extremity injuries as nondisabled athletes in the same sports (25). However, there is some indication that the risk may be higher for blind, single lower extremity amputees, or perambulating cerebral palsy athletes. Burnham et al. (8) noted that among members of the Canadian team at the 1988 Paralympics blind athletes had a statistically higher proportion of lower extremity injuries than either cerebral palsy or amputee athletes, even when the proportion of blind athletes participating in lower extremity sports was taken into account. The reason for this difference is not known, although stability or avoidance problems have been suggested (17, 23). In disabled skiers and amputee soccer players, lower extremity injuries are more common than upper extremity injuries and in line with those experienced by nondisabled athletes (24, 25, 32).

## 4. Injury Severity

There is little evidence to indicate a definitive trend in the severity of injury sustained in disability sports as a whole, or within particular sports or disability classifications. The data that are available show most injuries in disability sports to be minor. Several authors have supported this conclusion based on the small percentage of athletes with disabilities who seek medical treatment for their injuries. However, the percentage of injured athletes that do not seek medical treatment because their injuries are minor (and self-treatment is appropriate) and the percentage that are unwilling or unable to access treatment for sports-related injuries is not known.

Likewise, the lack of any published reports of catastrophic injury is an oblique indication that athletes in disability sports may be at less risk than nondisabled athletes for permanent injury as a result of sports participation. However, it has not been determined whether this is due to some characteristic of the athletes themselves (such as not generating the momentum normally found when collisions cause catastrophic injuries), whether the risk is mediated by the fact that athletes with disabilities generally do not participate in high risk sports (such as American football or gymnastics) or some other factor.

### 4.1 Time Loss

Few authors have attempted to identify injury severity by presenting time-loss data. Ferrara and his colleagues (14-19) have been pioneers in this regard. Ferrara and Buckley (14) in a 2-year, cross-disability study found that minor injuries (0-7 days of missed practice) constituted 47% of the total number of injuries, moderate (8-21 days) 25%, and major (> 22 days) 28%. The mean time lost in this group of athletes was 17 days. A similar pattern was evident in the distribution of injury severity in a survey of wheelchair athletes (minor = 57%; moderate = 11%; major = 32%; 19), although the significance of the difference seen in the incidence of moderate injury is unknown. Burnham et al.(7) noted that 18% of reported injuries in 116 wheelchair basketball players in the preceding year resulted in time loss from participation, but no information was provided on the relative amount(s) of time away. In their analysis of injuries in 68 disabled skiers, Ferrara et al. (18) reported that 100 time-loss injuries had occurred in the 6 months previous to a national competition but no further breakdown was provided.

### 4.2 Catastrophic Injury

Although there have been no reports of catastrophic injuries in any population of disability-sports athletes, concern over congenital atlanto-axial instability in Down's Syndrome individuals has resulted in the Special Olympics precluding them from activities considered high risk for trauma to this area, for example, gymnastics or diving (39). Although the radiologic incidence of atlantoaxial instability in this population has been cited as approximately 15% (9), only 7% of 336 Down's Syndrome athletes were confirmed to have the condition at an international competition in Great Britain (39). Robson (39) reported that 6% of 1,512 athletes at the same competition had congenital cardiac lesions, mostly septal lesions. However, the possibility of catastrophic injury due to these congenital defects has not, as yet, led to action to restrict participation.

## 5. Injury Risk Factors

The physical and physiological characteristics of athletes in disability sports have been held as predisposing them to injury to a greater degree than the general sporting public. Although there is a greater prevalence of preexisting nonsport-related conditions in this population when compared to athletes without disabilities, athletic injury rates in disability-sport participants are similar to those in other athletic populations (14).

Although several studies have collected information related to possible risk factors (e.g., age, sex, training times, equipment, types of sports played, etc.), very little analysis has been done (4, 10, 17-19, 25, 31, 32). In those instances where possible risk factors have been identified, small sample sizes and other methodological problems limit the confidence that can be placed in the observations. In most cases, identification of possible risk factors has followed from the most obvious cause–effect relationships or simple comparisons of descriptive data.

### 5.1 Intrinsic Factors

#### 5.1.1 Physical Characteristics

Given the foundations of disability sports, it is not surprising to find a majority of proposed risk factors relate to the disability conditions of the athletes. While most observations have been directed toward wheelchair athletes (principally SCI individuals), a few have noted relationships in other disability groups.

In wheelchair sports, two groups of factors are identified as placing athletes at risk for injury as a result of athletic involvement: (a) the necessary stress of wheeling on the upper extremities common to all wheelchair athletes and (b) problems such as urinary tract infections, pressure sores, and thermoregulation abnormalities related to impaired sensation and autonomic function in SCI athletes.

Curtis (10) indicated that athletes involved in sports that required substantial wheeling (e.g., road racing, track, basketball) seemed to experience more hand numbness/weakness than athletes involved in less wheeling-intensive activities (e.g., field events). No data were provided to augment this observation but a prospective study by Aljure et al. (2) of 47 nonathlete paraplegic wheelchair users showed 40% had clinical carpal tunnel syndrome and 63% had electrophysiological evidence of it. The authors concluded that the neuropathy appeared to be purely mechanical and that the incidence seemed to be related to the length of time as a paraplegic. Although the cross-sectional design, lack of statistical analysis, and small sample size compromise the findings, the results raise the possibility that upper extremity neuropathy in wheelchair athletes is related to the amount (intensity) and duration of wheeling stress. Burnham et al. (8) also observed that the "backhand" wheeling technique used by quadriplegic athletes may result in an increased incidence of tendinitis of the wrist. However, empirical evidence is lacking. Similarly, the importance of the shoulder in locomotion as well as sport-specific motions in wheelchair athletes seems to place quadriplegic athletes at higher risk for shoulder pathologies (1, 8), but this has not been demonstrated conclusively.

Several authors have suggested that SCI athletes have an increased risk of developing pressure sores as a result of sport activity (21, 31, 45). The occurrence of pressure sores as a percentage of athletic injuries in this population ranges from approximately 10% to 20% (17, 31, 35, 45). However, some evidence suggests that wheelchair athletes have a lower incidence of and fewer complications from pressure sores than their sedentary counterparts (42).

As with pressure sores, the risk of UTI and complications in SCI athletes is unclear. Whereas 100% of the cases of UTI from a small sample of athletes of mixed disability classifications occurred in catheter-dependent SCI athletes (8), the rate in SCI athletes as a group appears to be approximately 20% (35, 45). The one study comparing SCI athletes to sedentary SCI individuals identified a significantly lower frequency of UTI and complications in SCI athletes (42).

Thermoregulatory dysfunction as a result of athletic participation is rarely included in the definition of athletic injury. However, as hyperthermia or hypothermia are common sports-related conditions and can cause significant disability or death, they need to be considered in the risk evaluation of sport participation. This seems particularly important for SCI athletes. For example, Wilson and Washington (45) in a study of adolescent wheelchair athletes, noted that 49% of track injuries and 9% of swimming injuries were thermal and possibly exacerbated by impairment of thermoregulatory mechanisms that is characteristic of spinal cord injuries (6, 21).

In cross-disability studies, research has indicated differences in the risk of injury for different disability groups. For example, blind athletes are considered to be at greater risk for lower extremity injuries than other athletes with disabilities (8, 23), and to sustain significantly more injuries than cerebral palsy athletes (17). Similarly, paraplegic and polio wheelchair athletes have been found to have significantly more sports-related medical problems than other wheelchair athletes (e.g., amputees; 21).

Of the two studies that mention gender in their discussions of injury rates (35, 38), neither found significant differences in the incidence of injury or illness between males and females, except for a slightly greater number of UTI in females (35).

Although the congenital disabilities and multiple physical disabilities that are prevalent in Special Olympic athletes have raised concerns over an increased risk of injury from engaging in physical activity in this population, the experience of medical personnel who cover Special Olympics is that participants seem to have the same types and number of athletic injuries as other athletes (3, 4) and that the majority of medical problems in Special Olympics athletes are illness related rather than injury related (33). Most conditions are minor but attributable to the impaired decision-making capacity of the athletes (for example, high rates of sunburn) (4, 39). Preemptive restrictions from activities with a high probability of cervical spine stress (e.g., diving, high jumping, gymnastics) on athletes with Down's Syndrome eliminate the possibility of spinal cord injury due to congenital atlantoaxial instability. Athletes with Down's Syndrome have also been found to have a relative risk of injury or illness 3.2 times greater than other Special Olympics athletes (33).

### 5.1.2 Motor/Functional Characteristics

As has been mentioned previously, few of the studies available on injuries in disability sports supply sufficient data on which to base well-founded conclusions regarding risk factors. Lack of analytic information has left researchers, coaches, and athletes to suggest common-sense explanations for a wide range of athletic injuries, particularly chronic musculoskeletal injuries. Poor flexibility, insufficient strength conditioning, low levels of muscular endurance and similar factors have been widely advanced as responsible for the rate and types of injuries seen in athletes in disability sports (10, 17, 19, 32, 45).

## 5.2 Extrinsic Factors

Although conclusive data are not available, the following observations have been made in regards extrinsic risk factors in disability sports.

### 5.2.1 Exposure

Several studies of wheelchair athletes have identified a relationship between athletic injury and the total amount of time spent in activity. Hoeberigs and Verstappen (22) noted a statistically significant relationship between muscle soreness and the number of tournament games played by wheelchair basketballers, and Burnham et al. (7) found increased training time and increased weightlifting time were also each significantly associated with injuries in wheelchair basketballers. In addition, they concluded a significant relationship exists between shoulder injuries and playing center in wheelchair basketball (7). Across wheelchair athletes as a group, it has been proposed that the risk of injury for those involved in more than one sport is up to 9 times greater than for those engaged in only one activity (1, 7, 31).

### 5.2.2 Environment

Specific environmental circumstances such as playing surface, physical terrain, and climatic conditions may affect the risk of injury in different groups of disability sports participants. In data from the 1980 Paralympics, poor creep module, or deformation characteristics, of the floor was associated with increased rates of muscle soreness in wheelchair basketballers (22). Terrain characteristics or instructor experience in teaching novice skiers with disabilities may be responsible for significant (approximately fourfold) differences in injury rates in that population at different ski areas (25). Finally, climatic conditions, especially hot and sunny weather, have caused both SCI athletes (21, 45) and Special Olympians (3, 4, 39) to suffer an increase in a variety of medical problems, ranging from minor (sunburn) to serious (heat exhaustion).

### 5.2.3 Equipment

Equipment intrinsic to participation in particular disability sports, including wheelchairs, skiing outriggers, and crutches for amputee soccer, pose significant hazards to the athletes. Chair design and performance characteristics have been directly implicated in a range of injury in wheelchair athletes: acute (e.g., hand and finger spoke injuries, spills); chronic (e.g., muscle strains and inflammation from poor ergonomics); and complications (particularly pressure sores from body positioning and inadequate cushioning) (2, 10, 19, 22, 31). Outriggers and crutches injuries, however, are generally acute (lacerations, fractures, sprains) (24, 25, 32).

## 6. Suggestions for Injury Prevention

Because so little research has been done on injuries in disability sports "current prevention strategies rely on intuitive interventions based on prevailing notions about athletes without disabilities" (17). Given that studies covering a wide range of disability sports have concluded that injury rates and types are not significantly different between the two groups (except for injuries related to underlying disability), the general recommendations applied to nondisabled athletes have equal utility for athletes in disability sports (14, 18, 24, 32, 38). However, specific recommendations for particular disability groups and sports have also been proposed based on both obvious and theoretical cause-effect relationships. The literature provides many recommendations for injury prevention.

### 6.1 Players

- Improve general and sport-specific conditioning, including strength, endurance, and flexibility. Specific requirements need to be guided by the particular needs of different disability groups (e.g., wheelchair athletes need to improve upper extremity strength and flexibility; blind athletes need to focus on lower extremity function; training athletes with cerebral palsy or amputees will depend on whether or not they use wheelchairs; 10, 17-19, 45).
- Encourage participants in disability sports to train consistently and appropriately. Many individuals with disabilities participate recreationally, usually at lower frequencies than the general sporting population, but enter competitions at state or regional levels without adequate preparation (3, 18, 31, 45).
- Monitor athletes and climatic conditions and take appropriate precautions, such as ensuring adequate hydration, to avoid complications in athletes at risk for thermoregulatory problems due to poor judgement (Special Olympics) or impaired physiological responses (SCI; 3, 4, 21, 45).

### 6.2 Sport

- Continue to improve sports wheelchairs, including seat and wheel design, padding restraints, ergonomics, and propulsion mechanics (10, 17, 19, 21, 45) and reduce their cost to allow more athletes to use the most appropriate equipment available (21).
- Improve the functionality and durability of gloves for wheelchair athletes (7, 10, 17, 19, 31, 45), and design gloves to protect the hands without interfering with performance (e.g., altering "feel" in basketball; 7). Encourage athletes to replace worn-out or damaged protective devices (31).
- Require proper fitting and adjustment of equipment, especially wheelchairs (22) and skiing equipment (32).

### 6.3 External Environment

- Ensure safe and appropriate physical environments for participation; for example, evaluate floor characteristics for wheelchair basketball (22) and terrain for skiers with disabilities (32).

### 6.4 Health Support System

- Conduct preparticipation examinations and other proactive evaluative procedures (8). For example, Aljure et al. (2) recommend early testing of median and ulnar nerve function (within 5 years of spinal cord injury) and periodic retesting as clinical signs and symptoms require "so that with early detection, preventive and/or curative measures may be undertaken" (2) to avoid development of CTS in SCI wheelchair users.

- Initiate educational programs for athletes that cover (a) strategies for avoiding complications related to disabilities that may be aggravated by activity, such as UTI or pressure sores (6, 10, 21, 35, 45) and (b) resources and options for advice and treatment of sport-related injuries and associated health care problems (10, 14, 17, 18).
- Expand the numbers of athletic health care professionals working with, or available to, athletes with disabilities.

## 7. Suggestions for Further Research

Study of the scope, nature and unique characteristics of athletic injuries in disability sports is in its infancy. A thorough search of the literature revealed few original investigations, the majority of which were basic descriptive studies. Thus, the scarcity of data and methodological problems inherent in most of the literature reduces the confidence that can be placed in the conclusions concerning the extent or etiology of sports-related dysfunction in athletes with disabilities. In order to develop efficacious interventions to reduce injuries, better information on rates and risk factors is needed. To achieve this end, the following issues must be addressed:

- A comprehensive and standardized definition of an injury must be established. The definition must involve a graded scale of severity (time loss) and include activity-related complications secondary to specific primary disabilities (e.g., pressure sores and UTI in SCI athletes).
- Populations at risk must be clearly delimited. Minimum characteristics to be considered include age, gender, type of disability, severity of disability, and activity under investigation. Researchers must avoid presenting mean data from mixed athlete samples that mask important group differences (17).
- A standardized and rational metric for assessing risk (i.e., exposure) must be developed to allow appropriate comparisons across samples. Incidence per 1,000 hours of measured activity time is the most accurate exposure information (33) but is not logistically feasible for large scale studies. Use of injury per 1,000 athlete exposures or per 1,000 hours of participation is recommended.
- Uniform data collection, recording, and reporting guidelines are needed (24, 25). The growing accessibility of Internet, the information superhighway, holds excellent potential in this regard, as well as being a means of increasing sample sizes by accepting and combining data from sources throughout the world.
- Prospective cohort studies using both sedentary disabled and active, able-bodied individuals as controls for athletes with disabilities need to be implemented. These controls should answer the questions: (a) Are athletes with disabilities at greater risk of harm because of their activity than sedentary individuals? and (b) Are they at greater risk of harm because of their disability than non-disabled individuals? (42)

The foregoing are the minimum requirements to accurately establish the extent of the problem of sports-related injuries in disability sports. As van Mechelen et al. (43) point out, establishing the extent of the problem is only the first step in a four-step "sequence of prevention" that subsequently requires establishing etiology and mechanisms of injury, introducing preventive measures based on identified mechanisms of injury, and assessing the effectiveness of the interventions by reevaluating the extent of the sports-injury problem after the introduction of the preventive measure.

Unless the methodological issues detailed above are resolved, sequential and productive research as outlined by van Mechelen et al. (43) is not possible and problems such as the role played by prosthetic devices (e.g., skiing outriggers) in sports injuries or the effects of athletic participation on particular subgroups of athletes with disabilities (e.g., adolescents) can not be adequately investigated. Thus, attention to the mechanics of research will provide answers to ultimately pragmatic concerns such as the relative risk of participating in one sport as opposed to another and better information from which to devise interventions to eliminate unnecessary injury and illness from disability sports and assess their effectiveness. In light of past efforts the future can only hold promise.

## References

1. Ahsoh, K. Unpublished proceedings (1987). Ref: McCann, B.C. The disabled athlete. In: Meuller, F.O. & Ryan, A.J. eds. Prevention of athletic injuries: the role of the sports medicine team. Philadelphia: Davis; 1991:174-197.

2. Aljure, J.; Eltorai, I.; Bradley, W.E.; Lin, J.E.; Johnson, B. Carpal tunnel syndrome in paraplegic patients. Paraplegia 23:182-186; 1985.

3. Bedo, A.V.; Demlow, M.; Moffit, P.; Kopke, K.W. Special Olympics athletes face special needs. The Physician and Sportsmedicine 4(9):51-56; 1976.

4. Birrer, R.B. The Special Olympics: an injury overview. The Physician and Sportsmedicine. 12(4):95-97; 1984.

5. Bloomquist, L. Injuries to athletes with physical disabilities: prevention implications. The Physician and Sportsmedicine 14(9):96-105; 1986.

6. Booth, D.W. Athletes with disabilities. In: Harries, M., Williams, C., Stanish, W.D. & Micheli, L.J., eds. Oxford textbook of sports medicine. New York: Oxford University Press; 1994:634-646.

7. Burnham, R.; Higgins, J.; Steadward, R. Wheelchair basketball injuries. Palaestra 10(2):43-49; 1994.

8. Burnham, R.; Newell, E.; Steadward, R. Sports medicine for the physically disabled: The Canadian team experience at the 1988 Seoul Paralympic games. Clinical Journal of Sports Medicine 1:193-196; 1991.

9. Chang, F.M. The disabled athlete. In: Stanitski, C.L., DeLee, J.C., & Drez, D., eds. Pediatric and adolescent sports medicine, vol. 3. Philadelphia: Saunders; 1994:48-76.

10. Curtis, K. Wheelchair sportsmedicine. part 4 : athletic injuries. Sports 'n Spokes 7(1):20-24; 1982.

11. Curtis, K.; Dillon, D.A. Survey of wheelchair athletic injuries: common patterns and prevention. Paraplegia 23:170-175; 1985.

12. Curtis, K.; Dillon, D.A. Survey of wheelchair athletic injuries: common patterns and prevention. In: Sherrill, C., ed. Sport and disabled athletes. Champaign, IL: Human Kinetics; 1986:211-216.

13. DePauw, K.P. Sport for individuals with disabilities: research opportunities. Adapted Physical Activity Quarterly 5:80-89; 1988.

14. Ferrara, M.S.; Buckley, W.E. Athletes with disabilities registry. Journal of Athletic Training 29(2): 152 (abstract); 1994.

15. Ferrara, M.S.; Buckley, W.E. Athletes with disabilities registry: practical implications. Medicine and Science in Sports and Exercise 25(5), Supplement: S150 (abstract); 1993.

16. Ferrara, M.S.; Buckley, W.E. Athletes with disabilities registry: an update. Medicine and Science in Sports and Exercise 24(5), Supplement: S87 (abstract); 1992.

17. Ferrara, M.S.; Buckley, W.F.; McCann, B.C.; Limbird, T.J.; Powell, J.W.; Robl, R. The injury experience of the competitive athlete with a disability: prevention implications. Medicine and Science in Sports and Exercise 24(2):184-188; 1992a.

18. Ferrara, M.S.; Buckley, W.E.; Messner, D.G.; Benedict, J. The injury experience and training history of the competitive skier with a disability. American Journal of Sports Medicine 20(1):55-60; 1992b.

19. Ferrara, M.S; Davis, R.W. Injuries to elite wheelchair athletes. Paraplegia 28:335-341; 1990.

20. Hoeberigs, J.H. Sports, disabled athletes and injuries. In: Vermeer, A., ed. Sports for the disabled. Haarlem, the Netherlands: Uitgeverij de Vrieseborch; 1987:35-44.

21. Hoeberigs, J.H.; Debets-Eggen, H.B.; Debets, P.M. Sports medical experiences from the International Flower Marathon for disabled wheelers. American Journal of Sports Medicine 18(4):418-421; 1990.

22. Hoeberigs, J.H.; Verstappen, F.T.J. Muscle soreness in wheelchair basketballers. International Journal of Sports Medicine 5:177-179 (supplement); 1984.

23. Jackson, R.W.; Fredrickson, A. Sports for the physically disabled - the 1976 Olympiad (Toronto). American Journal of Sports Medicine 7(5):293-296; 1979.

24. Kegel, B.; Malchow, D. Incidence of injury in amputees playing soccer. Palaestra 10(2):50-54; 1994.

25. Laskowski, E.R.; Murtaugh, P.A. Snow skiing injuries in physically disabled skiers. American Journal of Sports Medicine 20(5):553-557; 1992.

26. Madorsky, J.G.B.; Curtis, K.A. Wheelchair sports medicine. American Journal of Sports Medicine 12:128-132; 1984.

27. Mangus, B.C. Sports injuries, the disabled athlete, and the athletic trainer. Athletic Training 22(4):305-310; 1987.

28. Mangus, B.C. Medical care for wheelchair athletes. Adapted Physical Activity Quarterly 5:90-95; 1988.

29. Mangus, B.C.; French, R. Wanted: athletic trainers for Special Olympic athletes. Athletic Training 20(3):204-205, 259; 1985.

30. McCann, B.C. The disabled athlete. In: Meuller, F.O. & Ryan, A.J., eds. Prevention of athletic injuries: the role of the sports medicine team. Philadelphia: Davis; 1991:174-197.

31. McCormack, D.A.R.; Reid, D.C.; Steadward, R.D.; Syrotuik, D.G. Injury profiles in wheelchair athletes: results of a retrospective survey. Clinical Journal of Sports Medicine 1:35-40; 1991.

32. McCormick, D. Injuries in handicapped alpine ski racers. The Physician and Sportsmedicine 13(12):93-97; 1985.

33. McCormick, D.P.; Niebuhr, V.N.; Risser, W.L. Injury and illness surveillance at local Special Olympic games. British Journal of Sports Medicine 24(4):221-224; 1990.

34. Monahan, T. Wheelchair athletes need special treatment—but only for injuries. The Physician and Sportsmedicine 14(7):121-128; 1986.

35. Nilsen, R.; Nygaard, P.; Bjorholt, P.G. Complications that may occur in those with spinal injuries who participate in sport. Paraplegia 23:52-58; 1985.

36. Paciorek, M.J.; Jones, J.A. Sports and recreation for the disabled. (2nd ed.). Indianapolis: Benchmark; 1994.

37. Richter, K.J. Unpublished material (1988). Ref: McCann, B.C. The disabled athlete. In: Meuller, F.O. & Ryan, A.J., eds. Prevention of athletic injuries: the role of the sports medicine team. Philadelphia: Davis; 1991:174-197.

38. Richter, K.J.; Hyman, S.C.; Mushett, C.A.; Ellenburg, M.R.; Ferrara, M.J. Injuries in world class cerebral palsy athletes of the 1988 South Korea Paralympics. Journal of Osteopathic Sports Medicine. October:15-18; 1991.

39. Robson, H.E. The Special Olympic games for the mentally handicapped—United Kingdom 1989. British Journal of Sports Medicine 24(4):225-230; 1990.

40. Schaefer, R.S.; Proffer, D.S. Sports medicine for wheelchair athletes. American Family Physician 39(5):239-245; 1989.

41. Shephard, R.J. Sports medicine and the wheelchair athlete. Sports Medicine 4:226-247; 1988.

42. Stotts, K.M. Health maintenance: paraplegic athletes and non-athletes. Archives of Physical Medicine and Rehabilitation 67:109-114; 1986.

43. van Mechelen, W; Hlobil, H; Kemper, H.C.G. Incidence, severity, aetiology and prevention of sports injuries - a review of concepts. Sports Medicine. 14(2):82-89; 1992.

44. Wekesa, M.; Onsongo, J. Kenyan team care at the Special Olympics—1991. British Journal of Sports Medicine 26(3):128-133; 1992.

45. Wilson, P.E.; Washington, R.L. Pediatric wheelchair athletics: sports injuries and prevention. Paraplegia 31:330-337; 1993.

# 11

# Diving

*Benjamin D. Rubin and Steven J. Anderson*

## 1. Introduction

The sport of competitive diving has received relatively little attention in the medical literature. Much of the medical literature about diving has dealt with the unsupervised, recreational version of the sport. This has included diving into lakes, streams and shallow pools, and from roofs, balconies, tables, cars, and bridges (7, 17-21, 30, 58, 64). In many cases recreational diving accidents have involved the concomitant ingestion of alcohol (1, 5, 25, 55). Thus, an unacceptably high number of serious head and neck injuries, many involving death or paralysis, has plagued recreational diving (17, 19).

Despite the absence of similar head and neck injuries in organized diving, the safety issues of competitive and recreational diving are too often inappropriately linked. As a result, the medical literature on diving may be arguably unfocused or inappropriately focused on an activity that should be clearly distinct from competitive diving. With the recent difficulty in obtaining insurance for aquatic facilities with diving boards being based on many of these reports, it is easy to understand why it is essential to the future of the sport of competitive diving that safety issues be clarified (9). This chapter will therefore focus specifically on those injuries reported in *organized, competitive* diving.

A significant amount of information has been collected on mechanisms and types of injuries in competitive diving (4, 8, 10, 31, 40, 41, 48, 50-54). However, much of the relevant information on diving injuries has been presented at various diving seminars and remains unpublished (except as part of seminar proceedings). Although the authors of these papers were not specifically attempting to present epidemiological data, their presentations,

as well as the bibliographies in several published reports on injuries, represented a useful starting point for this review. Much of the information available represents case reports, injury trends, and recommended treatments. We were unable to identify a single published study specifically addressing the epidemiology of diving injuries.

This chapter documents all references pertaining to injuries in competitive diving and puts them in perspective based on our experience in providing medical care to these athletes. This includes all studies presented or published in English, as well as foreign data previously reviewed or translated into the English literature. To our knowledge, this chapter represents the first published literature review of the sport of competitive diving.

A number of procedures were used to accomplish a complete and up-to-date collection of data. First, previously presented or published material, including bibliographic references, were reviewed. Second, computer searches were performed utilizing the Medline and SPORT Discus databases from January 1975 to January 1994. Search words included diving, competitive diving, springboard diving, platform diving, and diving injuries. Finally, data from the United States Diving Injury Surveillance Study were reviewed.

## 2. Incidence of Injury

### 2.1 Injury Rates

This discussion will deviate from the standard presentation format of this book for a number of reasons. (a) Most diving studies were case series and do not allow for calculation of injury rates. (b) Only one prospective study (66) is available. (c) The definition of injury varied from inability to train for at least 1 week to any withdrawal from competition or training.

Zimmerman (66) reported injury rates in recreational divers and competitive divers of 4.0 and 8.8 injuries per 1,000 training hours, respectively. He prospectively studied 56 divers for only 3 months and considered any inability to train or compete as an injury. Thus, the reported injury rate would seem higher than expected. Coaches reported only 25% of injuries observed by the researcher.

Gabriel (16) collected data through the USA Diving Injury Surveillance Program. Information was based on reports submitted by coaches to the medical insurance carrier over a period of 3 years. The reported injury rate was 6.5 injuries per 100 participants per year. Given the number of athletes involved in diving, the number of injuries is significantly fewer than expected. Data collection was based on reports to the insurance carrier and therefore only injuries severe enough to require medical attention that involved an expense were included. This would skew the data toward fewer but more serious injuries.

The case series of Rubin and Richardson (50), Mutoh (47) and Anderson (3) indicate:

- an incidence of injury in divers ranging from 92% to 100%,
- a trend toward increasing numbers of injuries with increasing years of training and competition, and
- no male–female differences.

The review of literature clearly demonstrates the need for a more consistent definition of injuries and injury severity. Uniform definitions of injuries and injury severity are necessary for comparing risk between different sports and in prioritizing

medical coverage. Methods of reporting injuries are clearly inconsistent, with reporting rates and injury definitions varying between athletes, coaches, parents, trainers, and insurance carriers.

## 2.2 Reinjury Rates

No study to date has addressed the incidence of reinjury, although it has been observed (53, 54) that divers frequently reinjure their shoulders, especially if the underlying pathology is not corrected.

## 2.3 Dryland Training vs. Pool Training

Several studies have demonstrated a higher incidence of injuries during pool training than during dryland activities (Table 11.1). This is not surprising, because most American divers spend considerably more time training in pools than on dryland.

## 2.4 Springboard vs. Platform

Although no denominator-based studies regarding the relative incidence of springboard and platform injuries exist, Rubin (53, 54) has observed that injuries to the wrists, elbows, shoulders, cervical and lumbar spines, and ears, which prevented training for at least 1 week, occur more frequently on platform than on springboard.

## 2.5 Practice vs. Competition

Because considerably more dives are done in practice than during competition, it would be reasonable to expect the incidence of injury to be higher during training. The only such data available for

Table 11.1  Dryland Versus Pool Training

|  | # of athletes | # of injuries reported | % injuries from diving | % injuries on dryland | % diving related** |
|---|---|---|---|---|---|
| Gabriel (1992)* | 3,705 Junior Olympic | 8 | 75 | 5 | 12 |
|  | 524 senior | 4 |  |  |  |
|  | 294 masters | 0 |  |  |  |
| Zimmerman (1993) | 56 | 41 | 82.6 | 17.4 | 0 |
| Mizel (1993)*** | 517 | 55 | 59 | 13 | 28 |

*Data based on reports to insurance carrier.

**Walking on pool deck, showering, etc.

***Foot and ankle injuries in athletes ≥ 18 years of age only.

diving is that of Gabriel (16), which is based on medical insurance claims. She reported that for athletes 13 to 18 years of age, practice accounted for 60% of injuries, and for the 19- to 30-year age group, 43.3% occurred in practice. When the data were analyzed by gender, 50.7% of the injuries in males and 69.9% in females occurred in practice. Of the 37 injuries reported by Zimmerman (66) in which the circumstances of the injury were known, 92% occurred in training.

## 3. Injury Characteristics

### 3.1 Injury Onset

Zimmerman (66) determined that 62.2% of all the observed diving injuries in his series were the result of a single traumatic episode, and that 37.8% could be classified as "overuse" injuries.

### 3.2 Injury Type

Most of the information that has been collected on diving injuries has been classified by anatomical location and mechanism of injury, and not by injury type or diagnosis (3, 8, 31, 50, 51, 66). The aforementioned reports and clinical experience of the authors indicate that the most common injuries in competitive divers are strains, followed by sprains, contusions, subluxations and dislocations, lacerations, fractures, and concussions.

### 3.3 Injury Location

Only Rubin and Richardson (50) and Mutoh (47) have collected reportable statistics regarding incidence of injuries by anatomical location (Table 11.2). Unfortunately these studies included only 37 and 10 divers, respectively.

**Table 11.2   Incidence of Injury in Diving by Anatomical Location**

| Location | Rubin and Richardson (1981) ($n = 37$) | Mutoh (1988) ($n = 10$) |
| --- | --- | --- |
| Spine/trunk | | |
| Neck | 40% | 10% |
| Back | 61% | 28% |
| Upper extremity | | |
| Shoulder | 32% | 21% |
| Hand/wrist | 29% | 24% |
| Lower extremity | | |
| Knee | 27% | |
| Ankle | 19% | |

### 3.3.1 Head/Spine/Trunk

**3.3.1.1 Cervical Spine.**   There has not been a single reported fracture or dislocation of the cervical spine in organized diving. While catastrophic injuries may be preventable through implementation of safety measures (15), the potential still exists for noncatastrophic injuries from repetitive impact loading to the cervical spine.

**3.3.1.2 Lumbar Spine.**   Low back pain is a common complaint among male and female competitive divers of all ages (51, 52). Table 11.3 shows the studies of lumbar spine injuries in competitive divers.

Diving demonstrated the highest incidence of global isthmic lesions (83.3%) when compared to weightlifting (44.8%), wrestling (33.3%), gymnastics (37.9%), and athletics (24.5%; 49). Mangine (40) found the most common physical findings to be decreased lumbar extension, tightness of the hip flexors, and hyperlordosis. Radiculopathy was uncommon.

Strupler and Saxer (60) could not show any correlation between the number of dives from 7.5 and 10 meters over a diver's lifetime and the degree of back pain; however, there was a correlation between the degree of difficulty and intensity of training programs and back complaints. Groher (23), however, theorized that back pain resulted from the strain on the lumbar spine from missed entries with resultant fatigue fractures.

### 3.3.2 Upper Extremity

The sport of diving requires repetitive impact at high loads to the upper extremities. These forces are transmitted proximally from the wrist to the elbow and ultimately to the shoulder. It is not surprising that 80% of national team members have had shoulder injuries (54). Table 11.4 reveals the reported cases, case studies, and published observations on upper extremity injuries in competitive divers. Rubin (51) and Rubin et al. (54) have reported the only data on incidence of upper extremity injuries.

In summary, the most common diagnoses and precipitating factors are:

- shoulder—instability secondary to required multidirectional laxity, weakness of rotator cuff and scapular stabilizers, tendinitis secondary to traction from instability or impingement;
- elbow—triceps strains, tendinitis, or both usually due to failure to lock the elbows in extension for entry; more frequent in younger divers and platform divers; and

**Table 11.3  Case Series of Injuries Occurring in the Cervical or Lumbar Spine of Divers**

| Study | Design | Type of study | # subjects | Age | Competitive level | Diagnosis/condition |
|---|---|---|---|---|---|---|
| Schneider et al. (1962) | Case series | Clinical evaluation; X ray | 6 | — | Cliff divers (Acapulco) | None of the divers had cervical abnormalities |
| Groher and Heindensohn (1970) | Case series | Clinical evaluation | 60 | 8-49 18-27 | Competitive | Back pain (50%) Back pain (81.3%) |
| | | X ray | 17 | — | | Spondylolysis (34%); lumbosacral arthrosis (100%) |
| Groher (1978) | Case series | Clinical evaluation; X ray | 45 | — | > 5 years training | Changes of spinous processes (50%); arthritis of small joints (55%); spondylolysis (20%) |
| Rossi (1978) | Case series | X ray | 30 | 15-27 | Competitive | "Isthmic modifications" (83.3%); spondylolysis (63.3%); spondylolisthesis (16%) |
| Krejcova et al. (1981) | Case series | Clinical evaluation; X ray | 40 | 7-68 | Competitive SB and PF | Decreased mobility of cervical spine (61%); scoliosis (47.5%); lumbar discogenic and spondylitic changes 70% of high divers, 83% of all X ray changes in cervical spine (79%, 7-16 yrs; 90%, 13-19 yrs; 53%, 20-68 yrs) divers |
| Mangine (1981) | Case series | Clinical evaluation; questionnaire | 66 | — | Competitive SB and PF | Back pain (89%) |
| Strupler and Saxer (1982) | Case series | — | 49 | — | Olympic caliber SB and PF | Back pain requiring medical attention (61%) |
| Rubin (1983) | Case series | Questionnaire | 37 | 11-26 | Competitive SB and PF | Neck injury (40%); back injury (61%) |
| Anderson et al. (1993) | Case series | Clinical evaluation; X ray | 14 | — | Competitive | All subjects had some degree of symptomology in the cervical spine, but only 2 met radiographic criteria for "disease" |

SB = springboard.

PF = platform.

- wrist—carpal subluxations, dorsal impaction syndrome, stress fractures of the carpus and distal radial epiphysis due to repetitive impact on the water; sprained ulnar collateral ligament of the thumb from missing the grab; fractures of the metacarpals and phalanges from striking the board during flight.

### 3.3.3 Lower Extremity

Lower extremity injuries in divers are usually related to jumping and can be divided into those of the knee and leg and those of the foot and ankle. In summary, knee and leg injuries include patellar and quadriceps tendinitis, patellar tracking problems, and stress reactions of the lower leg. Foot and ankle problems are primarily sprains and fractures, most of which occur during the hurdle or press, or from striking the board in the pike position (46). Table 11.5 details studies discussing lower extremity injuries.

### 3.3.4 Nonorthopedic

Most nonorthopedic injuries sustained by divers affect the eyes and ears and are related to the forces exerted by entry into the water. The most common injuries can be summarized as follows:

- Vestibular abnormalities
- Ocular abnormalities
- Head lacerations
- Tympanic membrane ruptures
- Otitis externa
- Pulmonary contusion (see Table 11.6)

**Table 11.4   Case Reports, Case Series, Observations of Injuries Occurring in the Upper Extremity of Competitive Divers**

| Study | Design | # subjects | Age | Competitive level | Diagnosis/condition/observation |
|---|---|---|---|---|---|
| Kendall (1964) | Observation | — | — | — | Triceps strain |
| Hunter and O'Connor (1980) | Case report | 1 | 15 | Competitive | Olecranon apophysitis |
| Merinu et al. (1981) | Observation | — | — | — | Triceps tendinitis and strains |
| Rubin (1983) | Case series | 37 | 11-26 | Competitive | Shoulder-multidirectional instability; traction tendinitis; elbow-triceps strains/tendinitis in younger divers; wrist-dorsal impaction syndrome; stress fractures carpus and distal radial epiphysis; carpal instabilities; hand-sprain thumb ulnar collateral ligament; fractures phalanges and metacarpals |
| Rubin (1989) | Case series arthroscopic | 15 | 17-24 | Competitive senior | Labral pathology (88%); rotator interval/biceps tendinitis (33%); rotator cuff tears (8%) |
| Mathis (1990) | Case report | 1 | 23 | Recreational | Bilateral shoulder dislocation |
| McClure (1991) | Observation | — | — | — | Carpal subluxations, especially volar subluxation of lunate |
| Dawson (1992) | Case report | 1 | 17 | Recreational | Rupture extensor pollicis longus tendon |
| Rubin et al. (1993) | Case series | 20 | 17-28 | Senior national team | Shoulder-instability 45%; inflammation 45% |

**Table 11.5   Case Reports, Case Series, Observations of Injuries Occurring in the Lower Extremity of Competitive Divers**

| Study | Design | # subjects | Age | Competitive level | Diagnosis/condition/observation |
|---|---|---|---|---|---|
| Darda (1971) | Observation | — | — | Competitive | Shin splints |
| Krackow (1980) | Case report | 1 | 34 | Recreational | Acute rupture flexor hallicus longus |
| Rubin (1983) | Case series | 37 | 11-26 | Competitive | Patellar tendinitis; quadriceps tendinitis; patellar maltracking |
| Wieder (1992) | Case report | 1 | 16 | Recreational | Myositis ossificans of quadriceps femoris after diving onto swimmer below |
| Mizel et al. (1993) | Case series questionnaire, record review | 120 (41 sustained 55 injuries) | > 18 | Competitive | Ankle sprain (33%); fracture (31%); Achilles contusion (9%); midfoot strain (7%) |

Landing flat on the water surface from the 10-meter platform has been associated with chest and pulmonary contusion with resultant disruption of pulmonary blood vessels and hemoptysis (48, 52). All divers have returned to practice or competition within 48 hours. Pneumothorax has not been observed.

Scalp lacerations occur most commonly on inward dives and reverse dives when the diver leans toward the board while spinning in that direction (31). These injuries are quite dramatic. Occasionally there is temporary loss of consciousness (61);

however, neurologic sequelae other than headache are rarely observed.

## 4. Injury Severity

### 4.1 Time Loss

The only data that have been collected on time loss from injury are those of Zimmerman (66). Of the 40 injuries for which the time loss was recorded, 31 divers (77.5%) missed 4 hours of practice or less.

**Table 11.6    Case Reports, Case Series, and Observations of Nonorthopaedic Injuries in Divers**

| Study | Design | Subjects | Area studied | Condition/diagnosis |
|---|---|---|---|---|
| Lee (1971, 1978) | Observations | — | Otology | Reported observation of tympanic membrane ruptures and otitis externa (swimmer's ear) |
| Strauss and Cantrall (1979) | Observations | — | Otology | Otitis externa (swimmer's ear) |
| Schneider and Bratzke (1979) | Case report | 1 | Abdomen | 13-year-old boy: traumatic rupture of aorta secondary to jump from 3-meter board |
| Krejcova et al. (1981) | Case series | 40 | Neurologic and vestibular | Vestibulo-ocular and X ray abnormalities (42.5%); vestibulo-ocular, X ray, EEG abnormalities (42.5%); vestibular abnormalities (75%); gaze nystagmus (40%); positional nystagmus (60%) |
| Reilly and Miles (1981) | Observations | — | Otology, pulmonary | Reported observation of tympanic membrane ruptures and pulmonary contusions with hemoptysis |
| Fabiani et al. (1982) | Case series record review | 24 | Otology | Otitis media (15%); perforated tympanic membrane (10%) |
| Krejci and Rezek (1982) | Case series | 34 | Ophthalmology | Microdefects on corneal epithelium and changes in composition and "continuance" of tear film; no permanent ocular injuries or changes of intraocular pressure |
| Kimball et al. (1985) | Observations | — | Ophthalmology, neurology | Reported observation of retinal detachment and scalp lacerations |
| Rubin (1987) | Observations | — | Pulmonary | Reported observation of pulmonary contusion with hemoptysis |

Ninety percent of the divers returned to practice within 2 weeks. Ten injuries (25%) forced divers to modify their training by performing only foot-first entries. Clearly, there is a significant need in the diving literature for information on time-loss-from-injury data.

### 4.2 Catastrophic Injury

Two cases of fatal head injury have occurred in the history of competitive diving. In both cases, the divers were attempting to do a reverse 3-1/2 somersault in the tuck position and struck their heads on the 10-meter platform (31). As stated previously, there have been no catastrophic cervical spine injuries (including paralysis) in competitive divers, nor has a significant spine injury occurred in a pool meeting the recommended dimensions for diving facilities advocated by the National Collegiate Athletic Association (NCAA), United States Diving, or the Federation Internationale de Natation Amateur (FINA) (12).

### 4.3 Injury Outcome

There are no reported data regarding the residual effects of injuries after retirement, types of injuries associated with forced retirement, or clinical outcome of injuries. It is the authors' experience that few injuries are severe enough to require withdrawal from participation; however, some athletes with shoulder or cervical spine injuries have discontinued platform diving and limited their participation to springboard competition in order to minimize the physical stress.

## 5. Injury Risk Factors

Diving injuries, like injuries from other sports, are felt to result from a combination of intrinsic and extrinsic risk factors (28, 37, 39, 44). Understanding the intrinsic and extrinsic causes of injury is a prerequisite for injury treatment and prevention.

Until further scientific studies are available, the discussion of injury risk factors will rely primarily on inferences from current injury data and from the cumulative experience of the authors.

### 5.1 Intrinsic Factors

Intrinsic risk factors for diving include physical, motor, and functional characteristics. The relation between diving injury and age, sex, fitness, and injury history awaits further investigation.

### 5.5.1 Physical Characteristics

Variation related to joint laxity, biomechanics, and muscle balances has been implicated in the cause of sports injury (62). However, it should also be noted that variable physical characteristics do not necessarily have a positive or negative effect on risk. For example, excessive joint laxity may increase the risk of joint dislocations, but may also be necessary for performing certain aspects of the sport.

Studies from sports other than diving provide insights into the role of biomechanics in injury. Lower extremity malalignment is an accepted risk factor for injury in jumping sports (13,63). With the significant jumping demands of springboard and platform diving, anatomic variations such as flat feet, genu valgum, and patellar malalignment should be considered as possible contributing factors for injury in divers.

### 5.1.2 Motor/Functional Characteristics

Deficiencies in strength, particularly shoulder girdle and upper extremity strength (58, 62), coordination, spatial orientation, previous injury (38, 39), and skill are potential risk factors for diving injury. Lack of skill and technical competence as a risk factor warrants illustration. The relationship between suboptimal performance and injury is more obvious in diving than in many other sports. A runner who fails to win a race, a pitcher who fails to throw a strike, or a basketball player who fails to make a shot do not expose themselves to greater injury risk simply by failing to perform. Conversely, a diver who fails to perform optimally, resulting in a nonvertical entry into the water, suffers negative consequences both on the scoreboard and physically.

## 5.2 Extrinsic Factors

Extrinsic risk factors for injury in divers include exposure, coaching, environmental conditions, and equipment. Each factor may contribute to injury independently or in combination with other risk factors.

### 5.2.1 Exposure

In diving, exposure is determined by the number of hours and days per week of training and competition and how that time is allocated between dryland training and diving from the 1-, 3-, and 10-meter heights. The practice sessions of platform divers demonstrates how exposure is modified to prevent injury. Most platform divers limit their training on the 10-meter platform to 2 to 3 days per week and typically do each dive on their list just two or three times per workout session.

It should be pointed out that divers with poor technique or low skill level are not sheltered from injury by having their "playing time" or exposure limited. The number of required dives on a list and the force of impact on water entry is the same for both high- and low-skilled divers.

### 5.5.2 Coaching/Supervision

Studies relating injury rates to coaching experience have not been done in diving. In the sport of football, studies have shown an inverse relation between injury rate and coaching experience (6). Given the coaches' high level of involvement with all aspects of training and competition in divers, a similar relationship might be expected in diving.

Overtraining, inadequate technique, and inappropriate skill progressions are all risk factors whose impact on injury can vary according to the experience and attentiveness of the coach.

### 5.2.3 Environment

The environment is an obvious factor in injury when a diver slips off a diving surface or strikes the bottom of a shallow pool. Less obvious environmental factors in injury relate to facility design and use:

- Divers who are concurrently training on a diving tower with platforms at 1, 3, 5, 7.5, and 10 meters are at risk of collisions with other divers or divers in the process of emerging from underwater.
- Divers must be able to adequately spot the water surface to maintain orientation while spinning and twisting. The presence of a surface agitator (bubbles or spray) or a dark-colored pool bottom can help divers maintain their orientation to the surface and properly time their entry.

### 5.2.4 Equipment

Dryland equipment such as trampolines, landing pits, spotting harnesses, spotting belts, and weights may be factors in injury. Discussion of these risks and further discussion of environment and equipment related risks is available in the U.S. Diving Safety Manual (15).

# 6. Suggestions for Injury Prevention

The discussion of injury prevention in diving logically follows the discussion of injury risk factors. The guidelines for enhancing safety in diving are presently based on logical inferences from available epidemiologic and injury data and not on intervention studies. The U.S. Diving Safety Manual (15) details what is known and what is recommended for promotion of diving safety by those most closely involved with the sport.

## 6.1 Players

Flexibility, strength, power, balance, and agility are the functional and motor characteristics required for both optimal performance and safety in diving. Conditioning programs that address these characteristics as they apply to diving may augment performance and help minimize the breakdown that occurs from strenuous training (4, 26).

## 6.2 Sport

The rules and regulations for the sport of diving as well as guidelines for training and skill progression are formulated, in large part, with safety in mind. Such guidelines should be considered as a starting point for safety promotion. For the sport to maintain a good safety record, safe training regimens need to be followed, monitored, and continually updated.

## 6.3 External Environment

Environmental risk can be minimized by proper facility design, maintenance, and use. Guidelines for facility design are summarized in the U.S. Diving Safety Manual (15). Compliance with design standards is required for construction of new facilities and may be a prerequisite for obtaining liability insurance.

## 6.4 Health Support System

The presence and active involvement of a health support system can further enhance safety for divers. A preparticipation examination and early recognition and treatment of minor injuries can decrease the risk of developing more severe or chronic problems.

First aid training by coaches and the presence of an athletic trainer can help with appropriate initial management and treatment of the injuries that do occur. All diving facilities should have a spine board available and a practiced protocol for performing deep water rescues.

# 7. Suggestions for Further Research

This exhaustive review of the literature regarding competitive diving injuries clearly demonstrates the need for organized prospective epidemiologic studies. It is imperative to conduct studies of larger populations in which the data are collected over multiple seasons, in a consistent manner, and that address epidemiologic variables (Table 11.7).

**Table 11.7   Suggestions for Further Research**

| Research component | Research directions/questions |
| --- | --- |
| Literature | |
| Injury definition | A medical condition that occurs as a result of participation in an organized diving training session or competition and results in the inability of the diver to participate in full practice or competition for at least one day |
| Study population | Male vs. female, springboard vs. platform, skeletally immature vs. mature, senior divers vs. masters divers |
| Study design | Prospective<br>Three to 5 years<br>Controlled (compared with other sports)<br>Correlates injury risk with exposure (years training, dives/training session, training sessions/day, week, month, year)<br>Correlates injury with physical characteristics (strength, flexibility, alignment) |
| Data collection | Standardized reporting form<br>Insurance claims information<br>Trainers on site<br>Surveys at regional and national competitions<br>Incentives for compliance with injury reporting requests |
| Research team | Physician, athletic trainer and/or physical therapist, biomechanist, epidemiologist, statistician, coach, and (possibly) a sports psychologist |
| Incidence of injury | |
| Injury rates | Include information about the population of divers who are not injured for accurate calculation; prospective studies best identify the part of the dive during which injury occurred; define the setting—practice vs. competition, springboard vs. platform, dryland vs. pool. |
| Reinjury rates | Calculate rates; study the contribution of reinjury to new injury. |

*(continued)*

**Table 11.7**  *(continued)*

| Research component | Research directions/questions |
| --- | --- |
| **Injury characteristics** | |
| Injury onset | Systematic rates for gradual vs. sudden onset injuries. |
| Injury type | Classify injury (sprain, strain, fracture, concussion, medical problem, etc.). |
| Location | Design studies to provide meaningful injury rates to the head, spine/trunk (cervical, thoracic, lumbar), upper extremity (shoulder, elbow, wrist, hand), lower extremity (hip, knee, leg, foot/ankle). |
| Injury severity | Time loss from training, modification of training program, medical expenditure, forced retirement from diving, permanent disability, catastrophic injury—all need further research attention. |
| Injury risk factors | Analytical research into factors that may predispose divers to injury is needed. |
| Injury prevention | Design intervention studies that provide reliable information to both divers and their coaches about injury prevention modalities and their expected effectiveness. |

# References

1. Albrand, O.W.; Corkill, G. Broken necks from diving accidents: A summer epidemic in young men. AJSM 4(3):107-110; 1976.
2. Anderson, S.J.; Gerard, B.; Ziatkin, M. Cervical spine problems in competitive divers. Proceedings, U.S. Diving Sport Science Seminar, Los Angeles, CA: 144-157; September 1993.
3. Anderson, S.J. Sport, medical and injury background of JO divers. Proceedings, 1993 U.S. Diving Sports Science Seminar, Los Angeles: 4-49; September, 1993.
4. Anderson, S.J.; Rubin, B.D. The evaluation and treatment of injuries in competitive divers. In: Buschsbacher, B. and Braddom, R.L., eds. Sports medicine and rehabilitation: a sport specific approach. Philadelphia: Hanley & Belfus; 1994: 95-106.
5. Bailes, J.E.; Herman, J.M.; Quigley, M.R.; Cerullo, L.J.; Meyer, R.R. Diving injuries of the cervical spine. Surgical Neurology 34(3):155-158; 1990.
6. Blyth, C.S.; Mueller, F.O. Injury rates vary with coaching. Phys. Sport Med. 2:45-50; Nov. 1974.
7. Bowerman, J.W. Water Sports. In: Bowerman, J.W., ed. Radiology and injury in sport. New York: Appleton Century Crofts; 1977:270-276.
8. Carter, R.L. Prevention of springboard and platform diving injuries. Clin. in Sports Med. 5(1):185-194; 1986.
9. Clement, A. Current trends in aquatic litigation. Council For National Cooperation in Aquatics National Conference. Indianapolis, IN; Nov, 1989.
10. Darda, G. Encyclopedia of sportsmedicine. Larson, LA: 520-521, 610-611, 673-675; 1971.
11. Dawson, W.J. Sports-induced spontaneous rupture of the extensor pollicis longus tendon. J. Hand Surg. 17A:457-458; 1992.
12. DeMers, G. Competitive diving and swimming. In: Adams, S.H. et al., eds. Catastrophic injuries in sports: avoidance strategies. Salinas, CA: Coyote Press; 1984:22-37.
13. Dufek, J.S.; Bates, B.T. Biomechanical factors associated with injury during landing in jump sports. Sports Medicine 12:326-337; 1991.
14. Fabiani, M.; Bolasco, P.; Barbara, M. Incidence of otorhinolaryngological diseases in water sports. J. Sports Med. and Physical Fitness 22:108-112; 1982.
15. Gabriel, J.L., ed. U.S. Diving Safety Manual. Indianapolis, IN: U.S. Diving Publications; 1990.
16. Gabriel, J. USA Diving Injury Surveillance Data; 1992.
17. Gabrielsen, A.; Rubin, B.D., eds. Prevention of the most catastrophic sports-related injuries. Indianapolis, IN: Council for National Cooperation in Aquatics; 1981.
18. Gabrielsen, M.A.; Clayton, R.D. Diving injuries: a critical insight and recommendations. Indianapolis: Council for National Cooperation in Aquatics; 1984.
19. Gabrielsen, M.A. Spinal cord injuries resulting from diving. In: Priest, E.L., ed. Aquatics in the 80's, Conservation, Education, and Research, November 20-23, 1980, Atlanta Biltmore Hotel, Georgia Institute of Technology. Indianapolis: Council for National Cooperation in Aquatics; 1984.
20. Gabrielsen, M.A. Proceedings of the National Pool and Spa Safety Conference. Co-Sponsored by the U.S. Consumer Product Safety Commission and The National Spa and Pool Institute, Arlington, CA; 1985.
21. Good, R.P.; Nickel, V.L. Cervical spine injuries resulting from water sports. Spine 5(6):502-506; 1980.
22. Groher, W.; Heindensohn, P. Backache and x-ray changes in diving. Z. Orthop. 108:51-61; 1970.
23. Groher, W. Low back pain in divers. Brit. J. Sports Med. 7:100-103; 1973.
24. Groher, W. Damage to a diver's motor system. Diving World 8-10; February/March, 1978.
25. Herman, J.M.; Sonntag, V. Diving accidents: mechanism of injury and treatment of the patient. Crit. Care Nurs. Clin. North Am. 3(2):331-337; 1991.
26. Hess, G.P.; Capiello, W.L.; Poole, R.M.; Hunter, S.C. Prevention and treatment of overuse tendon injuries. Sports Med. 8:371-384; 1990.
27. Hunter, L.Y.; O'Connor, G.A. Traction apophysitis of the olecranon. AJSM 8(1):51-52; 1980.
28. Jackson, D.W.; Jarrett, H.; Bailey, D.; Kausek, J.; Swanson, J.; Powell, J.W. Injury prediction in the young athlete: a preliminary report. AJSM 6:6-11; 1978.
29. Kendall, P.H. Swimming. In: Armstrong, J.R. & Tucker, W.E., eds. Injuries in sport. London: Staples; 1964.

30. Kewalramani, L.S.; Taylor, R.G. Injuries to the cervical spine from diving accidents. Journal of Trauma 15(2):130-142; 1975.

31. Kimball, R.J.; Carter, R.L.; Schneider, R.C. Competitive diving injuries. In: Schneider, R.C., ed. Sports injuries: mechanisms, prevention, and treatment. Baltimore: Williams & Wilkins; 1985:192-211.

32. Krackow, K. Acute, traumatic rupture of a flexor hallicis tendon: a case report. Clin Orthop. 150: 261; 1980.

33. Krejci, L.; Rezek, P. Ocular changes in competition divers. Ceskoslovanska Optalmologie 38(2):96-99; 1982.

34. Krejcova, H.; Krejci, L.; Jirout, J.; Stracarova, G.; Rezek, P. Vestibular and neurological disorders in diving competitors. Ann. N.Y. Acad. Sci. 839-845; 1981.

35. Lee, S. Clinical examination: diving. In: Larson, L.D., ed. Encyclopedia of sports sciences and medicine. New York: MacMillan; 1971.

36. Lee, S. Aquatic hazards related to otolaryngology. In: Craig, T.T., ed. Medical Aspects of Sports; 1978:52-55.

37. Lysens, R.; Steverlynck, A.; van den Auweele, Y.; et al. The predictability of sports injuries. Sports Med. 1:6-10; 1984.

38. Lysens, R.J.; Ostyn, M.S.; van den Auweele, Y.; Lefevre, J.; Vuylsteke, M.; Renson, L. The accident-prone and overuse-prone profiles of the young athlete. AJSM 17:612-619; 1989.

39. Lysens, R.J.; deWeerdt, W.; Nieuwboer, A. Factors associated with injury proneness. Sports Med. 12:281-289; 1991.

40. Mangine, B. Back injuries in diving: a preliminary report. In: Golden, D., ed. Proceedings United States Diving Sports Sciences Seminar. Indianapolis: U.S. Diving; 1981:123-130.

41. Mangine, R. Wrist and thumb taping in diving. In: Golden D., ed. Proceedings of the United States Diving Sports Science Seminar. Indianapolis: U.S. Diving; 1983:59-63.

42. Mathis, R.D. Bilateral shoulder dislocation: an unusual occurrence. J. Emerg. Med. 8(1):41-43; 1990.

43. McClure, D. Personal Communication, 1991.

44. Meeuwisse, W.H. Predictability of sports injuries: what is the epidemiologic evidence? Sports Med. 12:8-15; 1991.

45. Merinu, J.A.; Dragan, I.; Escalas, R.; Dominguez, R. Traumatic lesions in swimming, water polo and diving. International Swimming and Water Polo 3:52-53, 56; 1981.

46. Mizel, M.S.; Rubin, B.D.; Decker, E.; Trepman, E.; O'Brien, R.; LaFace, K. Foot and ankle injuries in U.S. divers. Proceedings of the U.S. Diving Sports Science Seminar. Los Angeles, CA: September 1993:129-131.

47. Mutoh, Y.; Takamoto, M.; Miyashita, M. Chronic injuries in elite competitive swimmers, divers, water polo players, and synchronized swimmers. In: Ungerechts, B.E. et al., eds. Swimming science V.

Champaign, IL: Human Kinetics Publishers; 1988: 333-337.

48. Reilly, T.; Miles, S. Background to injuries in swimming and diving. In: Reilly, T., ed. Sports fitness and sports injuries. London: Faber and Faber; 1981: 159-167.

49. Rossi, F. Spondylolysis, spondylolisthesis and sports. J. of Sports Med. and Physical Fitness 18(4): 317-340; 1978.

50. Rubin, B.D.; Richardson, A.B. Injuries in competitive divers. AOSSM Meeting, Las Vegas, NV: February 1981.

51. Rubin, B. Orthopaedic aspects of competitive diving injuries. In: Golden, D., ed. Proceedings of the United States Diving Sports Sciences Seminar. Indianapolis: U.S. Diving; 1983:65-78.

52. Rubin, B.D. Injuries in competitive diving. Sports Medicine Digest 9(4):1-3; 1987.

53. Rubin, B.D. Shoulder injuries in competitive divers. Presented at the 6th annual meeting, Arthroscopic Surgery of the Shoulder, San Diego, CA: 1989.

54. Rubin, B.D.; Chandler, J.; Anderson, S.J.; Kibler, W.B. A physiological and shoulder injury profile of elite divers. Proceedings, U.S. Diving Sports Science Seminar, Los Angeles, CA: September, 1993:158-164.

55. Samples, P. Spinal cord injuries: the high cost of careless diving. Phys. & Sportsmed. 17(7):143-148; 1989.

56. Schneider, R.C.; Papo, M.; Alverez, C.S. The effects of chronic recurrent spinal trauma in high diving: a study of Acapulco's divers. J. Bone and Joint Surg. 44-A:648-656; 1962.

57. Schneider, V.; Bratzke, H. Traumatic rupture of the aorta after a jump from the 3M board. Zeitschrift Fuer Rechtsmedizin. 83(2):169-177; 1979.

58. Shields, C.L.; Fox, J.M.; Stauffer, E.S. Cervical cord injuries in sports. Phys Sportsmed. 6:71-76; 1978.

59. Strauss, M.B.; Cantrall, R.W. Swimmer's ear. Physician and Sportsmedicine 7(6):101-103; 1979.

60. Strupler, M.; Saxer, U. Verletzungen und Schaden am Bewegungsapparat beim Wasserspringen. Ztschr. Sportmed. 30:13-17; 1982.

61. Stubbs, D. Diver hits board and misses chance for Olympic team. Swimming World & Junior Swimmers 21(8):12-13; 1980.

62. Taimela, S.; Kujala, U.M.; Osterman, K. Intrinsic risk factors and athletic injuries. Sports Med. 9:205-215; 1990.

63. Taunton, J.E.; Clement, D.B. The role of biomechanics in the epidemiology of injuries. Sports Med. 6:107-120; 1988.

64. Torg, J.S. Epidemiology, pathomechanics and prevention of athletic injuries to the cervical spine. Medicine and Science in Sports and Exercise 17(3):295-303; 1985.

65. Wieder, D.L. Treatment of traumatic myositis ossificans with acetic acid iontophoresis. Phys. Ther. 72(2):133-137; 1992.

66. Zimmerman, W. Registration of injuries in springboard and platform diving in The Netherlands. Medical School Thesis, University of Leiden, The Netherlands; 1993.

# 12

# Fencing

*Eric D. Zemper and Peter A. Harmer*

## 1. Introduction

Although the sport of fencing has a long history, there is very little research on fencing injury rates and patterns. In an effort to review and summarize the literature on fencing injury epidemiology, a search of English language articles published since 1975 was undertaken (i.e., Medline and SPORT Discus searches using [fencing and (injury or accident) and language=english] for the search request). This search found only three published studies from the United States. Search efforts beyond the U.S. literature turned up a very small number of additional studies, three of which are included in this analysis. Only articles providing data about injury occurrence or rates were selected for this review. In addition, some unpublished data from the authors were included. Differing definitions of a reportable injury (no two studies used the same definition) and the fact that only three of the studies reported any exposure data make analysis of even this small number of studies difficult.

Five of the studies collected injury data on site and thus can be considered prospective studies (6, 8, 10, 11, 15). All of these, except Lanese et al. (10), involved only competitions; the Lanese data covered both competition and practices, but not enough detail was provided to differentiate between them. Only three studies provided any exposure data (8, 10, 15). The Harmer (8) and Roi and Fasci (15) studies provide data on the number of participants and number of bouts, making it possible to calculate rates per 100 fencers and per 1,000 athlete exposures. In this case, an athlete exposure (AE) is one fencer participating in one bout; each bout results in two AE. The Lanese study (10) provided data on the number of participants and was the only study to provide data on the hours of exposure, but since the study covered only one men's and one women's collegiate team (18 men, 6 women) for one season, and involved only eight total injuries, the size of the study was not sufficient to provide any significant data in relation to injury rates based on time of exposure.

The studies by Moyer and Konin (11) and Crawfurd (6) were prospective, collecting data on site at competitions, but the researcher did not provide any information on numbers of participants in these competitions or any other exposure data. Thus, the studies are essentially case series reports. The article published by Moyer and Konin provided only a narrative summary of some of their data analyses, without any tables or other presentation of data. The raw data tabulations from this study were provided to the authors and were used for the analyses of injury sites and types for this review. The remaining two studies (2, 12) were retrospective studies, collecting data by means of surveys requesting information from fencers about previous injuries. Because no exposure data were collected, these studies also are essentially case series reports. The Müller-Sturm article (12) did not state the time period of the survey. The survey of the United States Fencing Association (USFA) membership by Carter, Heil, and Zemper (2) was undertaken as a pilot project to assess the need for a full-scale prospective study of fencing injuries, but it has provided by far the largest current database on fencing injuries.

## 2. Incidence of Injury

Only two published studies (10, 15) present true injury rates (i.e., recorded exposure data). In addition, as yet unpublished data collected by Dr. Peter Harmer (8) provide injury rates during four major national and international competitions. The remaining published studies (2, 6, 11, 12) do not provide exposure data and present only distributions of types and sites of injuries.

## 2.1 Injury Rates

The study by Lanese et al. (10) involved only one university team for one season, and 18 men and 6 women. With five injuries to the men and three to the women, the injury rates shown in Table 12.1 cannot be considered very representative because of the extremely small study sample. The data reported by Roi and Fasci (15) tabulated 58 "requests for medical attention" or "intervention" in fencing competitions involving 1,365 fencers and 6,802 bouts in 47 competitions during one year in the Lombard region of Italy. From their data it is possible to calculate the injury rates presented in Table 12.1.

Harmer's unpublished data (8) covered four major competitions in 1 year, including the 1989 Pan American and World Championships, and involved 1,031 participants in 7,798 bouts. The injury rates presented in Table 12.1 were based on any request for assistance from the medical staff during the period of the competitions.

While the USFA survey (2) did not provide exposure data, the survey instrument did ask the respondents to provide the total number of injuries they incurred during the previous 12 months, from which it is possible to calculate an injury rate of 92 per 100 fencers per year. This is considerably higher than the rates provided by the other studies in Table 12.1. However, those studies (except for the Lanese study where the rate is distorted by the very small sample size) cover only an extremely limited time frame from a few competitions, while the data from the USFA survey includes the much longer time frame of a full year of participation in both practices and competitions. This illustrates one of the problems of using injury rates per 100 participants rather than a rate based on numbers of exposures or actual amount of time exposed (18).

## 2.2 Practice vs Competition

Although the small amount of data provided in the Lanese et al. study (10) included exposure in both practices and competition, no distinction was made between them. The larger Roi and Fasci (15) and Harmer (8) data sets involved competitions only, so the rates in Table 12.1 for these studies should be considered competition injury rates. No specific data are available for practice injury rates, although if fencing follows the pattern of most other sports (18), the practice injury rate per 1,000 AE could be projected to be no greater than one third to one fourth of the competition rate.

## 3. Injury Characteristics

The compilations of data on injury type in fencers are presented in Table 12.2. Table 12.2 and Table 12.3 present data from the Roi and Fasci (15) and Harmer (8) studies included in Table 12.1, as well as studies by Crawfurd (6) on injuries "sufficient

**Table 12.1    Injury Rates in Fencing**

| Study | Duration | # participants | # bouts | # athlete-exposures | # injuries | Injuries/100 participants | Injuries/ 1,000 A-E |
|---|---|---|---|---|---|---|---|
| Lanese et al. (1990) | 1 yr | | | | | | |
| Men | | 18 | — | — | 5 | 27.8[a] | — |
| Women | | 6 | — | — | 3 | 50.0[a] | — |
| Roi & Fasci (1988) | 47 local and regional competitions during one year | | | | | | |
| Men | | 952 | 4,696 | 9,392 | 35 | 3.7 | 3.7 |
| Women | | 413 | 2,106 | 4,212 | 23 | 5.6 | 5.5 |
| Harmer (unpublished) | 4 major national and international competitions during one year | | | | | | |
| Men | | 685 | 5,173 | 10,346 | 80 | 11.7 | 7.7 |
| Women | | 346 | 2,625 | 5,250 | 27 | 7.8 | 5.1 |

*Note.* All studies in this table were prospective in design, collecting data on-site as the injuries occurred.

[a]The rates per 100 participants for the Lanese et al. study differ greatly from the other studies because it involved an extremely small sample and because it covered daily practices as well as competitions. The other studies covered only the restricted time frame of competitions.

to cause a fencer to stop a bout" (i.e., the most serious injuries) at competitions during a 4-year period in England, by Moyer and Konin (11) on "acute" injury reports collected at USFA competitions during a two year period, by Müller-Sturm and Biener (12) on "accidents and injuries" reported in a retrospective survey of 105 Swiss and German international competitors, and by Carter, Heil, and Zemper (2) from a retrospective survey of the USFA membership.

### 3.1 Injury Onset

The only data on the nature of onset of fencing injuries comes from the Carter, Heil, and Zemper study (2), where survey respondents indicated that 67.6% of their worst injuries in the previous year were sudden onset (acute) injuries and the remaining 32.4% were gradual onset in nature. Of the 67.6% sudden onset injuries, 28.5% occurred in competition, 28.7% occurred in practice, and the remaining 10.3% occurred in related training activities (weight lifting, running, etc.). A slightly

larger percentage of injuries from this case series appears to occur during practice activities (considerably more time is spent in practices than in competition), but the implication is that the injury rate for competition would be higher than for practice, if exposure data were available. Higher injury rates in competition than in practice is a common pattern seen in nearly all sports (18).

### 3.2 Injury Type

The distribution by type of injury for the six studies that provided this type of data is presented in Table 12.2. As is the case with most other sports, ligament sprains and muscle strains are the predominant types of injuries, accounting for nearly half the recorded injuries. In several of the studies, contusions accounted for at least one fourth of all recorded injuries. Punctures and lacerations are of concern in fencing, and in the prospective studies in Table 12.2 together account for at least 10% of the injuries. These types of injuries usually are caused by the weapon, with punctures being of

**Table 12.2   A Percent Comparison of Injury Types in Fencers**

| Injury type | # injuries<br>Study type[b]<br># participants | Harmer<br>(unpubl.)<br>n = 107<br>Prosp.<br>N = 1,031 | Roi &<br>Fasci, 1988<br>n = 58<br>Prosp.<br>N = 1,365 | Crawfurd,<br>1990<br>n = 25<br>Prosp., CS<br>N = ??? | Moyer &<br>Konin, 1992<br>n = 322<br>Prosp., CS<br>N = ??? | Carter et al.,<br>1993[a]<br>n = 842<br>Retro., CS<br>N = 1,603 | Müller-Sturm<br>& Biener, 1991<br>n = 148<br>Retro., CS<br>N = 105 |
|---|---|---|---|---|---|---|---|
| Abrasion | | 3.7 | 3.4 | — | 0.0 | 0.0 | — |
| Blister | | 14.0 | 8.6 | — | 0.0 | 0.0 | — |
| Bursitis | | 0.0 | — | — | — | 2.0 | — |
| Cartilage tear | | 0.0 | — | — | — | 5.3 | 1.0 |
| Contusion | | 24.3 | 24.1 | 28.0 | 6.2 | 0.0 | 8.0 |
| Fatigue/cramp | | 0.9 | 8.6 | — | — | 0.0 | — |
| Fracture | | 0.0 | 1.7 | — | 0.9 | 2.1 | 2.0 |
| Heat | | 0.0 | 1.7 | — | 18.0 | 0.0 | — |
| Laceration | | 10.3 | 32.8 | 36.0 | 17.4 | 3.0 | 6.0 |
| Puncture | | 1.9 | 1.7 | 16.0 | 0.0 | 3.3 | 2.0 |
| Separation/dislocation | | 0.0 | — | — | — | 2.7 | — |
| Sprain | | 23.4 | 10.3 | 16.0 | 33.2 | 23.9 | 24.0 |
| Strain | | 10.3 | 5.2 | 4.0 | 23.9 | 26.6 | 26.0 |
| Stress fracture | | 0.0 | — | — | — | 2.1 | — |
| Subluxation | | 0.9 | — | — | — | 0.0 | — |
| Systemic | | 0.0 | 1.7 | — | 0.3 | 0.4 | — |
| Tendinitis | | 4.7 | — | — | — | 14.5 | 8.0 |
| Torn tendon | | 0.0 | — | — | — | 2.4 | 11.0 |
| Other | | 5.6 | — | — | — | 12.0 | 12.0 |

[a]The data from the survey by Carter, Heil, and Zemper (1993) represent only the worst injury sustained during the previous 12-month period (therefore, mild injuries such as contusions were not noted). The average number of injuries sustained by the respondents during this period was 0.9.

[b]Study type: Prosp. = prospective, data collected on-site as injuries occur; definitions of a reportable injury may vary. Retro. = retrospective, data collected by questionnaire after the fact; subject to recall error. CS = case series, no exposure data collected to allow calculation of injury rates.

particular concern since they often are the result of those occasions when the weapon blade breaks, leaving a sharp unprotected tip capable of piercing protective gear. Another type of injury occasionally noted in fencers, particularly in the Moyer and Konin study (11), is heat illness or heat exhaustion caused by the heavy protective gear that fencers wear during long periods of competition. Tendinitis and torn tendons are relatively common problems for fencers, primarily in the forearm and wrist of the weapon arm and in the Achilles tendon.

## 3.3 Injury Location

A summary of the distribution of the site of injuries in fencers is presented in Table 12.3. This table indicates that approximately one half of all injuries to fencers occur in the lower extremities, with the ankle and the knee being the predominant sites. The hand and fingers also account for a major proportion of the injuries. Fencing is an asymmetri-

cal sport involving rapid lunges and retreats that put strain on the legs and lengthy periods of extension and quick movements of the weapon arm, wrist, and hand. The hand and fingers holding the weapon, as well as the nonweapon hand, also are vulnerable to lacerations and contusions from the opponent's weapon.

The head and trunk are reasonably well protected by the equipment a fencer wears, although these areas occasionally sustain injuries from collision contact with an opponent or lacerations from an opponent's weapon. The great majority of injuries occur in the upper and lower extremities, which have the most stress placed upon them during fencing activity and which generally are less well protected.

# 4. Injury Severity
## 4.1 Time Loss

Only three of the studies used in this review noted whether or not an individual injury was

**Table 12.3   A Percent Comparison of Injury Location in Fencers**

| Injury location | # injuries Study type[b] | Harmer (unpubl.) N = 107 Prosp. | Roi & Fasci, 1988 N = 58 Prosp. | Crawfurd, 1990 N = 15[a] Prosp., CS | Moyer & Konin, 1992 N = 322 Prosp., CS | Carter et al., 1993 N = 842 Retro., CS | Müller-Sturm & Biener, 1991 N = 148 Retro., CS |
|---|---|---|---|---|---|---|---|
| Head | | 2.8 | 10.3 | — | 5.9 | 0.6 | 2.0 |
| Spine/trunk | | 9.3 | 3.4 | 46.7 | 9.0 | 13.8 | 23.0 |
| Neck | | 0.0 | — | 26.7 | 2.2 | 1.4 | — |
| Back | | 2.8 | 1.7 | — | 6.5 | 8.1 | — |
| Chest/rib | | 5.6 | 1.7 | 6.7 | — | 2.3 | — |
| Abdomen | | 0.0 | — | — | — | 0.4 | — |
| Groin | | 0.9 | — | 13.3 | 0.3 | 1.7 | — |
| Upper extremity | | 41.1 | 55.2 | 6.7 | 32.9 | 30.4 | 20.0 |
| Shoulder | | 1.9 | 3.4 | — | 6.2 | 5.0 | — |
| Upper arm | | 1.9 | 1.7 | — | 1.6 | 1.5 | — |
| Elbow | | 3.7 | — | — | 2.8 | 6.8 | — |
| Forearm | | 2.8 | 10.3 | — | 1.2 | 1.5 | — |
| Wrist | | 0.0 | 1.7 | — | 4.7 | 5.9 | — |
| Hand/finger | | 30.8 | 37.9 | 6.7 | 16.5 | 9.6 | — |
| Lower extremity | | 46.7 | 27.6 | 46.7 | 40.7 | 54.6 | 55.0 |
| Pelvis/hip | | 3.7 | 1.7 | — | 0.9 | 2.5 | — |
| Thigh | | 8.4 | 1.7 | 20.0 | 5.0 | 9.0 | — |
| Knee | | 4.7 | 10.3 | — | 8.1 | 17.3 | — |
| Lower leg | | 1.8 | 3.4 | — | 3.4 | 4.8 | — |
| Ankle | | 17.8 | 6.9 | 26.7 | 15.8 | 14.5 | — |
| Heel/Achilles | | 1.9 | — | — | 1.2 | 0.0 | — |
| Foot/toe | | 8.4 | 3.4 | — | 6.2 | 6.5 | — |
| Systemic | | 0.0 | 3.4 | — | 1.6 | 0.6 | — |

[a]Only 15 of the 25 recorded injuries specified the site in Crawfurd (1990).

[b]Study type: Prosp. = prospective, data collected on-site as injuries occur; definitions of a reportable injury may vary. Retro. = retrospective, data collected by questionnaire after the fact; subject to recall error. CS = case series, no exposure data collected to allow calculation of injury rates.

of sufficient severity to cause any time loss from participation; one retrospective study provided a total of days lost from all reported injuries. The Roi and Fasci study (15) indicated that 3 of their 58 recorded injuries caused the fencer to withdraw from the tournament. The data from Harmer (8) included 5 of 107 injuries that caused the fencer to withdraw from the competition. The remaining 95.2% of the injuries were not of sufficient severity to cause any loss of participation time. Both of these studies involved competition only, and because they both provided exposure data, it is possible to calculate time-loss injury rates of 0.33 per 100 participants and 0.27 per 1,000 AE in competition.

The survey by Müller-Sturm and Biener (12) of 105 German and Swiss international fencers indicated that 36% of the fencers never had an injury and that the 64% who had been injured accumulated 203 days of missed work (average of 1.4 days/injury), 64 days in hospital, and 9 injuries requiring surgery. A more detailed breakdown of these injuries was not presented, and no time frame for the study was given.

The survey of the USFA membership (2) involved both competition and practice injuries, although no exposure data was collected. Survey respondents were asked how many injuries they had sustained in the previous 12 months, how many days of participation were lost due to all injuries, and the impact of injuries on their fencing success. Of 1,603 respondents, 761 (47.5%) said they had sustained no injuries during the previous year. The remaining 842 reported 1,470 injuries, for a mean of 0.92 injuries per fencer (92/100 participants/year) and 1.75 injuries per participant who had an injury. Of the 842 who reported injuries, 181 (21.5%) said they lost no participation time, 30.8% lost 1 to 6 days of participation, 18.7% lost 7 to 14 days, 13.0% lost 15 to 30 days, and the remaining 16.2% lost more than 30 days. Of those who were injured, 61.4% said their injuries caused no interference or only mild interference with their fencing success. In general, it appears from these reports that fencing injuries during competition most often are not severe enough to cause any time loss and that throughout the year in practices and competitions the majority of injuries are not severe enough to cause any significant loss of participation time.

## 4.2 Catastrophic Injury

Injuries resulting in death or permanent disability rarely occur in modern competitive fencing. Only seven fatalities have been recorded since 1937, and most of these have occurred in highly skilled competitors in elite competition (5, 7, 13, 14, 16). All fatalities have been male fencers; five of seven deaths involved epée, with foil and sabre one each, and broken blades were responsible for the fatal wound in six of the seven cases. Four fatalities resulted from penetration of the thorax, with one or both lungs punctured and laceration of at least one major blood vessel in each case. The other three deaths involved neck (one case) and head (two cases) wounds. The two head wounds resulted from broken blades penetrating the mask (13, 16), whereas the mortal neck wound followed a broken blade slipping under the mask and penetrating the trachea and left common carotid artery (5). Two of the thoracic fatalities occurred before plastrons (underarm protectors) were mandatory. The second incident was, in fact, the impetus for the introduction of the plastron (13). Changes in equipment standards (design, strength, type of materials) generally have followed catastrophic incidents. However, all fatalities subsequent to the introduction of the plastron have occurred to fencers utilizing equipment that met at least the minimum standards set by the Fédération Internationale d'Escrime (FIE), the international governing body for the sport. Unfortunately, the force generated by elite athletes seems to be increasing even beyond the accelerating standards for the structural integrity of fencing equipment (4, 7). In the most recent death, the athlete was using the highest standard equipment available (14).

Several characteristics or mechanisms that may contribute (either singly or in combination) to blade breakage, force of penetration, or both and result in death have been postulated based on the seven incidents discussed here. Most often noted are a right-handed fencer fencing a left-handed fencer, the use of orthopaedic grips, and the propensity to make counterattacks (4, 13). Each of these characteristics was present in a majority of the fatalities (although in different combinations). Further research is needed to determine if modifying one or more of these characteristics would decrease the risk of sustaining a catastrophic injury.

Although anecdotal evidence suggests that penetrating wounds (especially thoracic) of varying severity occur more frequently than is generally realized, fatalities or permanent disabilities are extreme aberrations. Without adequate exposure data, it is not possible to calculate accurately the risk of catastrophic injuries in fencing. Given seven fatalities over the tens of thousands of athlete exposures in elite competition during the past 60 years, it seems reasonable to argue that the risk is minimal. During the 25 years from the late 1930s to the early 1960s only three deaths occurred, and none were reported during the next 20 years (early 1960s-early 1980s). However, four catastrophic incidents have been noted in the last 13 years (1982-1994) despite increasingly stringent structural standards applied to fencing equipment. With a fine line separating penetrating wounds and catastrophic injuries, careful monitoring (reporting and recording) of penetrating wounds of all types must be undertaken on an international level to determine whether the risk of significant or mortal injury is changing.

# 5. Injury Risk Factors

The data for this section comes from the USFA survey (2). These data relate to the most severe injury sustained by the fencer during the previous 12 months. Responses to the question about what factors contributed significantly to the fencer's worst injury during the previous year are summarized in Table 12.4. The reader should be aware

**Table 12.4  Factors Contributing to Fencing Injuries**

|  | Percent |
| --- | --- |
| Personal factors | 48.3 |
| Inadequate warm-up | 13.2 |
| Poor technique | 12.2 |
| Fatigue | 11.0 |
| Dangerous tactics | 2.4 |
| Other (e.g., inadequate conditioning, overtraining) | 9.5 |
| Equipment and facilities | 27.9 |
| Fencing strip | 9.6 |
| Shoes | 9.5 |
| Weapon | 4.5 |
| Jacket | 0.8 |
| Mask | 0.4 |
| Lighting | 0.4 |
| Other | 2.7 |
| Behavior of others | 12.7 |
| Dangerous tactics by opponent | 8.5 |
| Poor officiating | 1.6 |
| Poor coaching | 1.0 |
| Other | 1.6 |
| No identifiable contributing factors | 11.1 |

*Note.* Data from Carter, Heil, and Zemper (1993). Percent breakdown of factors contributing to the most significant injury during the previous 12 months, as indicated by survey respondents.

that what is presented here about risk factors in fencing is derived from this minimally descriptive data and that the proposed factors have not been subjected to risk factor analysis.

## 5.1 Intrinsic Factors

Nearly half of the factors identified in Table 12.4 were personal factors under direct control of the fencer, therefore implying that these injuries were preventable. Most of the factors identified involved inadequate warm-up, poor fencing technique, and fatigue. The use of dangerous tactics was identified 2.4% of the time as causing the fencer's own injury. Other factors mentioned included lack of adequate general conditioning, overtraining, and repetitive movements leading to overuse injuries.

## 5.2 Extrinsic Factors

Just over one quarter of the factors mentioned in Table 12.4 were problems with equipment and facilities. Problems with the fencing strip and with shoes were the predominant factors at nearly 10% each. Problems with the fencing strip appear to be related to injuries in the lower extremities, particularly ankle and knee injuries. The most common problems with the fencing strip were the use of hard concrete floors, dust and dirt causing slipperiness on wood or rubber floors, lack of adequate means of securing copper fencing strips that tend to "bunch up" and trip the fencer, and raised fencing strips that cause ankle injuries. Problems with shoes most frequently mentioned included lack of adequate cushioning and heel support, and the lack of shoe designs to protect against stresses specific to the sport, such as lunging. The weapon was mentioned less frequently as a causative factor; the grip of the weapon and the bell were the parts most likely to cause injury. There was only occasional mention of other equipment factors such as the fencing jacket, mask, or lighting.

In the factors grouped under the heading of "Behavior of Others," the most frequently mentioned factor was dangerous tactics by an opponent. In written comments, fencers often mentioned the tendency for some fencers to depend more on aggression and brute strength rather than skill and finesse. Poor officiating or poor coaching were seldom mentioned as factors leading to injury.

## 6. Suggestions for Injury Prevention

While major injuries or injuries causing any significant time loss in fencing appear to be relatively rare, there is a real risk of sustaining numerous minor injuries that may be preventable. Because so little research has been done on fencing injuries, at the moment it is impossible to provide injury prevention suggestions derived from solid empirical or analytical data. These suggestions (Table 12.5) for preventing fencing injuries follow directly from information presented in Table 12.4 and from written comments and observations of fencers responding to the survey of USFA members (2). They are essentially common-sense suggestions that should have a reasonable chance of being confirmed in the future by appropriate research. The suggestions fall into three primary areas: actions that can be taken by participants; improvements in equipment and facilities; and administration of fencing competitions.

### 6.1 Players

It is evident from data that the most predominant types of injuries are sprains and strains (Table 12.2), occurring most frequently in the lower extremities (Table 12.3), and that because the most frequently cited cause of injury was inadequate warm-up (Table 12.4), that proper warm-up and stretching may help prevent fencing injuries. The comments of fencers in the USFA survey provide two important reasons for this. Many admit to "laziness" in doing warm-up and stretching, while a significant number state that instructors and coaches do not place enough emphasis on them or never mention them at all. Therefore, the first recommendation for preventing fencing injuries is to educate fencing instructors and coaches (and thereby the fencers) on the importance of proper techniques of warming up and stretching prior to practice and competition (9). Related to this is the suggestion that instructors and coaches emphasize the need for adequate general physical conditioning before and during the fencing season to prevent injuries caused by fatigue and inadequate conditioning.

Although sometimes related to fatigue and improper conditioning, the problem of injuries caused by poor technique is probably best addressed by ensuring the availability of adequately trained and experienced instructors and coaches who can identify and correct faulty technique in this technique-oriented sport, particularly in the novice fencer. Overtraining seems to be a problem

**Table 12.5   Recommendations for Preventing Injuries in Fencing**

Participants
1. Educate fencing instructors, coaches, and fencers as to the importance and proper techniques of warm-up and stretching prior to practice and competition.
2. Instructors and coaches should emphasize the need for adequate general physical conditioning before and during the fencing season.
3. Ensure availability of adequately trained and experienced instructors and coaches who can identify and correct faulty technique, particularly in novice fencers.
4. Develop sports psychology mental training routines to reinforce use of appropriate fencing technique, especially in the face of fatigue or overly aggressive tactics by opponents.

Equipment and facilities
5. Do not allow practices or competitions on concrete surfaces without adequate cushioning.
6. When raised fencing strips are used, they should be of low height and adequate width to reduce risk of ankle injuries.
7. In practices and competitions, wooden and rubber surfaces should be cleaned at regular intervals, and fencers should wipe shoes on a damp towel before beginning each session of activity, to reduce the risk of slipping due to dusty or dirty surfaces.
8. Copper fencing strips should be fully stretched and firmly anchored to prevent "bunching."
9. Electric cord reels and other potential hazards (including officials) should be placed so they do not present a hazard to a fencer during a rapid retreat or when leaving the confines of the fencing strip during action.
10. The national governing body sports medicine committees should work with shoe manufacturers to develop an affordable fencing shoe that is designed specifically for the stresses of fencing.
11. Continue research on better breaking characteristics of weapon blades.

Administration of competitions
12. The national governing bodies should establish and enforce minimum standards for fencing strips, for spacing between fencing strips, and for medical coverage at all sanctioned competitions.
13. The national governing bodies should make a concerted effort to instruct competition officials to enforce existing rules against dangerous or overly aggressive conduct, and, if necessary, institute new rules against such inappropriate or dangerous tactics.
14. In order to prevent the possible spread of HIV and HBV infections, the national governing bodies should immediately institute and enforce rules requiring that action be halted any time a laceration or puncture draws blood, until the wound is covered and the weapon is cleaned.

limited to elite fencers who train on a daily basis throughout the year.

### 6.2 Sport

National governing bodies for fencing, through their sports medicine committees, should establish and enforce minimum standards for fencing strips in competitions to reduce the risk of injury in relation to factors noted previously (e.g., prohibit placement of strips on concrete floors without adequate cushioning). Standards should be established and enforced with regard to factors such as minimum spacing between fencing strips and availability of medical coverage.

From the comments of fencers in the USFA survey and from published comments that began appearing more than 10 years ago (4), there is a growing concern about the tendency of some fencers to depend more on aggression and brute strength instead of traditional fencing skills and finesse. The resulting use of dangerous tactics by opponents was a factor frequently listed as causing injuries (Table 12.4), and a common complaint was that officials often ignore these tactics even when rules against their use exist. As a result of this concern, it is suggested that national governing bodies make a concerted effort to instruct officials (and coaches) to enforce existing rules against such conduct and, if necessary, institute new rules against inappropriate or dangerous tactics.

Although not mentioned in any of the recent literature, because there are occasions when lacerations and punctures draw blood, there must be concern about prevention of the transmission of the HIV and the Hepatitis B Virus (HBV). Even though the possibility of HIV or HBV transmission in this sport may be relatively remote, it is suggested that national governing bodies immediately institute and enforce policies and competition rules requiring that, any time a participant's skin is broken by laceration or puncture, action be immediately stopped to treat and cover the wound (this should include practices as well as competitions). These policies and rules also should require that any areas where blood has been spilled must be cleaned and, to prevent the possibility of HIV or HBV transmission to later opponents or fencing partners, the blade of any unbroken weapon causing a laceration or puncture should be appropriately cleaned.

### 6.3 External Environment

The primary equipment and facility problems are related to the fencing strip, shoes, and weapon (Table 12.4). It is recommended that fencing strips provide adequate cushioning for all practices and competition, and specifically that the common use of concrete surfaces for practices and competition be discontinued. Fencing on concrete floors was

the most frequent complaint by respondents in the USFA survey and has begun to receive more attention in fencing publications and by sports safety committees such as that of the American Society for Testing and Materials (cf., 3, 17). If raised fencing strips must be used, they should be of low height and of sufficient width to not create a hazard to a fencer who inadvertently leaves the designated competition area of the strip during an attack or retreat. Wooden or rubber surfaces should be cleaned at regular intervals during practices or competition, and fencers should wipe their shoes on a damp towel before beginning each session in order to avoid injuries caused by slipping on dusty or dirty surfaces. Copper fencing strips must be adequately stretched and firmly anchored to prevent injuries caused by the "bunching" of the strip surface. Electric cord reels that are part of the electric touch scoring apparatus must be placed where they do not create a hazard to the retreating fencer and, in general, there must be adequate room between fencing strips during competitions so that placement of scoring tables, officials, equipment bags, etc., do not pose a hazard if fencers leave the strip during the heat of action.

It is suggested that sports medicine committees of fencing's national governing bodies work with shoe manufacturers to develop a fencing shoe with better support and cushioning specifically designed for the stresses of fencing movements. With regard to the weapons, the greatest concern among fencers is puncture wounds, which potentially are fatal, when the tip of a weapon breaks. These breaks occur when a blade is bent beyond its limit during a touch, and the force of the lunge often is more than sufficient to cause the broken tip to penetrate protective gear. Research is now being conducted on blade composition and ways of modifying breaking characteristics that will reduce the risk of penetration by broken blade tips (1), and this research should be continued.

## 7. Suggestions for Further Research

It is obvious from the summary presented here that little research has been completed on the epidemiology of fencing injuries and therefore, as with most other sports, there is much to be done. The studies reviewed illustrate the usual problems of lack of a common definition of a reportable injury, inadequate collection and use of exposure data to generate true injury rates, and the use of a variety of rates that hinder the ability to compare results across studies. The great majority of the data reviewed here comes from studies that essentially are case series, which is the weakest form of epidemiological study.

It is recommended that a basic, large-scale, prospective study of injuries in fencers be conducted to develop initial reliable data on fencing injury rates and patterns in both practices and competitions. None of the studies presented in this review provide an ideal model of what is needed, although the study by Lanese et al. (10) probably comes closest in overall design. Its major shortcomings are the extremely small size of the sample and the fact that it only lasted one year. This future study of fencing injuries should cover a large representative sample of fencers over a sufficient period of time to provide stable results. It should be prospective in design, collecting exposure and injury data as they occur in both practice and competition. Preferably the data should be collected by medically trained personnel, such as on-site athletic trainers, although in this sport the only place where such a situation regularly exists is with collegiate teams. Data still can be collected by medical staff at competitions, as was the case with several of the existing studies, but exposure data must be included in the data collected. Competition data are relatively easy to collect; it is more difficult to collect practice data, and this type of data is needed because essentially no practice-injury data are available. Included in the data should be information on the nature of onset of the injury and information on reinjury, which also are not currently available for fencing.

Future studies should use a common definition of a reportable injury. There finally seems to be a growing consensus to use a definition based on time loss (i.e., an injury that occurs during sports participation, requires some level of medical treatment, and causes the athlete to stop or reduce level of participation for one day or more). As illustrated in this review, most injuries in fencing do not result in loss of participation time. In this case it might be reasonable to collect data on any injury requiring medical attention and analyze total injury rates and time-loss injury rates separately.

Finally, injury rate reports should be based on some measurement of exposure. The minimum standard should be reporting based on number of athlete exposures (injuries/1,000 AE), with one AE being one athlete participating in one practice session or one competition bout. Injury rates based on time of exposure (injuries/100 hours or 1,000 hours) are preferred, although it is difficult to collect such detailed exposure data in large-scale studies. The use of rates per 100 participants does not provide an adequate means for comparisons, since it does not compensate for differing amounts of exposure in practice or competition from one group to the next, as illustrated in this review and as noted previously (18).

Some special areas that need attention in future research on fencing injuries include reinjury and research on the characteristics that seem to be related to risk of catastrophic injury (e.g., right-handed fencer competing against a left-handed fencer, the use of orthopaedic grips, and the propensity to make counterattacks).

In the absence of a large-scale prospective study of fencing injuries, an alternative method for developing information on injury rates and patterns is to combine results from smaller, local studies. However, the only way it will be possible for results from smaller individual studies to be combined will be to use a common definition of a reportable injury, provide adequate exposure data, and use an injury rate based on some measurement of exposure, as suggested here. Still, the most reliable data will come from a well-designed, prospective study of a large, representative population of fencers.

The implementation of such a study would provide a solid basis for confirming or expanding the above suggestions for preventing injuries in fencers and would provide clues as to what specialized studies might be needed to investigate specific types of injuries common or unique to fencers or studies related to specific pieces of fencing equipment.

# References

1. Carter, C.; Heil, J. Safer fencing for everyone. American Fencing 42(3):13-14; 1992.
2. Carter, C.; Heil, J.; Zemper, E. What hurts and why: data from the 1992 USFA fencing injury survey. American Fencing 43(3):16-17, 29; 1993.
3. Carter, C.; Heil, J.; Zemper, E. Fencing surfaces. American Fencing (in press).
4. Clery, R. Apropos d'un accident. American Fencing Sept.-Oct. pp. 7-11, Nov.-Dec. pp. 7-11; 1983.
5. Crawfurd, A.R. Death of a fencer. Br. J. Sports Med. 18(3):220-222; 1984.
6. Crawfurd, A.R. The medical hazards of fencing. In: Payne, S.D.W., ed. Medicine, sport and the law. London: Blackwell Scientific Publication; 1990.
7. Crawfurd, A.R. Rapport sur l'accident mortel d'Howard Travis, le 25 Avril 1990, a t'Harde, Pays Bas. Unpublished report; 1991.

8. Harmer, P. Unpublished data. Willamette University; 1994.

9. Heil, J.; Zemper, E.; Carter, C. Behavioral factors in fencing injuries. In: Proceedings of the VIII world congress of sport psychology. Lisbon, Portugal: International Society for Sport Psychology; 1993.

10. Lanese, R.R.; Strauss, R.H.; Leizman, D.J.; Rotondi, A.M. Injury and disability in matched men's and women's intercollegiate sports. Am. J. Publ. Health 80:1459-1462; 1990.

11. Moyer, J.; Konin, J. An overview of fencing injuries. American Fencing 42(4):25; 1992.

12. Müller-Sturm, A.E.; Biener, K. Fechtsportunfalle— Epidemiologie und Pravention (Fencing accidents— epidemiology and prevention). Deutsche Zeitschrift fur Sportmedizin 42(2):48-52; 1991.

13. Parfitt, R. The fencer at risk. In: Armstrong, J.R.; Tucker, W.E., eds. Injury in sport. London: Staples; 1964: 173-190.

14. Poux, D. Personal communication with P. Harmer: 1994.

15. Roi, G.S.; Fasci, A. Indagine sulle rechieste di intervento del medico durante le gare di scherma (Requests for medical assistance during fencing matches). Ital. J. Sports Traumatol. 10(1):55-62; 1988.

16. Safra, J-M. La securite en question aprés l'accident de Vladmir Smirnov. Escrime. 42 (Aout-Septembre):26-28; 1982.

17. Soter, P. Competitions on concrete surfaces. American Fencing. 42(4):30-31; 1992.

18. Zemper, E. Epidemiology of athletic injuries. In: McKeag, D.; Hough, D.; Zemper, E., eds. Primary care sports medicine. Dubuque, IA: Brown and Benchmark; 1993: 63-73.

# 13

# Field Events

## M.J.L. Alexander

## 1. Introduction

The skills of running, jumping, throwing, and swimming are all survival skills that are the most basic of human skills. The field events in the sport of track and field include the throwing events: shot, hammer, discus, and javelin; as well as the jumping events: high jump, long jump, pole vault, and triple jump. The jumping events were essential for fighting and defense, and the throwing sports were essential for the activities of war (16). These events can all be classified as maximum-force events, in which the maximum distance thrown or jumped is the criterion for success, and they will often produce force-related injuries. Whenever an athlete is asked to produce maximum-force output during training and competition, resulting injuries will be due to the high stresses of maximal muscle contractions.

An *injury* has been defined as a condition that produces symptoms and delays, modifies, or stops participation in athletic activities (74). Athletic injuries to field athletes are usually of two types: acute injuries that are sudden, rapid injuries such as a fracture, ligament tear, or dislocation or chronic overuse injuries that are due to repeated microtrauma and will eventually produce tissue damage (67). It is essential that an athlete adopt a technique that keeps the loads on the body within bounds that can be tolerated, or injury will occur (51). However, research that examines the tolerance limits of human tissues in maximum-force movements is almost nonexistent, so descriptions of tolerance limits in specific activities are not available. There is evidence that joint and tendon forces during running can exceed the ultimate strength measured in cadaver studies, but we are unable to specify the limits to which intact tissues can be stressed without injury (159).

The purpose of this review is to examine the types and incidence of injuries to athletes competing in track and field events. These field athletes are athletes of all ages and skill levels including school children, high school and college students, and elite athletes. The literature search consisted of computerized searches of the SPORT Discus and Medline databases, as well as sports medicine books and track-coaching periodicals. The most extensive information describing field injuries appears in case studies and case series, which provide the best insight into causes and types of injuries. The study was limited to those periodicals that were available to the author and several foreign articles for which an English abstract was available in the database. There were no review studies that described only athletes in field events; the majority of the retrospective studies in this sample described the incidence of injuries in the track events as well (40, 41, 154, 155, 163). It has been suggested that only 10% to 20% of track and field injuries occur in field events (127), so the frequencies reported for track and field may be misleading when applied to field events only.

## 2. Incidence of Injury

### 2.1 Injury Rates

To determine the risk in a sport, it is necessary to calculate the rate of injury. The rate is determined by comparing the number of injured athletes to the number of athletes at risk (82). Very few track and field injury studies have included number of exposures or length of exposure in the calculation of the injury rates.

The frequency or incidence of reported injuries from surveys of all track and field events is summarized in Table 13.1. Because the track, or running,

**Table 13.1  A Comparison of Injury Rates in Track and Field Events**

| Study | Study design | Information collection | Duration | Events | # of participants | # of injuries | Rate/period |
|---|---|---|---|---|---|---|---|
| Kosek, 1973 | R | Trainer's report | 2 years | All | HS, 17 F | | 25/10 athletes/100 exposures |
| Garrick & Requa, 1978 | R | Trainer's report | 2 years | All | HS, 308 M, 208 F | 52 M, 55 F | 31/100 males 32/100 females |
| Zaricznyj et al., 1980 | R | School report | 1 year | All | GS, 289 Ss | 50 | 7.9/100 athletes |
| Requa & Garrick, 1981 | R | Trainer's report | 2 years | All | HS, 308 M, 208 F | | 35/100 athletes |
| Shively et al., 1981 | R | Telephone interview | 1 year | All | HS, 1,682 M, 1,141 F | 28 M 8 F | 16.6/1,000 athl (m) 7.0/1,000 athl (f) |
| Watson, 1984 | R | Teacher's report | 1 year | All | GS, 3,527 M, 3,272 F | | 15/season |
| Watson & Dimartino, 1987 | P | Coach/trainer report | 1 season | All | HS, 174 M, 83 F | | 1/5.8 males, 1/7.5 females |
| Backx et al., 1989 | R | Questionnaire | 6 weeks | All | GS, HS, 78 M, 78 F | | 1.54 |
| McLennan & McLennan, 1990 | R | Questionnaire | 10 years | Scottish heavy athletics | Elite, 170 M | 729 | 42.9% |
| Backx et al., 1992 | R | Questionnaire | 7 months | All | GS, 1,000 M, 818 F | | 295/1,000 athletes 1/1,000 hr practice |

*Note.* R = retrospective; P = prospective; HS = high school; GS = grade school; All = all track and field.

events produce a high number of overuse injuries, the injury rates for the whole sport of track and field are moderately high.

Incidence studies in track and field have nearly all been at the school levels and were generally part of injury studies across sports (5, 41, 78). A few reports have been specifically about track and field injuries (88, 127, 155). Watson and Dimartino (155) recorded the injury incidence of 257 high school track and field athletes, and they reported that most injuries occurred during running events, with 46.3% occurring during sprinting events. Pole vaulting was the only field event in which a high incidence of injury was apparent, and the jumping and weight events produced few injuries during the year of the study (155). No injuries were reported for female athletes in field events.

A survey of injuries at Special Olympics events suggests that track and field events provide the least activity time and the most injuries (88), but this comparison is with a limited number of sports, with a special group of athletes.

No studies were located that focused on the incidence of injuries to athletes in the jumping events (long jump, high jump, triple jump, pole vault) or in the throwing events (javelin, discus, shot put, hammer throw) in track and field. However, one survey described the injury patterns in Scottish

heavy athletics (91). It was suggested that field events of modern track and field evolved in part from the seven events of the "heavy athletics," and since many of the events are similar to the throwing events, the injuries are likely to be similar.

Some of the findings about the incidence of injuries in track and field events are summarized below.

- Compared to track events, field events have a relatively low incidence of injury (127, 155).
- Four out of every five injuries occur during a track event, as opposed to a field event (127).
- The incidence of injury in the field events has been reported anecdotally as 10% of all track and field injuries, and the pole vault has the highest reported risk (91).
- Among field events, pole vaulters sustain one of the highest injury rates (13.3%; 22, 155).
- Field-events injuries also cluster in the long jump for boys, where 45% of the field-event problems occurred (127).

## 2.2 Reinjury Rates

No data were located that reported reinjury rates for field events. This is an important area of research and requires further study. DuRant et al.

(24) reported a survey of 674 high school athletes who completed a preparticipation athletic examination and then were monitored for injury incidence. Athletes who were previously injured were more likely to be reinjured: Knee injuries were associated with previous knee injuries and knee surgery, ankle injuries were associated with previous ankle injuries, and both arm and leg injuries were associated with previous fractures (24).

One case series of stress fracture of the olecranon tip in javelin throwers reported that one of the four patients had a refracture 11 months after the primary operation; the reinjury was successfully treated (59). Stanish (138) suggested that a muscle strain injury will leave a collagenous scar within the injured tendon or muscle, which may render these tissues vulnerable to reinjury.

## 2.3 Practice vs Competition

It is useful to compare the injury rates in practices to those incurred in competitive situations. In the sport of track and field where there is little scientific information on injury rates in practice versus competition, the total injury rate for males was 0.33 per participant overall and 0.12 during competition; and for females it was 0.35 overall and 0.04 during competition (41). In a survey of Australian pole vault injuries, 72% of those surveyed suffered their injuries during practice, which is reasonable since most of the vaulting takes place in training (118).

## 3. Injury Characteristics

### 3.1 Injury Onset

Injury onset in field events can occur as either a sudden, acute injury or a chronic overuse injury. Most field events injuries are chronic in nature, due to the many hours of practice in a single jumping or throwing event requiring maximum-force output. Chronic overuse injuries develop with time and include stress fractures, various types of tendinitis, bursitis, and apophysitis. The tissue is stressed repeatedly over time, and the time between exposures is not sufficient for healing to occur. Gradual degeneration of the tissue and loss of strength produce the overuse injury. These injuries are often related to overtraining, when the athlete suddenly increases the length and intensity of workouts.

Acute injuries are sudden in onset and occur during one specific forceful movement performed in competition or practice. There is some question regarding the presence of chronic conditions in many occurrences of sudden onset injuries. Although the tissues may fail in one dramatic incident, they have been stressed over a long term and the final failure occurs as an acute injury. Hamstring strains and spinal spondylolytic stress injuries are likely the result of repeated stresses to the tissue involved, so the breakdown is gradual but is manifested in a sudden injury that is the final failure of the tissue. Examples of acute injuries include neck hyperflexion injuries in high jump and hamstring strains during the long jump approach. Groin and lower back injuries in the long jump often occur from repeated imperfect landings in the sand (126). Pole vaulting is the only field event with a significant number of injuries in this group (37), which can include a fall from a height landing on a hard surface, such as the track or infield; or injury from a broken pole.

## 3.2 Injury Types

Few current data describe the incidence of injury types in the field events, but several studies have reported injury types in track and field. Since the sport includes all of the running events, in which most of the injuries occur, overuse injuries to the lower limb are most common. Parker (115) suggested that the most common type of injury to track and field athletes is muscle strain, which can be prevented by thorough warm-up and endurance training. He noted that ankle sprains are also common in the sport. A summary of the types and percentages of injuries in track and field from several studies is presented in Table 13.2.

### 3.2.1 Muscle Injuries

Muscle overload injury is the most common type of athletic injury, comprising up to 67% of injuries, depending on the sport (74). Muscle injuries most often take the form of strain injuries (106) frequently occurring with eccentric contractions, due to the higher forces produced in the muscle during these lengthening contractions (39). Muscle injuries occurring during the deceleration phase of the javelin throw, during the run up for the jump events, and during the explosive eccentric contraction prior to takeoff for a jump and when decelerating the swing leg during the airborne phase of the long jump are examples (126). The lumbar spine is also extended in midflight and flexed forward

**Table 13.2  Percentage of Injuries in Track and Field Events by Location**

| Site | McLennan & McLennan, 1990* N = 170 | Watson & Dimartino, 1987 N = 257 | Payton, 1981 (pole vault) N = 25 |
|---|---|---|---|
| Shoulder, rotator cuff | | | 12.5 |
| Impingement | 12 | | |
| Supraspinatus tear | 1 | 2.4 | |
| Biceps tendinitis | 5 | | |
| Elbow, epicondylitis | | | |
| Lateral | 11 | | |
| Medial | 2 | 2.4 | |
| Wrist | | | |
| DeQuervains | 8 | | |
| Carpal tunnel | 2 | | |
| Back/abdominal | | | 3.1 |
| Musculoligamentous | 14 | 2.4 | |
| Facet syndrome | 2 | | |
| Undiagnosed pain | | 7.3 | 10.9 |
| Head/neck | | | |
| Unspecified injuries | | | 14.1 |
| Hip | | | |
| Bursitis | 1 | 2.4 | |
| Iliac apophysitis | | 2.4 | |
| Thigh, strain | | | |
| Quadricep strain | 4 | 2.4 | 7.8 |
| Hamstring strain | 7 | 4.9 | |
| Adductor strain | | 7.3 | 9.4 |
| Knee | | | |
| Iliotibial band | 1 | | |
| Patellar tendinitis | 3 | 9.8 | |
| Prepatellar bursitis | | 4.9 | |
| Chondromalacia | 8 | 2.4 | |
| Menisci tear | 5 | | |
| Tibial tuberosity pain/avulsion | | 2.4 | 10.9 |
| Lower leg | | | |
| Posterior tibial syndrome | | 19.5 | 4.7 |
| Ankle | | | |
| Achilles tendinitis | 7 | 2.4 | |
| Ligament sprain | 2 | 17.1 | |
| Foot | | | |
| Foot pain/stress fracture | | | 21.8 |
| Metatarsalgia | | 2.4 | |

*Scottish heavy athletics.

for landing, leading to lumbar strain injuries and psoas strain (145).

A common type of muscle injury to the upper extremity (especially to javelin throwers) is rotator cuff injury to the muscles of the shoulder joint (66). A less common injury to throwing athletes is partial rupture of the pectoralis major muscle occasionally sustained when training with heavy weights (128).

### 3.2.2 Tendon and Ligament Injuries

Tendon injuries are very common sports-related injuries, because vigorous physical activity focuses much stress and force on the tendinous part of the muscle–tendon unit (63, 77, 108). The strength of a tendon is related to thickness and collagen content, rather than to the maximum tension its muscle can exert, and the tensile strength of a healthy tendon is usually greater than twice the strength of its attached muscle (36).

Tendinitis, a result of microscopic tearing of the collagen and connective tissue fibers of the tendon, is produced by repeated high intensity contractions of skeletal muscle. Common types of tendinitis in jumping events include patellar tendinitis (jumper's knee) (16, 23, 80) involving the upper or lower poles of the kneecap or the tibial tuberosity (32), quadriceps tendinitis (137), and Achilles tendinitis (68, 92, 108). Injuries to throwing athletes include supraspinatus tendinitis (83, 92), biceps tendinitis (120, 160), subscapular and levator scapulae tendinitis (27, 54), and triceps tendon inflammation (136).

Patellar tendon rupture is fairly common in elite high jumpers due to the high repetitive forces on this tendon (30, 98, 149), and Achilles tendon rupture is a sport injury that commonly occurs in athletes between 30 and 40 years of age and is more common in men than women (63). A survey of Achilles tendon injuries showed that 5% were due to jumping activities including those sustained in jumping field events (68).

Of the ligament injuries, the most troublesome in the shoulder is the coracoacromial ligament, which impinges on the supraspinatus tendon during the overhand throwing motion (134). Elbow ligament injuries are common in throwing athletes in baseball pitching and javelin throwing with stretching or tearing of the medial ligaments being the most common types (94, 147, 161). The most frequently seen throwing injury to the lateral side of the elbow is the subluxation of the head of the radius, which requires surgical tightening of the annular ligament (161).

### 3.2.3 Nerve Injuries

Throwing athletes often experience nerve problems in the throwing limb, especially in the elbow joint. It has been suggested that most of these are compressive in nature, resulting from overuse or overload on the joint (156) and producing inflammation, lesions, and progressive compression of the ulnar nerve (45). Entrapment, dislocation, or both, of the ulnar nerve are conditions seen in throwing athletes (including javelin throwers) whose arms repeatedly perform a throwing motion that results in valgus stress at the elbow (65), excessive laxity of the ulnar collateral ligament, ulnar traction spurs medially, and secondary ulnar neuritis (10).

In nerve injuries to throwing athletes, the neurogenic syndromes are usually incomplete, indicating the absence of severe motor or sensory deficits (156). The symptoms of ulnar neuritis at the elbow joint begins with intermittent paresthesias in the ring and small fingers, and as the inflammation progresses, pain and paresthesias will occur down the ulnar aspect of the forearm and hand (45).

### 3.2.4 Bone and Articular Cartilage Injuries

Apophyseal injuries are most common in adolescents, who are undergoing a growth spurt so that the muscle insertions on the bone, which often is still undergoing ossification (48), are placed under tension as the bone grows rapidly and the muscle is unable to keep up. This constant tensile force on the bone will produce pain, tenderness, or even avulsion of the apophysis under extreme forces. The most common types of injury to jumping athletes are calcaneal apophysitis (Sever's disease), which is an inflammation of the insertion of the Achilles tendon on the calcaneus (92) due to rapid growth of the tibia without accompanying growth of the tendon, and Osgood-Schlatter's disease (apophysitis of the tibial tuberosity; 96).

Medial epicondylitis is an apophyseal injury which occurs in adolescents who participate in maximum force throwing events, such as javelin throwing (92, 116). A relatively uncommon apophyseal fracture can occur to the lumbar spine, to an area of the vertebrae known as the ring apophysis, a narrow mound of cartilaginous tissue that almost completely encircles the rims of the superior and inferior surface of the vertebrae (14). This is the site of attachment of the long intervertebral ligaments and is one site of lumbar apophyseal fractures in adolescents, especially during heavy activities such as weight lifting. Adolescents training for field events must have strict supervision regarding amount of weight and types of exercises.

One of the most common injuries to adolescent athletes is the avulsion fracture, in which the bony apophysis to which a muscle is attached is avulsed from high tensile forces. A common example in adolescent jumpers is an avulsion fracture of the tibial tuberosity during vigorous jumping events (30, 61, 69, 96). Avulsion fractures of the tibial tuberosity can occur when the knee is bent by high

forces at landing from a jump, accompanied by strong contraction of the quadriceps group (69).

Another type of adolescent injury to the bone is injury to the epiphysis, or the growth plate of the bone, in which forces on a bone produce a fracture at the growth plate. Fractures of the tibia through the proximal tibial epiphysis are rare; however, four adolescent males engaged in jumping sports presented with five avulsion fractures at this site (13, 60).

Avulsion fractures can occur to almost any of the insertion points of major muscle groups. A common avulsion fracture occurs to the rectus femoris tendon attachment to the anterior inferior iliac spine during vigorous exercise such as track and field training (86). In adolescents, prior to complete fusion of the apophysis, excess exertion on the rectus femoris tendons may result in avulsion of the anterior inferior iliac spine.

Stress fractures are a common overuse injury in athletes who train at high intensities for extended periods of time. A stress fracture is a partial or complete fracture of the bone due to its inability to withstand the nonviolent stress that is applied in a rhythmic subthreshold manner (87, 151). Stress fractures may occur in the bones of the feet, the metatarsals, the bones of the lower leg, tibial or fibular stress fractures (42), or the femur and femoral neck (112).

High jumpers experience extreme foot stress during the flop takeoff, due to the angle of foot placement relative to the direction of the velocity of the jumper. These high forces produce stress fractures of the tarsal navicular, which is the cornerstone of the longitudinal foot arch (72, 73, 76, 79), as well as other tarsal bones (58) mainly in the takeoff leg (33). Jumping athletes also experience a specific type of tibial stress fracture produced by jump training (139) believed to be associated with excessive pronation (160).

The femoral shaft is another common site of stress fractures in athletes, which may occur with alterations in training or increases in training intensity (87). Stress fractures of the femoral shaft are uncommon in athletes, with the incidence of these fractures reported between 2.8% and 3.5% in various series (53). Other forms include stress fractures to the femoral neck in high jumpers (112) and olecranon stress fractures in throwers (38, 59, 94, 107).

Athletes in throwing sports such as the javelin throw may suffer a spiral stress fracture of the humerus during maximal throws (1, 49, 105, 119), due to the repeated high velocity of medial rotation that occurs during the release, while transverse fractures can occur in response to the high-impact forces in landing from the long jump or triple jump (153).

## 3.3 Injury Location

A listing of injury locations in field events is reported in Table 13.3 for jumping events and Table 13.4 for throwing events. As might be expected, the majority of the jumping injuries occurred to the lower extremity, and throwing injuries occurred to the upper extremity.

### 3.3.1 Head/Spine/Trunk

Javelin throwers have an unusually high incidence of spondylolysis (9, 103) due to the extreme ranges of hyperextension during the backswing, followed by rapid and forceful flexion during the delivery of the implement. The high jumper is also at risk for spondylolytic fractures, as the position at bar clearance for a skilled flopper is an extreme hyperlordotic position (95) that places high stresses on the neural arch. Pole vaulters have a high incidence of spondylolytic fractures, which occur due to the extreme range of motion in the lumbar spine during the takeoff and bar clearance phases of the skill (8, 37). The discus throw may lead to back injuries, due to the rapid and forceful trunk rotation during the delivery. The lower back is subjected to high stresses during the delivery, as the lumbar spine is rotated and extended, and this position will lead to facet opposition and locking, as well as ligamentous and annular strains of the disc (145).

The landing phase of the Fosbury flop high jump event has some risk of cervical spine fracture because the jumper has to land on the back of the head and neck after clearing the bar (110, 113). The majority of pole vault injuries are the result of a fall during attempted bar clearance, as the drop is from a considerable height (118), and the vaulter is at risk of a head or neck injury.

Many degenerative spine injuries to throwing athletes are a result of overuse and repeated high stresses produced when the athlete assumes a position at the end of the range of motion, such as in the lumbar spine of the javelin thrower. The extreme range of hyperlordosis and trunk rotation places extreme stresses on the apophyseal joints, the discs, and the vertebral bodies attached to the discs, causing increased rates of degenerative alterations (103) and possibly fatigue fractures of the apophyseal joints, as well as spondylolytic changes in the neural arch. The high compressive forces from heavy weight training on the vertebrae can produce compressive injuries to the discs of throwing athletes (14).

The momentum of the follow-through in shot, hammer, and discus throws places tremendous traction stress on the anchoring structures, and certain lesions ,such as muscle tears to the muscles attached to the scapulae, especially the rhomboids (7), are particular to these sports. Hammer throwers in particular throw from a position of extreme trunk tilt to balance the forces of the hammer, and this position causes near-maximal stresses on the lower back (20). The right quadriceps is strongly contracted, pulling the right iliac crest anteriorly, while L5 is rotating to the left. This produces lower back stresses, which will produce right-sided low back pain (145). The repeated high stresses of hammer throwing may also produce muscle strains at the myotendinous junctions of the back muscles, including the insertions of the lumbodorsal fascia, latissimus dorsi, rhomboids, and trapezius (121).

### 3.3.2 Upper Extremity

The muscles of the shoulder joint, rotator cuff musculature—especially the infraspinatus muscle (26)—deltoid, and long head of the biceps brachii (157), play an important role in glenohumeral stabilization during the throwing motion. If a weakened, inflamed rotator cuff fails to hold the humeral head down during abduction, the deltoid muscles will pull it up (102). Associated injuries to elite throwing athletes include rotator cuff impingements, biceps tendinitis, and lateral elbow epicondylitis (91), and the development of shoulder asymmetry in which there is a depression or droop of the dominant shoulder with an apparent scoliosis (123). Impingement of the supraspinatus tendon between the undersurface of the acromion and the coraco-acromial arch and the greater humeral tuberosity occurs as soon as the upper arm is elevated above 80 degrees of abduction. Impingement occurs more frequently when there is weakness or fatigue in the shoulder girdle musculature (144) in individuals with a narrow space between the glenoid and the acromion (102), and in individuals using their upper arms at or above shoulder level for prolonged periods (83), such as javelin, discus, and hammer throwers. It has been suggested that 90% of shoulder complaints in javelin throwers are the result of bicipital groove tendinitis secondary to tendinitis (134, 162). Another common shoulder injury in throwers is spiral fracture of the humerus, due to the high rates of shoulder rotation (49, 89, 119).

The glenohumeral joint becomes unstable when the humerus is abducted, externally rotated, and extended, as during the backswing phase of the

**Table 13.3    Case Series and Case Reports of Injury Locations in Jumping Events**

| Study | Design | Subjects | Age | Level | Condition/diagnosis |
|---|---|---|---|---|---|
| Spine/trunk | | | | | |
| Gainor et al., 1983 | Case series | 3 pole vaulters | 20, 20, 15 | College | Unilateral defect of pars interarticularis of L4, L5, L5 (spondylolysis) |
| Paley & Gillespie, 1986 | Case study | 1 high jumper | 17 | International | Cervical spine instability with anterior subluxation of C5 on C6 |
| Olerud & Karlstrom, 1990 | Case study | 1 high jumper | 13 | School | Cervical spine fracture in the facets of C5-C6 |
| Beattie, 1992 | Case study | 1 pole vaulter | 22 | International | Pain and restricted motion at levels of L3/L4 |
| Lower extremity | | | | | |
| Blazina et al., 1973 | Case series | 1 high jumper | 20 | Elite | Patellar tendinitis, surgically treated |
| Liemohn, 1978 | Case series | 6 long/triple jumpers, 6 pole vaulters | — | College | Hamstring strains, usually to take-off leg |
| Orava et al., 1978 | Case series | 1 high jumper | — | — | Stress fracture of the femoral neck |
| Krahl & Knebel, 1979 | Case series | 4 high jumpers | — | International | Stress fractures of the tarsal navicular |
| Ferretti et al., 1993 | Case series | 1 high jumper | 21 | Elite | Patellar tendinitis with pain over insertion of tendon |
| Kameyama et al., 1983 | Case series | 43 high jumpers, 6 long jumpers | 13-18 | School | Avulsion fractures of the tibial tuberosity |
| Ciullo & Jackson, 1985 | Case report | 1 high jumper | 20 | College | L2 wedge and compression fractures and Schmorl's nodes |
| Hughes, 1985 | Case study | 1 high jumper | 13 | School | Avulsion fracture of body of patella during bar clearance |
| Vainionpaa et al., 1985 | Case study | 1 high jumper | 19 | International | Patellar tendon rupture |
| Wang, 1986 | Case series | 3 long jumpers | — | — | Transverse fracture of middle one third of the femoral shaft |
| Bracker & Siekmann, 1987 | Case study | 1 high jumper | Adolescent | School | Fracture of a proximal tibial epiphysis during takeoff |
| Schwobel, 1987 | Case series | 7 jumpers | 13-16 | School | Avulsion of the tibial tuberosity |
| Hulkko & Orava, 1987 | Case series | 27 field athletes | 21.5 | — | Stress fractures, primarily lower leg and tarsal |
| Mirbey et al., 1988 | Case series | 4 high jumpers | 15-17 | High school | Avulsion fracture of the tibial tuberosity with moderate displacement |
| Jozsa et al., 1989 | Cross-section | 14 jumpers | — | Recreation | Achilles tendon ruptures |
| Inoue et al., 1991 | Case series | 1 long jumper, 1 high jumper | 16 | School | Bilateral avulsion fractures of tibial physis, avulsion of the anterior tibial epiphysis |
| Falster & Hasselbach, 1992 | Case study | 1 long jumper | 15 | High school | Avulsion fracture of tibial tuberosity with medial ligament and meniscal tear |
| Moore, 1992 | Case series | 1 high jumper | — | International | Ruptured patellar tendon |
| Khan et al., 1992 | Case series | 1 long jumper | 16 | School | Navicular stress fracture of proximal navicular |
| | | 1 long jumper | 24 | International | Navicular stress fracture with displaced fragment |
| Micheli & Fehlandt, 1992 | Case series | 2 jumpers | 8-19 | School | 2 Achilles tendinitis |

throw (43). This position places the anterior capsule under stress, and this repeated stress may produce weakness of the anterior capsule. This may be accompanied by hypertrophy of the internal rotators, which will produce anterior displacement of the humeral head (43) and even dislocation (98).

Injuries to the elbow are very common in javelin and hammer-throwing and shot-putting athletes as large traction stresses are on the medial muscles of

**Table 13.4   Case Series and Case Studies of Injury Location in Throwing Events**

| Study | Design | Subjects | Age | Level | Condition/diagnosis |
|---|---|---|---|---|---|
| Spine/trunk | | | | | |
| Roncardi, 1988 | Case study | 1 shot putter | 20 | College | Bilateral lower leg and ankle pain, due to spina bifida occulta at L5 |
| Browne et al., 1990 | Case study | 1 weight lifter | 16 | High school | Lumbar ring apophyseal fracture (L3), displaced by posterior longitudinal ligament |
| Roi et al., 1990 | Case series | 1 shot putter | — | — | Partial rupture of pectoralis major muscle while weight training |
| Upper extremity | | | | | |
| Yokoe et al., 1959 (cited in Hill, 1983) | Case series | 29% of javelin throwers | — | College | Bicipital tendinitis secondary to impingement |
| Miller, 1960 | Case study | 1 javelin thrower | 18 | International | Medial ligament strain and fracture of the olecranon tip |
| Peltokallio et al., 1968 | Case study | 1 javelin thrower | 28 | Elite | Spiral fracture to middle third of humerus |
| Tullos et al., 1972 | Case series | 1 javelin thrower | — | — | Acute rupture of the medial collateral ligament |
| Haw, 1981 | Case report | 1 javelin thrower | Adolescent | School | Avulsion fracture of the medial epicondyle of the elbow |
| Moore, 1983 | Case report | 1 shot putter | — | International | Pulled hamstring |
| Hulkko et al., 1986 | Case series | 4 javelin throwers | 21-22 28 | Elite | Stress fractures of the olecranon process; 2 at the tip, 2 oblique and more distal |
| Hartonas & Verettas, 1987 | Case study | 1 shot putter | 19 | College | Spiral fracture of the distal third of the humerus |
| Priest, 1988 | Case study | 1 shot/javelin | — | College | Hypertrophy and depression of throwing shoulder with apparent scoliosis |
| Horrigan & Shaw, 1989 | Case study | 1 shot putter | — | International | Patellar tendon rupture during training |
| Lo et al., 1990 | Case series | 3 throwers | — | — | Impingement of the rotator cuff |
| Moore, 1992 | Case series | 1 javelin thrower | 36 | International | Dislocation of throwing shoulder |
| Micheli & Fehlandt, 1992 | Case series | 2 throwers | 8-19 | School | 1 rotator cuff tendinitis; 1 medial epicondylitis |

the elbow and shoulder as a result of the momentum of the follow-through and the heavy projectile (2). It is often weakness of muscles surrounding the elbow joint that leads to bony injuries to the joint, including medial epicondylitis (100) and early degenerative arthritis. Nerve injuries are also common in throwing athletes, especially ulnar neuritis (45).

In the javelin event the stress at the beginning of the acceleration phase is on the medial elbow musculature, the medial collateral ligament, the medial joint capsule, and the joint itself (94, 146, 148). The valgus force may produce avulsion fractures of the medial epicondyle in children (84) or ligament sprains in adult throwers. Acute rupture of the medial collateral ligament has been reported in javelin throwers (10) and may occur in other throwing events. Elbow injuries in javelin throwers are often of the whiplash type and are due to hyperextension of the elbow joint, causing the ole-

cranon process to impinge upon the olecranon fossa of the humerus (158) or producing loose bodies in the joint (3). Stress fractures of the olecranon are common in javelin throwers, and the strong pull of the triceps often produces wide separation between the fragments and requires surgical intervention (59, 94, 158).

Excessive valgus stress at the elbow joint during the javelin throw leads to arthritic alterations in the medial aspect of the joint (103), traction injuries medially, and compression injuries (including avascular necrosis) laterally (143). Miller (94) described the symptoms of javelin-thrower's elbow as including the following injuries: constriction of the ulnar nerve, stretching or tearing of the ulnar collateral ligament, and fracture of the olecranon process. The majority of the pain and irritation to the elbow is likely due to the stretching and irritation of the medial ligament (35, 94).

The lateral aspect of the elbow joint is subjected to compressive and rotational forces during javelin throwing, which affects the articular surfaces of the radius and capitellum (21) and can lead to degeneration of the articular cartilage of the radial head, capitellum, or both (116).

Shot putters often strain the flexor muscles of the wrist and fingers during the delivery of the shot, as it rests on the fingers, not the palm of the hand, and its inertia produces hyperextension of the wrist stretching flexor tendons of the fingers. The final stage of the put requires a powerful push to propel the shot, as the flexor muscles of the wrist and fingers are stretched prior to the forceful contraction that propels the shot forward (145). Shot putting also places high compression loads on the wrist joint, which may produce ligament sprains and exostosis on the posterior aspect of the wrist, usually at the base of the second metacarpal bone (Lister's tubercle).

Hand injuries frequently prevent pole vaulters from practicing and competing and are due to the high friction created by the powder and resin vaulters use on their hands to improve grip for takeoff. When the pole is planted and the high forces of the run up are transmitted to the pole via the hands, abrasions and cuts in the palms often occur due to the high coefficient of friction.

### 3.3.3 Lower Extremity

Injuries to the knee are less common in field events athletes than in athletes in other sports (80). There are reports of torn meniscal cartilage in a long jumper (30) and a top high jumper (122), and knee meniscal injuries and ligament injuries may occur in the triple jump due to the compressive and rotatory forces during landing (16). Other common types of knee injuries in jumpers include patellar tendinitis, or jumper's knee (31, 56), and avulsion fracture of the tibial tuberosity (30, 57, 69), including bilateral avulsion fractures (130). It has been suggested that a large proportion of knee injuries are due to malalignments at the knee joint, such as varus, valgus, or recurvatum, and that these malalignments will predispose the athlete to injuries (138). Retropatellar knee pain is common in young athletes, especially during jumping or descending stairs, and is often caused by maltracking of the patella and consequent irritation of the patellofemoral joint (44).

Jumping athletes suffer from a number of leg, foot and ankle problems that result from the high forces produced during takeoff. These include calcaneal and metatarsal stress fractures (42), ankle sprains, and peroneal and Achilles tendinitis (68, 92). These type of injuries can seriously affect performance, as immobilization or injury of distal segments interrupts the normal generation, summation, and transmission of muscular forces across joints (104). Krahl and Knebel (79) have described the foot stress present in high jumpers during the flop takeoff, as when the foot is planted and the body is leaning inward toward the center of the arc of the run up. This lean produces extreme eversion of the takeoff foot, with excessive traction on the medial aspect of the foot and ankle joint. This position produces very high stresses on the tarsal navicular, which may produce stress fractures, especially in young female jumpers (79), for whom there appears to be a higher incidence than in males (76). It has been suggested that these high forces take effect when the foot plant is out of the approach direction and that in the optimal jump the longitudinal axis of the takeoff foot must be exactly tangential to the impulse curve. Stress injuries to the takeoff foot are also common in high jumpers, due to the angle of foot placement relative to the velocity vector (76, 79).

## 4. Injury Severity

### 4.1 Time Loss

There is very little published information on the severity of field events injuries, the time lost due to injury, and incidence of catastrophic injuries. The majority of injuries include muscle strains and ligament sprains, which are not serious and heal quite quickly. Achilles tendinitis and patellar tendinitis are also common and take several weeks of treatment before full activity can be resumed. More serious conditions such as jumper's knee, tibial tuberosity avulsions, medial epicondyle avulsions, and stress fractures of the lower back and humerus take several months to heal and may require surgical intervention.

### 4.2 Catastrophic Injury

Few of the injuries reported in field events can be described as catastrophic. The exceptions are in the pole vault event where there have been seven high school fatal injuries from 1983 to 1992. In addition to the fatalities there were also three permanent disabilities and four severe injuries. All 14 of these accidents involved the vaulter bouncing out of or landing out of the pit area (101). Casselman (15) suggested that the throwing events are inherently dangerous to participants, as they could involve impact with the projectiles, producing concussion, skull fractures, and stabbing wounds. Mueller and Cantu (101) reported that there were five accidents, including one fatality, involving participants being struck by a thrown discus, shot, or javelin from 1982 to 1992. Another aspect of injury in the throwing events is the danger to spectators when the implement is released prematurely and flies off sideways into spectators or other athletes. This has occurred in the javelin (90, 99), discus (29), and hammer-throwing (136) events.

## 5. Injury Risk Factors

The appropriate design for predicting injuries is the prospective study that attempts to identify possible deficits in strength and flexibility before the actual occurrence of the injury. In retrospective studies, where athletes are evaluated after the injury has occurred, it is not possible to determine whether the deficit predisposed the athlete to the injury, or the injury caused the deficit (75). Several published studies describe the methodologies for studying sport injuries (85, 152). Most information concerning sport-related injuries is presently derived from case series, in which all patients with a specific type of injury are described (152), but this type of study does not provide much information on risk factors.

Injury risk factors can be divided into two main categories: internal personal factors (intrinsic factors) and external environmental factors (extrinsic factors; 150). Some of the major potential injury risk factors in the field events are summarized in Table 13.5.

### 5.1 Intrinsic Factors

Intrinsic factors include anatomical and morphological characteristics of the athlete and may not be subject to change. Examples of these factors include: body composition, growth characteristics of the adolescent, the presence of growth cartilage and its susceptibility to injury, soft tissue flexibility, muscular strength, muscular imbalances, muscular weakness, leg length discrepancies, abnormal joint structures, bone density, previous injury, and training level of the athlete (19, 63, 135). Other risk factors sometimes mentioned in relation to injuries are taut muscles and faulty running technique (140).

**Table 13.5  Potential Risk Factors in Field Events**

Intrinsic factors
- Younger athletes may suffer injuries to the growth plates, the weakest areas of the growing bone. Excessive exercise loads can cause growth-plate injury and lead to permanent bony deformity (Stanish, 1984).
- In adolescent athletes, apophyseal injuries are common as the bones are incompletely ossified; in mature athletes overuse injuries more often take the form of tendinitis (Jarvinen, 1992).
- In younger athletes, the articular cartilage is susceptible to shear stresses, especially at the elbow, knee, and ankle (Stanish, 1984).
- Musculotendinous imbalance of strength, flexibility, or bulk (Micheli & Fehlandt, 1992).
- The more highly skilled athletes are injured more often than other athletes, regardless of greater exposure time (Watson & Dimartino, 1987).
- Anatomic malalignment of the lower extremities, including differences in leg length, abnormalities of rotation of the hips, position of the knee cap, and bow legs, knock knees, or flat feet (Micheli & Fehlandt, 1992).
- Athletes who were previously injured were more likely to be reinjured: Knee injuries were associated with previous knee injuries and knee surgery, ankle injuries were associated with previous ankle injuries, and both arm and leg injuries were associated with previous fractures (DuRant et al., 1992).
- Associated disease state of the lower extremity, including arthritis, poor circulation, old fractures, or other injury (Micheli & Fehlandt, 1992).
- The high mechanical forces seen in the field events can produce greater bone cross-sectional areas and greater resistance to fracture injuries.
- Muscle imbalance between the agonist and antagonist muscles crossing a joint is possible cause of sports-related injuries (Kibler et al., 1992).

Extrinsic factors
- Training errors, including rapid changes in intensity, duration, or frequency (Micheli & Fehlandt, 1992).
- Poor footwear, including improper fit, inadequate impact-absorbing material, excessive stiffness of the sole, and/or insufficient support of the heel.
- Excessively hard or bumpy playing surfaces.
- Pole too light for the weight and speed of the vaulter (Craig, 1973; Ecker, 1970).

The age of the athlete is associated with the type of injuries that occur in field events. Young athletes who are in a rapid growth period may suffer from traction apophysitis conditions, such as Osgood-Schlatter disease and Sever's disease, in which an abnormally tight muscle will place high tensile loads on an attachment that is weak (74). Juvenile osteochondritis dissecans of the elbow or knee is thought to be due to abnormal compressive loads, with bony and (eventually) cartilaginous fracture (74). World class throwers are relatively older athletes, with an average age of 28.5 years necessary to develop the potential for maximum-force capacity (109). Older athletes, over the age of 50 years, are more likely to suffer injuries to the bone, such as ligament avulsion fractures, due to the decreased mineralization of bone that occurs in the aging skeleton.

There is some question regarding whether males or females have a higher incidence of injury in field events. Watson and Dimartino (155) found a slightly higher incidence of injuries in male high school track and field athletes than in female athletes. In a survey of adolescent athletes' exertion injuries, it was found that 45% of these occurred in girls (< 20 years), but only 9.5% of exertion injuries among older athletes were sustained by women (> 20 years) (111). In a study of injury incidence of women midshipmen at the U.S. Naval Academy, it was found that women had higher incidences of stress-related problems such as shin splints and stress fractures than males (17). Males had a slightly higher incidence of injury in track and field than females, and this has been reported to be true in other sports (155). In a contrary finding, DuRant et al. (24) reported that one of the high school sports with the highest incidence of injury (15.8%) was female track and field. A similar finding was reported by Garrick and Requa (41) on high school track and field athletes for whom the injury rate was 33% for males and 35% for females. More emphasis is currently being placed on the study of psychosocial and behavioral aspects of the occurrence of sports injuries and how injury risk depends on the interaction between athletes and their personal characteristics (150).

Factors relating to body structure and body composition that contribute to injury include bone size and density (124), muscle mass and composition (70) and associated drug abuse (28), muscle group imbalances (74), body and limb size (29, 74, 141, 159), lower extremity malalignments (138, 142), and body fat and obesity (28, 29, 55).

## 5.2 Extrinsic Factors

External factors that may lead to injuries include equipment, footwear, playing surface, weather conditions, and most prominently training schedule (19, 63, 135). The most important risk factor for injuries is training errors and includes changes in the rate or intensity of training or in the type of training (93). Training should not be increased suddenly, as this will produce overuse injuries and overtraining in young athletes. Exercise and training must be demanding in intensity, frequency,

and duration, but these factors must be increased gradually to produce improvements in cardiovascular performance and strength (6). The rate, duration, or intensity of training should not be increased more than 10% per week. Training errors have been reported with 60% to 70% of the running injuries, with injuries following rapid increase in mileage, increased interval training, and running on sloping and slippery roads (63). Other training errors that produce injuries are errors in technique, in which poor biomechanical technique is used to perform skills such as throwing or landing from a jump (93). It has been suggested that a thrower can open up too soon, so that the athlete turns the body while allowing the arm to lag behind. This forces the elbow to descend, resulting in a rapid acceleration through the shoulder and producing excessive force on the rotator cuff (138, 157).

The training terrain can also affect the athlete, and a bumpy or muddy field may lead to acute injuries. Excessively hard training surfaces (e.g., concrete pavement or asphalt) are also important in injuries, especially stress fractures (58). The material of the run up runways is important in the high jump, pole vault, and long jump events; it must be smooth and free of cracks or bumps. The landing mats in the pole vault have been a problem in the past, and beginning with the 1987 season, all individual units in the pole vault had to include a common cover or pad extending over all sections of the pit (101). The size of the cage is an ongoing problem in the hammer throw, as the length of the arms and wire place the hammer at least 2 m from the thrower. Since the thrower is moving through the middle of the circle, the thrower must aim for the left sector line in order to clear the cage on the right. Paradoxically what is required for safety is a widening of the cage mouth so the thrower can use the whole throwing sector without hitting the side of the cage (117). Fencing the back and sides of the discus circle will help eliminate accidents in which other athletes and spectators are struck by the discus (101).

In the realm of equipment, athletic footwear is one of the key risk factors for athletes in field events. Problems include: improper fit, inadequate impact-absorbing material, excessive stiffness of the sole, and insufficient support of the heel (92). Wires and handles on the hammer must be checked regularly to ensure that they are safe for throwing (15). The jumping pits must be of sufficient size, have adequate cushioning, and be soft enough to allow the falling athlete's velocity to decrease to zero over the greatest possible distance (25). The type of pole used by the vaulter is one of the most controversial issues in track and field; the standard fiberglass pole is difficult to control and vulnerable to breakage (18). The forces on the pole at the time of pole bend are a combination of the vaulter's weight and the forward speed, which may be up to 1.5 times body weight (25). Hand position on the pole will also affect the forces applied to the pole by the athlete, and these should be considered when selecting a pole (18). It is obvious that poles cannot be classified by the body weight of the vaulter without also allowing for hand-hold height, take-off speed, and other variables (25).

# 6. Suggestions for Injury Prevention

## 6.1 Players

It is generally agreed that strength increases are probably the most effective method of injury prevention, as high strength values will assist in resisting the extreme forces produced during throwing and jumping events. Strength increases will also help to resist overuse injuries, which are caused by repeated submaximal forces that break down tissues over the long term. Flexibility increases allow the athlete to maximize the range of motion of the joints without injury to the surrounding tissues. Many of the injuries reported as case studies likely occurred through overtraining or improper technique. These can be prevented through closer monitoring of the athlete. There should be implementation of a national injury reporting registry, in which all injuries to track and field athletes are reported by the coach or trainer to a central registry, such as US Track and Field or Athletics Canada, for tabulation.

All competitive athletes should use a detailed training diary to prevent rapid increases in training volume that may not be reported by the athlete or noticed by the coach. Injuries that result from training errors should be reported to the proposed injury registry.

## 6.2 Sport

Injuries resulting from mishaps can be prevented by selecting proper equipment and by proper field maintenance practices. The high ground-reaction forces during jumping should be reduced with good quality athletic shoes and the judicious selection of training surfaces (58). Table 13.6 summarizes injury prevention techniques.

## 6.3 External Environment

Coaches and field events administrators must have knowledge of the safety requirements in field events, and these events must be closely monitored. Close attention must be paid to environmental aspects such as: clear throwing areas, throwing cages in good repair, safe wires and handles on the hammer, jumping pits of sufficient depth and width, jumping runway surfaces in good repair, and pole vault poles matched to weight of vaulter.

**Table 13.6   Injury Prevention for Field Events**

General conditioning
- Resistance training programs must be sport-specific and designed to prevent and correct muscle imbalance. Detailed information on designing effective resistance training programs is available in several references (Bozeman et al., 1986; Fleck, 1986; Grace, 1985; Read & Bellamy, 1992).
- Long-term participation in a particular field event will prevent injuries by increasing skill, efficiency, strength, and flexibility (Jobe, 1983).

Throwing events
- Isolate throwing events from running events to avoid incidental contact of bystanders or other athletes (Moore, 1982).
- There are 35 rules for javelin safety, including keeping the throwing area clear (Schmidt, 1979).
- Modify throwing implements. For example, make the high-school hammer 12 inches in diameter with the outer two inches of foam rubber (Held, 1970).
- Use rubber-tipped practice javelins in both practices and meets (Held, 1970).
- Use rubber disci for safety in practice throws (Ganslen, 1979).

Jumping events
- Use 1-m wide rubberized surfaces for approach ramps and aprons to provide greater traction (Ciullo & Jackson, 1985).
- Replace long jump and triple jump landing boards regularly.
- The shoe for the flop high jump should be modified medial sole elevation, medially extended heel cap, and individual foot padding to reduce stress-related foot injuries (Knebel & Krahl, 1981).
- Landing pits for high jump and pole vault should be at least 1-m high and firm enough that the jumper does not contact the ground through the mat. Use higher density mats (Kay, 1975).
- Minimum standards for landing pits must be long enough and wide enough to ensure that the jumper will land on them; 4-m (13 ft) long and 3-m (10 ft) wide (Kay, 1975).
- Place sawdust or sand in the pole vault landing boxes to lessen the impact (Ciullo & Jackson, 1985).
- Vaulting poles must be matched to the weight and speed of the vaulter; lighter poles should not be used (Payton, 1981).

Injuries due to environmental problems should be reported to the proposed injury registry so they do not recur.

## 7. Suggestions for Further Research

Little published research examines the epidemiology of injuries in field events, even though the sport has participants at all school, club, national, and international levels. There is need for a well-controlled survey of coaches, athletes, and sports medicine personnel, to determine the type, frequency, and causes of injuries to field athletes at all levels of performance and by gender, age, and level of competition. There is a problem with injury definition among the studies available, and this aspect must be more closely defined. Closer monitoring of field athletes is necessary to determine injury rates by field event, by number of athletes, and by number of practice hours. No information that reported injury rates specifically in field events was located. Reinjury rates are also of interest and need to be examined more closely by more detailed monitoring of field events athletes.

If the loads exerted on an athlete's body exceed his or her ability to control or withstand them, an injury is very likely to result. It is essential to an athlete's welfare to use techniques that keep the loads on the body within the bounds that can be tolerated. It is therefore essential that the loads to which the body is exposed in field events, especially in triple jumping which produces the largest loads to the legs, be well understood (51). There is great need for research on this topic (51).

## References

1. Allen, M.E. Stress fracture of the humerus: a case study. Am. J. Sports Med. 19:244-245; 1974.
2. Allman, F.L.; Carlson, C.A. Rehabilitation of elbow injuries. In: The upper extremity in sports medicine. Nicholas, J.A., and Hershman, E.B., eds. St. Louis, MO: C.V. Mosby; 1990.
3. Arnheim, D.; Arnheim, H. Modern principles of athletic training. St. Louis, MO: C.V. Mosby; 1989.
4. Backx, F.J.; Erich, W.B.; Kemper, A.B.; Verbeek, A.L. Sports injuries in school aged children. Am. J. Sports Med. 17:234-240; 1989.
5. Backx, F.J.; Beijer, H.J.; Bol, E.; Erich, W.B. Injuries in high-risk persons and high-risk sports. Am. J. Sports Med. 19:124-130; 1992.
6. Bale, P. The functional performance of children in relation to growth, maturation and exercise. Sports Med. 13:151-159; 1992.
7. Bateman, J.E. Athletic injuries about the shoulder in throwing and body-contact sports. Clin. Orthop. 23:75-83; 1962.
8. Beattie, P. The use of an eclectic approach for the treatment of low back pain: a case study. Physical Therapy 72:923-928; 1992.
9. Bejjani, F.J. Occupational biomechanics of athletes and dancers: a comparative approach. Clin. Pod. Med. Surg. 4:671; 1987.
10. Bennett, J.B.; Tullos, H.S. Acute injuries to the elbow. In: The upper extremity in sports medicine. Nicholas, J.A., Hershman, E.B. (eds.). St. Louis: C.V. Mosby; 1990.
11. Blazina, M.E.; Kerlan, R.K.; Jobe, F.W.; Carter, V.S.; Carlson, G.J. Jumper's knee. Orthop. Clin. N. Am. 4:665-678; 1973.
12. Bozeman, M.; Mackie, J.; Kaufmann, D.A. Quadriceps, hamstrings, strength and flexibility. Track Technique. 96(Summer):3060-3061; 1986.
13. Bracker, W.; Siekmann, W. Epiphysiolysis of the proximal tibia in high jumping. Sportverletz Sportschaden 1:150-151; 1987.
14. Browne, T.D.; Yost, R.P.; McCarron, R.F. Lumbar ring apophyseal fracture in an adolescent weight lifter. Am. J. Sports Med. 18:533-535; 1990.
15. Casselman, R. Track and Field. In Catastrophic injuries in sport—avoidance strategies. Adams, S.; Adrian, M.; Bayless, M. eds. Indianapolis, IN: Benchmark Press; 213-222; 1987.
16. Ciullo, J.V.; Jackson, D.W. Track and field. In: Sports injuries: mechanisms, prevention and treatment. Schneider, R.W., ed. Baltimore: Williams & Wilkins; 212-246; 1985.
17. Cox, J.S.; Lenz, H.W. Women midshipmen in sports. Am. J. Sports Med. 12:241-243; 1984.
18. Craig, T.T. Comments in sports medicine. Chicago, IL: American Medical Association; 1973.
19. Dalton, S.E. Overuse injuries in adolescent athletes. Sports Med. 13:58-70, 1992.
20. Dapena, J.; McDonald, C. A three-dimensional analysis of angular momentum in the hammer throw. MedSci Sports Exer. 21:206-220; 1989.
21. DeHaven, K.E.; Evarts, C.M. Throwing injuries of the elbow in athletes. Orthop. Clin. N. Am. 4:801-808; 1973.
22. Dominguez, R.H. The complete book of sports medicine. New York: Warner Books; 1979.
23. Dufek, J.S.; Bates, B.T. Biomechanical factors associated with injury during landing in jump sports. Sports Med. 12:326-337; 1991.
24. DuRant, R.H.; Pendergast, R.A.; Seymore, C.; Gaillard, G.; Donner, J. Findings from the preparticipation athletic examination and athletic injuries. Am. J. Dis. Child 146:85-91; 1992.
25. Ecker, T. Poles and pits. Track Technique 39; March:1228-1230; 1970.
26. Ellenbecker, T.S.; Derscheid, G.L. Rehabilitation of overuse injuries of the shoulder. Clin. Sports Med. 8:583-604; 1989.

27. Estwanik, J.J. Levator scapulae syndrome. Phys. Sportsmed 17:57-68; 1989.

28. Faber, M.; Spinnier-Benade, A.J.; Daubitzer, A. Dietary intake, anthropometric measurements and plasma lipid levels in throwing field athletes. Int. J. Sports Med. 11:140-145; 1990.

29. Faber, M.; Spinnier-Benade, A.J. Mineral and vitamin intake in field athletes (discus, hammer, javelin throwers and shotputters). Int. J. Sports Med. 12:324-327; 1991.

30. Falster, O.; Hasselbach, H. Avulsion fracture of the tibial tuberosity with combined ligament and meniscal tear. Am. J. Sports Med. 21:82-83; 1992.

31. Ferretti, A.; Ippolito, E.; Mariani, P.; Puddu, G. Jumper's knee. Am. J. Sports Med. 11:58-62; 1993.

32. Ferretti, A.; Papandrea, P.; Conteduca, F. Knee injuries in volleyball. Sports Med. 10:132-138; 1990.

33. Fitch, K.D.; Blackwell, J.D.; Gilmour, W.N. Operation for non-union of navicular stress fracture of the tarsal navicular. J. Bone Joint Surg. 71B:105-110; 1989.

34. Fleck, S.J. Value of resistance training for the reduction of sports injuries. Sports Med. 3:61-68; 1986.

35. Fricker, P.A. Injuries to the shoulder girdle and upper limb. In: Textbook of science and medicine in sport. Bloomfield, J.; Fricker, P.A.; Fitch, K.D.; eds. Champaign, IL: Human Kinetics Publishers; 356-380; 1992.

36. Fyfe, I.; Stanish, W.D. The use of eccentric training and stretching in the treatment and prevention of tendon injuries. Clin. Sports Med. 11:601-624; 1992.

37. Gainor, B.J.; Hagen, R.J.; Allen, W.C. Biomechanics of the spine in the pole vaulter as related to spondylolysis. Am. J. Sports Med. 11:53-57; 1983.

38. Ganslen, R.V. Tips for the throwing events. Athletic J. (January):54-57, 66-68; 1979.

39. Garrett, W.E. Muscle strain injuries: clinical and basic aspects. MedSci Sports Exer. 22:436-443; 1990.

40. Garrick, J.G.; Requa, R. Medical care and injury surveillance in the high school setting. Phys. Sportsmed. 9:115-120; 1981.

41. Garrick, J.G.; Requa, R.K. Injuries in high school sports. Pediatrics 61:465-469; 1978.

42. Garrick, J.G.; Requa, R.K. Aerobic dance. A review. Sports Med. 6:169-179; 1988.

43. Garth, W.P.; Allman, F.L.; Armstrong, W.S. Occult anterior subluxations of the shoulder in noncontact sports. Am. J. Sports Med. 15:579-589; 1987.

44. Gerrard, D.F. Overuse injury and growing bones: the young athlete at risk. Brit. J. Sports Med. 27:14-18; 1993.

45. Glousman, R.E. Ulnar nerve problems in the athlete's elbow. Clin. Sports Med. 9:365-377; 1990.

46. Glousman, R.E.; Barron, J.; Jobe, F.W.; Perry, J.; Pink, M. An electromyographic analysis of the elbow in normal and injured pitchers with medial collateral ligament insufficiency. Am. J. Sports Med. 20:311-317; 1992.

47. Grace, T.G. Muscle imbalance and extremity injury: a perplexing relationship. Sports Med. 2:77-82; 1985.

48. Gregg, J.R.; Torg, E. Upper extremity injuries in adolescent tennis players. Clin. Sports Med. 7:371-383; 1988.

49. Hartonas, G.D.; Verettas, D.J. Fracture of the humerus in a shotput athlete. Injury 18:68-69; 1987.

50. Haw, D.W. Avulsion fracture of the medial epicondyle of the elbow in a young javelin thrower. Case report. Brit. J. Sports Med. 15:47; 1981.

51. Hay, J.G. The biomechanics of the triple jump: a review. J. Sports Sci. 10:343-378; 1992.

52. Held, D. The hammer and javelin for high school. Track Technique 41(Sept):1306; 1970.

53. Hershman, E.B.; Lombardo, J.; Bergfeld, J.A. Femoral shaft stress fractures in athletes. Clin. Sports Med. 9:111-119; 1990.

54. Hill, J.A. Epidemiologic perspective on shoulder injuries. Clin. Sports Med. 2:241-246; 1983.

55. Hollings, S.C.; Robson, G.J. Body build and performance characteristics of male adolescent track and field athletes. J. Sports Med. Phys. Fit. 31:178-182; 1991.

56. Horrigan, J.; Shaw, D. Plyometrics: think before you leap. Track and Field Quart. Rev. 89:41-43; 1989.

57. Hughes, A.W. Case report avulsion fracture involving the body of the patella. Brit. J. Sports Med. 19:119-120; 1985.

58. Hulkko, A.; Orava, S. Stress fractures in athletes. Int. J. Sports Med. 8:221-226; 1987.

59. Hulkko, A.; Orava, S.; Nikula, P. Stress fractures of the olecranon in javelin throwers. Int. J. Sports Med. 7:210-213; 1986.

60. Inoue, G.; Kuboyama, K.; Shido, T. Avulsion fractures of the proximal tibial epiphysis. Brit. J. Sports Med. 25:52-56; 1991.

61. Israeli, A.; Ganel, A.; Blankstein, A.; Horoszowski, H. Stress fracture of the tibial tuberosity in a high jumper: a case report. Int. J. Sports Med. 5:299-300; 1984.

62. Jackson, D.W. Chronic rotator cuff impingement in the throwing athlete. Am. J. Sports Med. 4:231-239; 1976.

63. Jarvinen, M. Epidemiology of tendon injuries in sports. Clin. Sports Med. 11:493-503; 1992.

64. Jobe, C.M. Special properties of living tissue that affect the shoulder in athletes. Clin. Sports Med. 2:271-281; 1983.

65. Jobe, F.W. Ulnar neuritis and medial collateral ligament instabilities in overarm throwers. In Current therapy in sports medicine. Welsh, R.P.; Shephard, R.J.; eds. St. Louis: C.V. Mosby; 1985.

66. Jobe, F.W.; Bradley, J.P. Rotator cuff injuries in baseball: prevention and rehabilitation. Sports Med. 6:378-387; 1988.

67. Jobe, F.W.; Jobe, C.M. Painful athletic injuries of the shoulder. Clin. Orthop. Rel. Res. 173:117-124; 1983.

68. Jozsa, L.; Kvist, M.; Balint, B.J. The role of recreational sport activity in Achilles tendon rupture. Am. J. Sports Med. 17:338-344; 1989.

69. Kameyama, O.; Oka, H.; Hashimoto, F.; Nakamura, K.; Hatano, I. Avulsion of the tibial tuberosity as

a result of violent muscle contraction. In Biomechanics VIII-A. Matsui, H.; Kobayashi, K.; eds. Champaign, Il: Human Kinetics Publishers; 157-162; 1983.

70. Karayannis, M. The biomechanics of the triple jump. Track and Field Quart. Rev. 87(Spring):45-50; 1987.

71. Kay, D. Picking safe high jump pits. Track Technique 61(Sept):1941-1942; 1975.

72. Khan, K.M.; Brukner, P.D.; Kearney, C.; Fuller, P.J.; Bradshaw, C.J.; Kiss, Z.S. Tarsal navicular stress fractures in athletes. Sports Med. 17:65-76; 1994.

73. Khan, K.M.; Fuller, P.J.; Brukner, P.D.; Kearney, C.; Burry, H.C. Outcome of conservative and surgical management of navicular stress fracture in athletes. Am. J. Sports Med. 20:657-666; 1992.

74. Kibler, W.B.; Chandler, T.J.; Stracener, E.S. Musculoskeletal adaptations and injuries due to overtraining. In: Exercise and sport sciences reviews. Holloszy, J.O., ed. Baltimore: Williams & Wilkins, 99-126; 1992.

75. Knapik, J.J.; Jones, B.H.; Bauman, C.L.; Harris, J.M. Strength, flexibility and athletic injuries. Sports Med. 14:277-288; 1992.

76. Knebel, K.P.; Krahl, H. Movement analysis and the prevention of foot problems in the Fosbury flop. Track and Field Quart. Rev. 81:40-43; 1981.

77. Komi, P.; Fukashiro, S.; Jarvinen, M. Biomechanical loading of the Achilles tendon during locomotion. Clin. Sports Med. 11:521-531; 1992.

78. Kosek, S. Nature and incidence of traumatic injury to women in sports. In: Current issues in sports medicine. Craig, T.T., ed. Cincinnati, Ohio: American Association for Health, Physical Education and Recreation, 50-53; 1973.

79. Krahl, H.; Knebel, K. Foot stress during the flop takeoff. Track Technique 75(Spring):2384-2386; 1979.

80. Kujala, U.M.; Kvist, M.; Osterman, K. Knee injuries in athletes: review of exertion injuries and retrospective study of outpatient sports clinic material. Sports Med. 3:447-460; 1986.

81. Liemohn, W. Factors related to hamstring strains. J. Sports Med. 18:71-76; 1978.

82. Lindenfield, T.N.; Noyes, F.R.; Marshall, M.T. Components of injury reporting systems. Am. J. Sports Med. 15:S69-S80; 1987.

83. Lo, Y.P.C.; Hsu, Y.C.S.; Chan, K.M. Epidemiology of shoulder impingement in upper arm sports events. Brit. J. Sports Med. 24:173-177; 1990.

84. Loomer, R.L. Elbow injuries in athletes. Can. J. Applied Sport Sci. 7:164-166; 1992.

85. Lysens, R.; Lefevre, J.; Renson, L.; Ostyn, M. The predictability of sports injuries—a preliminary report. Int. J. Sports Med. 5:153-155; 1984.

86. Mader, T.J. Avulsion of the rectus femoris tendon: an unusual type of pelvic fracture. Ped. Emerg. Care 6:198-199; 1990.

87. Masters, S.; Fricker, P.; Purdham, C. Stress fractures of the femoral shaft—four case studies. Brit. J. Sports Med. 20:14-16; 1986.

88. McCormick, D.P.; Niebuhr, V.N.; Risser, W.L. Injury and illness surveillance and local Special Olympic Games. Brit. J. Sports Med. 24:221-224; 1990.

89. McCue, F.C.; Gieck, J.H.; West, J.O. Throwing injuries to the shoulder. In: Injuries to the throwing arm. Zarins, B.; Andrews, J.R.; Carson, W.G.; ed. Philadelphia: W.B. Saunders; 95-111; 1985.

90. McFadden, P.M.; Ochsner, J.L. Javelin injury to the subclavian artery. Am. J. Sports Med. 9:400-404; 1981.

91. McLennan, J.G.; McLennan, J.E. Injury patterns in Scottish heavy athletics. Am. J. Sports Med. 18:529-532; 1990.

92. Micheli, L.J.; Fehlandt, A.F. Overuse injuries to tendons and apophyses in children and adolescents. Clin. Sports Med. 11:713-728; 1992.

93. Micheli, L.J. Pediatric and adolescent sports injuries: Recent trends. In Exercise and Sport Science Reviews, Pandolf, K.B. (Ed.). New York: Macmillan, 359-374; 1986.

94. Miller, J.E. Javelin thrower's elbow. J. Bone Joint Surg. 42B:788-792; 1960.

95. Miller, R.D. Spinal lordosis in the flop. Athletic J. 58:100-101; 106-107; 1978.

96. Mirbey, J.; Bescancenot, J.; Chambers, R.T.; Durey, A.; Vichard, P. Avulsion fractures of the tibial tuberosity in the adolescent athlete. Am. J. Sports Med. 16:336-340; 1988.

97. Moore, K. Splendor and agony in Helsinki. Sports Illustrated 59:26-29; 1983.

98. Moore, K. No pain, no Spain. Sports Illustrated 76:30-33; 1992.

99. Moore, M. Javelin fatality prompts concern over impact areas. Phys. Sportsmed. 10:24; 1982.

100. Morris, M.; Jobe, F.W.; Perry, J.; Pink, M.; Healy, B.G. Electromyographic analysis of elbow function in tennis players. Am. J. Sports Med. 17:241-247; 1989.

101. Mueller, F.O.; Cantu, R.C. National center for catastrophic sports injury research: tenth annual report. Chapel Hill, NC: University of North Carolina; 1992.

102. Nash, H.L. Rotator cuff damage: reexamining the causes and treatments. Phys. Sportsmed. 16:129-135; 1988.

103. Neusel, E.; Arza, D.; Rompe, G.; Steinbruck, K. Long-term roentgenologic studies in peak performance javelin throwers. Sportverletz Sportschaden 1:76-80; 1987.

104. Nicholas, J.A.; Marino, M. The relationship of injuries of the leg, foot, and ankle to proximal thigh strength in athletes. Foot and Ankle 7:218-228; 1987.

105. Noack, W.; Rottinger, H. Indirect humerus fracture in sport. Sportverletz Sportschaden 4:50-52; 1990.

106. Nordin, M.; Frankel, V.H. Basic biomechanics of the musculoskeletal system, second edition. Philadelphia: Lea & Febiger; 1989.

107. Nuber, G.W.; Diment, M.T. Olecranon stress fractures in throwers. A report of two cases and a review of the literature. Clin. Orthop. 278:58-61; 1992.

108. O'Brien, M. Functional anatomy and physiology of tendons. Clin. Sports Med. 11:505-519; 1992.

109. O'Shea, J.P. Super quality strength training for the elite athlete. In: Science in athletics. Terauds, J.; Dales, G.G.; eds. Del Mar, CA: Academic Press; 145-152; 1979.

110. Olerud, C.; Karlstrom, G. Cervical spine fracture caused by high jump. J. Orthop. Trauma 4:179-182; 1990.

111. Orava, S.; Hulkko, A.; Jormakka, E. Exertion injuries in female athletes. Brit. J. Sports Med. 15:229-233; 1981.

112. Orava, S.; Puranen, J.; Ala-Ketola, L. Stress fractures caused by physical exercise. Acta Orthop. Scand. 49:19-27; 1978.

113. Paley, D.; Gillespie, R. Chronic repetitive unrecognized flexion injury of the cervical spine (high jumper's neck). Am. J. Sports Med. 14:92-95; 1986.

114. Pappas, A.M.; Goss, T.P.; Kleinman, P.K. Symptomatic shoulder instability due to lesions of the glenoid labrum. Am. J. Sports Med. 11:279-288; 1983.

115. Parker, R.S. Getting started in track and field. Los Altos, CA: Track and Field News; 1976.

116. Parkes, J.C. Overuse injuries of the elbow. In: The upper extremity in sports medicine. Nicholas, J.B.; Hershman, E.B.; eds. St. Louis: C.V. Mosby; 1990.

117. Payne, A.H. Hammer Throwing "Bridging the Gap." In: Science in athletics. Terauds, J.; Dales, G.G.; eds. Del Mar, CA: Academic Press; 137-144; 1979.

118. Payton, J. Australian pole vault injuries. Modern Athlete Coach 19:33-35; 1981.

119. Peltokallio, P.; Peltokallio, V.; Vaalasti, T. Fractures of the humerus from muscular violence in sport. J. Sports Med. 8:21-25; 1968.

120. Perry, J. Anatomy and biomechanics of the shoulder in throwing, swimming, gymnastics and tennis. Clin. Sports Med. 2:247-270; 1983.

121. Peterson, L.; Renstrom, P. Sports injuries: their prevention and treatment. Chicago, IL: Yearbook Medical Publishers; 1983.

122. Physician and sportsmedicine: Jacobs overcomes heights but fears knife. Phys. Sportsmed. 6:130, 132; 1978.

123. Priest, J.D. The shoulder of the tennis player. Clin. Sports Med. 7:387-402; 1988.

124. Qu, X. Morphological effects of mechanical forces on the human humerus. Brit. J. Sports Med. 26:51-53; 1992.

125. Read, M.T.F.; Bellamy, M.J. Comparison of hamstring/quadriceps isokinetic strength ratios and power in tennis, squash and track athletes. Brit. J. Sports Med. 24:178-182; 1992.

126. Reilly, T. Some risk factors in selected track and field events. Brit. J. Sports Med. 11:53-56; 1977.

127. Requa, R.K.; Garrick, J.G. Injuries in interscholastic track and field. Phys. Sportsmed. 9:42-49; 1981.

128. Roi, G.S.; Respizzi, S.; Dworzak, F. Partial rupture of the pectoralis major muscle in athletes. Int. J. Sports Med. 11:85-87; 1990.

129. Roncardi, A. Congenital limitation in sport: it's role in performance—a case study. Track and Field Quart. Rev. (October):45-48; 1988.

130. Rosenberg, J.M.; Whitaker, J.H. Bilateral infrapatellar tendon rupture in a patient with jumper's knee. Am. J. Sports Med. 19:94-95; 1991.

131. Schmidt, V.J. The javelin throw. Athletic J. 59:26, 70; 1979.

132. Schwobel, M.G. Fracture of the tibial apophysis—a typical sports injury in adolescents. Z. Kinderchirurg 42:181-183; 1987.

133. Shively, R.A.; Grana, W.A.; Ellis, D. High school sports injuries. Phys. Sportsmed. 9:46-50; 1981.

134. Sin, R.F. Shoulder injuries in the javelin throw. J. Am. Orthop. Acad. 83:107-111; 1984.

135. Sommer, H.M. Patellar chondropathy and apicitis and muscle imbalances of the lower extremities in competitive sports. Sports Med. 5:386-394; 1988.

136. Sperryn, P.N. Sport and medicine. London: Butterworths; 1983.

137. Stanish, B.; Lamb, H.; Curwin, S. The biomechanical analysis of chronic patellar tendinitis and treatment with eccentric loading. In: Surgery and arthroscopy, 2nd congress of European society. Springer Verlag; 1989.

138. Stanish, W.D. Overuse injuries in athletes: a perspective. Med. Sci. Sports Exer. 16:1-7; 1984.

139. Sugiura, Y.; Mutoh, Y.; Fujimaki, E. Stress fractures of athletes in Japan: a clinical-roentgenological and biomechanical study. In Biomechanics VIII-A. Matsui, H.; Kobayashi, K.; ed. Champaign, IL: Human Kinetics Publishers; 165-170; 1993.

140. Swardt, de A. The role of the coach in the prevention, treatment and rehabilitation of injuries. Modern Athlete and Coach 30(2); 1992.

141. Taimela, S.; Kujala, U.M.; Osterman, K. Intrinsic risk factors and athletic injuries. Sport Med. 9:205-215; 1990.

142. Taunton, J.E.; Clement, D.B.; Webber, D. Lower extremity stress fractures in athletes. Phys. Sportsmed. 9:77-83; 1981.

143. Taunton, J.E.; McKenzie, D.C.; Clement, D.B. The role of biomechanics in the epidemiology of injuries. Sports Med. 6:107-120; 1988.

144. Thein, L.A. Impingement syndrome and its conservative management. J. Occup. Sports Phys. Therapy 11:183-191; 1989.

145. Tucker, C. The mechanics of sports injuries. Oxford: Blackwell Scientific Publications; 1990.

146. Tullos, H.S.; Erwin, W.D.; Woods, G.W.; Wukusch, D.C.; Cooley, D.A.; King, J.W. Unusual lesions of the pitching arm. Clin. Orthop. 88:169-182; 1972.

147. Tullos, H.S.; King, J.W. Lesions of the pitching arm in adolescents. J. Am. Med. Assoc. 220:264-271; 1972.

148. Tullos, H.S.; King, J.W. Throwing mechanism in sports. Orthop. Clin. N. Am. 4:709-720; 1973.

149. Vainionpaa, S.; Bostman, O.; Patiala, H.; Rokkanen, P. Megapatella following a rupture of patellar tendon. Am. J. Sports Med. 13:204-205; 1985.

150. van Mechelen, W.; Hlobil, H.; Kemper, H.C.G. Incidence, severity, aetiology and prevention of sports injuries. A review of concepts. Sports Med. 14:82-99; 1992.

151. Walter, N.E.; Wolf, M.D. Stress fractures in young athletes. Am. J. Sports Med. 5:165-169; 1977.

152. Walter, S.D.; Sutton, J.R.; McIntosh, J.M.; Connolly, C. The aetiology of sport injuries: a review of methodologies. Sports Med. 2:47-58; 1985.

153. Wang, J. The femoral fracture in the long jump. Chinese J. Sports Med. 5:140-141; 1986.

154. Watson, A.W. Sports injuries during one academic year in 6799 Irish school children. Am. J. Sports Med. 12:65-71; 1984.

155. Watson, M.D.; Dimartino, P.P. Incidence of injuries in high school track and field athletes and its relation to performance ability. Am. J. Sports Med. 15:251-254; 1987.

156. Weinstein, S.M.; Herring, S.A. Nerve problems and compartment syndromes in the hand, wrist and forearm. Clin. Sports Med. 11:161-188; 1992.

157. Wilk, K.E.; Andrews, J.R.; Arrigo, C.A.; Keirns, M.A.; Erber, D.J. The strength characteristics of internal and external rotator muscles in professional baseball pitchers. Am. J. Sports Med. 21:61-66; 1993.

158. Williams, J.G.; Sperryn, P.N. Sports medicine. London: Edward Arnold; 1976.

159. Williams, K.R. Biomechanics of running. In Exercise and sport science review. Terjung, R.L.; ed. New York: Macmillan; 389-435; 1985.

160. Winter, D.A.; Bishop, P. Lower extremity injury. Biomechanical factors associated with chronic injury to the lower extremity. Sports Med. 14:149-156; 1992.

161. Wirth, C.J. Secondary ligament instabilities in the area of the elbow joint. Orthopade 6:1-38; 1988.

162. Yokoe, K.; Nanajima, H.; Yamazaki, Y. Injuries of the shoulder in volleyball players and javelin throwers. Orthop. Trauma. Surg. 22:351-359; 1959.

163. Zaricznyj, B.; Shattuck, L.J.; Mast, T.A.; Robertson, R.V.; D'Elia, G. Sports-related injuries in school-aged children. Am. J. Sports Med. 8:318-324; 1980.

# 14

# Gymnastics

*Dennis J. Caine, Koenraad J. Lindner,*
*Bert R. Mandelbaum, and William A. Sands*

## 1. Introduction

Like many sports that involve children and adolescents, gymnastics has undergone a period of rapid growth during the last 2 decades. According to Garrick & Requa (46), the number of female interscholastic gymnastic participants in the United States increased 461% between 1974 and 1980. Since 1980, however, the number of interscholastic participants has been decreasing while the number of clubs, and consequently younger participants, has been increasing dramatically (68). Elite female and male gymnasts are reported to initiate training for their sport as early as ages 6 and 9 years, respectively, with peak performance being 10 or more years away (95).

Extraordinary levels of biomechanical loading during training and competition are associated with this trend toward earlier and increased participation. The biomechanical loads of gymnastics skills have been quantified for several skills. Lower extremity impact forces incurred from a double backward somersault, for example, resulted in peak vertical ground reaction forces (GRF) of 8.8 to 14.4 times body weight per foot (117). By way of comparison, high impact aerobic dance skills resulted in peak GRFs of 2.12 to 2.88 times body weight (104).

Frequency, duration, and intensity of training loads have also increased. Elite level gymnasts, for example, are reported to train 30 to 40 hours, 5 to 6 days per week and up to 12 months of the year (18, 36). National level gymnasts may average between 700 and 1,300 elements (e.g., vault, back handspring) per day. This corresponds to approximately 220,000 to 400,000 elements per year (134). The degree of difficulty of maneuvers practiced and performed has also increased (101). Increased involvement and difficulty of skills practiced at an early age and continued through the years of growth, with the extreme training intensity required, strongly suggests the possibility of a concomitant rise in the number of injuries. Given the uncertain long-term consequences of pediatric sports injuries and the rising costs of medical care, injury prevention is of utmost importance (101).

The purpose of this scientific overview of the epidemiologic literature on gymnastics injuries is to describe the qualitative and quantitative details of gymnastic injuries. In doing so, we elucidate possible risk factors with the hope of achieving specific recommendations for injury prevention and directing future research methodology. Data collection focused on the English literature; however, foreign publications that have been reviewed/translated elsewhere in the English literature were included. Data collection was limited to published articles and reports and was conducted using the following procedures:

- Ancestry approach (i.e., retrieval of research cited in published research such as clinical or research reports as well as past literature reviews)
- Computer searches (January 1975 to July 1994): SPORT Discus database (key words = gymnastics, injury, accident), and Medline database (key words = gymnastic, injury)
- Formal requests of scholars who were active in the field (e.g., solicitation letters)
- Manual search of abstract databases (e.g., physical fitness/sports medicine)
- Published reports available to the public (e.g., *NCAA News*)

Studies that did not distinguish between genders in reporting injury data were excluded from this review. We felt this to be an important exclusion criterion in view of the obvious differences in skill demands and hence injury risk between men's and women's events. Otherwise, all articles were included regardless of their methodological strength or research design.

Retrieval procedures produced a gymnastics injury literature that, for ethical or logistic reasons, has been limited to nonrandomized studies including case reports, case series, cross-sectional, retrospective, and prospective studies. While all of these approaches have contributed to our knowledge, some offer more valid and useful findings than others. Case-type studies have helped to generate hypotheses about possible causes of gymnastics injuries and stimulated research designed to uncover more information about the nature and rate of particular injuries and possible risk factors related to these injuries. A limitation of these data, however, is that they are usually not representative of the morbidity in the general population of gymnasts and therefore cannot be used to calculate absolute risks of injury, identify injury prone gymnasts, or detect factors that will increase the risk of injury (174).

Cross-sectional studies provided prevalence rate estimates for particular injury types. However, since this study design only records injuries actually present at the time of the survey, prevalent cases are more likely to be those with a pattern of slow, chronic onset and resolution (174). Further, gymnasts who have been injured and given up the sport may be missing from the sample (175). Prospective and retrospective studies provided information on the nature and rate of injuries in gymnastics and infrequently were used to explore the relationship between injury and possible injury risk factors. However, these studies were difficult to interpret and compare for the following reasons:

- Diversity of study populations and consequent differences in the nature and extent of exposure to injury risk (e.g., recreational, club and varying competitive levels within this category, high school, and college gymnasts)
- Instability of study results due to relatively short periods of data collection
- Insufficient sample size to warrant risk factor analysis in some studies
- Low response rates, short- and long-term recall bias, and response motivation bias associated with the frequent use of questionnaires in both prospective and retrospective studies
- Nonrandom selection (i.e., the possibility that some schools or clubs most concerned with

safety may be the ones to consent to involvement in an epidemiological study of injuries)
- No standard descriptive criteria for injury, reinjury, injury types, and injury onset (i.e., studies are limited in their categorical description of these injuries)
- Variability in study design and data collection methods across studies

Unfortunately, these methodological shortcomings and study differences preclude an analysis of the diverse properties and findings of the various studies through a common statistical treatment. However, by summarizing the gymnastics injury data in table form, it was possible to consider the methodological and interpretative aspects of the research reviewed across studies rather than on a study-by-study basis. Study designs are indicated in the tables to help readers distinguish level of epidemiologic evidence. Summary comments derived from these tables should be interpreted cautiously, however, due to the methodological weaknesses discussed above.

## 2. Incidence of Injury

### 2.1 Injury Rates

A comparison of injury rates derived from prospective and retrospective injury studies in women's and men's gymnastics is shown in Tables 14.1 and 14.2, respectively. A review of these tables indicates that most injury rates were calculated with reference to participant-seasons and thus do not account for differences in exposure to injury risk. A review of the limited exposure data in Tables 14.1 and 14.2 suggests much higher injury rates (range = 22.7 – 69.2) for college female gymnasts compared to their club-level counterparts (range = 0.5 – 3.7). This observation is generally supported by non-exposure data (i.e., participant-seasons) representing both prospective and retrospective studies. Exposure data also indicate higher injury rates for college female gymnasts compared to their male counterparts. Non-exposure data suggest higher injury rates for both male and female gymnasts at the club and high school level compared to their recreational counterparts. However, this observation awaits confirmation from injury rates calculated with reference to exposure units.

### 2.2 Reinjury Rates

While two studies (18, 82) reported reinjuries as a proportion (%) of the total number of injuries, only

**Table 14.1   A Comparison of Injury Rates in Women's Gymnastics**

| Study | Design pros/retro (P) (R) | Data collection interv/question (I) (Q) | Duration inj. surv. | # of injuries | Sample # participants (1 participant = 1 gymnast participating in one season) | # teams | Rate: # injuries /100 particip. seasons | Rate: # injuries /1,000 hours of exposure | Rate: # injuries /1,000 athletic exposures* |
|---|---|---|---|---|---|---|---|---|---|
| **Recreational** | | | | | | | | | |
| Pettrone & Ricciardelli, 1987 | P | Q | 7 months | 33 | 2016 | 15 | 1.6 | — | — |
| Goodway et al., 1989 | P | Q | 1 year | 7 | 5929 | — | 0.1 | — | — |
| Lowry & Leveau, 1982 | R | Q | 11 months | 128 | 3042 | 14 | 4.2 | — | — |
| **Club** | | | | | | | | | |
| Garrick & Requa, 1980 | P | Q | 1 season | 16 | 72 | 3 | 22.2 | — | — |
| Weiker, 1985 | P | Q | 9 months | 95 | 766[a] | 6 | 12.4 | — | — |
| Vergouwen, 1986 | P | I | 3 seasons | 353 | 42 | — | 840.5 | — | — |
| Pettrone & Ricciardelli, 1987 | P | Q | 7 months | 29 | 542 | 15 | 5.3 | — | — |
| Caine et al., 1989 | P | I | 1 year | 147 | 50 | 2 | 294.0 | 3.7 | — |
| Goodway et al., 1989 | P | Q | 1 year | 93 | 725 | — | 12.8 | — | — |
| Lindner & Caine, 1990a | P | QI | 3 seasons | 90 | 362 | 5 | 24.9 | 0.5 | — |
| Lowry & Leveau, 1982 | R | Q | 11 months | 260 | 370 | 14 | 70.3 | — | — |
| Steele & White, 1983 | R | Q | 2 seasons | 146 | 268 | 9 | 54.5 | — | — |
| Backx et al., 1991 | R | Q | 7 months | — | 220 | — | — | 3.6[b] | — |
| Dixon & Fricker, 1993 | R | I | 10 years | 325 | 162 | 1 | 200.0 | — | — |
| **High school** | | | | | | | | | |
| Garrick & Requa, 1980 | | | | | | | | | |
|   1973-75 | P | IQ | 2 seasons | 39 | 98 | — | 39.8 | — | — |
|   1973-74 | P | I | 1st season | — | — | 3 | 56.0[c] | — | — |
|   1974-75 | P | Q | 2nd season | — | — | 2 | 28.0 | — | — |
| Garrick & Requa, 1980 | P | Q | 1 season | 73 | 221 | 12 | 33.0 | — | — |
| McLain & Reynolds, 1989 | P | I | 1 season | 11 | 24 | 1 | 45.8 | — | — |
| **College** | | | | | | | | | |
| Clarke & Miller, 1977 | P | I | 1 season | — | 117 | 9 | 42.7[d] | — | 3.2[e] |
| Eisenberg & Allen, 1978 | P | I | 1 season | 27 | 10 | 1 | 270.0 | — | — |
| Snook, 1979 | P | I | 5 seasons | 66 | 70 | 1 | 94.3 | — | — |
| Garrick & Requa, 1980 | P | I | 1 season | 17 | 24 | 2 | 70.8 | — | — |
| Clarke & Buckley, (NAIRS) 1980 | P | I | 3 seasons | — | — | 9[f] | — | — | 2.7 |
| Sands et al., 1987 | | | | | | | | | |
|   1984-85 | P | S[g] | 1 season | 54 | 10 | 1 | 540.0 | — | 86.5 |
|   1985-86 | P | S[g] | 1 season | 70 | 13 | 1 | 538.0 | — | 69.2 |
| Sands et al., 1993 | P | S[g] | 5 seasons | 509 | 37 | 1 | 1375.7 | 22.7 | 90.9 |
| Wadley & Albright, 1993 | P | I | 4 seasons | 106 | 53 | 1 | 200.0 | — | — |
| NCAA Injury SS[h] | | | | | | | | | |
|   1983-84 | P | I | 1 season | 91 | — | 8 | — | — | 10.23 |
|   1984-85 | P | I | 1 season | 121 | — | 15 | — | — | 7.94 |
|   1985-94 | P | I | 9 seasons | 2260 | — | 212 | — | — | 9.05 |
| Jackson et al. 1980 | R | I | 2 seasons | 9 | 30 | 2 | 30.0 | — | — |

*An athletic exposure (AE) is one athlete participating in one practice or game in which the athlete is exposed to the possibility of athletic injury.

[a]Includes 477 recreational gymnasts.

[b]Includes data from 25 male gymnasts.

[c]Rate inflated due to high incidence of trampoline injuries; trampoline was eliminated as a scholastic event after this year.

[d]Number of reportable injuries per 100 athletes; reportable = an injury that caused at least 1 day absence from participation.

[e]Number of reportable injuries per 1,000 exposures.

[f]11 teams during first year, 5 teams in the second, 11 teams in the third year; average = 9 teams/yr.

[g]Self-report at the time of injury; athletes received instructions on the recording of injury information at the start of each season.

[h]SS = surveillance system.

**Table 14.2   A Comparison of Injury Rates in Men's Gymnastics**

| Study | Design Pros/Retro (P) (R) | Data Collection Interv/Question (I) (Q) | Duration inj. surv. | # of injuries | Sample # participants (1 participant = 1 gymnast participating in 1 season) | # teams | Rate # injuries/ 100 particip. seasons | Rate # injuries/ 1,000 hours of exposure | Rate # injuries/ 1,000 athletic exposures* |
|---|---|---|---|---|---|---|---|---|---|
| Recreational | | | | | | | | | |
| Lowry & Leveau, 1982 | R | Q | 11 months | 1 | 377 | 14 | 0.3 | — | — |
| Club | | | | | | | | | |
| Weiker, 1985 | P | Q | 9 months | 10 | 107[a] | 6 | 9.3 | — | — |
| Kerr, 1991 | P | Q | 8 months | 61 | 24 | 2 | 254.0[b] | — | — |
| Lowry & Leveau, 1982 | R | Q | 11 months | 16 | 21 | — | 76.2 | — | — |
| Dixon & Fricker, 1993 | R | I | 10 years | 247 | 121 | 1 | 204.0 | — | — |
| High School | | | | | | | | | |
| Garrick & Requa, 1978 | P | I | 2 seasons | 5 | 18 | 1 | 13.9 | — | — |
| McLain & Reynolds, 1989 | P | I | 1 season | 8 | 20 | 1 | 40.0 | — | — |
| College | | | | | | | | | |
| Clarke & Miller, 1977 (NAIRS) | P | I | 1 season | — | 140 | 7 | 39.2[c] | — | 3.5[d] |
| Clarke & Buckley, 1980 (NAIRS) | P | I | 3 seasons | — | — | 6 | 16.4 | — | 1.5 |
| NCAA Injury SS 1985-94 | P | I | 9 seasons | 536 | — | 61 | — | — | 5.33 |
| Jackson et al., 1980 | R | I | 2 seasons | 3 | 21 | — | 7.1 | — | — |

*Injuries per 1,000 athletic exposures (AE); an athletic exposure is one athlete participating in one practice or game in which the athlete is exposed to the possibility of athletic injury.

[a]Includes 70 recreational gymnasts.

[b]Includes data from 8 female gymnasts.

[c]Number of reportable cases per 100 athletes; reportable = at least one day absence from participation.

[d]Number of reportable cases per 1,000 exposures.

the NCAA (113) reported reinjury rates. During the 1993-1994 season college females suffered 2.19 reinjuries per 1,000 athletic exposures (AE) compared to 0.53 reinjuries per 1,000 AE for their male counterparts. These results reflect the reoccurrence of injury from the previous and current seasons.

## 2.3 Practice vs Competition

Several studies calculated injury rates for practice and competition in women's and men's gymnastics. The rates for women's gymnastics are shown in Table 14.3.

As might be expected the proportion of injuries occurring in practice is greater than in competition. This is true for all competitive levels studied and both genders. However, when the number of in-

juries are computed with reference to exposure data, the injury rate for college females is almost three times greater in competition. Similarly, the average competition injury rate for college males in 1986-1994 was 15.77 injuries per 1,000 AE compared to a practice injury rate of 4.67 injuries per 1,000 AE during the same period (113). Since study design and data collection methods are consistent across practice and competition, as well as genders, these NCAA comparisons may be considered reliable.

## 3. Injury Characteristics

### 3.1 Injury Onset

A percent comparison of injury onset in women's gymnastics is shown in Table 14.4. A review of

**Table 14.3    A Comparison of Injury Rate in Practice vs. Competition in Women's Gymnastics**

| Study | Study design Pros/Retro (P)    (R) | # of injuries | # of participant seasons[a] | Practice Percent of total # of injuries | Practice Injuries/ 1,000 AE[b] | Competition Percent of total # of injuries | Competition Injuries/ 1,000 AE[b] |
|---|---|---|---|---|---|---|---|
| **Club** | | | | | | | |
| Pettrone & Ricciardelli, 1987[c] | P | 29 | 542 | 80.0 | — | 20.0 | — |
| Caine et al., 1989 | P | 147 | 50 | 96.6 | — | 3.4 | — |
| Lindner & Caine, 1990a[d] | P | 362 | 362 | 87.0 | — | 7.4 | — |
| Kerr & Minden, 1988 | R | — | 82 | 79.0 | — | 21.0 | — |
| **High school** | | | | | | | |
| Garrick & Requa, 1980 | P | 16 | 72 | 95.0 | — | 5.0 | — |
| **College** | | | | | | | |
| NCAA Injury SS | | | | | | | |
| 1983-84 | P | 91 | — | — | 8.67 | — | 28.49 |
| 1984-85 | P | 121 | — | — | 6.55 | — | 21.87 |
| 1986-90 | P | 748 | — | 79.0 | 6.9 | 21.0 | 20.1 |
| 1986-94 | P | 2260 | — | — | 7.9 | — | 21.88 |
| Wadley & Albright, 1993 | P | 106 | 53 | 85.0 | — | 15.0 | — |

[a]A participant season is one gymnast participating in one season.

[b]Number of injuries per 1,000 athletic exposures (AE); an athletic exposure is one athlete participating in one practice or game in which the athlete is exposed to the possibility of athletic injury.

[c]Includes data for recreational gymnasts.

[d]4.4% of injuries occurred in warm up for practice or competition.

**Table 14.4    A Percent Comparison of Nature of Injury Onset in Women's Gymnastics**

| Study | Study design Pros/Retro (P)    (R) | # of injuries | # participant seasons[a] | Injury Onset Gradual | Injury Onset Sudden |
|---|---|---|---|---|---|
| **Club** | | | | | |
| Weiker, 1985[b] | P | 95 | 766 | 42.9 | 57.1 |
| Pettrone & Ricciardelli, 1987[b] | P | 29 | 2558 | 17.7 | 82.3 |
| Goodway et al., 1989 | P | 93 | 725 | 48.0 | 52.0 |
| Caine et al., 1989 | P | 147 | 50 | 55.8 | 44.2 |
| Lindner & Caine, 1990a | P | 90 | 362 | 21.9 | 78.1 |
| Steele & White, 1983 | R | 146 | 268 | 33.0 | 67.0 |
| Dixon & Fricker, 1993 | R | 325 | 162 | 36.9 | 63.1 |
| Jones, 1992 | R | — | — | 38.0 | 62.0 |
| Mackie & Taunton, 1994 | R | 279 | — | 44.0 | 56.0 |
| **College** | | | | | |
| Snook, 1979 | P | 66 | 70 | 33.0 | 67.0 |
| Sands et al., 1987 | | | | | |
| 1984-85 | P | 54 | 10 | 16.6 | 83.4 |
| 1985-86 | P | 70 | 13 | 24.3 | 75.7 |
| Sands et al., 1993 | P | 509 | 37 | 31.2 | 69.8 |
| Wadley & Albright, 1993 | P | 106 | 53 | 43.0 | 57.0 |

[a]A participant season is one gymnast participating in one season.

[b]Includes data on recreational gymnasts.

values for prospective studies indicates that the majority of injuries at the club and collegiate levels are sudden onset injuries. This was also the finding in retrospective studies. A limitation of these data, however, is that injuries that involve both categories of injury onset have not been distinguished (e.g., when an acute injury has been superimposed on a chronic mechanism).

Several gymnastics injury studies cross-tabulated injury onset with injury location to obtain more specific information regarding injury distribution (18, 36, 82). For example, the majority of wrist and low back injuries in these studies were gradual onset. Similarly, most ankle injuries were sudden onset injuries (e.g., sprains).

### 3.2 Injury Types

A percent comparison of injury types sustained in women's gymnastics is shown in Table 14.5. A review of the prospective studies in Table 14.5 indicates that sprains (range = 15.9-43.6%), strains (range = 6.4-47.1%), or both are consistently among the three most common injury types reported. This was also the finding in the retrospective study (87). Sprains (range = 23.5-33.0%; rate = 3.84 injuries per 1,000 AE) and strains (range = 9.1-47.1%; rate = 3.2 injuries per 1,000 AE) were the top two injury types occurring among college female gymnasts (113). Table 14.5 indicates that fractures, contusions, and inflammation were also reported among the top three injury types, but were not consistent across the various competitive levels and study designs.

The limited data on injury types in men's gymnastics suggest an injury distribution similar to that reported for female gymnasts. In men's collegiate gymnastics, both frequency (29, 113) and rate (113) data indicate that sprains occur most often, followed by strains.

The frequent occurrence of sprains and strains is perhaps not surprising when one considers the high frequency of dismounts in gymnastics, including the repetitive landings associated with floor routines. The occurrence of these injuries among physically immature gymnasts is a concern, however, in view of the growing gymnast's susceptibility to physeal injury, especially during rapid periods of growth (21, 107). The young gymnast is more likely to sustain a fracture through the physis than to dislocate the joint or rupture the ligaments or tendons about the joint. Although cases of acute physeal injuries affecting the lower extremities of gymnasts have been reported (1, 49, 76), there is no reliable evidence

of the incidence of this problem due to lack of denominator data.

### 3.3 Injury Location

A percent comparison of injury location in women's club gymnastics is shown in Table 14.6. A review of prospective data in this table indicates that the lower extremity was the most frequently injured body region (range = 54.1-70.2%) followed by the upper extremity (range = 18.1-25%), and spine/trunk (range = 0-16.7%). Retrospective data suggested a similar injury distribution except that injuries appear evenly distributed among the spine/trunk (range = 13.7-22.3%) and upper extremity (range = 14.4-21.7%) regions. The most frequently injured body part in the spine/trunk region was the lower back; this finding was consistent for both prospective and retrospective studies. Common injury locations in the upper extremity were the wrist, elbow, and hand/fingers; among these, order of frequency varied within and between study designs. The ankle was the top body part injured in the lower extremity, followed by the knee in all but one prospective study (176). This trend was also apparent in the retrospective studies. The heel/Achilles tendon and foot/toes were also frequently mentioned lower extremity injury sites in both prospective and retrospective studies.

The injury distribution for Garrick and Requa's (46) mixed study of high school gymnasts is consistent with that reported above. By contrast, their interscholastic study results showed that the spine/trunk was the most frequently injured body region. Notably, a preponderance of these injuries occurred on the trampoline, which was eliminated as a competitive event after the 1st year of this study.

Review of injury location data for female collegiate gymnasts (Table 14.7) shows the lower extremity was the most frequently injured body region followed by the upper extremity and spine/trunk in all but one study (172). Wadley & Albright's results (172) indicate the knee was the most frequently injured body part followed by the ankle and lower back. NCAA (113) data for 1985 to 1994 show a somewhat different injury distribution; during most of these years, the ankle was the most frequently injured body part followed by the knee and lower back.

The ankle was shown to have the greatest incidence of injury in two studies of female collegiate gymnasts (113, 138). Sands et al. (139) reported injury location by side of body and anatomical

**Table 14.5   A Percent Comparison of Injury Types in Women's Gymnastics**

| Level/study | # injuries/ part seas* | Abrasion | Concussion | Contusion | Dislocation | Fracture | Inflammation | Laceration | Nonspecific | Sprain | Strain | Other |
|---|---|---|---|---|---|---|---|---|---|---|---|---|
| **Recreational** | | | | | | | | | | | | |
| Retrospective Study: | | | | | | | | | | | | |
| Lowry & Leveau, 1982 | 128/3042 | 0 | 0 | 27.3 | 1.6 | 3.0 | 11.7 | 2.3 | 0 | 32.0 | 21.9 | 0 |
| **Club** | | | | | | | | | | | | |
| Prospective Studies: | | | | | | | | | | | | |
| Garrick & Requa, 1980 | 16/72 | — | — | 0 | — | 31.2 | — | — | — | 15.9 | 16.2 | 18.7[a] |
| Pettrone & Ricciardelli, 1987** | 29/542 | 0 | 0 | 9.7 | 6.4 | 27.4 | 8.1 | 0 | 0 | 41.9 | 6.4 | 0 |
| Caine et al., 1989 | 147/50 | 0 | 0.7 | 4.1 | 0.7 | 3.4 | 10.2 | 0 | 40.1 | 19.0 | 17.7 | 4.1 |
| Lindner & Caine, 1990a | 90/362 | 2.2 | 0 | 6.5 | 4.3 | 24.8 | 6.5 | 1.1 | 11.8 | 19.4 | 11.8 | 9.7 |
| Retrospective Study: | | | | | | | | | | | | |
| Lowry & Leveau, 1982 | 260/370 | 0 | 0 | 34.2 | 1.5 | 8.1 | 13.8 | 0 | 0 | 41.9 | 6.4 | 0 |
| **High School** | | | | | | | | | | | | |
| Prospective Studies: | | | | | | | | | | | | |
| Garrick & Requa, 1980 | | | | | | | | | | | | |
| 1 year (mixed study) | — | — | — | 4.1 | — | 8.2 | — | — | — | 39.7 | 31.5 | 16.4[a] |
| 2 year (interscholastic study) | — | — | — | 20.5 | — | 0 | — | — | — | 43.6 | 17.9 | 17.9[a] |
| **College** | | | | | | | | | | | | |
| Prospective Studies: | | | | | | | | | | | | |
| Snook, 1979 | 66/70 | 0 | 0 | 4.5 | 6.1 | 16.7 | 25.8 | 7.6 | 0 | 30.3 | 9.1 | 0 |
| Garrick & Requa, 1980 | 17/24 | — | — | 11.8 | — | — | — | — | — | 23.5 | 47.1 | 17.6[a] |
| Clarke & Buckley, 1980 | — | — | — | — | — | 3.7 | — | — | — | 18.8 | 4.8 | — |
| Wadley & Albright, 1993 | 106/53 | 0 | 0 | 3.8 | 0 | 5.7 | 14.1 | 0 | 8.5 | 33.0 | 35.0 | 0 |

*A participant season is one gymnast participating in one season.

**Includes data for recreational as well as club gymnasts.

[a]Information concerning categories within "other" category not available.

**Table 14.6  A Percent Comparison of Injury Location in Women's Club and High School Gymnastics**

| | Club: prospective studies | | | | Club: retrospective studies | | | High school: prospective studies | |
|---|---|---|---|---|---|---|---|---|---|
| # injuries<br># participant seasons | Garrick<br>1980<br>16<br>72 | Weiker<br>1985<br>95<br>766[a] | Caine<br>1989<br>147<br>50 | Lindner<br>1990a<br>90<br>362 | Steele<br>1983<br>146<br>268 | Kerr<br>1988<br>—<br>41 | Dixon<br>1993<br>325<br>162 | Garrick<br>1 year<br>(mixed) | Garrick<br>2 year<br>(interscholatic) |
| Head | (6.0) | (3.2) | (0.7) | (4.1) | (1.4) | — | (1.5) | (3.0) | (7.7) |
| Skull | — | 2.1 | — | 1.0 | — | — | — | — | — |
| Face | — | 1.1 | — | 2.1 | — | — | — | — | — |
| Teeth | — | 0.0 | — | 1.0 | — | — | — | — | — |
| Spine/Trunk | (0.0) | (7.5) | (15.0) | (16.7) | (13.7) | — | (22.3) | (13.0) | (43.6) |
| Neck | 0.0 | 1.1 | 0.7 | 6.3 | 2.7 | — | 3.9 | — | — |
| Upper back | 0.0 | 0.0 | 0.7 | 3.1 | 0.0 | — | 2.4 | — | — |
| Lower back | 0.0 | 6.4 | 12.2 | 5.2 | 11.0 | 13.0 | 13.3 | — | — |
| Ribs | 0.0 | 0.0 | 0.7 | 2.1 | 0.0 | — | 2.1 | — | — |
| Stomach | 0.0 | 0.0 | 0.7 | 0.0 | 0.0 | — | 0.6 | — | — |
| Upper Extremity | (25.0) | (18.1) | (20.5) | (22.9) | (14.4) | — | (21.7) | (36.0) | (12.8) |
| Shoulder | — | 1.1 | 0.7 | 4.2 | 0.0 | — | 1.2 | — | — |
| Arm | — | 0.0 | 0.7 | 1.0 | 0.7 | — | 0.0 | — | — |
| Elbow | — | 5.3 | 4.8 | 7.3 | 4.8 | — | 8.5 | — | — |
| Forearm | — | 1.1 | 0.7 | 0.0 | 0.0 | — | 0.6 | — | — |
| Wrist | — | 6.4 | 9.5 | 5.2 | 7.5 | — | 6.0 | — | — |
| Hand/fingers | — | 4.2 | 4.1 | 5.2 | 1.4 | — | 5.4 | — | — |
| Lower Extremity | (69.0) | (70.1) | (63.7) | (54.1) | (69.1) | — | (54.3) | (48.0) | (35.9) |
| Pelvis, Hips | — | 2.1 | 2.7 | 1.0 | 1.3 | — | 4.5 | — | — |
| Thigh | — | 1.1 | 8.7 | 1.0 | 1.3 | — | 3.0 | — | — |
| Knee | 19.0 | 24.5 | 14.3 | 19.8 | 18.5 | 15.0 | 10.9 | 7.0 | 5.1 |
| Leg | — | 8.5 | 6.8 | 0.0 | 7.5 | — | 1.5 | — | — |
| Ankle | 25.0 | 19.1 | 21.1 | 20.8 | 22.0 | 29.0 | 16.0 | 10.0 | 10.3 |
| Heel/Achilles | — | 4.2 | 5.4 | 4.2 | 0.0 | — | 6.9 | — | — |
| Foot/toes | — | 10.6 | 4.7 | 7.3 | 18.5 | 12.0 | 11.5 | — | — |

[a]Includes data for recreational gymnasts.

location for female collegiate gymnasts. The right side was injured more than the left ($p < 0.01$) possibly because the preferred side of performance tends to be the right in most gymnasts (139).

Few studies reported injury location data for men's gymnastics. A review of the club-level prospective studies in Table 14.8 shows that the upper and lower extremities were injured most often. Retrospective data indicate the upper extremity was injured most, followed by the lower extremity, then spine/trunk. Variability of percent values across studies precluded determination of top injury location for each body region; however, common injury sites included the lower back, shoulder, wrist, knee, and ankle. NCAA (113) injury location data show the top three injury sites for college male gymnasts varied each season; however, common sites in this category included ankle, knee, shoulder, wrist, lower back, and finger(s). NCAA (113) data show the ankle at greatest risk of injury,

followed by the finger(s), then lower back, wrist, and elbow during the 1993-94 season.

These findings differ from those in women's gymnastics and may reflect the different types of apparatus used in men's gymnastics that place greater physical demands on the upper body. For example, still rings and horizontal bar exercises include movements of great amplitude and speed, so the amount of stress placed on the shoulder is enormous (155).

One study reported injury location during competition. In a 17-month study of 206 competition injuries, Sands (130) reported the ankle (19.2%), knee (19.2%), foot (13.1%), and back (13.1%) as the most frequently injured locations. These data were United States Gymnastics Federation (USGF) insurance company data, however, and should be interpreted cautiously because data reflect only injuries submitted for insurance coverage, and not all injuries.

**Table 14.7  A Percent Comparison of Injury Location in Women's Collegiate Gymnastics**

| | Collegiate level: prospective studies | | | | | | |
|---|---|---|---|---|---|---|---|
| | Eisenberg 1978 | Snook 1979 | Clarke 1980 | Garrick 1980 | Sands 1984 | Sands 1986 | Wadley 1993 |
| # injuries | 27 | 66 | — | 17 | 54 | 70 | 106 |
| # participants* | 10 | 70 | — | 24 | 10 | 13 | 53 |
| Head | — | (4.8) | — | (6.0) | (1.9) | (1.4) | (1.9) |
| Face | — | — | — | — | — | — | 0 |
| Skull | — | — | — | — | — | — | 1.9 |
| Teeth | — | — | — | — | — | — | 0 |
| Spine/trunk | (12.3) | (16.7) | — | — | (13.0) | (15.7) | (16.0) |
| Neck | — | — | — | — | — | — | 2.8 |
| Upper back | — | — | — | — | — | — | 0 |
| Lower back | — | — | — | — | — | — | 13.2 |
| Ribs | — | — | — | — | — | — | — |
| Stomach | — | — | — | — | — | — | — |
| Upper extremity | (22.2) | (30.3) | — | (18.0) | (16.7) | (21.4) | (15.1) |
| Shoulder | — | — | — | — | — | — | 4.7 |
| Arm | — | — | — | — | — | — | — |
| Elbow | — | — | — | — | — | — | — |
| Forearm | — | — | — | — | — | — | 1.9 |
| Wrist | — | — | — | — | — | — | 4.7 |
| Hand/fingers | — | — | — | — | — | — | 3.8 |
| Lower extremity | (66.6) | (53.0) | (67.0) | (60.0) | (68.5) | (61.4) | (66.9) |
| Pelvis, hips | — | — | — | — | — | — | 5.7 |
| Thigh | — | — | — | — | — | — | 2.8 |
| Knee | — | — | — | — | — | — | 20.7 |
| Leg | — | — | — | — | — | — | 7.5 |
| Ankle | — | — | — | — | — | — | 17.0 |
| Heel/Achilles | — | — | — | — | — | — | 0 |
| Foot/toes | — | — | — | — | — | — | 13.2 |

*A participant is one gymnast participating in one season.

### 3.3.1 Head/Spine/Trunk

The young gymnast engaging in strenuous competition places demands on the lower back that are unparalleled in most other sports (64). Demands on the gymnast's back include repetitive flexion and hyperextension postures during vaulting, dismounts, and flips and specific postures directed at extreme hyperextension of the lumbar spine (48). It is the chronic repetitive flexion, rotation, and extension of the spine during these activities that may cause injuries to the spinal elements (53). In addition to the hyperlordotic posture, vertical impact loading occurs as the gymnast lands on both feet during dismount activities (173). Since the vertical forces of impact can be six times body weight, the human body must tolerate and absorb a great deal of stress when landing (163). A biomechanical study of the compression of the spine showed that spines of elite gymnasts were significantly more compressed than controls following training, and significantly more compressed following high impact training (166).

Tables 14.9 and 14.10 show the case reports, case series, and cross-sectional studies of injuries occurring in the spine/trunk of female and male gymnasts, respectively. A review of the case and case series data indicated most lower back injuries reported were gradual onset and involved primarily advanced level competitive gymnasts, implicating number of years of experience and competitive level in the pathogenesis of these injuries. Common injury sites reported include the vertebral bodies, intervertebral disks, and pars interarticularis. Common problems reported included vertebral endplate abnormalities and damage to the pars interarticularis with resultant spondylolysis and spondylolisthesis.

Perhaps most disturbing among these reports are those suggesting growth insult secondary to spinal injury (38, 52, 173). The body of the vertebra is subject to the same deforming factors that influence the growth of long bones elsewhere in the body (9). Repeated flexion at the thoraco-lumbar junction associated with landing from various

**Table 14.8    A Percent Comparison of Injury Location in Men's Gymnastics**

| | Club | | | | College |
|---|---|---|---|---|---|
| Design<br># injuries<br># participant seasons*** | Weiker<br>1985<br>Prospective<br>10<br>107 | Kerr*<br>1991<br>Prospective<br>61<br>24 | Lueken**<br>1993<br>Prospective<br>—<br>— | Dixon<br>1993<br>Retrospective<br>247<br>121 | Clarke<br>1980<br>Prospective<br>—<br>140 |
| Head | (18.2) | — | (3.2) | (0.4) | — |
| Skull | 18.2 | — | — | — | — |
| Face | — | — | — | — | — |
| Teeth | — | — | — | — | — |
| Spine/trunk | (9.1) | — | (17.1) | (13.3) | — |
| Neck | 9.1 | — | 3.5 | 2.0 | — |
| Upper back | — | — | 4.3 | 1.6 | — |
| Lower back | — | 20.0 | 6.1 | 9.3 | — |
| Ribs | — | — | 0 | 0 | — |
| Stomach | — | — | 0.3 | 0.4 | — |
| Chest | — | — | 2.9 | 0 | — |
| Upper extremity | (36.4) | — | (39.3) | (53.4) | — |
| Shoulder | 18.2 | 13.0 | 16.8 | 19.0 | — |
| Arm | — | — | 1.4 | 0 | — |
| Elbow | — | — | 4.3 | 11.3 | — |
| Forearm | — | — | 1.7 | 1.6 | — |
| Wrist | 18.2 | — | 8.4 | 13.8 | — |
| Hand/fingers | — | — | 6.7 | 7.7 | — |
| Lower extremity | (36.4) | — | (43.1) | (32.8) | — |
| Pelvis/hips | — | — | 3.2 | 1.6 | — |
| Thigh | — | — | 4.6 | 2.0 | — |
| Knee | 27.3 | 10.0 | 7.8 | 7.7 | 14.0 |
| Leg | — | 10.0 | 4.9 | 2.0 | — |
| Ankle | 9.1 | 27.0 | 13.9 | 9.7 | — |
| Heel/Achilles | — | — | 0 | 4.1 | — |
| Foot/toes | — | — | 8.7 | 5.7 | — |

*Competitive level Class VI to elite males training at the U.S. Olympic Training Center from January 1990 to July 1992.

**Includes data for 8 female gymnasts.

***A participant season is one participant participating in one season.

heights may create biomechanical compression forces sufficient to disrupt the growth potential of the vertebral growth plate (39). Growth disturbance of the vertebral bodies may result when disc material herniates either through the endplates or through the annulus fibrosis, resulting in a decrease in intradisc pressure, deterioration of the mechanical properties of the disc, and disturbed distribution of stress over the endplates (149).

Stress injury may also involve the pars interarticularis. Many authors believe that repeated loading in hyperflexion and hyperextension of the spine causes a stress reaction in the pars interarticularis of the neural arch (149). The initial response appears to involve microfractures with attempts at repair. This may be followed by overt fracturing (spondylolysis) occurring first on one side, resulting in overload and subsequent microfracture

and spondylolysis on the other side. With bilateral spondylolysis the stage is set for spondylolisthesis if excessive loading continues (78).

The cross-sectional studies in Tables 14.9 and 14.10 provide prevalence rate estimates for stress injuries of the spine with possible growth sequelae. Some studies indicated a higher prevalence of radiographic abnormalities of the thoraco-lumbar spine in highly competitive gymnasts versus nonathletes (56, 150, 152) and other athletes (50), although this finding was equivocal (154, 159).

Prevalence rates for spondylolysis ranged from 0% to 32.8% for females and were 11.5% for males (56, 153). Notably, Hellström and his coworkers (56) reported a spondylolysis prevalence rate of 3.3% for the control sample of 30 male and female nonathletes. These results lend credence to the supposition that gymnasts can and do suffer a greater

**Table 14.9  Case Reports, Case Series, and Cross-Sectional Studies of Injuries Occurring in the Spine/Trunk of Female Gymnasts**

| Study | Design | # Subjects | Age | Level | Condition/diagnosis |
|---|---|---|---|---|---|
| **Lower back** | | | | | |
| Knight et al., 1977 | Case | 1 | 20 | College | Bilateral spondylolysis at L2 |
| Walsh et al., 1984 | Case | 3 | 16 | — | Irregularity in wedging of the vertebral endplates at the thoracolumbar junction (1 case); spondylolysis L4-L5 and L5-S1 (2 cases) |
| Swärd et al., 1990a | Case | 2 | 13.75 16.33 | Elite | Traumatic injury of the vertebral ring apophysis followed by prolapse of disc material; reduction in disc height and disc degeneration |
| Li & Lloyd-Smith, 1991 | Case | 1 | 13 | Competitive | Stress fracture of the pars interarticularis |
| Wiltse et al., 1975 | Case series | 1 | 13 | — | Spondylolysis L5 |
| Jackson et al., 1981 | Case series | 3 | 12.3 | — | Stress reaction involving the pars interarticularis |
| Greene et al., 1985 | Case series | 1 | 14 | — | Acute localized kyphosis at the dorsolumbar junction (1 case); dorsolumbar vertebral changes without kyphosis (1 case) |
| Lishen & Jianhua, 1983 (cited in Caine, 1990) | Case series[a] | 18 | 11-16 | Regional | Vertebral epiphysitis in all gymnasts |
| Letts et al., 1986 | Case series | 3 | 15.7 | National, club | Stress fracture of the pars interarticularis |
| Bozdech & Dufek, 1986 | Case series[b] | 24 | 10-22 | — | Spondylolisthesis in 5 gymnasts |
| Tütsch & Ulrich, 1975 (cited in Caine, 1990) | Cross-sectional | 12 | 14.3 | Top level | Scheuermann's disease (41.7%); spondylolisthesis (8.3%) |
| Jackson et al., 1976 | Cross-sectional | 100 | 14.0 | Regional | Bilateral L5 pars interarticularis defects (11%); 6 of the 11 cases had coexisting spondylolisthesis at L5 |
| Knight et al., 1977 | Cross-sectional | 8 | — | College | No cases of spondylolysis |
| Rossi, 1978 | Cross-sectional | 132 | — | Olympic | 32.8% spondylolysis; 8.9% spondylolisthesis |
| Swärd et al., 1989 | Cross-sectional | 26 | 16-25 | National; jr. national | 19.2% spondylolysis, 4/5 with coexisting spondylolisthesis |
| Rossi & Dragoni, 1990 | Cross-sectional | 417 | 15-27 | Competition | 16.31% spondylolysis |
| Tertti et al., 1990 | Cross-sectional | 17 | 8-19 | District, national, internat. | Sacrilization of L5 (5.9%); Scheuermann's disease (5.9%); spondylolysis at L5 (5.9%); degenerated discs (11.8%) |
| | | 10 | 8-14 | Nonathletes | Abnormal discs (10%) |
| Hellström et al., 1990 | Cross-sectional | 26 | 14-25 | Nationally ranked | Scoliosis (11.5%); spondylolysis (19.2%); with coexisting spondylolisthesis in 4 of the 5 cases; abnormal configuration of the vertebrae (15.4%); disc height reduction (3.8%); Schmorl's nodes (11.5%); apophyseal abnormalities (15.4%) |
| | | 30 | 19-25 | Nonathletes | Scoliosis (3.3%); spondylolysis (3.3%); coexisting spondylolisthesis (3.3%); spina bifida occulta (13.3%); abnormal configuration of the vertebrae (10%); disc height reduction (6.7%); Schmorl's nodes (40%); apophyseal abnormalities (0) |
| Swärd et al., 1990b | Cross-sectional | 26 | 16-25 | National; jr. national | 42.3% radiological abnormalities of the thoraco-lumbar spine |
| Goldstein et al., 1991 | Cross-sectional | 8 | 25.7 | National | Spondylolysis (12.5%); abnormal disc (62.5%) |
| | | 14 | 16.6 | Elite | Spondylolysis (21.4%); abnormal disc (21.4%) |
| | | 11 | 11.8 | Pre-Elite | Spondylolysis (9.1%); abnormal disc (0) |
| | | 11 | 18.6 | National swimmers | Abnormal disc (9.1%) |
| | | 8 | 14.6 | AAA/AA swimmers | Abnormal disc (25%) |
| Swärd et al., 1993 | Cross-sectional | 26 | 14-25 | National | Abnormalities affecting the vertebral ring apophyses (30.8%) |
| | | 30 | 16-25 | Nonathletes | No abnormalities of the vertebral ring apophyses |

*(continued)*

**Table 14.9**  *(continued)*

| Study | Design | # Subjects | Age | Level | Condition/diagnosis |
|---|---|---|---|---|---|
| **Ribs** | | | | | |
| Proffer et al., 1991 | Case | 1 | 12 | — | Nonunion of a rib fracture |
| Holden & Jackson, 1985 | Case series | 1 | — | — | Posterolateral stress fracture of a rib |
| **Stomach** | | | | | |
| Danneker et al., 1979 | Case | 1 | 18 | High school | Intra-abdominal injury |
| Vaos et al., 1989 | Case | 1 | 10 | — | Intra-abdominal injury involving the small intestine |

[a]Obtained from the radiographic monitoring of the Hunan (China) gymnastics team over a period of 9 years.

[b]Obtained from the radiographic monitoring of a Czechoslovakian gymnastics team over a period of 10 years.

incidence of spondylolysis than nongymnasts. Therefore, it is likely that in some gymnasts fatigue loading of the pars interarticularis secondary to the rigorous demands of the sport plays a pivotal role in the pathogenesis of fresh defects (98).

Few researchers studied the incidence of pars defects among gymnasts. Caine et al. (18) reported one case among 50 club-level female gymnasts followed prospectively over 1 year (2 cases per 100 participant seasons). Dixon and Fricker (36) reported 6 cases of spondylolysis per 100 participant seasons for female gymnasts and 2.5 cases per 100 participant seasons among male gymnasts. Mackie and Taunton (90) reported 5 cases among 100 gymnasts over 40 months. These relatively low rates may reflect the recent change in practice habits of gymnasts that encourages dismounting into a polyurethane foam pit, or increasing the thickness of mats, or both, thus diminishing the overall stress on the lumbosacral spine.

This review indicates that competitive gymnasts are at risk of incurring stress injury to the spine during their competitive career. The radiological findings indicate the potential damaging effects of excessive mechanical loading on the immature spine of gymnasts, including damage to the pars interarticularis resulting in spondylolysis or spondylolisthesis, discogenic pathology, and vertebral endplate abnormalities. A spectrum of spinal abnormalities may thus be associated with gymnastics training, suggesting a dose–response gradient with an increased risk of severity of the outcome in association with an increased intensity or duration of exposure.

### 3.3.2 Upper Extremity

Unlike most other sports, gymnastics uses the upper extremities as weight-bearing limbs, causing high impact loads to be distributed through the elbow and wrist. Upper extremity forces have been quantified for several gymnastics events. Vaulting studies show forces on the upper extremity of 1.13 to 1.57 times body weight (156). Studies of peak forces on large hanging/swinging skills report 3.9 times body weight on the horizontal bar (75), 9.2 times body weight on still rings (132), and 3.1 times body weight on women's uneven parallel bars (180). Markhoff et al. (100) reported force magnitudes up to 2.0 times body weight during pommel horse activities. From a teleological perspective, however, the upper extremity is no longer adapted for these types of forces. Thus, it is not unexpected that injury occurs in this region.

The case reports, case series, and cross-sectional studies of upper extremity injuries among females and males are shown in Tables 14.11 and 14.12, respectively. Perusal of case data in these tables indicates that the majority of cases reported were gradual onset injuries and involved primarily advanced level competitive gymnasts. This pattern suggests the role of years of experience and competitive level in the pathogenesis of these injuries. Commonly reported injury sites include the distal radius and distal humerus. Common problems reported include stress injury of the distal radial growth plate and osteochondritis dissecans (OD) of the humeral capitellum (primarily females).

The case and case series data attest to the potential for growth insult involving the stress-injured distal radial growth plate in young gymnasts (2, 34, 43, 162, 169). Complications may include symmetrical or asymmetrical retardation in growth at the affected site and, in extreme cases, premature arrest of longitudinal growth and associated positive ulnar variance. Loss of the normal anatomic relationship between the radius and ulna (i.e., positive ulnar variance), in turn, may result in a range

**Table 14.10   Case Reports, Case Series, and Cross-Sectional Studies of Injuries Occurring in the Spine/Trunk of Male Gymnasts**

| Study | Design | No. of Subjects | Age | Competitive level | Condition/diagnosis |
|---|---|---|---|---|---|
| *Lower back* | | | | | |
| Weir & Smith, 1989 | Case | 1 | 12.0 | — | Bilateral spondylolysis at L-5 |
| Lishen & Jianhua, 1983 (cited in Caine, 1990) | Case series[a] | 10 | 12-16 | Regional | Gymnasts' vertebral epiphysitis (6 cases) |
| Dzioba, 1984 | Case series | 5 | — | Top level | Thoracolumbar deformity and associated low back pain |
| Letts et al., 1986 | Case series | 3 | 12.3 | National; club | Stress fracture of the pars interarticularis (3 cases) |
| Bozdech & Dufek, 1986 | Case series[b] | 19 | 10-22 | — | Spondylolisthesis in 3 cases |
| Szot et al., 1985 | Cross-sectional | 41 | 21.3 | National | Radiological changes of the spinal column (65.8%) (i.e., fracture and deformation of vertebral bodies, degeneration of the intervertebral discs, degenerative changes in the intervertebral articulations) |
| Swärd et al., 1989 | Cross-sectional | 26 | 16-25 | National; jr. national | Spondylolysis (11.5%); coexisting spondylolisthesis (11.5%) |
| Tertti et al., 1990 | Cross-sectional | 18 | 8-19 | District, national, international | Sacrilization of L5 (11.1%); Scheuermann's disease (11.1%); disc degeneration (5.6%) |
|  |  | 10 | 8-14 | Nonathletes | Degenerated disc (5.6%) |
| Hellström et al., 1990 | Cross-sectional | 26 | 16-25 | National | Scoliosis (19.2%); spondylolysis and spondylolisthesis (11.5%); abnormal configuration of the vertebrae (38.5%); disc height reduction (11.5%); Schmorl's nodes (26.9%), apophyseal abnormalities (11.5%) |
|  |  | 30 M/F | 16-25 | Nonathletes | Scoliosis (3.3%); spondylolysis (3.3%); coexisting spondylolisthesis (3.3%); abnormal configuration of the vertebrae (10%); disc height reduction (6.7%); Schmorl's nodes (40%); apophyseal abnormalities (0) |
| Swärd et al., 1991 | Cross-sectional | 24 | 19-29 | Elite | Reduced disc height (38%); posterior disc bulging (50%); Schmorl's nodes (71%); apophyseal ring abnormalities (17%); abnormal configuration of the vertebral bodies (33%) |
|  |  | 16 | 23-26 | Nonathletes | Reduced disc height (13%); posterior disc bulging (19%); Schmorl's nodes (71%); apophyseal ring abnormalities (0); abnormal configuration of vertebral bodies (0) |
| Swärd et al., 1993 | Cross-sectional | 26 |  | Nationally ranked | Abnormalities affecting the vertebral ring apophyses (19.2%) |
|  |  | 30 M/F |  | Nonathletes | No abnormalities affecting the vertebral ring apophyses |

[a]Obtained from the radiographic monitoring of the Hunan (China) gymnastics team over a period of 9 years.

[b]Obtained from the radiographic monitoring of a Czechoslovakian gymnastics team over a period of 10 years.

of pathoanatomical sequelae with associated chronic wrist pain and resultant compromise to training, participation, and performance (96).

Perhaps the most disabling condition among the chronic elbow injuries reported is OD of the humeral capitellum (63). This injury is believed to represent a disorder of endochondral ossification caused by vascular insufficiency and induced by repetitive shear and compressive forces to a stressed and vulnerable epiphysis (142). Based on a follow-up of gymnasts presenting with derangement of the articular surfaces of the elbow, Maffuli and his coworkers (91) described a possible continuum of stress-related changes that may affect the elbow. At an early age, when the radial head epiphysis is still not ossified, the compression exerted by the humeral capitellum may result in angulation deformity. Subsequently, chronic repetitive stress

**Table 14.11   Case Reports, Case Series, and Cross-Sectional Studies of Injuries Occurring in the Upper Extremity of Female Gymnasts**

| Study | Design | No. of subjects | Age | Competitive level | Diagnosis/condition |
|-------|--------|-----------------|-----|-------------------|---------------------|
| **Shoulder/arm** | | | | | |
| Jahn, 1982 | Case | 1 | 12 | — | Spontaneous reduced glenohumeral partial dislocation |
| **Elbow** | | | | | |
| Tayob & Shively, 1980 | Case | 1 | 13 | — | Bilateral epicondylar entrapment following fracture dislocation of the elbow |
| Priest & Weise, 1981 | Case series | 30 | 13.6 | — | Dislocations (17 cases); fractures (23 cases); radial nerve palsy (1 case); osteochondritis of the humeral capitellum (2 cases) |
| Hirasawa & Sakakida, 1983 | Case series | 4 M/F | — | — | Radial nerve injury (2 cases); ulnar nerve injury secondary to supracondylar and lateral condylar fracture of the humerus (2 cases) |
| Singer & Roy, 1984 | Case series | 5 | 11-13 | Elite, II | 7 cases of osteochondrosis of the humeral capitellum |
| Jackson et al., 1989 | Case series | 7 | 13.3 | Classes III, II, I, elite | 10 cases of osteochondritis dissecans of the humeral capitellum |
| Maffuli et al., 1992a | Case series | 6 | 11.8 | — | Osteochondritis dissecans of the humeral capitellum (7 cases) and radial head (1 case); flattened radial head (2 cases); loose body formation (5 cases); anterior inclination of the radial head (1 case) |
| Maffuli et al., 1992b | Case series | 2 | 14.7 | National; international | Widening of the olecranon physes and fragmentation of the epiphysis |
| Singer & Roy, 1984 | Cross-sectional | 37 | 13.3 | Class II | No cases of osteochondrosis dissecans of the humeral capitellum |
| Jackson et al., 1989 | Cross-sectional | 43 | 12.5 | Classes III, II, I; elite | No subclinical cases of osteochondritis dissecans of the humeral capitellum |
| **Forearm** | | | | | |
| Victor et al., 1993 | Case | 1 | 13 | — | Refracture of the radius and ulna |
| **Wrist** | | | | | |
| Read, 1981 | Case | 3 | 13.7 | — | Stress fractures involving the metaphyseal-epiphyseal interface of the distal radius |
| Murakami & Nakajima, 1984 | Case | 1 | 19.0 | College | Aseptic necrosis of the capitate bone |
| Fliegel, 1986 | Case | 1 | 14 | — | Stress-induced widening of the distal radial growth plate |
| Resnick, 1988 | Case | 1 M/F | 12 | — | Stress changes of the distal radial growth plate |
| Vender & Watson, 1988 | Case | 1 | 17 | — | Premature bilateral closure of the ulnar side of the distal radial growth plate leading to a Madelung-like deformity |
| Albanese et al., 1989 | Case | 3 | 13.3 | — | Chronic overuse leading to premature growth plate closure, resulting in shortening of the radius and alterations in the normal distal radioulnar articulation |
| Ruggles et al., 1991 | Case | 1 | 12 | Elite | Bilateral widening of the distal radial growth plate |
| Li & Lloyd-Smith, 1991 | Case | 1 | 13 | — | Widening and irregularities of the distal radial growth plate; flaring of the distal radial metaphysis with spurring along its palmar aspect |
| Carek & Fumich, 1992 | Case | 1 | 14 | — | Stress fracture (epiphysiolysis) of the distal radial growth plate |
| Lishen & Jianhua, 1983 (cited in Caine, 1990) | Case series | 18 | 11-12 | Top level | Stress changes leading to hindered radial growth and a relatively lengthened ulna (6 cases) |
| Roy et al., 1985 | Case series | 10 | 12.2 | Classes II, I; elite | Stress changes, possibly stress fractures of the distal radial growth plate |
| Carter & Aldridge, 1988 | Case series | 4 | 14 | National; club | Salter Type I stress fractures of the distal radial growth plate due to chronic repetitive force |
| Hermsdorfer et al., 1991 | Case series | 1 M/F | 16 | — | Traumatic separation of the triangular fibrocartilage complex from its peripheral origin |

| Study | Design | No. of subjects | Age | Competitive level | Diagnosis/condition |
|---|---|---|---|---|---|
| Tolat et al., 1992 | Case series | 5 | 16.8 | — | Symptomatic acquired positive ulnar variance due to premature physeal closure of the distal radial growth plate |
| DeSmet et al., 1993 | Case series | 6 | 16-23 | College | Positive ulnar variance and increased sagittal angle of the distal radial epiphysis (Madelung deformity) with ulnar wrist pain |
| Auberge et al., 1984 | Cross-sectional | 57 | 14-17 | Junior national | Chronic osteoarticular lesions involving the distal radial growth plate (85%) |
| Roy et al., 1985 | Cross-sectional | 26 | 9-14 | Class II | Minimal widening and irregularity of the distal radial growth plate (30.8%) |
| Mandelbaum et al., 1989 | Cross-sectional | 9 | 20 | College | Positive ulnar variance associated with "gymnast wrist pain syndrome"; female gymnasts averaged 1.44-mm positive ulnar variance |
| Caine et al., 1992 | Cross-sectional | 39 | 12.6 | Classes III, II, I | Minimal widening and irregularities of the distal radial growth plate (10%) |
| Teurlings & Mandelbaum, 1992 | Cross-sectional | 36 | 11.7 | — | Tendency (compared to control subjects) toward positive ulnar variance that increases with age and increasing levels of participation |
| DeSmet et al., 1994 | Cross-sectional | 156 | 15.9 | National | Enlargement of the distal radial growth plate with irregular borders in 10% of the cases |

may cause OD of either the humerus or the radius, with possible formation of loose bodies. Finally, if the athlete is relatively mature, Panner's disease may ensue.

Tables 14.11 and 14.12 show injury data derived from cross-sectional studies involving upper extremity injuries in female and male gymnasts, respectively. The prevalence rates of stress injury at the distal radial growth plate ranged from 10% to 85% for females, and from 4.8% to 80% in males. Incidence of stress injury involving the distal radial growth plate was reported by Caine et al. (21) and Dixon and Fricker (36) who reported rates of 2.7 and 1.9 injuries per 100 participant seasons, respectively.

The prevalence of OD and other stress-related injuries involving the gymnast's elbow is unclear. Singer and Roy (142) and Jackson et al. (63) found no cases of OD in their cross-sectional samples of female gymnasts. Szot et al. (155), on the other hand, found radiographic abnormalities of the elbow in 73.2% of their sample of national team male gymnasts. Nocini and Silvij (114) examined a select group of nine past and present Italian Olympic gymnasts with varying years of competitive experience. Radiographic changes indicated a cumulative effect of microtrauma in the elbows of five gymnasts.

Few researchers studied the incidence of OD of the humeral capitellum. Caine et al. (18) found no

cases among 50 female gymnasts followed prospectively for one year. Dixon and Fricker (36) reported 1.2 cases and 2.5 cases per 100 participant seasons for female and male gymnasts, respectively.

### 3.3.3 Lower Extremity

The lower extremity of gymnasts is also a site of tremendous physical loading. This involves the repetitive jarring impact of vault takeoffs and dismounts from a variety of heights and during tumbling activities. Lower extremity impact forces have been quantified in tumbling, vaulting and landings. For example, vault takeoffs resulted in GRFs of 5.1 times body weight (156) and a single-leg takeoff for an aerial walkover showed peak GRF of 3.3 times body weight (72). As discussed previously, GRF for landing may range from 8.8 to 14.4 times body weight per foot (117).

A review of the prospective and retrospective data in Tables 14.6 and 14.7 suggests the majority of injuries among female gymnasts were lower extremity injuries, and most of these involved the ankle and knee. In male gymnasts (Table 14.8) the limited research indicates lower extremity injuries occurred as often as upper extremity injuries. By contrast, perusal of Tables 14.13 and 14.14 reveals a relative paucity of case reports and no cross-sectional studies relating to lower extremity injuries among gymnasts.

**Table 14.12   Case Reports, Case Series, and Cross-Sectional Studies of Injuries Occurring in the Upper Extremity of Male Gymnasts**

| Study | Design | No. of subjects | Age | Competitive level | Diagnosis/condition |
|---|---|---|---|---|---|
| **Shoulder/arm** | | | | | |
| Postacchini & Puddu, 1975 | Case | 1 | 21 | — | Subcutaneous rupture of the distal biceps brachii tendon |
| Del Pizzo et al., 1978 | Case | 1 | 22 | College | Rupture of the long head of the biceps tendon |
| D'Alessandro et al., 1993 | Case series | 1 | 25 | — | Distal biceps tendon rupture |
| Fulton, 1979 | Cross-sectional | 16 | 21 | National team | Evidence of cortical desmoidlike lesions of the proximal humerus (50%) |
| Silvij & Nocini, 1982 | Cross-sectional | 9 | 22-41 | National team | Radiographic changes consistent with acromio-clavicular arthrosis (22.2%) |
| Szot et al., 1985 | Cross-sectional | 41 | 21.3 | National team | Cystlike formation of the humerus head and breaking of the acromioclavicular ligament (59.8%) |
| **Elbow** | | | | | |
| Wilkerson & Johns, 1990 | Case | 1 | 14 | — | Stress fracture of the olecranon epiphyseal plate |
| Svihlik, 1993 | Case | 1 | 13 | — | Osteochondritis dissecans of the humeral capitellum with osteocartilaginous loose bodies of the elbow |
| Chan et al., 1991 | Case series | 19 M/F (14 M) | 13.5 | Elite | Panner's disease (1 case); osteochondritis dissecans of the capitellum (5 cases); osteochondritis dissecans of the anterior aspect of the radial head (1 case); osteochondritis dissecans of the medial articular eminence of the distal humerus (1 case); a spectrum of olecranon changes from fragmentation of the epiphysis to chronic Salter Type I stress fractures of the growth plate (7 cases); flattening and anterior depression of the radial head epiphysis (3 cases) |
| Maffuli et al., 1992a | Case series | 6 | 15.2 | — | Osteochondritis dissecans of the humeral capitellum (1 case) and of the radial head (5 cases); flattened radial head (2 cases); intraarticular loose bodies (9 cases) |
| Maffuli et al., 1992b | Case series | 8 | 11-19 | National | Widening of the olecranon physis and fragmentation of the epiphysis (9 cases); stress fractures through the olecranon growth plate (2 cases) |
| Nocini & Silvij, 1982 | Cross-sectional | 9 | 22-41 | National team | Enthesitis of the brachial biceps and coracobrachialis at the inferior insertion; gymnasts elbow lesion (55.5%) |
| Szot et al., 1985 | Cross-sectional | 41 | 21.3 | National team | Degenerative exostoses of olecranon and coronoid processes; disturbances in ossification centers of the distal epiphyses of the humerus (73.2%) |
| **Wrist** | | | | | |
| Manzione & Pizzutillo, 1981 | Case | 1 | 16 | Nationally ranked | Stress fracture of the scaphoid waist |
| Murakami & Nakajima, 1984 | Case | 1 | 18 | College | Aseptic necrosis of the capitate bone |
| Roy et al., 1985 | Case | 1 | 12 | Upper-level club | Stress changes, possibly stress fracture of the distal radial growth plate |
| Fliegel, 1986 | Case | 1 | 14.2 | — | Stress-induced widening of the distal radial growth plate |
| Yong-Hing et al., 1988 | Case | 1 | 13 | National | Stress-related widening of the growth plates of the distal radius and ulna |
| Mandelbaum et al., 1988 | Case | 1 | 23 | College | Positive ulnar variance associated with tears of the ulnar triangular fibrocartilage and erosions of the lunate and triquetrum |
| Hanks et al., 1989 | Case | 2 | 18 | Jr. olympic; college | Stress fracture of carpal scaphoid |

| Study | Design | No. of subjects | Age | Competitive level | Diagnosis/condition |
|---|---|---|---|---|---|
| Stuart & Briggs, 1993 | Case | 1 | 16 | — | Delayed closed rupture of the extensor indicis proprius tendon following greenstick fracture of the distal radius |
| Lishen & Jianhua, 1983 (cited in Caine, 1990) | Case series | 10 | 13-15 | Top level | Stress changes leading to hindered radial growth and a relatively lengthened ulna (8 cases) |
| Carter & Aldridge, 1988 | Case series | 17 | 13.5 | National | Salter Type I stress fracture of the ranked distal radial growth plate |
| Auberge et al., 1984 | Cross-sectional | 41 | 17-33 | Jr. national | Chronic osteoarticular lesions of the distal radial growth plate (80%) |
| Szot et al., 1985 | Cross-sectional | 41 | 21.3 | National | Distal radial epiphyseal irregularities (58.5%) |
| Mandelbaum et al., 1989 | Cross-sectional | 29 | 20-21 | College | Positive ulnar variance associated with "gymnast wrist pain syndrome"; average of 2.82-mm positive ulnar variance in 11 males and 1.28-mm positive ulnar variance in 18 males) |
| Caine et al., 1992 | Cross-sectional | 21 | 12.6 | Classes IV, III, II, I | Definite changes of subchondral sclerosis, physeal widening, marginal new bone formation, and distortion of the distal end of the radius (4.8%) |
| Teurlings & Mandelbaum, 1992 | Cross-sectional | 7 | 11.7 | — | Tendency (compared to control subjects) toward positive ulnar variance that increases with age and level of competition |

A review of Tables 14.13 and 14.14 reveals twelve reports of lower extremity nerve injury. In three cases (13, 47, 157) there was femoral nerve palsy secondary to injury of the iliacus muscle. In nine cases (58, 89) the neuropathy was caused by direct compression (as a result of "beating" on the lower of the asymmetric bars; 89) and repeated trauma to a peripheral nerve. Usually these injuries appeared as an entrapment neuropathy and the symptoms improved with conservative management. However, several cases were complicated by fractures and surgical exploration was necessary (58).

## 4. Injury Severity

### 4.1 Time Loss

Time loss due to injury is difficult to measure in gymnastics due to the tendency for injured gymnasts, depending on the severity of injury, to continue to train on selected apparatus with some modifications. In addition, many subjective and objective factors may influence performance time lost due to injury (e.g., personal motivation, peer influence, coaching staff reluctance/encouragement, approaching competition) and consequently bias the studies. This bias is minimized when numerical definitions are used (161).

Two prospective studies of club-level gymnasts reported time loss using numerical definitions to represent injury severity. Caine et al. (18) reported that 40.8% of injuries in their study required less than 8 days at reduced training. By comparison, Lindner and Caine (82) reported only 3.4% of the injuries in their study required less than 8 days absence from full training and 60.2% of injuries resulted in more than 21 days at reduced training. These contrasting results may reflect different definitions of *injury*.

NCAA data (113) indicate that from 1985 to 1994 (1986-1994 for males) 60.7% of injuries affecting female gymnasts and 62.7% of injuries to male gymnasts resulted in 1 to 6 time-loss days due to injury. During this same period almost 30% of injuries for both female and male collegiate gymnasts resulted in 10 or more time-loss days as a result of injury.

### 4.2 Catastrophic Injuries

The worst case scenario of gymnastic injury is catastrophic injury. This type of injury is a concern in view of the increasing difficulty of gymnastics maneuvers (e.g., Yurchenko vault). A summary of the case report and case series data on catastrophic injuries in women's and men's gymnastics is

**Table 14.13   Case Reports and Case Series of Injuries Occurring in the Lower Extremity of Female Gymnasts**

| Study | Design | No. of subjects | Age | Competitive level | Diagnosis/condition |
|---|---|---|---|---|---|
| **Pelvis, Hips** | | | | | |
| Guiliani et al., 1990 | Case | 1 | 14 | — | Iliacus hematoma syndrome as a result of compression; neuropathy of the femoral nerve subsequent to hemorrhage in the iliac fossa |
| **Thigh** | | | | | |
| MacGregor & Moncur, 1977 | Case | 2 | 14 18 | — | Mild neuropathy of the lateral femoral cutaneous nerve (i.e., meralgia paresthetica) |
| **Knee** | | | | | |
| Abrams et al., 1986 | Case | 1 | 15 | High school | Salter-Harris Type III fracture of proximal fibula |
| Donati et al., 1986 | Case | 1 | 21 | College | Bilateral simultaneous patellar tendon rupture |
| Hunter & Torgan, 1983 | Case series | 12 | 17 | High school (9) College (3) | Anterior cruciate tear (9 cases); meniscus tear (5 cases) |
| Andrish, 1985 | Case series | 170[a] | — | — | Patello-femoral (102 cases); sprains (30 cases); meniscal tears (24 cases); contusions (12 cases); Osgood-Schlatter syndrome (8 cases); strains (4 cases) |
| **Leg** | | | | | |
| Burks et al., 1992 | Case | 1 | 14 | Class I | Occult tibial fracture |
| **Ankle** | | | | | |
| Barron & Yocum, 1993 | Case | 1 | 30 | — | Achilles tendon rupture associated with an ipsilateral medial malleollar fracture |
| Bruijn et al., 1993 | Case | 1 | 12 | — | Sleeve fracture of the patella |
| **Foot** | | | | | |
| Mahler & Fricker, 1992 | Case | 1 | 20 | Elite | Stress fracture of the cuboid tarsal bone |

[a]Analysis included data from 28 male gymnasts.

shown in Table 14.15. The data in Table 14.15 indicate that most catastrophic injuries were nonfatal and resulted in permanent severe functional disability such as quadriplegia. Most of the maneuvers leading to these injuries were back or front somersaults performed on the trampoline (164). Although the trampoline and minitramp were often associated with catastrophic injury, other apparatus, including the springboard, were also implicated (22, 26, 115, 140). Noteworthy among these reports are the many cases involving experienced, expert and elite gymnasts and/or trampolinists (164). The greater skill of these advanced level athletes may not compensate for the extra risks they take. In addition many skilled gymnasts are beginners in many of the newly invented, highly complex exercises that they attempt (140).

Table 14.16 summarizes data from studies that report rates for catastrophic injuries in men's and women's gymnastics. The data suggest risk of catastrophic injury was greater at the college level than in high school, and higher for male than female gymnasts. No rate data are given for club-level gymnasts, but recent cohort studies report no catastrophic injuries among club-level gymnasts (18, 36, 82).

## 4.3 Clinical Outcome/Residual Symptoms

### 4.3.1 Non-Participation

Caine et al. (18) reported that 21 female gymnasts in their study (42%) dropped out during the course of one year. Of these, 11 gymnasts were injured when they withdrew from gymnastics and 11 were from out-of-state, or both, suggesting the possible role of injury and absence from home as potential sources of motivation for dropping out. Dixon and Fricker (36) reported 7 females (9.5% of sample) and 1 male (2.4%) retired as a result of injury during a 10-year retrospective study of elite gymnasts. Lindholm et al. (81) followed 22 elite level female gymnasts over 5 years. By the end of this period, only 5 gymnasts remained in elite level training, 11 were involved in a less strenuous form of gymnastics (five of these due to injury), 5 had changed to another sport, and 1 discontinued training.

**Table 14.14    Case Reports and Case Series of Injuries Occurring in the Lower Extremity of Male Gymnasts**

| Study | Design | No. of subjects | Age | Competitive level | Diagnosis/condition |
|---|---|---|---|---|---|
| *Hips, pelvis* | | | | | |
| Takami et al., 1983 | Case | 1 | 15 | — | Traumatic rupture of the iliacus muscle with femoral nerve paralysis |
| *Thigh* | | | | | |
| Brozin et al., 1982 | Case | 1 | 15 | — | Traumatic closed femoral nerve neuropathy |
| *Knee* | | | | | |
| Levi & Coleman, 1976 | Case | 1 | 12 | — | Fracture of the tibial tubercle |
| Lepse et al., 1988 | Case | 1 | 14 | — | Simultaneous bilateral avulsion fracture of the tibial tuberosity |
| Bruijn et al., 1993 | Case | 1 | 14 | — | Sleeve fracture of the tibial tuberosity |
| Andrews et al., 1994 | Case | 1 | 13 | — | Peripheral lateral meniscal tear with partial meniscal tear and an ACL tear at the femoral insertion |
| *Leg* | | | | | |
| Hirasawa & Sakakida, 1983 | Case series | 2 | 20 | — | Peripheral nerve injury associated with a medialcondylar fracture of the left tibia (1 case) |
| | | | 19 | — | Entrapment of the lateral cutaneous nerve of the left femur (1 case) |
| *Ankle* | | | | | |
| Mulligan, 1986 | Case | 1 | 27 | — | Horizontal fracture of the talar head |
| Biedert, 1993 | Case | 1 | 18 | — | Dislocation of the tibialis posterior tendon |
| *Foot/toes* | | | | | |
| Maffuli et al., 1989 | Case | 1 | 24 | — | Total anterolateral dislocation of the talus |

Several authors reported nonparticipation related to specific injury types. Maffuli et al. (91) reported 11 of 12 gymnasts (6F, 6M) with derangement of the articular surfaces of the elbow who discontinued competitive gymnastics because of incapacitating elbow pain, associated with shock loading and hyperextension of the elbow in routines such as vaulting and tumbling. Jackson et al. (63) reported 7 female gymnasts with osteochondritis in the elbow who withdrew from participation. Similarly, some gymnasts with positive ulnar variance have been unable to continue with competitive gymnastics because of chronic wrist pain (34, 162).

Dixon and Fricker (36) also reported on injuries that resulted in retirement of gymnasts. These were as follows: chronic rotator cuff injury, navicular stress fracture, loose bodies in an ankle joint, medial and lateral meniscus lesions, anterior cruciate ligament rupture, and osteochondritis of the elbow joint. With the exception of OD, all of these injuries required surgery. Overall, 8 (7F, 1M) of 116 gymnasts retired from gymnastics as a result of injury.

### 4.3.2 Long-Term Symptoms

To our knowledge few studies have investigated long-term symptoms related to gymnastics injuries. Maffuli et al. (91) reported the long-term follow-up (mean = 3.6 years) of lesions of the articular surface of the elbow joint in a group of 12 gymnasts (6F, 6M). In this group there was a high frequency of osteochondritic lesions, intraarticular loose bodies, and precocious signs of joint aging. Residual mild pain in the elbow at full extension occurring after activity was present in 10 patients, and all patients showed marked loss of elbow extension compared with their first visit. On the other hand, Jackson et al. (63) reported minimal limitation in range of motion in 7 patients with previous cases of osteochondritis in the elbow.

Wadley and Albright (172) investigated injury patterns in female gymnasts over a 4-year period. To identify which injuries resulted in persistent impairment, these same athletes were contacted again 3 years later. Responding gymnasts reported 41 of 92 previous gymnastics-related injuries (45%) still bothered them at that time, especially low back, ankle, great toe, shoulder, and knee injuries. However, most former gymnasts continued to be active despite complaints of pain and stiffness.

## 5. Injury Risk Factors

Results of analytic gymnastic injury studies are summarized in Table 14.17 and discussed below

**Table 14.15    Case Reports and Case Series of Catastrophic Injuries Occurring in Men's and Women's Gymnastics**

| Study | Design | No. of subjects | Age | Competitive level | Apparatus | Condition/diagnosis |
|---|---|---|---|---|---|---|
| Evans, 1979 | Case | 2 F | 13, 14 | — | Trampoline | Nonfatal[a] |
| Hammer et al., 1981 (cited in Torg, 1987) | Case | 2 M | 18, 30 | Elite | Minitramp | Nonfatal |
| Ferrandez et al., 1989 | Case | 1 F | 14 | — | — | Serious[b] |
| Swärd et al., 1990a | Case | 2 F | 15 | Elite | — | Serious |
| Noden, 1994 | Case | 1 F | — | — | Vaulting | Fatal[c] |
| Rapp & Nicely, 1978* | Case series | 34 M/F | — | — | Trampoline | 31 nonfatal; 3 fatal |
| Christensen & Clarke, 1982 | Case series | 1 F | 16 | Skilled[d] | Minitramp | Nonfatal |
|  |  | 13 M | 14-35 | Skilled[d] | Minitramp (4); trampoline (9) | Fatal (1); nonfatal (12) |
| Silver et al., 1986** | Case series | 35 M 3 F | — | Club, school, service, recreation | Trampette, springboard, trampoline | Most injuries led to paralysis and total incapacity |
| Noguchi, 1994 | Case series | 7 F/1 M | — | — | — | Spinal injuries resulting in paralysis |

*Proportion of competitive gymnasts not provided; however, one of the fatalities involved a national team male gymnast using a minitramp.

**Proportion of competitive gymnasts not provided.

[a]Permanent, severe functional disability such as quadriplegia.

[b]Permanent, functional disability such as a fractured vertebra with no permanent paralysis.

[c]Resulting in death.

[d]Skilled novice, skilled, highly skilled, expertly skilled.

with reference to intrinsic or extrinsic risk factors. The data should be interpreted cautiously due to the methodological problems and study differences mentioned earlier. Further, risk factors may interact differently with the categories of injury onset, a possibility which was not accounted for in most of the studies reviewed. Risk factors identified should be viewed as initial steps in the important search for predictor variables and may provide interesting characteristics for manipulation in other experimental designs.

## 5.1 Intrinsic Factors

### 5.1.1 Physical Characteristics

Results of cross-sectional studies indicated that female gymnasts were characterized by more musculoskeletal symptoms in the wrist, low back, hip, shin, and foot regions (73) and averaged greater ulnar variance (35, 96) than control subjects. Because these data were cross-sectional, one cannot determine with absolute certainty whether observed group differences resulted from gymnastics

participation or if children with more musculoskeletal symptoms and positive ulnar variance are more likely to become and continue to be gymnasts. Intuitively, however, it seems reasonable to expect a greater prevalence of musculoskeletal symptoms and positive ulnar variance in gymnasts. Similarly, due to greater impact loads, it is reasonable that taller, heavier gymnasts would be at increased risk of physeal injury at the distal radius given the same training loads (e.g., hours training) as their shorter, lighter counterparts (35).

A review of the prospective studies in Table 14.17 indicates that in comparison with low injury risk or injury-free gymnasts, the injured or injury-prone gymnasts tended to be characterized by rapid growth, with greater body size, age, and body fat. Thus, it would seem that the tall, heavy, early-maturing gymnast (with a high percent body fat) is especially susceptible to injury (103). Steele & White's (146) retrospective analyses generally support this hypothesis; however, their results should be viewed cautiously because the measures were taken after injury occurred, creating the possibility that injury itself caused the observed difference (104).

**Table 14.16    A Comparison of Catastrophic Injury Rates in Men's and Women's Gymnastics**

| Study | Duration | Injuries | Condition | Rate # of cases/injuries per 1,000 athletes | Rate # cases/injuries per 100,000 participants |
|---|---|---|---|---|---|
| High school | | | | | |
| Clarke, 1977 | 3 years | 1 M | Permanent[a] | 0.1 | — |
| | (1973-1975) | 1 F | Permanent | 0[b] | — |
| Mueller & Cantu*, 1994 | 11 years | 1 M | Fatal[b] | — | 1.66 M |
| | (1982-1993) | 6 M/F | Nonfatal[c] | — | 1.66 M |
| | | | | — | 1.49 F |
| | | 3 F | Serious[d] | — | 0.9  F |
| College | | | | | |
| Clarke, 1977 | 3 years | 6 M | Permanent | 0.8 | — |
| | (1973-1975) | 3 F | Permanent | 0.3 | — |
| Mueller & Cantu, 1994 | 11 years | — | Fatal | — | — |
| | (1982-1993) | | | | |
| | | 2 M/F | Nonfatal | — | 10.46 M |
| | | | | — | 5.53 F |
| | | 1 M | Serious | — | 10.46 M |
| NCAA, 1994 | 9 years | 1 F | Nonfatal | — | — |
| | (1985-1994) | | | | |

*National Center for Catastrophic Sports Injury Research.

[a]Refers to permanent disability, including death, secondary to spinal cord injury.

[b]Not zero, but not rounding to 0.1/1000 athletes.

[c]Refers to permanent, severe functional disability such as quadriplegia.

[d]Refers to no permanent, functional disability such as a fractured vertebra with no permanent paralysis.

It is also possible that factors such as greater height, weight and age tend to characterize older gymnasts who tend to have more years training and participate in higher levels of training and competition. Older gymnasts may be more likely to sustain injury because they may attempt more risky movements and have greater exposure due to more prolonged practice. Age-related changes in body dimensions and composition may also place older gymnasts at higher injury risk (85). Notably, injury rates for female gymnasts were highest at the college level (see Table 14.1).

Somatotype and physical maturity may also be important variables for determining susceptibility to injury. Although somatotype was not a significant predictor of injury proneness, gymnasts characterized by endomorphic mesomorphy and balanced ectomorphy experienced the greatest time loss due to injury in one study (16). Steele and White (146) found mesomorphy to be negatively related to injury ($p < 0.05$); however, as mentioned previously their analyses were based on injury data obtained retrospectively; thus, the possibility that the injury itself caused the difference. It seems reasonable to expect that gymnasts characterized by somatotypes most congruent to the physical demands of their sport would also be most protected from injury. However, determination of the true nature of this relationship awaits confirmation by three-dimensional somatotype analyses comparing injured to noninjured gymnasts.

Due to such factors as increased moments of inertia (67), increased muscle–tendon tightness (107), and decreased physeal strength (12) the rapidly growing gymnast, regardless of age, may be at increased risk of injury. Studies of the incidence of growth plate injuries show a peak clinical occurrence at pubescence (7, 118). Caine (16) reported an increased injury risk ($p < 0.05$) associated with periods of rapid growth in his study of female gymnasts. However, these results were based on Tanner staging and await confirmation from height velocity data obtained longitudinally and related to individual injury rates.

### 5.1.2 Motor Characteristics

Lindner and Caine (83) reported speed (−), balance (−), endurance (+), and flexibility (+) to be significant injury predictors; however, these were not significant at all age and competitive levels studied. Further, the number of gymnasts in each

**Table 14.17   A Comparison of Analytical Epidemiologic Injury Studies in Women's Gymnastics**

| Study | Duration | Design | Method | n | Purpose | Results |
|---|---|---|---|---|---|---|
| Kirby et al., 1981 | | Cross-sectional | Interview; flexibility measurement | 95 | To determine if gymnasts have different musculoskeletal symptoms than nonathletic controls; to determine if gymnasts are more flexible | Gymnasts had significantly more musculoskeletal symptoms in the wrist, low back, hip, shin, and foot regions than the controls ($p < 0.01$). Gymnasts have greater shoulder flexion and horizontal abduction, lumbar flexion, hip extension, and toe-touching abilities ($p < 0.001$). |
| Mandelbaum et al., 1989 | | Cross-sectional | Radiographic | 38 | To determine ulnar variance differences between collegiate gymnasts and controls | College gymnasts had significantly greater ulnar variance (1.28-2.82 mm) than the controls who averaged −0.52 mm ($p < 0.0001$). |
| Teurlings & Mandelbaum, 1992 | | Cross-sectional | Radiographic | 43 | To determine ulnar variance differences between club-level gymnasts and controls | A tendency towards ulnar variance in gymnasts is observed beginning at an early age (11.7 yr; $p < 0.01$). |
| DeSmet et al., 1994 | | Cross-sectional | Radiographic | 201 | To determine the nature of the relationship between ulnar variance and selected host and environmental variables | Ulnar variance parameters were significantly correlated with height and weight ($p < 0.01$). Taller and heavier gymnasts have a longer ulna related to the radius. |
| Steele & White, 1986 | 2 years | Retrospective | Questionnaire | 40 | To determine whether high and low injury risk gymnasts could be identified. | High and low injury risk gymnasts could be classified with 70% and 79% accuracy; significant differences ($p < 0.05$ or better) were found in the following variables:<br><br>weight................high > low<br>height................high > low<br>age................high > low<br>mesomorphy................high < low<br>quetelet index................high < low<br>shoulder flexion................high < low<br>lumbar extension................high > low<br><br>Variables associated with injury risk ($p < .05$ or better): weight (+), mesomorphy (−), lumbar curvature (+), age (+), height (−). |
| Kerr & Minden, 1988 | 2 years | Retrospective | Questionnaire | 41 | To determine whether selected psychological variables (trait anxiety, locus of control, self-concept, and stressful life events) were related to number or severity of injuries | Moderately strong relationship between stressful life events and injury number ($r = 53$; $p < 0.01$) and between stressful life events and injury severity ($r = 53$; $p < 0.01$). |
| Pettrone & Ricciardelli, 1987 | 7 months | Prospective | Questionnaire | 542 | To identify physical parameters that predispose the athlete to injury | Duration and frequency of workouts in clubs with high injury rates were significantly greater ($p < 0.05$) than in clubs with low injury rates (20-30 hr/wk vs. 4-6 hrs/wk). |

| Study | Duration | Design | Method | n | Purpose | Results |
|---|---|---|---|---|---|---|
| Caine et al., 1989 | 1 year | Prospective | Interview | 50 | To identify the nature of the relationship between injury status and selected host and environmental factors | No significant canonical relationship between the predictor variables and the injury measures ($p = 0.11$); separate (Caine, 1988) multiple regression tests ($p < .05$) showed maturation rate associated with injury rate (+) and competitive level associated with time loss (+). |
| | | | | | To determine the extent to which group classification into high and low injury risk groups could be predicted | The results of discriminant analysis involving the criterion variable injury rate were not significant ($p = .10$); for the criterion variable individual proportion time loss, the groups were significantly different ($p < 0.05$) and could best be distinguished as a result of the contribution of competitive level (high > low) and maturation rate (high > low). 84.6% of high risk and 69.3% of low injury risk gymnasts were correctly classified. |
| Goodway et al., 1989 | 1 year | Prospective | Questionnaire | 6654 | To gain statistical verification for trends identified by descriptive means | Trends associated with increased injury risk: higher competitive level, smaller, less well-equipped facilities, and lower gymnast/coach ratio. |
| Lindner & Caine, 1990b | 3 years | Prospective | Interview | 68 | To distinguish injured from uninjured gymnasts | 85.2% of uninjured and 75.6% of the injured gymnasts were correctly classified; the best discriminating component variables were age/body size (injured > uninjured), gymnastic-specific flexibility (varied by competitive and age levels) and body fat (injured > uninjured). |
| | | | | | To identify injury predictors | Significant predictors ($p < 0.05$) of the injury measures (injury rate, time lost, previous injuries) were identified among the anthropometric and performance components, but were specific to the components and various age and competitive levels. Overall, training hr/wk was a positive predictor of time lost ($p < 0.01$). |
| Lindner & Caine, 1992 | 3 years | Prospective | Interview | 68 | To distinguish high- from low-level competitive gymnasts | 80% of low level and 100% of high-level gymnasts were correctly classified; time loss due to injury ($p < 0.001$) and number of previous injuries ($p < 0.05$) were significantly higher for the high-level gymnasts. |

age and competitive level were small, thus limiting the precision of analysis within subgroups (175).

Steele and White (146) found that injury proneness was associated with relatively low shoulder flexion and high lumbar extension. Since these measures were taken after the injury occurred, however, there is a possibility that the injury itself caused the observed difference (i.e., lower flexibility with higher injury) and could result in a misleadingly high statistical correlation (104). No doubt success in gymnastics depends on a certain minimum of joint looseness; yet flexibility is specifically difficult to define, and its relationship to injury remains conjectural.

Several studies, while not relating physiological characteristics to injury, have reported data that suggest the potential role of physiological variables in increased injury risk. Muscle weakness (106, 136) and poor bilateral and anterior posterior symmetry (61, 135, 137) have been shown in elite male and female gymnasts and young female gymnasts ages 9 to 11 years.

### 5.1.3 Psychological and Psychosocial Characteristics

An intriguing, but relatively unexplored area of injury research in gymnastics, is the role of psychological and psychosocial factors in injury occurrence. Kerr & Minden (71) reported a moderately strong positive relationship between the number of stressful life events and injury number and severity. They suggested that an accumulation of stressful life events may result in a lack of concentration that in turn is related to performance decrement and increased risk of injury. The difficulty with Kerr and Minden's study, however, is that the psychosocial measures were taken after the injury occurred; thus the possibility exists that the stress profile of the gymnasts was different at the time of injury than prior to injury.

## 5.2 Extrinsic Factors

### 5.2.1 Exposure

Number of years training since competitive initiation may be a risk factor for the development of certain chronic injuries. Based on a small case series, Dzioba (38) observed that the earlier children began serious training, the more serious the radiologic findings of the thoracolumbar spine. Teurlings and Mandelbaum (160) reported a tendency toward increased ulnar variance in gymnasts who begin training at an early age ($p < 0.01$). DeSmet et al. (35) did not find this relationship in

their radiographic study of European gymnasts but did report a positive correlation between carpal angle and age at which gymnasts began their training ($p < 0.05$). These results and the data shown in Tables 14.9-14.12 suggest that some chronic injuries may be more prevalent among advanced level gymnasts; however, determination of the relationship between age of competitive initiation and chronic injury awaits clarification from prospective cohort research that examines the presence of this risk factor longitudinally in both injured and noninjured gymnasts.

The number of injuries would naturally tend to increase with increasing competitive levels because as gymnasts become more skilled, there are more hours of practice and, thus, more exposure time and an increased opportunity for injury. One would also expect exposure injury rates to increase with higher levels of competition because advanced level gymnasts have more years training since competitive initiation and the technical difficulty of the skills they perform is also greater. The data for female gymnasts support this notion in all (18, 90, 108, 113, 176) but one study (83). Only one study subjected competitive level to statistical tests for correlation and predictive value. Interestingly, Caine (16) reported competitive level as a positive predictor of time loss due to injury, but not for injury rate. When time loss was used as a criterion variable, competitive level also surfaced as one of the best discriminators between high- and low-injury risk gymnasts (18).

Events associated with injury have attracted considerable attention in the gymnastics injury literature. Of concern has been whether a particular event(s) is disproportionately associated with injury. Unfortunately, most data in Table 14.18 represent both sudden and gradual onset injuries. In view of the difficulty determining the precise event associated with many overuse injuries, only studies relating sudden onset injuries to events will be addressed (18, 82, 119). Review of these studies indicates floor exercise was the event most often associated with injury in women's club-level gymnastics. This would seem a reasonable finding in view of the many elements practiced at floor exercise. Depending on the gymnastic club and the skill development needs of gymnasts, however, more time may be spent on some events than others. Thus, determination of injury incidence would provide a more reliable estimate of injury risk associated with various events. Notably, three recent studies involving college-level female gymnasts adopted this approach. In two studies (113, 139) floor exercise was associated with the greatest

**Table 14.18   A Percent Comparison of Events Associated With Injury in Women's Gymnastics**

| Study/event | Study design | No. of injuries | No. participant seasons* | Balance beam | Floor exercise | Uneven bars | Vaulting | Other |
|---|---|---|---|---|---|---|---|---|
| Club | | | | | | | | |
| Garrick & Requa, 1980 | P | 16 | 72 | 19.0 | 37.0 | 6.0 | 13.0 | 25.0 |
| Weiker, 1985 | P | 95 | 766 | 41.7 | 20.0 | 21.7 | 6.7 | 10.0 |
| Pettrone & Ricciardelli, 1987** | P | 29 | 2,558 | 25.5 | 41.2 | 11.8 | 21.6 | — |
| Caine et al., 1989** | P | 147 | 50 | 23.1 | 35.4 | 20.0 | 13.8 | 7.7 |
| Lindner & Caine, 1990** | P | 90 | 362 | 17.4 | 37.7 | 18.8 | 13.0 | 13.0 |
| Steele & White, 1983 | R | 146 | 268 | 11.6 | 20.5 | 15.0 | 31.5 | 21.4 |
| Kerr & Minden, 1988 | R | 41 | — | 31.0 | — | - | — | — |
| Mackie & Taunton, 1994 | R | 156 | 32.0 | 39.0 | 18.0 | 6.0 | 5.0 | — |
| High school | | | | | | | | |
| Garrick & Requa, 1980 (2 years) | P | — | — | 21.0 | 38.0 | 18.0 | 5.0 | 18.0 |
| Garrick & Requa, 1980 (1 year) | P | — | — | 12.0 | 49.0 | 10.0 | 11.0 | 18.0 |
| College | | | | | | | | |
| Garrick & Requa, 1980 | P | — | 24 | 6.0 | 47.0 | 12.0 | 12.0 | 23.0 |
| Clarke & Buckley, 1980 | P | | | | | | | |
| 1975-76 | | — | — | 15.0 | 59.0 | 12.0 | 15.0 | 0 |
| 1976-77 | | — | — | 25.0 | 25.0 | 38.0 | 13.0 | 0 |
| 1977-78 | | — | — | 23.0 | 33.0 | 25.0 | 17.0 | 2.0 |
| Sands et al., 1987 | | | | | | | | |
| 1984-85 | P | 54 | 10 | — | — | 24.0 | — | 22.2 |
| 1985-86 | P | 70 | 13 | — | 27.1 | — | — | 24.3 |
| Wadley & Albright, 1993 | P | 106 | 53 | 26.7 | 28.3 | 31.7 | 13.3 | 0 |
| NCAA injury SS (1985-94) | P | 2,260 | — | 14.5 | 33.6 | 21.3 | 14.5 | 16.1 |

*A participant in one gymnast participating in one season.

**Sudden onset injuries only.

*Note.* P = prospective study; R = retrospective study.

incidence of injury. In the third report, which was a 2-year study (138), uneven bars caused the highest injury rate during the 1st year and floor exercise during the 2nd year.

Only two studies reported events associated with injury in men's gymnastics. Lueken et al. (88) reported on 345 injuries affecting club level gymnasts attending the U.S. Olympic Training Center over a 1.5-year period. Floor exercise was most often associated with injury (24.9%), followed by still rings (19.2%), horizontal bar (16.9%), parallel bars (16.4%), pommel horse (14.7%), and vault (7.9%). NCAA results (113) indicate that floor exercise was the event associated with the highest injury rate during the 1993-1994 season, followed by the horizontal bar and pommel horse.

### 5.2.2 Training Conditions

Insufficient spotting or no spotting have been suggested as risk factors for acute and catastrophic injury (27, 140). Several studies indicate a greater proportion (82, 119, 176) and rate (113) of injuries occurring when the injured gymnasts were unassisted. No doubt spotting is of great value in preventing injuries, particularly in the early stages of skill learning and for off-apparatus landings. Indeed, hand-spotting is performed by the majority of coaches every day (133). Yet it is the nature of gymnastics to progress to a point where spotting is no longer needed. Thus exposure to injury is likely greater when the gymnast is unassisted.

Training errors or inappropriate control of volume and intensity, placement of conditioning volume and intensity, and general poor planning have been shown to occur in women's gymnastics (133). The prevalence of on-apparatus trauma in catastrophic injuries suggests premature attempts to execute advanced maneuvers (27, 116). Other coaching techniques may also be implicated, especially long practices with few rotations that may lead to lack of concentration and inattentiveness. Notably, Lindner & Caine (82) found that many injuries happened with moves that were basic or of moderate difficulty and that had been well established.

### 5.2.3 Environment

Two studies (18, 82) analyzed time elapsed in practice when sudden onset injuries occurred. The results showed a disproportionate number of injuries occurring early in practice contrary to a cumulative fatigue effect and suggesting the possibility of a qualitatively or quantitatively insufficient warm-up in the gymnasts studied. Other possible explanations include the possibility that appropriate progressions were not provided and that gymnasts may practice difficult skills earlier in practice when they are freshest.

Several women's injury studies reported time of season when injury occurs (18, 36, 71, 130, 138, 139). This is relevant information because the training emphasis varies according to time of year. The results of these analyses indicate a relative increase in injury rates

- following periods of reduced training or a short vacation (18, 138, 139)—perhaps due to the shock of increased workload demands on relatively untrained athletes (139);
- during competitive routine preparation (18, 138, 139)—perhaps due to increased fatigue during performance of longer combinations and routines or hurried attempts to prepare routines with skills that were not thoroughly learned (138);
- during the weeks just prior to competition (71, 139)—perhaps due to heightened competitive anxiety or stress (71, 139) or performing skills that are not thoroughly learned (129); and
- during competition (18, 139; see also Table 14.3)—perhaps due to the fact that gymnasts were much better protected in training than in competition because of spotting, and the opportunity to land on softer mats or in foam pits (139).

### 5.2.4 Equipment

Intuitively, it seems reasonable that a poorly equipped facility would be associated with an increased incidence of injury, as reported by Goodway et al. (51). However, there may also be a tendency for gymnasts and coaches at more well-equipped facilities to attempt more difficult and dangerous skills that they would not have tried under less (apparently) safe circumstances. This has been shown in the elevated levels of difficulty with equipment and matting enhancements. When spring floors, spring beams, thicker landing mats, and fiber glass rails were instituted, there was a marked increase in performance difficulty. In spite of the fact that these changes in equipment were instituted for safety/injury prevention reasons, the level of skill difficulty increased and perhaps reduced the long-term effectiveness of safer equipment.

## 6. Suggestions for Injury Prevention

The purpose of this manuscript is to suggest ways to facilitate performance, minimize injury morbidity, and prevent injury in the future. It is of course desirable to suggest methods for injury prevention that are based on risk factors whose predictive value has been demonstrated. Unfortunately, our overview of the gymnastics injury literature reveals that few risk factors have been subjected to statistical tests for correlation or evaluated for predictive value. Further, risk factors that were subjected to risk factor analysis are of limited value due to the methodological problems discussed earlier in this chapter. Yet because the institution of a preventive strategy based on intuition may still prevent injury (104), it is incumbent upon us to offer our best data-based recommendations for injury prevention. We acknowledge that many of these suggestions were derived from somewhat unwieldy data and await confirmation from more controlled epidemiologic studies to evaluate their effectiveness in preventing injuries.

Recommended preventive measures are organized around the gymnasts, the sport, the gymnastics environment, and the health support system. Recommendations are referenced, where appropriate, to indicate source and any available supporting evidence. While it is useful to organize preventive measures in this way, it is important to emphasize that prevention of gymnastics injury is a complex phenomenon that requires interaction among gymnast, parent, coach, gymnastics federation, and medical support staff. A multidisciplinary team including coach, conditioner, rehabilitator, psychologist, and physician is essential to optimizing the preventive strategies.

### 6.1 The Gymnasts

The first line of protection from injury lies with the gymnast. A well-educated and thoroughly trained gymnast will often detect and avoid many potentially injurious situations (131). Gymnasts should be educated from an early age to detect the early signs of stress injury and to seek appropriate treatment and modification of training. They should know when they are performing skills that are beyond their current capacity and voice their concerns to the coach. Finally, they should understand the importance of general fitness and warm-up procedures in relation to later performance and injury avoidance, the importance of proper nutrition, and the need to avoid excess weight gain or loss.

## 6.2 Sport

The knowledge of a coach is logically assumed to be related to injury prevention. Coaches at all levels should be required to meet a minimum level of qualification necessary to meet the responsibilities of coaching (20, 143). Further, coaches should be required to enroll in continuing education programs. Examples of important knowledge and principles that should be included in the education of coaches are as follows:

- alternate loading types during workouts (e.g., alternate swinging and support movements to reduce stress on the wrist; 95);
- emphasis on quality of workouts rather than chronic repetitiveness at all times; utilization of aerobic, anaerobic and cross-training techniques, as well as imagery techniques that cause no physical impact, may allow a gymnast to work more hours without increased injury risk;
- excessive pressure from coaches and parents should be avoided (143);
- training should be done in a cyclically progressive manner so the athlete is not increasing the dose of load bearing in a progressive stepwise fashion but rather in a cyclical manner; every escalation is followed by a decrease in overall load for a week's time, followed by another increase, thereby allowing reparative time for connective tissue structures (95);
- individualize training and skill development to accommodate possible size, build, strength, performance, and maturity differences among chronological age peers (19, 20);
- knowledge of skills development, safety rules, and equipment maintenance (143);
- pain is a signal in an important process and should be regarded as a warning, not something to get used to (103); "no pain–no gain" is inappropriate;

- reduce duration of rotations and increase their number per workout to avoid lack of concentration and inattentiveness (82);
- reduce training loads during periods of rapid growth (12, 17, 18, 67, 107)
- the existence or potential for growth plate injury and the importance of referring the gymnast for medical evaluation as soon as symptoms occur (21, 128);
- the importance of protecting gymnasts from premature attempts to execute advanced maneuvers (27);
- the importance of fitness development and warm-up procedures in relation to later performance and injury avoidance; and
- the importance of encouraging gymnasts to share with their coach and parents any concerns they have about difficulty of skills practiced or pain experienced.

## 6.3 External Environment

The training environment of gymnasts has progressed slowly to its current state of foam pits, thick mats, bungee tumbling and trampoline systems, multiple-use spotting belts, and other safety equipment. Several decades ago there were large differences in the quality of training facilities. Most of these differences have vanished today. Protective equipment, both personal and gymnasium based, is in common use by most gymnasts. Because injury rates appear much greater during competition (see Table 14.3), it seems reasonable to suggest using some types of safety equipment during competitive events. Goldstein et al. (50), for example, suggested using thicker landing mats during competition to reduce mechanical loading on the spine.

## 6.4 Health Support System

The health support system of gymnastics has never been more important than in modern gymnastics training. However, medical monitoring of gymnasts is rare in gymnastics settings below the college level. We recommend that a preparticipation physical examination (PPE) be administered to each gymnast prior to entry into competitive gymnastics, before any change in competitive level, and before returning to practice following injury (20). The medical history and physical examination can define underlying conditions that require special protection or treatment or that predispose the gymnast to injury unless special training programs or precautions are followed (143). In conjunction with the PPE, it would be helpful to encourage dialogue on important health issues between parents, coaches, gymnasts and physician.

We further recommend that gymnastic clubs include within their cost structure sufficient funds to hire an athletic trainer or physical therapist, at least on a part-time basis (20, 143). The functions of this individual should include the following:

- early detection of developing stress injuries;
- identification of potential injury-provoking practices (143);
- act as liaison between gymnasts, coaches, and physician (143);
- development of special rehabiliation programs for injured gymnasts or injury-prone gymnasts identified in the PPE; and
- supervision of cross-training techniques.

It would also be ideal to have a sport psychologist and nutritionist present for multiple lectures,

counseling sessions, or both with individual athletes. In addition to enhancing performance, these individuals may prove of particular value in counseling gymnasts for psychological or nutritional problems that could lead to an injury or retard recovery from injury (143). The presence of the sport psychologist may be particularly important around the time of competitions (71).

# 7. Suggestions for Further Research

An important purpose of this chapter has been to identify methodological weaknesses in the literature and provide suggestions for further research. This is an integral component of the epidemiology of sports injuries because informed decisions related to the establishment of injury prevention programs depend on accurate and reliable data. Above all, this scientific overview of the gymnastics injury

**Table 14.19    Suggestions for Further Research**

| Research component | Research directions/questions |
| --- | --- |
| **Incidence of injury** | |
| Injury rates | • Define injury as any damaged body part that interferes with training and is recorded on the first day of onset and every day thereafter until it does not interfere with training |
| | • Injury rates should be expressed as # injuries per 1,000 hrs. training or per athletic exposure (AE) |
| | • Explore using more sensitive indicators of exposure (e.g., # of elements per unit time) in determining injury rates |
| | • Determine injury rates for the various competitive levels |
| Reinjury rates | • Classification criteria for reinjury should include same body part, body side, type, nature of onset, and history of injury the previous year; at least 2 injury-free days must intervene between an injury and reinjury |
| | • Cross-tabulate reinjury data with injury location, injury types, injury onset, and competitive level |
| | • Define reinjury as injury involving same body side, location, injury type, injury onset, occurring during current or previous year |
| Practice vs. competition | • Videotape competitive events to obtain a clearer picture of injury mechanisms |
| | • Determine separate injury rates for practice and competition |
| | • Cross-tabulate with injury type, location, and severity |
| **Injury type and location** | |
| Injury onset | • Determine injury proportions (%) and incidence of chronic and acute injuries |
| | • Cross-tabulate with injury types, location, and severity |
| | • Determine injury proportion and incidence for acute injuries that are superimposed on chronic mechanisms |
| Injury types | • Determine injury proportions and incidence |
| | • Cross-tabulate injury types with injury location and severity |
| | • Include classifications to accommodate childhood injury types (e.g., apophyseal, physeal) |
| Injury location | • Determine injury proportions and incidence for the various injury locations |
| | • Cross-tabulate location with injury onset, injury types, and injury severity |
| Spine/trunk | • Determine incidence and mechanism(s) of stress injuries affecting the growing spine [e.g., vertebral endplate abnormalities, spondylolysis (see Tables 14.9-14.10)] |
| Upper extremity | • Determine incidence and mechanism(s) of stress injuries affecting the elbow and wrist [e.g., positive ulnar variance, OD of the humeral capitellum (see Tables 14.11 and 14.12)] |
| Lower extremity | • Determine incidence and mechanisms for chronic and acute injuries affecting the apophyses and physes of the lower extremities [e.g., calcaneal apophysitis, distal tibial growth plate fracture) |
| | • Determine incidence and mechanisms for compression neuropathies (see Tables 14.13 and 14.14) |

| Research component | Research directions/questions |
|---|---|
| **Injury severity** | |
| Time loss | • Determine time loss rates due to injury (i.e., number of exposure units lost per 1,000 exposure units) |
| | • Determine mean time loss per injury and per individual |
| | • Categorize time loss injuries at < 8 days, 8-21 days, and > 21 days |
| | • Cross-tabulate injury onset, injury types, and injury location with time loss |
| Catastrophic injury | • Determine incidence and mechanism(s) for club-level male and female gymnasts |
| Clinical outcome | • Determine proportion of gymnasts who withdraw from gymnastics permanently due to injury |
| | • Determine medical costs associated with injury |
| | • Follow up on previous surveillance samples to determine residue and complaints associated with previous injury |
| **Injury risk factors** | |

Since risk factors for chronic and acute injuries may be different it seems reasonable to suggest separate as well as combined risk factor analyses for these injury categories. With sufficient numbers of injuries/subjects, one might also wish to pursue the relationship between certain risk factors and specific injury types (e.g., physeal injury).

| | |
|---|---|
| Intrinsic factors | |
| Physical factors | • Growth rate, anthropometric characteristics, previous injury, body composition, overall somatotype, body symmetry, eating disorders, dietary intake, and bone density |
| Motor/fitness factors | • Strength, aerobic and anaerobic capacity, flexibility, power, speed, balance, and reaction time. |
| Psychological factors | • Stressful life events, cautiousness, trait anxiety, locus of control, extroversion, acting out, risk-taking behavior, and self-concept |
| Extrinsic factors | |
| Exposure | • Training hours, training elements, competitive level, years since competitive initiation, duration and frequency of practice sessions |
| Training conditions | • Gymnast/coach ratio, coach qualifications, skill difficulty, nature and extent of warmup, and training techniques for skill and fitness development |
| Environment | • Time into practice and time at station |
| Equipment | • Type and condition of apparatus, type of matting, thickness of matting, and protective equipment used |
| **Injury prevention** | • Evaluate effectiveness of injury prevention programs by conducting further prospective study, ideally with a control group |

literature underscores the need for well-designed epidemiologic studies.

We recommend large-scale prospective cohort studies of injuries involving male and female gymnasts, particularly at the club level. Populations of gymnasts should be assembled prior to being exposed to injury and followed longitudinally to study their outcome. Injury data should be analyzed according to gender. Suggestions for further research that are specific to our chapter headings are shown in Table 14.19. It is hoped that these suggestions will prove helpful in guiding future research initiatives.

In closing, it is important to stress that optimal results can be achieved only through concerted collaborative efforts. The research team must include the parent, coach, athlete, physician, nutritionist, psychologist, athletic trainer, and epidemiologist who interact in a very dynamic and fluid manner.

# References

1. Abrams, J.; Bennett, E.; Kumar, S.J.; Pizzutillo, P.D. Salter-Harris type III fracture of the proximal fibula. A case report. Am. J. Sports Med. 14:514-516; 1986.

2. Albanese, S.A.; Palmer, A.K.; Kerr, D.R.; Carpenter, C.W.; Lisi, D.; Levinsohn, E.M. Wrist pain and distal growth plate closure of the radius in gymnasts. J. Ped. Orthop. 9:23-28; 1989.

3. Andrews, M.; Noyes, F.R.; Barber-Westin, S.D. Anterior cruciate ligament allograft reconstruction in the skeletally immature athlete. Am. J. Sports Med. 22(1):48-54; 1994.

4. Andrish, J.T. Knee injuries in gymnastics. Clin. Sports Med. 4:111-121; 1985.

5. Auberge, T.; Zenny, J.C.; Duvallet, A.; Godefroy, D.; Horreard, P.; Chevrot, A. Study of bone maturation and osteo-articular lesions in top level sportsmen: a review of 105 cases. Journal de Radiologie (Paris) 65:555-561; 1984.

6. Backx, F.J.G.; Beijer, H.J.M.; Bol, E.; Erick, W.B.M. Injuries in high-risk persons and high-risk sports. A longitudinal study of 1818 school children. Am. J. Sports Med. 19:124-130; 1991.

7. Bailey, D.A.; Wedge, J.H.; McCulloch, R.G.; Martin, A.D. The relationship of fractures of the distal radius to growth velocity in children. Can. J. Sport Sci. 13:40-41; 1988.

8. Barron, J.L.; Yocum, L.A. Unrecognized achilles tendon rupture associated with ipsilateral medial malleolar fracture. Am. J. Sports Med. 21(4):629-631; 1993.

9. Bick, E.M.; Copel, J.W. Longitudinal growth of the human vertebra. J. Bone Jt. Surg. 32-A:803-814; 1950.

10. Biedert, R. Which investigations are required in stress fracture of the great toe sesamoids? Arch. Orthop. Trauma Surg. 112:94-95; 1993.

11. Bozdech, Z.; Dufek, P. Spondylolisthesis in young gymnasts. Acta Universitatis Carolinae Medica 32:405-409; 1986.

12. Bright, R.W.; Burnstein, A.H.; Elmore, S.W. Epiphyseal plate cartilage: A biomechanic and histological analysis of failure modes. J. Bone Jt. Surg. 56A (4):688-703; 1974.

13. Brozin, I.H.; Martfel, J.; Goldberg, I.; Kuritzky, A. Traumatic closed femoral nerve neuropathy. J. Trauma 22:158-160; 1982.

14. Bruijn, J.D.; Sanders, R.J.; Jansen, B.R.H. Ossification in the patellar tendon and patella alta following sports injuries in children. Complications of sleeve fractures after conservative treatment. Arch. Orthop. Trauma Surg. 112:157-158; 1993.

15. Burks, R.T.; Lock, T.R.; Negendank, W.G. Occult tibial fracture in a gymnast: diagnosis by magnetic resonance imaging. A case report. Am. J. Sports Med. 20:88-91; 1992.

16. Caine, D. An epidemiological investigation of injuries affecting young competitive female gymnasts. Doctoral Dissertation. University of Oregon Microform Publications; 1988.

17. Caine, D.; Broekhoff, J. Maturity assessment: a viable preventive measure against physical and pschyological insult to the young athlete? Phys. Sportsmed. 15:67-80; 1987.

18. Caine, D.; Cochrane, B.; Caine, C.; Zemper, E. An epidemiological investigation of injuries affecting young competitive female gymnasts. Am. J. Sports Med. 17:811-820; 1989.

19. Caine, D.; Lindner, K. Overuse injuries of growing bones: the young female gymnast at risk? Phys. Sportsmed. 13:51-64; 1985.

20. Caine, D.; Lindner, K. Preventing injury to young athletes. Part 2: Preventive measures. CAHPER J. 56(5):24-30; 1990.

21. Caine, D.; Roy, S.; Singer, K.; Broekhoff, J. Stress changes of the distal radial growth plate. A radiographic survey of 60 young competitive gymnasts and an epidemiologic review of the related literature. Am. J. Sports Med. 20:290-298; 1992.

22. Cantu, R.C. Catastrophic injuries in high school and collegiate athletes. Surg. Rounds Orthop. 2:62-66; 1988.

23. Carek, P.J.; Fumich, R.M. Stress fracture of the distal radius. Not just a risk for elite gymnasts. Phys. Sportsmed. 20(5):115-118; 1992.

24. Carter, S.R., Aldridge, M.J. Stress injury of the distal radial growth plate. J. Bone Jt. Surg. 70-B(5):834-836; 1988.

25. Chan, D.; Aldridge, M.J.; Maffuli, N.; Davies, A.M. Chronic stress injuries of the elbow in young gymnasts. Brit. J. Radiol. 64:1113-1118; 1991.

26. Christensen, C.; Clarke, K. Fourth annual national gymnastic catastrophic injury report 1981-82. Urbana-Champaign, IL; College of Applied Life Studies, University of Illinois, 1982:1-35.

27. Clarke, K.S. A survey of sports-related spinal cord injuries in schools and colleges, 1973-1975. J. Safety Res. 9:140-146; 1977.

28. Clarke, K.S. Women's injuries in collegiate sports. Am. J. Sports Med. 8(3):187-191; 1980.

29. Clarke, K.S.; Buckley, W.E. Women's injuries in collegiate sports. A preliminary comparative overview of three seasons. Am. J. Sports Med. 8:187-191; 1980.

30. Clarke, K.S.; Miller, S.J. The national athletic injury/illness reporting system (NAIRS). In: Morehouse, C.H., ed. Sports safety II. Proceedings of the second national sports safety conference. Washington: The American Alliance for Health, Physical Education and Recreation; 1977:41-53.

31. D'Allessandro, D.F.; Shields, C.L.; Tibone, J.E.; Chandler, R.W. Repair of distal biceps tendon ruptures in athletes. Am. J. Sports Med. 21(1):114-119; 1993.

32. Danneker, D.A.; Mandetta, D.F.; Rockower, R. Case report: intra-abdominal injury in a gymnast. Phys. Sportsmed. 7:119-120; 1979.

33. Del Pizzo, W.; Norwood, L.A.; Jobe, F.W.; Blazina, M.E.; Fox, J.M. Rupture of the biceps tendon in gymnastics. Am. J. Sports Med. 6:283-285; 1978.

34. DeSmet, L.; Claessens, A; Fabrey, G. Gymnast wrist. Acta Orthopaedica Belgica 59(4):377-380; 1993.

35. DeSmet, L; Claessens, A.; Lefevre, J.; DeCorte, F.; Beunen, G.; Stijnen, V.; Maes, H.; Veer, F.M. Gymnast wrist: an epidemiological survey of the ulnar variance in elite female gymnasts. Am. J. Sports Med. 22(6):846-850; 1994.

36. Dixon, M.; Fricker, P. Injuries to elite gymnasts over 10 yr. Med. Sci. Sports Exer. 25:1322-1329; 1993.

37. Donati, R.B.; Cox, S.; Echo, B.S.; Powell, C.E. Bilateral simultaneous patellar tendon rupture in a female collegiate gymnast. A case report. Am. J. Sports Med. 14:237-239; 1986.

38. Dzioba, R.B. Irreversible spinal deformity in olympic gymnasts. Orthop. Trans. 8:66; 1984.

39. Dzioba, R.B. Gymnastics. In Schneider, R.C.; Kennedy, J.C.; Plant, M.L., eds. Sports injuries. Mechanisms, prevention, and treatment. Baltimore: Williams and Wilkins; 1985:139-162.

40. Eisenberg, I.; Allen, W.C. Injuries in a women's varsity athletic program. Phys. Sports Med. 6:112-121; 1978.

41. Evans, R.F. Tetraplegia caused by gymnastics. Brit. Med. J. 2(6192):732; 1979.

42. Ferrandez, L.; Usabiaga, J.; Curto, J.M.; Alonso, A.; Martin, F. Atypical multivertebral fracture due to hyperextension in an adolescent girl. A case report. Spine 6:645-646; 1989.

43. Fliegel, C.P. Stress related widening of the radial growth plate in adolescents. Annales de Radiologie 29:374-376; 1986.

44. Fulton, N.; Albright, J.P.; El-Khoury, G.Y. Cortical desmoid-like lesion of the proximal humerus and its occurrence in gymnasts (Ringman's shoulder lesion). Am. J. Sports Med. 7:57-61; 1979.

45. Garrick, J.G.; Requa, R.K. Injuries in high school sports. Pediatrics 61:465-469; 1978.

46. Garrick, J.G.; Requa, R.K. Epidemiology of women's gymnastics injuries. Am. J. Sports Med. 8:261-264; 1980.

47. Giuliani, G.; Poppi, M.; Acciarri, N.; Forti, A. CT scan and surgical treatment of traumatic iliacus hematoma with femoral neuropathy: case report. J. Trauma 30:229-231; 1990.

48. Goldberg, M.J. Gymnastic injuries. Orthop. Clin. N. Am. 11(4):717-726.

49. Goldberg, V.M.; Aadalen, R. Distal tibial epiphyseal injuries: the role of athletics in 53 cases. Am. J. Sports Med. 6:263-268; 1978.

50. Goldstein, J.D.; Berger, P.E.; Windler, G.E.; Jackson, D.W. Spine injuries in gymnasts and swimmers: an epidemiologic investigation. Am. J. Sports Med. 19:463-468; 1991.

51. Goodway, J.D.; McNaught-Davis, J.P.; White, J. The distribution of injuries among young female gymnasts in relation to selected training and environmental factors. In: Beunen, G., ed. Children and exercise XIV. Band 4. Schriftenreihe der Hamburg-Mannheimer-Stiftung fur Informationsmedizeft Enke Verlag; 1989.

52. Greene, T.L.; Hensinger, R.N.; Hunter, L.Y. Back pain and vertebral changes simulating Scheuermann's disease. J. Ped. Orthop. 5:1-7; 1985.

53. Hall, S.J. Mechanical contribution to lumbar stress injuries in female gymnasts. Med. Sci. Sports Exer. 18:599-602; 1986.

54. Hammer, A.; Schwartzbasck, A.L.; Darre, E. Svaere neurologiske skader some folge af trampolinspring. Ugeske Laeger 143: 2970-2974; 1981. In: Torg, J.S. Trampoline-induced quadriplegia. Clin. Sports Med. 6(1):73-85; 1987.

55. Hanks, G.A.; Kalenak, A.; Bowman, L.S.; Sebastianelli, W.J. Stress fractures of the carpal scaphoid. J. Bone Jt. Surg. 71-A:938-941; 1989.

56. Hellström, M.; Jacobsson, B.; Swärd, L.; Peterson L. Radiologic abnormalities of the thoraco-lumbar spine in athletes. Acta Radiol. 31:127-132; 1990.

57. Hermsdorfer, J.D.; Kleinman, W.B. Management of chronic peripheral tears of the triangular fibrocartilage complex. J. Hand Surg. 16A(2):340-346; 1991.

58. Hirasawa, Y.; Sakakida, K. Sports and peripheral nerve injury. Am. J. Sports Med. 11:420-426; 1983.

59. Holden, D.L.; Jackson, D.W. Stress fracture in the ribs of female rowers. Am. J. Sports Med. 13:342-348; 1985

60. Hunter, L.Y., & Torgan, C. Dismounts in gymnastics: should scoring be reevaluated? Am. J. Sports Med. 11:208-210; 1983.

61. Irvin, R.; Major, J.; Sands, W.A. Lower body and torso strength norms for elite female gymnasts. In: McNitt-Gray, J.L.; Girandola, R.; Callaghan, J., eds.

1992 USGF sport science congress proceedings. Indianapolis: USGF Publications; 1992:5-12.

62. Jackson, D.S.; Furman, W.K.; Berson, B.L. Patterns of injuries in college athletes: a retrospective study of injuries sustained in intercollegiate athletics in two colleges over a two-year period. Mount Sinai J. Med. 47:423-426; 1980.

63. Jackson, D.W.; Silvino, N.; Reiman, P. Osteochondritis in the female gymnast's elbow. Arthroscopy 5:129-136; 1989.

64. Jackson, D.W.; Wiltse, L.L.; Cirincione, R.J. Spondylolysis in the female gymnast. Clin. Orthop. 117:68-73; 1976.

65. Jackson, D.W.; Wiltse, L.L.; Dingeman, R.D.; Hayes, M. Stress reactions involving the pars interarticularis in young athletes. Am. J. Sports Med. 9:304-312; 1981.

66. Jahn, W.T. Spontaneously reduced partial shoulder dislocation: a case report and literature review. J. Manipulative Phys. Therap. 5:21-24; 1982.

67. Jenson, R.K. The growth of children's moment of inertia. Med. Sci. Sports Exerc. 13:238-242; 1986.

68. Johnson, K.M. Where have all the gymnasts gone? JOPERD March:28-29; 1985.

69. Jones, A. Training of young athletes study. London: The Sports Council; 1992.

70. Kerr, G.A. Injuries in artistic gymnastics. J. Can. Athlet. Ther. Assoc. April:19-21; 1991.

71. Kerr, G.A.; Minden, H. Psychological factors related to the occurrence of athletic injuries. J. Sport Exer. Psych. 10:167-173; 1988.

72. Kinolik, Z.; Garhammer, J.; Gregor, R.J. Kinetic and kinematic factors involved in the execution of front aerial somersaults. Med. Sci. Sports Exer. 12(5):352-356; 1980.

73. Kirby, R.L.; Simms, F.C.; Symington, V.J.; Garner, J.B. Flexibility and musculoskeletal symptomatology in female gymnasts and age-matched controls. Am. J. Sports Med. 9:160-164; 1981.

74. Knight, N.A.; Burleson, R.J.; Higginbotham, J.A. Spondylolysis of the L-2 vertebra in a female gymnast. J. Med. Assoc. State Ala. 47:25-27; 1977.

75. Kopp, P.M.; Reid, J.G. A force torque analysis of giant swings on the horizontal bar. Can. J. Appl. Sport Sciences 5(2):98-102; 1980.

76. Krueger-Franke, M.; Siebert, C.H.; Pfoerringer, W. Sports-related epiphyseal injuries of the lower extremity. J. Sports Med. Phys. Fit. 32(1):106-111; 1992.

77. Lepse, P.S.; McCarthy, R.E.; McCullough, F.L. Simultaneous bilateral avulsion fracture of the tibial tuberosity: a case report. Clin. Orthop. Related Res. 229:232-235; 1988.

78. Letts, M.; Smallman, T.; Afanasiev, R.; Gouw, G. Fracture of the pars interarticularis in adolescent athletes: a clinical-biomechanical analysis. J. Ped. Orthop. 6:40-46; 1986.

79. Levi, J.H., & Coleman, C.R. Fracture of the tibial tubercle. Am. J. Sports Med. 4:254-263; 1976.

80. Li, D.K.B.; Lloyd-Smith, R. Wrist pain in an adolescent gymnast. Clin. J. Sports Med. 1:259-261; 1991.

81. Lindholm, C.; Hagenfeldt, K.; Ringertz, B. Pubertal development in elite juvenile gymnasts. Effects of physical training. Acta Obstet. Gynecol. Scand. 73:269-273; 1994.

82. Lindner, K.J.; Caine, D. Injury patterns of female competitive club gymnasts. Can J. Sport Sci. 15:254-261; 1990a.

83. Lindner, K.J.; Caine, D. Injury predictors among female gymnasts' anthropometric and performance characteristics. In: Hermans, G.P.; Mosterd, W.L., eds. Sports, medicine and health. Amsterdam: Excerpta Medica; 1990b:136-141.

84. Lindner, K.J.; Caine, D. Physical and performance differences between female gymnasts competing at high and low levels. J. Hum. Move. St. 23:1-15; 1992.

85. Lindner, K.J.; Caine, D. Physical and performance characteristics of injured and injury-free female gymnasts. J. Hum. Mov. Stud. 25:69-83; 1993.

86. Lishen, Q.; Jianhua, O. Epiphyseal injury in gymnasts. Chin. J. Sports Med. (China) 2:7-12; 1983. In: Caine, D. Growth plate injury and bone growth. An update. Pediatr. Exer. Sci. 2:209-229; 1990.

87. Lowry, C.B.; Leveau, B.F. A retrospective study of gymnastic injuries to competitors and noncompetitors in private clubs. Am. J. Sports Med. 10:237-239; 1982.

88. Lueken, J.; Stone, J.; Wallach, B.A. Olympic training center report men's gymnastics injuries. Gymnastics Safety Update 8(1):4-5; 1993.

89. MacGregor, J., Moncur, J.A.. Meralgia paraesthetica—a sports lesion in girl gymnasts. Brit. J. Sports Med. 11(1):16-19; 1977.

90. Mackie, S.J.; Taunton, J.E. Injuries in female gymnasts. Trends suggest prevention tactics. Phys. Sportsmed. 22(8):40-45; 1994.

91. Maffuli, N.; Chan, D.; Aldridge, M.J. Derangement of the articular surfaces of the elbow in young gymnasts. J. Ped. Orthop. 12:344-350; 1992a.

92. Maffuli, N.; Chan, D.; Aldridge, M.J. Overuse injuries of the olecranon in young gymnasts. J. Bone Jt. Surg. 74-B:305-308; 1992b.

93. Maffuli, N.; Francobandiera, C.; Lepore, L.; Cifarelli, V. Total dislocation of the talus. J. Foot Surg. 28:208-212; 1989.

94. Mahler, P.; Fricker, P. Case report: cuboid stress fracture. Excel 8:147-148; 1992.

95. Mandelbaum, B.R. Gymnastics. In: Reider, B., ed. Sports medicine. The school-age athlete. Philadelphia: W.B. Saunders; 1991:415-428.

96. Mandelbaum, B.R.; Bartolozzi, A.R.; Davis, C.A.; Teurlings, L.; Bragonier, B. Wrist pain syndrome in the gymnast. Pathogenetic, diagnostic, and therapeutic considerations. Am. J. Sports Med. 17:305-317; 1989.

97. Mandelbaum, B.R.; Grant, T.T.; Nichols, A.W. A case conference. Wrist pain in a gymnast. Phys. Sportsmed. 16:80-84; 1988.

98. Mandelbaum, B.; Gross, M.L. Spondylolysis and spondylolisthesis. In: Reider, B., ed. Sports medicine. The school-age athlete. Philadelphia: W.B. Saunders; 1991:144-156.

99. Manzione, M., Pizzutillo, P.D. Stress fracture of the scaphoid waist. A case report. Am. J. Sports Med. 9:268-269; 1981.

100. Markhoff, K.L; Shapiro, M.S.; Mandelbaum, B.R.; Teurlings, L. Wrist loading patterns during pommel horse exercises. J. Biomech. 23(10):1001-1011; 1990.

101. McAuley, E.; Hudash, G.; Shields, K.; Albright, J.P.; Garrick, J.; Requa, R.; Wallace, R.K. Injuries in women's gymnastics: the state of the art. Am. J. Sports Med. 15:558-565; 1987.

102. McLain, L.G.; Reynolds, S. Sports injuries in a high school. Pediatrics 84:446-450; 1989.

103. Meeusen, R.; Borms, J. Gymnastics injuries. Sports Med. 13(5):337-356; 1992.

104. Meeuwisse, W.H. Predictability of sports injuries: what is the epidemiological evidence? Sports Med. 12(1):8-15; 1991.

105. Michaud, T.J.; Rodriquez-Zayas, J.; Armstrong, C.; Hartnig, M. Ground reaction forces in high impact and low impact aerobic dance. J. Sports Med. Phys. Fit. 33(4):359-366; 1993.

106. Micheli, L.J. Low back pain in the adolescent: differential diagnosis. Am. J. Sports Med. 7(6):362-366; 1979.

107. Micheli, L.J. Overuse injuries in children's sports: the growth factor. Orthop. Clin. North. Am. 14:337-360; 1983.

108. Mueller, F.O.; Cantu, R.C. National Center for Catastrophic Sports Injury Research. Personal communication, August 30, 1994.

109. Mulligan, M.E. Horizontal fracture of the talar head. Am. J. Sports Med. 14:176-177; 1986.

110. Murakami, S.; Nakajima, H. Aseptic necrosis of the capitate bone in two gymnasts. Am. J. Sports Med. 12:170-173; 1984.

111. National Collegiate Athletic Association Injury Surveillance System Report 1982-86. Kansas: NCAA Report; Nov. 17, 1986.

112. National Collegiate Athletic Association News. Kansas: NCAA Report; May 9, 1990.

113. National Collegiate Athletic Assocation 1993-94 men's and women's gymnastics injury surveillance system. Kansas: NCAA Report; 1994.

114. Nocini, S.; Silvij, S. Clinical and radiological aspects of gymnast's elbow. J. Sports Med. Phys. Fitness. 22:54-59; 1982.

115. Noden, M. Dying to win. Sports Illust. August 8:52-60; 1994.

116. Noguchi, T. A survey of spinal cord injuries resulting from sport. Paraplegia 32:170-173; 1994.

117. Panzer, V.P.; Wood, G.A.; Bates, B.T.; Mason, B.R. Lower extremity loads in landings of elite gymnasts. In: de Groot, G., Hollander, A.P., Huijing, P.A., van Ingen Schenau, G.J., eds., Biomechanics

XI-B. Amsterdam: Free University Press; 1988: 727-735.

118. Peterson, C.A.; Peterson, H.A. Analysis of the incidence of injuries to the epiphyseal growth plate. J. Trauma 12:275-281; 1972.

119. Pettrone, F.A.; Ricciardelli, E. Gymnastic injuries: the Virginia experience 1982-83. Am. J. Sports Med. 15:59-62; 1987.

120. Postacchini, F.; Puddu, G. Subcutaneous rupture of the distal biceps brachii tendon. A report on seven cases. J. Sports Med. Phys. Fit. 15:81-90; 1975.

121. Priest, J.D.; Weise, D.J. Elbow injury in women's gymnastics. Am. J. Sports Med. 9:288-295; 1981.

122. Proffer, D.S.; Patton, J.J.; Jackson, D.W. Nonunion of a first rib fracture in a gymnast. Am. J. Sports Med. 19(2):198-201; 1991.

123. Rapp, G.F.; Nicely, P.G. Trampoline injuries. Am. J. Sports Med. 6:269-271; 1978.

124. Read, M.T. Stress fractures of the distal radius in adolescent gymnasts. British J. Sports Med. 15:272-276; 1981.

125. Resnick, D.L. A 12-year-old gymnast with intermittant pain in the wrist. Radiographics 8:246-248; 1988.

126. Rossi, F. Spondylolysis, spondylolisthesis and sports. J. Sports Med. 18(4):317-340; 1978.

127. Rossi, F.; Dragoni, S. Lumbar spondylolysis: occurrence in competitive athletes. J. Sports Med. Phys. Fit. 30(4):450-452; 1990.

128. Roy, S.; Caine, D.; Singer, K. Stress changes of the distal radial epiphysis in young gymnasts. A report of twenty-one cases and a review of the literature. Am. J. Sports Med. 13:301-308; 1985.

129. Ruggles, D.L.; Peterson, H.A.; Scott, S.G. Radial growth plate injury in a female gymnast. Med. Sci. Sports Exer. 23:393-396; 1991.

130. Sands, W.A. Competition injury study. A preliminary report. USGF Technical J. 1:7-9; 1981.

131. Sands, W.A. Coaching women's gymnastics. Champaign, IL: Human Kinetics Publishers; 1984.

132. Sands, W. A.; Cheetham, P.J. Velocity of the vault run: junior elite female gymnasts. Technique 6:10-14; 1986.

133. Sands, W.A.; Crain, R.S.; Lee, K.M. Gymnastics coaching survey—1989. Technique 10:22-27; 1990.

134. Sands, W.A.; Henschen, K.P.; Shultz, B.B. National women's tracking program. Technique 9:14-20, 1989.

135. Sands, W.A.; Major, J.A. The time course of fitness acquisition in women's gymnastics. FIG Scientific/Medical Symposium Proceedings 1:9-13; 1991a.

136. Sands, W.A.; Major, J.A.; Irvin, R.C.; Hauge Barber, L.S.; Marcus, R.L.; Paine, D.D.; Cervantez, R.D.; Ford, H.R.; McNeal, J.R. Physical abilities profiles: U.S. men's national team. Technique 14(2):34-37; 1994.

137. Sands, W.A.; Milesky, A.E.; Edwards, J.E. Physical abilities field tests U.S. gymnastics federation women's national teams. USGF Sport Science Congress Proceedings 1:39-47; 1991b.

138. Sands, W.A.; Newman, A.P.; Harner, C.; Paulos, L.E. A two year study of injury in collegiate women's gymnastics. Technique 7(3):4-10; 1987.

139. Sands, W.A.; Shultz, B.B.; Newman, A.P. Women's gymnastics injuries. A 5-year study. Am. J. Sports Med. 21(2):271-276; 1993.

140. Silver, J.R.; Silver, D.D.; Godfrey, J.J Injuries of the spine sustained during gymnastic activities. Brit. Med. J. 293:861-863; 1986.

141. Silvij, S.; Nocini, S. Clinical and radiological aspects of gymnast's shoulder. J. Sports Med; 22:49-53; 1982.

142. Singer, K.M.; Roy, S.P. Osteochondrosis of the humeral capitellum. Am. J. Sports Med. 12:351-360; 1984.

143. Smith, A.D.; Andrish, J.T.; Micheli, L.J. Current comment: the prevention of sport injuries of children and adolescents. Med. Sci. Sports Exer. (Special Supplement) 25(8):1-7; 1993.

144. Snook, G.A. Injuries in women's gymnastics. A 5-year study. Am. J. Sports Med. 7:242-244; 1979.

145. Steele, V.A.; White, J.A. Injury amongst female gymnasts. Proceedings of the Society of Sports Sciences: Sport and Science Conference. Liverpool: School of Physical Education and Recreation; 1983.

146. Steele, V.A.; White, J.A. Injury prediction in female gymnasts. Brit. J. Sports Med. 20:31-33; 1986.

147. Stuart, P.R.; Briggs, P.J. Closed extensor tendon rupture and distal radial fracture with use of a gymnast's wrist support. Br. J. Sports Med. 27(2):92-93; 1993.

148. Svihlik, L.W. Osteochondritis dissecans of the right capitellum with osteocartilaginous loose bodies of the elbow in a male gymnast: a case report. Chiro. Sports Med. 7(3):79-82; 1993.

149. Swärd, L. The thoracolumbar spine in young elite athletes. Current concepts on the effects of physical training. Sports Med. 13(5):357-362; 1992.

150. Swärd, L; Hellström, M.; Jacobsson, B.; Karlsson, L. Vertebral ring apophysis injury in athletes. Is the etiology different in the thoracic and lumbar spine? Am. J. Sports Med. 21(6):841-845; 1993.

151. Swärd, L.; Hellström, M.; Jacobsson, B.; Nyman, R.; Peterson, L. Acute injury of the vertebral ring apophysis and intervertebral disc in adolescent gymnasts. Spine 15:144-148; 1990a.

152. Swärd, L.; Hellström, M.; Jacobsson, B.; Nyman, R.; Peterson, L. Disc degeneration and associated abnormalities of the spine in elite gymnasts. Spine 16(4):437-443; 1991.

153. Swärd, L; Hellström, M; Jacobsson, B.; Peterson, L. Spondylolysis and the sacro-horizontal angle in athletes. Acta Radiol. 30:359-364; 1989.

154. Swärd, L.; Hellström, M.; Jacobsson, B.; Peterson, L. Back pain and radiologic changes in the thoracolumbar spine of athletes. Spine. 15(2):124-129; 1990b.

155. Szot, Z.; Boron, Z.; Galaj, Z. Int. J. Sports Med. 6:36-40; 1985.

156. Takai, Y. A comparison of techniques used in performing the men's compulsory gymnastic vault at 1988 Olympics. Int. J. Sport Biomech. 7(1):54-75; 1991.

157. Takami, H.; Takahashi, S.; Ando, M. Traumatic rupture of iliacus muscle with femoral nerve paralysis. J. Trauma 23:253-254; 1983.

158. Tayob, A.A.; Shively, R.A. Bilateral elbow dislocations with intra-articular displacement of the medial epicondyles. J. Trauma 20:332-335; 1980.

159. Tertti, M.; Paajanen, H.; Kujula, U.M.; Alanen, A.; Salmi, T.T.; Kormano, M. Disc degeneration in young gymnasts. A magnetic resonance imaging study. Am. J. Sports Med. 18:206-208; 1990.

160. Teurlings, L.; Mandelbaum, B.R. Wrist pain in gymnasts. Technique 12(3):8-9; 1992.

161. Thompson, N.; Halpern, B.; Curl, W.W.; Andrews, J.R.; Hunter, S.C.; McLeod, W.D. High school football injuries: evaluation. Am. J. Sports Med. 15:117-124; 1987.

162. Tolat, A.R.; Sanderson, P.L.; De Smet, L.; Stanley, J.K. The gymnast's wrist: Acquired postive ulnar variance following chronic epiphyseal injury. J. Hand Surg. 17B(6):678-681; 1992.

163. Too, D.; Adrian, M. Relationship of lumbar curvature and landing surface to ground reaction forces during gymnastic landing. In: Terauds, J.; Gowitzke, B.A.; Holt, L.E., eds. Biomechanics in Sports III & IV. Del Mar, CA: Academic Publishers; 1987:29-34.

164. Torg, J.S. Trampoline-induced quadriplegia. Clin. Sports Med. 6:73-85; 1987.

165. Tütsch, C.; Ulrich, S.P. Wirbelsäule und hochleistungsturnen bei mädchen (beobachtungen der entstehung einer spondylolisthesis). Sportarzt und Sportmedizin (Germany) 26:7-11; 1975. Cited in Caine, D. Growth plate injury and bone growth. An update. Pediatr. Exer. Sci. 2:209-229; 1990.

166. Vain, A. Dynamics of the deformations of the vertebral column and foot of gymnasts. In: Morecki, A.; Fidelus, K.; Kedizior, K.; Wit, A., eds. Biomechanics VII-B. Baltimore: University Park Press; 1981:566-570.

167. van Mechelen, W.; Hlobil, H.; Kemper, C.G. Incidence, severity, aetiology and prevention of sports injuries. A review of concepts. Sports Med. 14(2):82-99; 1992.

168. Vaos, G.C.; Maridaki, M.; Eston, R.G. Case report: Unusual intra-abdominal injury in a female gymnast. Australian J. Sci. Med. Sport March:20-21; 1989.

169. Vender, M.I.; Watson, K. Acquired Madelung-like deformity in a gymnast. J. Hand Surg. 13A:19-21; 1988.

170. Vergouwen, P. Epidemiologie van blessures bij topturnsters. Geneeskunde en Sport 18(2):27-33; 1986.

171. Victor, J.; Mulier, T.; Fabry, G. Refracture of radius and ulna in a female gymnast. A case report. Am. J. Sports Med. 21(5):753-754; 1993.

172. Wadley, G.H.; Albright, J.P. Women's intercollegiate gymnastics. Injury patterns and "permanent" medical disability. Am. J. Sports. Med. 21(2):314-320; 1993.

173. Walsh, M.W.; Huurman, W.W.; Shelton, G.L. Overuse injuries of the knee and spine in girl's gymnastics. Clin. Sports Med. 3:829-850; 1984.

174. Walter, S.D.; Hart, L.E. Application of epidemiological methodology in sports and exercise science research. In: Pandolf, K.B.; Holloszy, J.O., eds. Exercise and sports science reviews. Baltimore: Williams and Wilkins; (18):417-448; 1990.

175. Walter, S.D.; Sutton, J.R.; McIntosh, J.M.; Connelly, C. The aetiology of sport injuries. A review of methodologies. Sports Med. 2:47-58; 1985.

176. Weiker, G.G. Injuries in club gymnastics. Phys. Sportsmed. 13:63-66; 1985.

177. Weir, M.R.; Smith, D.S. Stress reaction of the pars interarticularis leading to spondylolysis. A cause of adolescent low back pain. J. Adol. Health Care 10:573-577; 1989.

178. Wilkerson, R.D.; Johns, J.C. Nonunion of an olecranon stress fracture in an adolescent gymnast. Am. J. Sports Med. 18:432-434; 1990.

179. Wiltse, L.L.; Widell, E.H.; Jackson, D.W. Fatigue fracture: the basic lesion in isthmic spondylolisthesis. J. Bone Jt. Surg. 57A:17-22; 1975.

180. Witten, W.A.; Witten, C.X.; Brown, E.W.; Wells, R. The back giant swing on the uneven parallel bars: a biomechanical analysis. USGF Sport Science Congress Proceedings. 1:12-18; 1991.

181. Yong-Hing, K.; Wedge, J.H.; Bowen, C.V. Chronic injury to the distal ulnar and radial growth plates in an adolescent gymnast. J. Bone Jt. Surg. 70-A:1087-1089; 1988.

# 15

# Ice Hockey

*William J. Montelpare,*
*Robert L. Pelletier, and Ryan M. Stark*

## 1. Introduction

Ice hockey is Canada's national sport (22), with an average annual participation rate of over 500,000 registered, amateur players. Although Canada is considered to be the birthplace of ice hockey (22), the sport is extremely popular in Europe and other countries around the world (30, 64, 69, 91). For example, the United States has over 300,000 registered amateur participants per year (16, 24).

Often described as a violent game, ice hockey is a fast-paced, contact sport (22, 30, 63, 64, 67, 83, 84, 91). In some leagues aggressive play is encouraged, while in others, even minimal body contact is not permitted. Yet, despite the style of play, the rate of reported injuries that are serious, catastrophic, or both is unknown because there is no complete register of injuries and the number of participants exposed to the risk of injury during games and practices has never been estimated accurately (64). The purpose of this review of ice hockey injury research is to provide a quantitative description of the injuries reported for the game of ice hockey within a variety of cohorts and across several levels of participation.

Information for this chapter was collected from on-line library searches, based on the SPORT Discus and Medline electronic databases, and from extensive searches of the reference lists of the research articles that were published between 1960 and 1993. However, since most ice hockey injury research was conducted during the 1970s and 1980s, most of this chapter is based on studies from that time period.

Although ice hockey injury research has been reported in several languages, this chapter is limited to those articles that were reported in English and French. The key words used to search the electronic databases included general terms, such as ice hockey injuries, epidemiology of injuries; injury specific terms, such as concussions, spinal trauma, eye injuries, retinal detachment, head and neck injuries, hematoma, and dental injuries; and key words associated with hockey play or the types of equipment such as hockey helmet, face shield, and mouth protectors. In addition, the electronic library databases provided lists of different study types, including case studies, large-scale epidemiological studies, and community-based reports.

Limitations of on-line searches have been reported previously (61); however, additional reviews of reference lists (the ancestral approach), in combination with multiple database searches, have yielded a comprehensive review of ice hockey injuries. Yet it remains unfortunate that despite the several reports of ice hockey injuries, the ability to ascertain valid and reliable descriptions of injuries and to estimate incidence and prevalence rates is difficult because of the following limiting factors:

- A lack of compliance by recorders (i.e., trainers, coaches, physiotherapists, and physicians) to report ice hockey injuries to a national, standardized, reporting system (23).
- A lack of compliance in reporting injury prevalence and incidence, that is, lack of standardization (e.g., using number of injuries per 1,000 hours of athlete exposure; 73, 83, 102).
- Differences in rules and differing policies with regard to rule enforcement, both within and between different levels of participation (23, 88).
- Changes in specific rules governing the mandatory use of protective equipment and styles of play over the past 2 decades (30). For example, Pashby (76) reported a reduction

across all types of eye injuries, with the exception of the "ruptured globe" type of injury, as a result of increased use of face masks and because the amateur leagues introduced new rules that penalized players who were caught high sticking.

- Inadequate descriptions of the sample at risk. Most ice hockey injury studies have been reviews of the number of specific injury reports accumulated over a single season. The risk of incurring an ice hockey injury may be inflated artificially (64).
- Inconsistent definitions used to identify an ice hockey injury. Lorentzon et al. (64) indicated that a strict definition of an injury is critical to the epidemiological description of sports injuries; however, definitions used to describe injuries are inconsistent across studies. For example, Lorentzon (63, 64) did not include facial lacerations in reports of the distribution of injury type, because the individuals did not miss participating in subsequent games or practices.

## 2. Incidence of Injury

### 2.1 Injury Rates

The term *incidence* refers to the number of new cases measured between two specific times for a designated sample at risk (54, 83). Estimates of the sample at risk differ across leagues and between cohorts. For example, the sample at risk in Canadian amateur ice hockey during the 1992-1993 season can be based on over 450,000 players registered in over 28,000 teams (62). However, the Canadian Old-Timers Hockey Association (COHA) that registers players over the age of 35 years, estimates that more than 60,000 eligible individuals participate annually in amateur old-timer leagues. In addition to the registered amateur players, across all cohorts there is a large group of ice hockey players who participate at least weekly in leagues that are not part of the jurisdiction of the accredited associations such as the NCAA, CAHA, NAIA, etc. and, therefore, would not be included in the estimation of the sample at risk nor included in determining injury rates.

Studies reporting specific rates of injuries are presented in Table 15.1. The inability to provide a single approximation for the rate of ice hockey injuries can be attributed to factors relating to study design and accepted definitions for terms. Most ice hockey injury studies were designed as retrospective investigations intended to identify

the injury prevalence within a specific team or league. Several studies, however, identified the number of injuries per game or per season, but used a retrospective design and therefore were less accurate in identifying the true population at risk. Other studies reported the frequency of injuries related to a specific body part. Few studies used the prospective design, which provides a specific incidence rate based on a predefined denominator.

Important considerations from the reports of the frequencies of ice hockey injuries reported in Table 15.1 are summarized as follows:

- Reports of injury rates are related to the type of league from which the data were collected (noncontact vs. contact; professional vs. amateur; junior vs. senior).
- In general, injury rates are low relative to the number of participants in a game or practice across the season.
- Although some types of soft tissue injuries (e.g., lacerations, contusions, and strains) occur at all levels of participation, this type of injury may not be reported.
- Legislation relating to the use of protective equipment in some leagues has reduced the number of reported injuries within those leagues that have adopted such rule changes.

### 2.2 Injury Rates in Practice vs Competition

Few studies have considered the type of hockey being played when the injury occurred; Figure 15.1 illustrates the distribution of injuries reported for games versus practices, expressed as a percentage of the total number of injuries reported per season. The results indicate that in all studies injuries occurred more often during games versus practices. According to Lorentzon et al. (64), the individual player incidence of injury was 1.4 per 1,000 player-practice hours versus 78.4 per 1,000 player-game hours. This large difference between practice-incidence injury rates versus game-incidence injury rates can be attributed to at least two related factors:

- There were more practices than games in the leagues studied; therefore, the number of injuries related to games may be skewed.
- However, most important, practice sessions do not always include the type of play that predisposes an athlete to an injury.

According to Bancroft (7), the NCAA data showed a sixfold increase in game injuries versus injuries that were reported for practices in each of the seasons studied.

**Table 15.1  Reports of Injury Rates**

| Authors | Study design | Number of participants | Description of participants | Injury rates |
|---|---|---|---|---|
| Lorentzon et al. (1988a) | P | 24-25 | Swedish National Team, 40 international games [240 player-game hrs; (AE)] | 19 injuries causing absence; 17 lacerations (no absence); injury rate causing absence: 79.2/1,000 AE |
| Lorentzon et al. (1988b) | P | 24-25 | 3-yr study of one Swedish elite ice hockey team | Injury rate for games = 78.4/1,000 AE; for practices = 1.4/1,000 AE; minor injury rate = 57.7/1,000 AE; moderate injury rate = 14.2/1,000 AE; major injury rate = 6.5/1,000 AE |
| Bancroft (1993) | P | 28 | American college players, 2 seasons (1988-1989 and 1989-1990) at U. North Dakota | Home games rate = 5.95/1,000 AE; away games rate = 7.58/1,000 AE; total contests rate = 6.80/1,000 AE; total practices rate = 1.32/1,000 AE; total rate = 2.69/1,000 AE |
| Dick (1993) | P | 120 teams/ season | American colleges and amateur athletes in the NCAA (1986-1990) | Game injury rate of 16.2/1,000 AE; practice injury rate of 2.4/1,000 AE |
| Hayes (1975) | P | 21 Cdn teams, 9 U.S. teams | Survey of U.S. and Canadian colleges and universities; 30 teams observed for 1 season | 328 injuries reported for 280 games; per game rate of 1.14 injuries in Canada; per game rate of 1.28 injuries in U.S.; total average per game rate of 1.17 |
| Bouchard (1977) | P | | 1 Canadian major jr. team over 3 seasons (257 games) | 238 injuries reported = 0.926 injuries per game; time loss due to injuries: 345 practices and 299 games |
| Downs (1979) | P | $n_1$ = 129; $n_2$ = 46 | Greater Lansing Amateur Hockey Association ($n_1$); Michigan State Univ ($n_2$) | Injury rates converted to 1,000 AE; $n_1$ = 26.3/1,000 AE; $n_2$ = 119/1,000 AE |
| Park & Castaldi (1980) | P | | 1 Jr B team for the 1977-1978 season: age 15-19 | 83 injuries recorded for 53 games = 1.57 injuries/game; predicted injury rate based on 83/(n = 20 x 53) = 78.3/1,000 AE |
| Pelletier et al. (1993) | P | 340 | Canadian Athletic Injury Reporting System, 17 university teams (1979 and 1986) | 188 ice hockey injuries total injury rate = 19.95/1,000 AE; injury rate for forwards = 20.83/1,000 AE; injury rate for defence = 18.14/1,000 AE; injury rate for goalies = 20.16/1,000 AE |
| Sutherland (1976) | P | 357; 350 | Minor amateur leagues in U.S. 1974 and 1975 seasons | 17 injuries for 707 players for 1,672 hr of ice time; injury rate of 10.17 injuries/1,000 AE |
| Rielly (1982) | R | 125 | 5-year injury data for a U.S. intercollegiate team | 104 injuries reported for 125 players over 5 years; injury rate of 78.67/1,000 AE |
| Arber & Biener (1985) | R | 2,462 | Swiss professional players | 2,462 injuries reported for 218 respondents; 232 injuries caused time loss |
| Rovere et al. (1978) | R | | 1 professional team, over 3 seasons | 233 injuries reported for 234 games; based on a team size of 20 players; 233/(n = 20 x 234) = 49.79 injuries/ 1,000 AE |
| Toogood & Love (1966) | R | 2,469 | Toronto minor hockey, ages 7-18 yrs: (2 seasons) | Overall injury proportion of 3.4%; 85 injury reports for 2,469 players; 56 of 85 were head and facial injuries |
| Feriencik (1979) | R | 62 | Review of players on the Slovan ChZJD team, 1965 to 1977 | 1,116 injuries reported/treated for 62 players |

*(continued)*

**Table 15.1**   *(continued)*

| Authors | Study design | Number of participants | Description of participants | Injury rates |
|---|---|---|---|---|
| Goodwin-Gerberich et al. (1987) | R | 263* | 12 secondary schools during the 1982-1983 season; coaches and players were surveyed | 75 injuries/100 players; 5 injuries/1,000 AE; 36,561 man-hours of exposure (games and practices) |
| Kropp et al. (1980) | R | 35,435 registered participants | British Columbia Amateur Hockey Association (1972-1973 season) | 8.1/1,000 AE; an injury ratio < 1:100 players; greater proportion of head and facial injuries |
| MacIntosh & Shephard (1971) | R | | 10,216 intercollegiate and intramural injuries, 1951 to 1969 | All sports, overall injury rate of 84/1,000 AE; ice hockey reported 102.7/1,000 athlete years |
| Kraus et al. (1979) | E | [C] = 69 teams; [E] = 73 teams, estimate of 18 players per team | Intramural college, 2 yr; 238 games; 4,223 AE | Unhelmeted control year game injury rate = 16.1/100 games or 8.2 injuries/1,000 AE; helmeted experimental year game injury rate = 8.8/100 games or 5.9 injuries/1,000 AE |
| Biener and Muller (1973) | XS | | Sample of insurance records over 5 yr from the Swiss professional league | 1,800 injuries reported for games vs. 800 in practice; 2,680 injuries/38,693 players = 6.92% |
| Bernard et al. (1993) | XS | 5 leagues > 44 teams > 300 games | Comparison across 2 levels of bantam aged players: AA vs. CC players; from 2 regions of Quebec (1987-1988 and 1988-1989) | Major injuries: 1/5.3 games; 1/10.8 games; 1/5.4 games; 1/15 games; minor injuries: 3.26/game; 0.45/game; 3.36/game; 1.21/game |
| Clayton (1993) | XS | 30 teams | Major junior hockey from Ontario and Western Canada leagues | 514 reported injuries for 424 games and 62 practices; 1,200 AE and 1,440 AE |
| Hastings et al. (1974) | XS | 20,000 | Survey of minor amateur leagues within Ontario, across 2 seasons | 542 injuries reported for 530 players within 2 seasons |
| Hornof & Napravnik (1973) | XS | 3,895 | Based on case reports from 65,881 registered players in Czechoslovakia | Injury incidence of 29.6 injuries/1,000 AE; 55% of injuries occurred in games vs. practice (45%) |
| Hayes (1978) | XS | 510 | U.S. and Canadian players; 14 professional players; 21 colleges and universities; 19 minor teams | Average number of injuries per game across the age levels: age 9-10 = 0.008; age 11-12 = .013; age 13-14 = .025; age 15-16 = .052; age 17-18 = .125; univ = 1.17; pro = 1.15 |
| Hovelius (1978) | XS | 63 | Swedish ice hockey players from 2 leagues; $n_1$ = 23 in 1st league (higher quality players); $n_2$ = 30 in 2nd level league | Shoulder injury rates per league based on the responses to the questionnaires within each league; 1st league shoulder injury rate = 23/300 players; 2nd league shoulder injury rate = 30/1,000 players |
| Jorgensen & Schmidt-Olsen (1986) | XS | 266 | Sample based on 210 survey responses from 266 players | Injury incidence rate of 4.7 injuries per 1,000 AE; game rate = 38/1,000 AE; practice rate = 1.5/1,000 AE |
| Pforringer & Smasal (1987) | XS | 88 | West German Bundesliga 1 (professional league) | Prevalence rate of 5.6 injuries per study participant |
| Reeves & Mendryk (1975) | XS | 6,890 | Edmonton amateur players 1969-1970 season; 5 age levels; minor, junior, inter-collegiate, and intramural | 446 injuries reported for 345 players; estimated injury rate of 36/1,000 AE; actual injury rate of 50.1/1,000 AE |

*Response rate of 12 coaches and 251 players was reported by Goodwin-Gerberich et al. (1987).

*Note.* AE denotes athlete exposures; E denotes experimental study; R denotes retrospective; P denotes prospective; XS denotes cross-sectional.

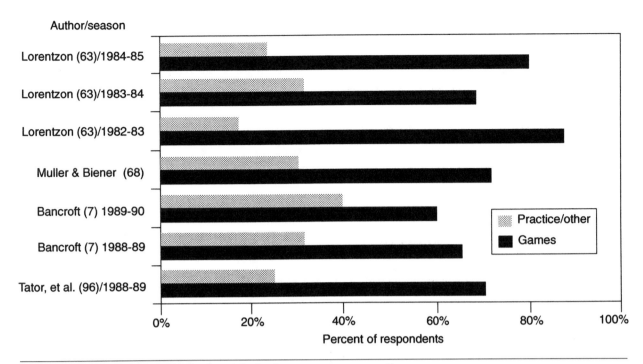

**Figure 15.1** Distribution of ice-hockey injuries in games versus practices.

## 3. Injury Characteristics

### 3.1 Injury Onset

Generally, ice hockey injury studies are based on reports of sudden onset injury statistics (9, 13, 49, 82, 91). This does not suggest that chronic injuries, such as those related to overuse, do not exist in the sport of ice hockey. For example, Lorentzon et al. (64) reported that of 96 ice hockey injuries recorded over 3 years, 19 injuries were classified as adductor or patellar tendinitis. However, the nature of the sport and the limitations in injury reporting influence the lack of availability of information about chronic/overuse injury. Therefore, comparisons of studies between sudden versus gradual onset injuries are not available.

### 3.2 Injury Types

The types of ice hockey injuries are presented in Table 15.2. The information reported in Table 15.2 refers to studies that have reviewed injuries to the entire body, rather than a single anatomic location such as head or facial injuries. A review of these data suggest that reports of injury type can be summarized as follows:

- When referring to the most common injuries across the entire body, contusions and sprains alternate as the most frequently reported injury type. For example, in the Canadian Athletic Injury Reporting System,(CAIRS), Pelletier and coworkers (83) reported that sprains were recorded most often; however, Lorentzon et al. (63) reported that contusions were recorded more often than sprains.
- The reports of lacerations were high, but a current profile of the prevalence of lacerations across all injury reports from 1960 to the present would be skewed by the introduction of specific equipment and rule changes.
- The data reported by Roy et al. (88) is especially important because there are so few studies that show a comparison between injury rates in amateur leagues that allow body contact versus leagues that restrict body contact. Yet the percentages of injury types reported by Roy et al. (88) are similar across the two leagues. For example Roy et al. (88) showed that 72% of injuries were contusions in the body checking league, likewise 69% of injuries were contusions in the nonbody checking league. However, a fourfold difference in the number of reports of injuries per game was reported for the contact versus noncontact league.

### 3.3 Injury Location

Several considerations underlie the risk for a body part to be involved in an injury. Using Hoyt's

**Table 15.2   Reports of Injuries by Injury Type***

| Authors | # of players | # of injuries | Concussion | Contusion | Sprains | Strains | Fractures | Dislocations | Lacerations | Unknown |
|---|---|---|---|---|---|---|---|---|---|---|
| Rovere, Gristina, & Nicastro (1978) | 1 team | 233 (234 games) | | 15 | 20 | 17 | 9 | 1 | 21 | 4 |

Study type: prospective study of an American semi-professional team, followed for three seasons

| Authors | # of players | # of injuries | Concussion | Contusion | Sprains | Strains | Fractures | Dislocations | Lacerations | Unknown |
|---|---|---|---|---|---|---|---|---|---|---|
| Lorentzon et al. (1988b) | 24-25 | 95 | 4 | 24 | 11 | 12 | 9.5 | 9.5 | 30 | |

Study type: prospective study of a Swedish national team; results based on data for three years

| Authors | # of players | # of injuries | Concussion | Contusion | Sprains | Strains | Fractures | Dislocations | Lacerations | Unknown |
|---|---|---|---|---|---|---|---|---|---|---|
| Bancroft (1993) | | | | | | | | | | |
| [1988 season] | 3,453 AE | 9 | | 22 | 33 | | 22 | | | |
| [1989 season] | 3,602 AE | 10 | | | 40 | 30 | 20 | | | |

Study type: prospective study of an American intercollegiate team across two seasons (1988-1989 and 1989-1990)

| Authors | # of players | # of injuries | Concussion | Contusion | Sprains | Strains | Fractures | Dislocations | Lacerations | Unknown |
|---|---|---|---|---|---|---|---|---|---|---|
| Hornof & Napravnik (1973) | 65,881 registrants | 3,895 | | | | | | | 37 | |

Study type: retrospective evaluation of ice hockey injuries in Czechoslovakia for the 1967-1968 season

| Authors | # of players | # of injuries | Concussion | Contusion | Sprains | Strains | Fractures | Dislocations | Lacerations | Unknown |
|---|---|---|---|---|---|---|---|---|---|---|
| Feriencik (1979) | 62 | 1,116 | 2 | 40 | | | 5 | 25 | 18 | 10 |

Study type: retrospective study of players on team Slovan ChZJD; data from injury reports for 62 players (1965-1977)

| Authors | # of players | # of injuries | Concussion | Contusion | Sprains | Strains | Fractures | Dislocations | Lacerations | Unknown |
|---|---|---|---|---|---|---|---|---|---|---|
| Rielly (1982) | 125 | 104 | 6 | 19 | 8 | 7 | 14 | 10 | 29 | |

Study type: retrospective study of an American intercollegiate team over 5 years

| Authors | # of players | # of injuries | Concussion | Contusion | Sprains | Strains | Fractures | Dislocations | Lacerations | Unknown |
|---|---|---|---|---|---|---|---|---|---|---|
| Goodwin-Gerberich et al. (1987) | 251 | 75 (100 players) | 12 | 29 | 9 | | 11 | 10 | 12 | |

Study type: retrospective study of 12 secondary schools; data based on responses from 12 coaches and 251 players

| Authors | # of players | # of injuries | Concussion | Contusion | Sprains | Strains | Fractures | Dislocations | Lacerations | Unknown |
|---|---|---|---|---|---|---|---|---|---|---|
| Pelletier et al. (1993) | 340 | 188 | 8 | 21 | 31 | 11 | 10 | | 13 | 6 |

Study type: retrospective study of data from the CAIR system; results based on injuries reported from 1979-1986

| Authors | # of players | # of injuries | Concussion | Contusion | Sprains | Strains | Fractures | Dislocations | Lacerations | Unknown |
|---|---|---|---|---|---|---|---|---|---|---|
| Biener & Muller (1973) | 38,693 | 2,680 cases | 6 | | | | 13 | | 28 | |

Study type: cross-sectional review of insurance records from the Swiss professional league

| Authors | # of players | # of injuries | Concussion | Contusion | Sprains | Strains | Fractures | Dislocations | Lacerations | Unknown |
|---|---|---|---|---|---|---|---|---|---|---|
| Reeves & Mendryk (1975) | 6,890 | 446 (345 players) | 4 | 20 | 6.5 | 6 | 13 | 4 | 38 | |

Study type: Cross-sectional review of amateur players in Edmonton, Canada, across 5 age levels

| Authors | # of players | # of injuries | Concussion | Contusion | Sprains | Strains | Fractures | Dislocations | Lacerations | Unknown |
|---|---|---|---|---|---|---|---|---|---|---|
| Jorgensen & Schmidt-Olsen (1986) | 266 | 189 | | 26 | 20 | 8 | 7 | 3 | | 36 |

Study type: Cross-sectional evaluation of players on 14 randomly chosen teams in the Danish ice hockey league

| Authors | # of players | # of injuries | Concussion | Contusion | Sprains | Strains | Fractures | Dislocations | Lacerations | Unknown |
|---|---|---|---|---|---|---|---|---|---|---|
| Roy et al. (1989) | | | | | | | | | | |
| Body contact | 744 | 54 | 2 | 72 | | 4 | | | 9 | |
| Noncontact | | 16 | 6 | 69 | | 6 | | | 13 | |

Study type: Cross-sectional evaluation of players, parents, coaches, administrators, and arena managers, across 2 leagues

| Authors | # of players | # of injuries | Concussion | Contusion | Sprains | Strains | Fractures | Dislocations | Lacerations | Unknown |
|---|---|---|---|---|---|---|---|---|---|---|
| Bernard et al. (1993) | | | | | | | | | | |
| Minor injuries | 304 teams | 632 | 8 | 66 | | | | 14 | | 22 |
| Major injuries | 44 teams | 132 | 15 | | 40 | | 28 | | | 17 |

Study type: Cross-sectional evaluation of bantam-age amateurs across 2 leagues, across 2 seasons

*Data are percentages of total injuries reported.

review of the etiology of shoulder injuries (53), one could consider that the type and severity of any injury will depend on (a) the position of the body part during the trauma, (b) the amount of muscle recruitment within the body part during the trauma, and (c) the momentum and direction of the athlete during the trauma. In addition, the correct use of protective equipment may also determine whether or not an individual receives an injury while playing hockey. Table 15.3 presents injury reports across the entire body, and Tables 15.4 and 15.5 present injury reports classified by body location. A review of data presented in these tables suggests the following observations:

- The findings of Lorentzon et al. (63) depict the trend of many studies that reported the head and face as the most frequently involved body part. This trend was also reported by Daly (29) for several epidemiological studies.

**Table 15.3   Reports of Injuries by Body Part**

| Author | Study design | Sampling frame | # in study | # of injuries | Proportion of injuries by body part |
|--------|--------------|----------------|------------|---------------|-------------------------------------|
| Hayes (1975) | P | Survey of U.S. and Cdn colleges and universities | 21 Cdn teams, 9 US teams | Avg. rate = 1.17/game | 45.1% head; 8% hand; 9% shoulder; 8.8% thigh (groin); 9.7% ribs/back/ foot/ankle; 10.4% knee; 8.9% trunk |
| Pelletier et al. (1993) | P | Canadian Athletic Injury Reporting System (CAIRS) | 340 | 188 injuries; 19.95/1,000 AE | 17.6% face, eye, jaw teeth; 10.6% head, neck; 5% neck/back; 7% hand/fingers; 4% arm/elbows; 15% other upper extremities; 18.6% knee; 4% leg/ankle/foot; 11% hip/ groin/abdomen/chest/back; 9% thigh/hamstrings |
| Toogood & Love (1966) | R | Toronto township amateur league | 2,469 | 85 | 21/85 mouth and teeth; 12/85 eye related; 8/85 nose; 15/85 head and face; 10/85 wrist and hand; 2/85 neck related; 3/85 ribs; 8% knee; 3.5% ankle; 2% other lower extremities |
| Feriencik (1979) | R | A review of players on the Slovan ChZJD team between 1965 to 1977 | 62 | 1,116 injuries reported/ treated | 17% head and neck; 25% arms; 34.5% legs; 6.5% trunk |
| Hornof & Napravnik (1973) | R | Czechoslovakian Ice Hockey Union | 65,881 | 3,895 | 37.1% head and neck; 22% shoulder; 35.7% thigh (groin); 5.3% ribs/back/foot/ankle |
| Goodwin-Gerberich et al. (1987) | R | 12 secondary schools during the 1982-1983 season; coaches and players were surveyed | 263** | 5 injuries/ 1,000 AE | 22% head and neck; 16% shoulder; 13% arm/hand; 12% chest/ribs/ back; 16% leg/ankle/foot; 4% hip/ pelvis; 14% chest/ribs/back/ abdomen |
| Pollard (1967) | R | U.S. college varsity 1934 to 1966 | 448 | 245 injury reports based on 387 records (55%) | 2.5% eyeball; < 1% ear; 13% nasal Fx; 2% facial bone Fx; 8% concussions; 8% arm/hand/ fingers; 9.4% shoulder, chest, and A-C joint; 21.6% thigh/knee/low leg; 5% foot/ankle; 3.7% pelvis/back |
| Reilly (1982) | R | 5-yr injury data for a U.S. intercollegiate team | 125 | 104 injuries; 78.67/1,000 AE | 17.3% face; 11.5% mouth/lip; 5.7% dental; 14.4% shoulder; 5% elbow/ forearm; 10% wrist/hand; 2.9% back; 10.6% hip/groin/thigh; 13.6% knee; 9.6% leg/ankle/foot |
| Sutherland (1976) | XS | Minor amateur hockey, Ohio high school, Bowling Green, Toledo (IHL) professional | 707, 207, 25 | 17, 41, 62, 51 | Average proportion = 7% head, 46% scalp and face, 2% eye; average proportion across groups combined = 8.6% shoulder, 2% hand; average proportion across groups combined = 18.4% thigh (groin); 11.6% knee; 3.8% ribs/ back/foot/ankle |
| Biener & Muller (1973) | XS | Sample of insurance records over 5 yr; Swiss professionals | 38,693 players | 2,680 | 42% head; 18% shoulder; 21% thigh (groin); 19% ribs/back/foot/ ankle |
| Pforringer & Smasal (1987) | XS | First Division Federal Republic of Germany | 88 | 496 total injuries reported for the sample | 49.6% head injuries; 5.8% shoulder; 17.7% upper extremity; 7.5% leg/ hips; 3.8% trunk; 10% knee; 5.8% ankle/foot |

*(continued)*

**Table 15.3   Reports of Injuries by Body Part**

| Author | Study design | Sampling frame | # in study | # of injuries | Proportion of injuries by body part |
|---|---|---|---|---|---|
| Reeves & Mendryk (1975) | XS | Edmonton amateur players 1969-1970 season, 5 age levels; minor, junior, intercollegiate and intramural | 6,890 | 446/345 players, actual injury rate of 50.1/ 1,000 AE | 16.4% mouth; 13.7% eye; 8.1% nose; 4.7% head; 4.5% forehead; 4.3% cheek; 3.8% jaw; 7.4% shoulder; 1.6% neck/upper back; 12.1% arm/hand; 2.5% chest/ abdomen; 7.4% knee; 5.4% ankle/ foot; 8.3% leg related |
| Hastings et al. (1974) | XS | Survey of minor amateur leagues within Ontario | 20,000 | 542/530 players, 1.02 injuries/ player | 7.5% head; 34.6% face and teeth; 4.8% neck/back; 9.2% hand/ fingers; 7.5% arm elbow; 16.5% other upper extremities; 9.2% ankle/foot; 7.5% knee/groin; 3.1% other lower extremities |

*The column labeled "# of injuries" refers to the total number of injuries reported by the author. As such, the reports of injuries describe the percentage of the total number of injuries reported.

*Data also published as Rontal et al., 1977.

**Response rate of 12 coaches and 251 players reported by Goodwin-Gerberich et al. (1987).

*Note.* Rv = review; E = experimental study; XS = cross-sectional study; R = retrospective, longitudinal study; P = prospective study; Fx = fracture.

- However, studies that reviewed injury rates across all body parts typically reported a high prevalence of injuries to the knee, followed by injuries to the shoulder, hands, and ankles.

### 3.3.1 Head and Face

Head and facial injuries resulting from ice hockey participation are well documented in the sports epidemiology literature (81, 94, 97). Most of the ice hockey injury studies reviewed for this chapter described trauma to the head and facial areas. Likewise, as shown in Tables 15.3 and 15.4, head and facial injuries appear to account for the greatest proportion of reported injuries. Perhaps this is because head and facial injuries are not only among the most likely to require immediate treatment, but also because injuries to the head and face are among the more severe of the reported injuries (81, 94).

In several studies conducted before the generally accepted use of face shields, Pashby (75, 81) and others (3, 46, 47, 85, 103) showed that the injuries to the face and eyes led the list of injury reports. A description of the effectiveness of rule and equipment changes on reports of injuries is presented later in this chapter.

The data reported by Hayes (46) is typical of injuries reported for this area of the body. Similarly, the study by Goodwin-Gerberich, Finke,

Madden, et al. (38) of high school age players within a metropolitan area of Minnesota during the 1982-1983 season demonstrated that head and facial trauma continues to be a problem in spite of attempts to eliminate these injuries. Reports of injuries to the head and face are included in Table 15.3 and Table 15.4. A summary of these findings indicates that

- most of the reported injuries were soft tissue trauma resulting in contusions and lacerations (46, 47),
- most of the injuries were accidental with no penalty being administered (46, 47; Sutherland in 11 stated that only 26.6% of injuries were penalty-related),
- injuries to the head and neck accounted for the largest proportion of injuries reported (38),
- all of the injuries to the head resulted from direct blows to the face mask or to the top of the helmet (38),
- in spite of the use of helmets, Goodwin-Gerberich et al. (38) reported a high rate of concussions from head trauma (12%), and,
- likewise, head trauma caused other symptoms, such as double vision, blurred vision, and a loss of motor coordination (38).

### 3.3.2 Upper Extremity

Injuries to the upper extremity include injuries to the neck, shoulder, clavicle, chest/ribs, arms, and

**Table 15.4  Head and Facial Injuries**

| Author | Study design | Sampling frame | # in study | # of injuries | Porportion of injuries by body part |
|---|---|---|---|---|---|
| Antaki et al. (1977) | P | Prospective study over 15 years at a retina clinic | 1,600 | 33 cases | 13.2% of all injuries (1,600) related to hockey; 2% of retinal detachments related to hockey |
| Vinger (1976) | R | Patient records from emergency room treatments | 38 | 38 | 9/38 ocular lacerations; 4/38 fractures to eye skeleton; 13/38 hyphema; 7/38 angle recession; 12/38 traumatic iritis; 9/38 corneal abrasion; 5/38 retinal edema |
| Kropp et al. (1975) | R | British Columbia Amateur Hockey Association (1972-1973 season) | 35,435 | 284 | 41% dental injuries; 59% head and face, not dental |
| Sane et al. (1988) | R | Part I: Finnish amateurs and 4 pro Finnish teams (1979-1982 season) | 108,921, 100 | 6,885 injuries reported | Maxillofacial and dental injuries; Part I: 11.5% |
| | R | Part II: All registered Finnish players (1984-1985) | 62,185 | 2,989 injuries reported | Part II: 10.7% |
| Kraus et al. (1979) | E | U.S. college intramural, 1968 control year [C], 1969 experimental year [E] | [C] 69 teams, [E] 73 teams | 8.2/1,000 AE 5.9/1,000 AE | % head injuries [C] vs. [E] 8.3% [C] 3.8% [E] |
| Horns (1976) | XS | Survey of members of Minnesota committee on ophthalmology (1974) | | 47 cases reported | 47 cases of eye injury due to ice hockey |
| Wilson et al. (1977)* | XS | Amateur; intercollegiate; professional | 853 | 460 to 562 | Facial bone fractures; dental loss; lacerations |
| Daffner (1977) | XS | Survey of youth (g1); adult (g2); and a semi pro team (g3) (1974-1975 and 1975-1976) | (g1) = 250; (g2) = 75; (g3) = 40 | (g1) = 2 cases; (g2) = 13 cases; (g3) = 44 cases | (g1) = 2 facial lacerations; (g2) = 12 facial lacerations, 1 facial Fx; (g3) = 43 facial lacerations, 1 facial Fx and 1 dental |
| Bolitho (1970) | XS | Survey of head injuries among college and junior players in Canada and U.S. (injury report forms) | 22 teams | 1,465 reported/ treated | 79% facial injuries; 12% cerebral trauma; 8% scalp; 1% skull fracture |
| Pashby (1979) | Rv | Review of 1972-1973 study, retrospective reports of COS physicians | 75 | 287 players | 211 intra-ocular; 255 extra-ocular |
| | | Review of 1974-1975 study, prospective reports by ophthalmologists | 114 | 253 players | 304 intra-ocular; 245 extra-ocular |

*The column labeled "# of injuries" refers to the total number of injuries reported by the author. As such, the reports of injuries describe the percentage of the total number of injuries reported.

*Data also published as Rontal et al., 1977.

**Response rate of 12 coaches and 251 players reported by Goodwin-Gerberich et al. (1987).

*Note.* Rv = review; E = experimental study; Xs = cross-sectional study; R = retrospective, longitudinal study; P = prospective study; Fx = fracture.

**Table 15.5  Upper Extremity Injuries**

| Author | Study design | Sampling frame | # in study | # of injuries | Proportion of injuries by body part |
|---|---|---|---|---|---|
| Lorentzon et al. (1988b) | P | 3-yr study of 1 Swedish elite ice hockey team | 25 | Game: 78.4/1,000 AE; practice: 1.4/1,000 AE | 7.4% shoulder; 17% arm/hand; 4.2% chest; 11.6% spine |
| Park & Castaldi (1980) | P | 1 Jr B team for the 1977-1978 season; age 15-19 yrs | 20 | 83; 1.57/game; 78.3/1,000 AE | 5% hand/wrist; 7% forearm/arm; 5% shoulder; 5% elbow; 6% chest/ribs/back |
| Rovere et al. (1978) | R | 1 professional team; 3 seasons | 20 | 233 for 234 games; 50/1,000 AE | 19% of injuries were major; 6.5% Fx hand/wrist; 1.3 shoulder related |
| Norfray et al. (1977) | R | Retrospective review of x-rays for amateur and professionals with previous shoulder injury | 87 | 10 amateur; 24 active pro players; 53 retired pro players | All clavicle |
| Finke et al.* (1988) | R | 12 secondary schools during the 1982-1983 season; coaches and players were surveyed | 263** | 45 shoulder | Breakdown of shoulder injuries: 38% A-C joint; 4% S-C joint; 4% fractures; 40% muscle strain/contusion; 14% other |
| Jorgensen & Schmidt-Olsen (1986) | XS | Sample based on 210 survey responses from 266 players | 266 | 4.7/1,000 AE | 19% attributed to upper extremity |
| Hovelius (1978) | XS | Swedish ice hockey players from 2 leagues: $n_1 = 23$; $n_2 = 30$ in 2nd level league | 300 | 63 | 48 respondents with 3 or more dislocations; 32 respondents had corrective surgery |

*The Finke report is from the Goodwin-Gerberich et al. (1987) study.

**Response rate of 12 coaches and 251 players reported by Goodwin-Gerberich et al. (1987).

*Note.* Rv = review; E = experimental study; XS = cross-sectional study; R = retrospective, longitudinal study; P = prospective study; CS = case study; Fx = fracture.

hands. The distribution of injuries to the upper extremity is presented in Table 15.5. The characteristics of upper extremity injury reports are summarized as follows:

- The causes of injuries to these body parts are not unlike those reported for other body parts; collisions with an opponent's stick, the boards, the goal posts, or other players are among the typical mechanisms of injuries (35, 36, 86).
- In those studies that reported upper extremity injuries, most authors indicated that the greatest proportion of injuries were classified as "minor" (36, 86, 87).
- There is a tendency for individuals to continue participating despite the prevalence of upper extremity injuries (52). In some cases then, depending on how the injury was defined, if no time was lost such injuries may have gone unreported.
- Case study reports of causes and types of upper extremity injuries are consistent with the larger sample studies.

### 3.3.3 Lower Extremity

Injuries to the lower extremities are included in Table 15.3. Reports of injuries to joints such as the knee and ankle typically involved ligament (55) or meniscus trauma (22). Using a biomechanical perspective, Nordin (71) examined the type and severity of ligament injuries during trauma. According to Nordin (71), the risks of injuries to ligaments depend on (a) the size and the shape of the ligament, (b) the speed of loading the ligament, and (c) the position of the joint in relation to the externally applied load.

The various types of ligament damage to the ankle were described by Hunter (55). According to Hunter (55), "hockey ankle" sprain occurs as a result of a severe dorsiflexion, eversion, external rotation of the ankle resulting from catching the skate blade in an ice rut. This sprain also can result from being involved in a forward fall over the ankle, while the ankle is caught in an external rotation, dorsiflexion position.

Tredget, Godberson, and Bose (98) presented case study research for two adolescent hockey players demonstrating the common problem of myositis ossificans. *Myositis ossificans traumatica* is a sequelae that arises from a severe contusion, hematoma, or fracture (98). In one individual the initial trauma resulted from a blow by a hockey stick; in the other individual the trauma resulted from a body check. In both cases, the players returned to hockey following treatment and therapy.

A summary of the findings reported in Table 15.3, which describes injuries to the lower extremities, suggests the following observations:

- The most prominent injury report refers to injuries to the thigh, followed by injuries to the knee and ankle/foot.
- Injuries to the lower extremity, on average, account for about one third of all injury reports in studies that surveyed injuries across all body parts.

# 4. Injury Severity

## 4.1 Time Loss

Few studies discussed the amount of time lost due to injury. This may be in part related to at least two factors: (a) study design and (b) definition used to report an injury. Most studies are retrospective descriptions of the numbers of "reported" injuries and, therefore, have not collected information about the participant's time lost as a result of incurring an injury. Similarly, because the injury reporting studies typically only count the number of injuries reported, there exists an implicit expectation that the injury definition is consistent for all individuals recording the injuries.

According to Pelletier et al. (83), the definition of a reportable injury for CAIRS is any event that causes cessation of an athlete's customary participation throughout the participation day and on the day immediately following the day of onset. This definition is consistent with Castaldi (23), who indicated that the American-based injury reporting system (NAIRS) used 1 week as the required absence from competition in order for an injury to be classified as more than minor in severity. While the use of these definitions is important to standardizing injury reports, strict use of these definitions may lead to underreporting some types of injuries. For example, facial lacerations were not included in Lorentzon's (63, 64) reports of the proportion of injuries by injury type because the player did not miss participating the following day. Hayes (46) indicated that on average time loss

due to an ice hockey injury was less than 2 days. However, in general, the epidemiological studies of ice hockey injuries do not report the amount of time loss within the cohorts studied.

## 4.2 Catastrophic Injuries

Catastrophic injuries were defined as those injuries that caused death or permanent disability (Table 15.6). Tator and Edmonds (94, 96) identified an alarming increase in the number of catastrophic injuries to the spine and head as a result of participation in ice hockey. In their 1984 study Tator and Edmonds (94) reported that between 1976 and 1983, there were 60 spinal injuries resulting from participation in ice hockey. The importance of this number of injuries is more distressing when one considers that in a previous report of 358 spinal injuries treated at two Toronto hospitals between 1948 and 1973 none of the injuries were related to participation in ice hockey (92).

By comparison, Pashby's (75-81) research of eye injuries has shown a reduction in catastrophic injuries since 1975. As stated previously, the reduction in eye injuries is directly attributable to the use of face masks and stricter enforcement of penalties for "high sticking." The distribution of catastrophic injuries to the eyes and spine are presented in Table 15.6.

**Table 15.6 Catastrophic Injuries (An Overview of the Work of Tator and Pashby)**

| Year | Tator et al.* number of spinal injuries | Pashby** number of eye injuries | % of injured players in study |
|---|---|---|---|
| 1975 | 1 | 258 | 43 |
| 1976 | 2 | 90 | 12 |
| 1977 | 2 | 52 | 8 |
| 1978 | 4 | 43 | 13 |
| 1979 | 2 | 85 | 21 |
| 1980 | 8 | 68 | 20 |
| 1981 | 12 | 119 | 18 |
| 1982 | 15 | 115 | 13 |
| 1983 | 15 | 124 | 12 |
| 1984 | 15 | 121 | 18 |
| 1985 | 12 | 123 | 22 |
| 1986 | 15 | 93 | 18 |
| 1987 | 9 | 62 | 11 |
| 1988 | 16 | 37 | 6 |
| 1989 | 13 | 33 | 6 |
| 1990 | 19 | 21 | 3 |
| 1991 | 14 | 28 | 7 |
| 1992 | Not available | 31 | 4 |

*Annual reports.

**Year begins at the start of hockey season.

Of all the epidemiological literature reviewed for this chapter, the most thorough descriptions of injuries are presented in the case study reports. The case studies are important because they add an element of personality to the rates and proportions of injuries. In general, the case studies follow a pattern in which the author documents events leading up to the injury, describes the injury, describes the outcomes from the injury, and presents several recommendations to prevent additional cases.

Typically, but not exclusively in ice hockey injury research, the case studies describe noteworthy events that were considered anomalous to the sport of ice hockey. Many of the injuries described in the case studies were either severe injuries or catastrophic injuries. For example, an early case study reported by Fekete (33) described the deaths of two minor league New Brunswick hockey players who were wearing "protective helmets" of the presuspension style. Even at the time this study was conducted, the author described this style of helmet as a "flimsy affair," with inadequate protection. A later report by Gibbs (37) was not only critical of the presuspension-style hockey helmets, but also described the ineffectiveness of the chin straps that were originally designed to hold the helmet in place.

Even though several rule and equipment modifications were intended to prevent catastrophic injuries, ice hockey players continue to sustain severe injuries that may be fatal. The causes of fatal injuries attributed to participation in ice hockey are sometimes difficult to identify and occasionally controversial. Unlike the case study reported by Bull (22) of a 12-year-old male who died after being struck by a hockey stick on his bare head, Aubry and Cantu (5) investigated the cause of death for a 17-year-old ice hockey player who was hit in the neck by an errant puck while he was sitting on the bench. According to Aubry and Cantu (5), the player was hit in the neck, fell backward, and lost consciousness. Not only was the player wearing a helmet but he was also wearing a neck protector. The coroner and the pathologist listed the cause of death as a "subarachnoid hemorrhage," not attributed to the blow in the neck. Aubry and Cantu (5) countered by providing strong evidence that the blow to the neck could have caused a traumatic rupture of the vertebral artery leading to a subarachnoid hemorrhage. Aubry and Cantu (5) promoted the need for a reassessment of neck protectors and the need for more comprehensive emergency medical support at hockey rinks.

# 5. Injury Risk Factors

As in all studies of sports injuries, ice hockey injury risk factors are classified, in general terms, as either intrinsic risk or extrinsic risk. According to Lysens, de Weerdt, and Nieuwboer (65), intrinsic risk factors refer to individual physical and psychological factors and extrinsic risk factors refer to the way an activity is performed, the environment in which it is performed, or the equipment used.

## 5.1 Intrinsic Risk Factors

The physiological events that occur during training/practice sessions or during the game of ice hockey are examples of intrinsic injury risk factors (11, 39, 51). Similarly, anthropometric differences between opposing players (19) might also be considered as important intrinsic risk factors, even though Kropp et al. (60) did not find a relationship between body size and risk of injury in the sample of "midget and bantam" aged players within their study. The studies by Roy et al. (88) and Bernard, Trudel, Marcotte, et al. (12) are of particular importance to the study of the epidemiology of ice hockey injuries, especially the role of body checking and aggressive play in amateur ice hockey. These studies reviewed differences in physical characteristics that could contribute to the prevalence of injuries. The critical results of the two studies are summarized as follows:

- Statistically significant differences were observed in measures of weight, height, grip strength, and the force of impact generated by a body check of the smallest versus the largest players within each age group (88).
- Significant differences were observed between the shortest and tallest players (41 cm), between the lightest and heaviest (47.7 kg), and between force of impact during body checking between the strongest and the weakest players (3.57%) (12).

However, as Houston and Green (51) stated, because hockey is a game of skill and not of size, coaches may differentiate between players by skill levels. Research by Trudel et al. (99) showed that within either a league or a team, there can be significant differences in performance relative to the players' position. For example, Trudel et al. (99) showed that within a league of bantam hockey players (aged 14 and 15 years), significant differences were observed in the number of shots on goal and the number of goals and assists obtained between forwards and defencemen (99). Further, Hastings (40) reported that there was no relationship between a player's position and his risk of injury. Therefore, when considering anthropometric characteristics, researchers should also consider the individual's performance skills, which include skating, shooting, and passing, as important covariates to differences in anthropometric measurements (51).

### 5.1.1 Motor/Functional Characteristics

Although no studies were found that document a direct relationship between an individual's level of fatigue and an ensuing injury, most descriptions of the intrinsic physiological factors refer to the individual's onset of fatigue and the influences of training on development of skill and adaptation (11, 39). During a round-table discussion among several leading researchers in the various aspects of ice hockey, Benton (11) and others discussed the physiological characteristics of the sport. Benton reported that through time/motion analyses and laboratory field tests that included heart rate telemetry, muscle biopsies, and venous blood sampling, exercise physiologists showed that several physiological events can lead to fatigue of the participant, and as such contribute to an increased risk of injury. According to Green (in 11), the participant's performance is limited by aerobic and anaerobic factors. For example, Green indicated that a participant's heart rate during a single shift could exceed 90% of the age-adjusted maximum heart rate. Such a large increase in cardiac rate within such a short period of time would limit the ability to deliver oxygen not only to the working muscles but also to the myocardium. During this event, the participant would have a far greater dependency on energy from anaerobic systems leading to an increase in the concentrations of metabolic end products. Green mentioned that the amounts of metabolic end products may not return to pregame levels until after the game. This latter point is more important when one considers the effect of the inhibitive action (due to increased muscle cell metabolite concentrations) on performance (36).

## 5.2 Extrinsic Factors

### 5.2.1 Exposure

A body check that leads to "contact" with an object or another participant is one of the more important extrinsic risk factors for either inflicting or receiving an injury in ice hockey. More specifically, the body check is one of the most commonly reported causes of both soft tissue and severe trauma injuries (96). Several researchers reported that body contact can lead to sprains, strains, contusions, ruptures and fractures (29, 46, 47, 57, 68, 96).

Aggressive play, which includes body contact, is an extrinsic risk factor for ice hockey injuries (8, 16, 86, 96). Studies that reported injuries related to body checking are included in Table 15.7. Considering the proportion of ice hockey injuries that are caused by collision, removing the element of legal body contact should lead to a reduction in the incidence of injuries. Further, considering that body contact is a primary cause for ice hockey injuries (26, 46, 47, 56, 83), it is of interest to note that some leagues continue to allow full contact (e.g., National Hockey League) while other leagues allow only limited or controlled contact (e.g., Canadian Colleges and Universities and CAHA) and some leagues strictly enforce no contact (e.g., COHA). Roy et al. (88) reported the following differences from comparisons of contact versus noncontact ice hockey leagues:

- Contact leagues registered an average of 2.84 injuries per game; the noncontact league reported a lower average of 0.67 injuries per game (88).
- Over 55% of injuries in the contact league were attributed to contact with an opponent (88).
- Data on injuries sustained over 2 seasons shows that body contact was associated with 46.2% of all minor injuries and 75% of all major injuries.
- Fewer penalties are called in those leagues in which a player can be ejected and suspended for a "major aggression" penalty.
- In addition, 20% of the total number of players on a team are responsible for nearly 46% of all penalties of aggression (99).

Even though aggressive play is apparent in many reports of injuries (38, 86), the findings of Trudel et al. (99) support the need for additional, prospective studies before concluding that all hockey leagues that allow body contact will have more reports of injuries than noncontact hockey leagues.

### 5.2.2 Training Methods or Conditions

Neron (70) conducted an extensive investigation of violence in ice hockey in the province of Quebec. The study included players of all age groups; parents; coaches; league officials; game officials; physical education professionals; medical, dental, and

**Table 15.7   Injuries Related to Body Checking**

| Author | Study design | # of players | # of injuries | % of total injuries related to body checking* | Notes |
|---|---|---|---|---|---|
| Hayes (1975) | P | 30 teams | 1.2/game | 38 | In most cases the injuries resulted from accidents with no assessment of a penalty |
| Dick (1993) | P | 120 teams/ season | 16.2/1,000 AE | 43 | Leading mechanism of injury to all body parts |
| Lorentzon et al. (1988b) | P | 24-25 | 78/1,000 AE | 57.9 | |
| Arber & Biener (1985) | R | 2,462 | 232/218 players | 18.6 | |
| Rielly (1982) | R | 125 | 104 | 43.3 | |
| Kropp et al. (1975) | R | 35,435 registrants | 8.1/1,000 AE | 24 | 34% of head injuries related to body checking |
| Goodwin-Gerberich et al. (1987) | R | 263** | 5/1,000 AE | 35 | 26% of injuries attributed to illegal activity |
| Toogood & Love (1966) | R | 2,469 | 85 | 50 | Recommend more stringent penalties for boarding |
| Biener & Muller (1973) | XS | 38,693 | 2,680 | 17 | |
| Reeves & Mendryk (1975) | XS | 6,890 | 446/345 players | 19.5 | 23% of injuries related to fighting, equipment, and litter |
| Hastings et al. (1974) | XS survey | 20,000 | 542/530 players | 64 | 3% of reported injuries related to fighting |
| Bernard et al. (1993) | XS | | | | |
| Minor injuries | | | | | |
| 1987-1988 | | 5 leagues > | | 46 | Proportion of injuries reported include |
| 1988-1989 | | 44 teams | | 47 | those that were associated with body |
| Major injuries | | | | | checks |
| 1987-1988 | | | | 65 | |
| 1988-1989 | | | | 68 | |

*Includes injuries related to collision with another player.

**A response rate of 12 coaches and 251 players was reported by Goodwin-Gerberich et al. (1987).

*Note.* XS = cross-sectional study; R = retrospective study; P = prospective study.

legal professionals; and the media. The comprehensive report recommended changes in the rules, changes in the roles and responsibilities of various organizations that promote safety in ice hockey, (e.g., the government of Quebec, the Ice Hockey Federation of Quebec, the municipalities, the Ministry of Education, the parents, and the media), and the adoption of a code of ethics based on the principle of fair play. One of the recommendations led to the establishment of La Régie de la Sécurité du Sport au Québec (Office for Safety in Sports in Quebec), a semijudicial body that subsequently had a profound affect on the way the game of ice hockey is played in the province of Quebec. Important findings from studies that this office has supported are summarized as follows:

- Coaches disagreed more with the referee when their teams were losing, yet these same

coaches would encourage their players to respect the rules of the game (27).
- Coaches did not encourage aggressive behaviors on the part of players, yet their own behavior changed in relation to the score differential (27).
- Changes in coaching behavior are important to the interaction between coaches and players in controlling the type of play. Overall there are fewer penalties in the National Hockey League, where players and coaches are elite, compared to junior and university leagues, where players and coaches may lack experience and skills (6).

### 5.2.3 Environment/Equipment

Studies that reported environmental and equipment related mechanisms for injuries are presented in Table 15.8. A review of the findings presented in Table 15.8 suggest the following observations.

- The hockey stick was the most often reported mechanism for ice hockey injuries.
- The puck and skates, although implicated as mechanisms of injury, were identified less often.
- The ice surface was reported by some authors as a mechanism of injury, but was not identified as often as the stick or the puck.
- The goal posts and the boards were typically associated with collision injuries resulting from a body check.

Examples of injury research leading to rule changes, and subsequent reductions in specific injuries, are shown in the work of Thomas Pashby (75-81). Pashby provided the most extensive reporting of injuries to the eye, especially before rule changes concerning the mandatory use of face masks were adopted. However, in a later review of eye injuries within several sports, Pashby (81) stated that the number of ice-hockey-related, post-mandatory face-mask injuries fell from an annual average of 273 to an average of 91, and cases of blind eyes fell from an average of 32 to an average of 17. Further, no blind eyes were reported in those leagues that instituted the use of full face protection. It is also interesting to note that professional leagues have refused to legislate the use of various forms of facial protection typically required by college and amateur leagues (23), despite the findings of researchers such as Audette and coworkers (6), who reported that the use of full face masks versus half visors could diminish the number of "major aggression" penalties assessed.

The benefits of facial protection were shown most profoundly in a comparison between two teams, where facial protection was required for one team but not in the other team. According to Downs (32), an intercollegiate ice hockey team that was required to wear helmets but not facial protection sustained 50 facial injuries, 52% of all reported injuries in one season. In comparison, an amateur team from the same geographic area, which was required to wear helmets and facial protection, similarly reported 52 facial injuries; however, facial injuries accounted for only 21% of all reported injuries during that season.

The use of improved protective head gear has also led to fewer reports like those of Fekete (33), who described the case studies of head-injury-related deaths in players who wore less than adequate protective head gear. Generally, researchers agree that the number of catastrophic injuries must be recognized and dealt with at all levels of hockey. The increase in the incidence of spinal cord injury was described by Benda (8) as a reflection of the changes in size of the players and changes in the

**Table 15.8  Equipment Related to Injury***

| Author | Stick | Puck | Goal post | Boards | Ice | Skates |
|---|---|---|---|---|---|---|
| Biener & Muller (1973) | 25 | 17 | | | | 5 |
| Reeves & Mendryk (1975) | 32.7 | 17.7 | 1.8 | 15.9 | 5.8 | 3.6 |
| Rielly (1982) | 14.4 | 27 | 5.7 | | | |
| Hastings et al. (1974) | 43 | 11 | 16.5 | 16 | 11 | 3 |
| Kropp et al. (1975) | 51 | 12 | 2 | 5 | 4 | |
| Goodwin-Gerberich et al. (1987) | | 7.5 | 10.2 | 19.8 | 8 | |
| Lorentzon et al. (1988b) | 11.8 | 14.5 | | 6.6 | | 2.6 |
| Toogood & Love (1966) | 25 | 19 | | 17 | 14.5 | 9 |
| Hayes (1975) | 29 | 15 | | | 14 | 3.5 |
| Bernard et al. (1993) | | | | | | |
| Minor injuries | | | | | | |
| 1987-1988 | 3 | 14 | Collision = 6 | | 7 | |
| 1988-1989 | 28 | 12 | Collision = 4 | | 6 | |
| Major injuries | | | | | | |
| 1987-1988 | 2 | 2 | Collision = 2 | | 13 | |
| 1988-1989 | 11 | 1 | Collision = 8 | | 2 | |
| Dick (1993) | | | 19 | | | |

*Data are percents of total injuries reported.

style of play. According to Benda (8), some researchers suggested that the developments in protective equipment have led to more aggressive play; other researchers indicated that the style and the weight of the protective equipment could lead to biomechanical changes in the postures of the players that predispose the player to an injury upon the point of impact. This latter perspective was investigated by Bishop, Norman, Wells, et al. (14a) who reported that the helmet and face shield does not predispose the participant to neck injury as a result of a modification in biomechanics (i.e., alteration of center of mass to accommodate the weight of the helmet and face shield). However, while the use of helmets and face masks may reduce the severity of injuries to the head and face, participants continue to report head and facial injuries. The following critical findings of Goodwin-Gerberich et al. (38) are typical of the epidemiological reports of injuries.

- Players with previous injuries were more likely to be reinjured than players who had never reported an injury (38).
- Wingers and defensemen were injured more often than centermen or goaltenders (38).
- Although most (74%) of the reported injuries resulted from legal activity, the causes of injuries included collisions with other players, the boards, or the frame of the net (38).

# 6. Suggestions for Injury Prevention

Continued reduction in ice hockey injuries is necessary. Any preventable injury is absolutely unacceptable. Several comprehensive injury studies reported in this chapter showed that rule changes and the designs of new equipment increased the safety of the game (15, 18, 46, 47, 75, 97).

## 6.1 Equipment

The benefits derived from the mandatory use of specific equipment, such as helmets (28, 43) and face guards (23, 28, 32, 43, 63, 81), are demonstrated by a natural experiment that evolved from the legislation for mandatory equipment use in several leagues. Studies conducted prior to the legislation of helmet and face mask use (15, 18, 97) reported a higher prevalence of specific types of injuries than survey-based studies conducted after specific rule changes (29, 38, 46, 47, 75, 77, 94, 95). In addition, enhancements in equipment, such as re-

designs of helmets to provide greater protection (14), safer designs for skate blades (23), and the establishment of the Canadian Standards Association/American Society for Testing and Materials (CSA/ASTM) standards have also contributed to a reduction in reports of ice hockey injuries.

## 6.2 Sport

Similar to rule changes regarding the use of specific equipment, changes in rules about style of play (43, 100), such as stricter rules concerning high sticking (29, 81) and checking from behind (96) as well as stricter enforcement of existing rules, have led to a reduction in specific ice hockey injuries. Attempts to change the rules to create a safer game are not uncommon, but as in most sports, the developments of more stringent rule enforcement frequently follows the occurrence of severe, and sometimes fatal, injuries (23).

Although legislated changes to the rules about body checking have affected the incidence of injury reports, hockey players at all levels continue to be injured. In order to prevent injuries in ice hockey, players, coaches, and officials must comply with specific rules about style of play. Based on the findings presented here, the following recommendations will create a safer game of ice hockey.

- Players must wear specific protective equipment at all times (i.e., while sitting on the bench and while playing in the game), including CSA/ASTM approved helmets, face shields, and throat protectors.
- Ice hockey governing bodies such as the CAHA, NHL, and USA Hockey must support (financially) the continued development of protective equipment and the on-going development of a safer playing environment.
- Ice hockey governing bodies must legislate that arenas establish and document appropriate plans to handle all forms of ice hockey related emergencies, injuries, and accidents at all levels of play. This will require specific staffing and equipment revisions for many arenas.
- Ice hockey governing bodies must approve and enforce stricter penalties for infractions of rules that predispose individuals to injuries.
- Ice hockey governing bodies must reconsider the need for specific types of play at various levels. For example, eliminating body checking and slapshots will prevent some injuries and should, therefore, be the norm for ice hockey.

- The media must avoid sensationalizing the contact aspect of ice hockey (e.g., showing videos that display the dangerous body checks that occur at the professional level).

# 7. Suggestions for Further Research

One of the more necessary additions to the continued monitoring of ice hockey injuries is the development of a standardized, commonly accepted, universal ice hockey injury reporting system. The reporting system will be a computer based, standardized instrument, which can be used easily to track injuries. Information collected within the system will be used for future epidemiological research reports.

The reporting system will require several stages of development as it evolves toward a comprehensive injury-data system. For example, attending physicians and therapists will be required to complete, in some detail, specific, standardized forms. Coaches and injured players will also have a set of forms to complete. The coach/injured player forms are intended to provide essential information that describes the characteristics of the participants, preparation for play, training regimens, previous injuries, and style of play. A standardized system, which is universally adopted, will increase the opportunity to conduct prospective studies that include the elements necessary to evaluate injury rates.

In addition, by creating a simple-to-use system volunteer recorders (i.e., trainers, coaches, team support personnel) will increase their injury-reporting compliance. Further, ice hockey leagues that adopt the standardized reporting system will designate an injury-reporting manager who will be trained in standardized data-collection procedures. Suggested definitions of terms for reportable injuries across the levels of injury severity and methods for computing injury rates are presented in Table 15.9.

Developing a data-collection system is, however, only one recommendation for future research in the area of the sport of ice hockey. There is a need to reconsider the types of injuries and problems that may arise from within the growing subgroups of the ice hockey population. For example, the number and size of old-timers hockey leagues are growing rapidly. The types of injuries and problems observed in these leagues will be different than injuries reported within the younger age groups. Problems such as recurring injuries or injuries that were caused by participation in other

**Table 15.9  Definitions for a Reportable Injury**

1. *Reportable injury/illness:* Injuries and illnesses meeting *any* of the following definitions are reportable. These definitions are meant to separate the nuisance injuries that warrant little attention and do not materially affect performance from the health problems that have potential or demonstrated significance.
   - Any injury/illness that causes cessation of an athlete's customary participation throughout the *participation day and following day of onset* is reportable. In other words: Could the player practice or play the next day without any restrictions?
   - Any *brain concussion* causing cessation of the athlete's participation for observation before return to play is permitted is reportable.
   - Any *dental injury* that *should* receive professional attention is reportable.
   - Any injury/illness that requires *substantive professional* attention before the athlete's return to participation is reportable (i.e., without such attention, the athlete would not have been permitted to return to participation the next participation day).

2. *Injury severity classification*
   - Minor case = any reportable injury/illness (other than dental injuries) that did not keep an athlete from participation longer than 1 week
   - Significant case = any injury/illness that kept an athlete from participation longer than 1 week, plus dental injuries regardless of time loss
   - Major case = any significant injury/illness that kept an athlete from participation longer than 3 weeks
   - Severe case = any significant injury/illness causing societally serious disability (e.g., death, quadriplegia, amputation)

3. *Injury rates classification*
   - Total athlete exposures = AE = (average squad size × # of practices) + (average squad size × # of games)
   - R/1,000 athlete exposures = # injuries ÷ total AE × 1,000
   - R/100 players = # injuries ÷ average squad size × 100

sports, at a younger age, may now become more prevalent. Further, problems related to aging physiological systems within the body may lead to injuries/problems not yet identified within this area of research. For example, the effects of progressive coronary heart disease, cigarette smoking, and adverse lifestyle will be more profound in the old-timer hockey player.

Likewise, as the professional game evolves toward a form of entertainment in which collisions are expected, participant selection will be based on size, strength, and the ability to initiate such collision-type play, while demonstrating an ability to receive a violent body check without interruption of play. Such an evolution will have ramifications within the leagues that feed the professional systems. The types of injuries observed in the feeder systems may be more profound than were observed previously and, in some cases, may be more likely to end careers before they ever begin.

Future research into the sport of ice hockey will require epidemiological evidence to substantiate recommendations for continued changes in rules and equipment. The research teams should include therapists, physicians, sport epidemiologists, behavioral scientists, and technical consultants who will develop a system of problem identification, injury/problem description, and injury/problem presentation. The research team will recommend ways to create a safer playing environment and a safer method of participation for those who play ice hockey.

# References

1. Adams, L.; Montelpare, W. Directions for research in old-timers hockey: a summary of findings on physical preparation and attitudes in the Jordan old-timers hockey league. In: Castaldi, C., Bishop, P.J., Hoerner, E.F., eds. Safety in ice hockey: second volume. ASTM STP 1212, C.R., Philadelphia: American Society for Testing and Materials; 1993:71-77.

2. Akermark, C. Prevention of ice hockey injuries. In: Törnquist, C., ed. Proceedings of the 3rd International Conference on the Coaching Aspects of Ice Hockey. Gothenburg, Sweden: The Swedish Ice Hockey Association; 1981.

3. Antaki, S.; Labelle, P.; Dumas, J. Retinal detachment following hockey injury. CMAJ 117(3):245-246; 1977.

4. Arber, W.; Biener, K. Accidents dus à la pratique du hockey sur glace. Macolin. 2:10-12; 1985.

5. Aubry, M.; Cantu, R. Sudden death of an ice hockey player. Physician Sportsmed. 17(1):53-64; 1989.

6. Audette, S.; Trudel, P.; Bernard, D. Comparison of penalties assessed in minor, junior, university and professional ice hockey leagues. In: Castaldi, C., Bishop, P.J., Hoerner, E.F., eds. Safety in ice hockey: second volume. ASTM STP 1212, C.R., Philadelphia: American Society for Testing and Materials; 1993:88-94.

7. Bancroft, R. Type, location and severity of hockey injuries occurring during competition and practice. In: Castaldi, C., Bishop, P.J., Hoerner, E.F., eds. Safety in ice hockey: second volume. ASTM STP 1212, C.R., Philadelphia: American Society for Testing and Materials; 1993:31-43.

8. Benda, C. Catastrophic head and neck injuries in amateur hockey. Physician Sportsmed. 17(12):115-122; 1989.

9. Benoit, B.; Russell, M.; Hugenholtz, R.; Ventureyra, E.; Choo, S. Epidural hematoma: report of seven cases with delayed evolution of symptoms. J. Can. des Sciences Neurologiques 9(3):321-324; 1982.

10. Benton, J. Epiphyseal fracture in sports. Physician Sportsmed. 10(11):62-71; 1982.

11. Benton, J. Hockey: optimizing performance and safety. A round table. Physician Sportsmed. 11(12):73-83; 1983.

12. Bernard, D.; Trudel, P.; Marcotte, G.; Boileau, R. The incidence, types and circumstances of injuries to ice hockey players at the bantam level (14 to 15 years old). In: Castaldi, C., Bishop, P.J., Hoerner, E.F., eds. Safety in ice hockey: second volume. ASTM STP 1212, C.R., Philadelphia: American Society for Testing and Materials; 1993:45-55.

13. Biener, K.; Muller, P. Les accidents du hockey sur glace. Cahiers de Medecine (Europa Medica) 14(11):959-962;1973.

14. Bishop, P.; Norman, R.; Pierrynowski, M.; Kozey, J. The ice hockey helmet: how effective is it? Physician Sportsmed. 7(2):97-106; 1979.

14a. Bishop, P.; Norman, R.; Wells, R.; Ranney, D.; Skleryk, B. Charges in the center of mass and moment of inertia of a head form induced by a hockey helmet and face shield. Can. J. Applied Sport Sciences 8(1):19-25; 1983.

15. Blackburn, M.M. One-year evaluation of twelve mouth protectors for Edmonton hockey players. Can. Dental Assoc. J. 30(9):561-564; 1964.

16. Blase, K. USA hockey: a vision for the 1990s. In: W. Grana, J. Lombardo, B. Sharkey, and J. Stone, eds. Advances in sports medicine and fitness, volume 3. Chicago: Year Book Medical Publishers, Inc.; 1990:245-257.

17. Boileau, R.; Marcotte, G.; Trudel, P.; Bernard, D. Final report on the implementation of an intervention strategy for reducing the number of injuries and acts of aggression in the bantam hockey division. FCAR Fund, Regie de la securitie dans les sports du Quebec, Jan 1990.

18. Bolitho, N. Head injuries in ice hockey at the amateur level. CAHPER 37(2):29-34; 1970.

19. Bouchard, C.; Landry, F.; Leblanc, C.; Mondor, J.C. Quelques-unes des caracteristiques physiques et physiologiques des jouers de hockey et leurs relations avec la performance. Mouvement 9(1):95-110; 1974.

20. Bouchard, C.; Roy, B. L'age osseux des jeunes participants du tournoi international de hockey pee-wee de Quebec. Mouvement 4:225-232; 1969.

21. Bouchard, F. Blessures au hockey majeur: 3 ans d'etude. CMAJ 117(6):640-643; 1977.

22. Bull, C. Hockey injuries. In: Schneider, R., Kennedy, J., Plant, M., eds. Sports injuries: mechanisms, prevention, and treatment. Baltimore: Williams and Wilkins; 1985:90-113.

23. Castaldi, C. Ice hockey. In: Adams, S., Adrian, M., and Bayless, M.A., eds. Catastrophic injuries in sports: avoidance strategies, 2nd edition. Indianapolis: Benchmark Press; 1987:81-99.

24. Chao, E.; Sim, F.; Stauffer, R.; Johannson, K. Mechanics of ice hockey injuries. In: Bleustein, J.L., ed.

Mechanics and sport. New York: The American Society of Mechanical Engineers; 1973:143-154.

25. Clayton, P. International Hockey Centre of Excellence, Injury Report System, 1990-91 season. Canadian Amateur Hockey Association. Distributed at Safety in Ice Hockey: Symposium for the American Society for Testing and Materials (ASTM), Pittsburgh, 1993.

26. Clayton, P. Western Hockey League 1989-90 Final Data Summary. International Hockey Centre of Excellence. Calgary, Alberta, 1990.

27. Côté, J.; Trudel, P.; Bernard, D.; Boileau, R.; Marcotte, G. Observation of coach behaviours during different game score differentials. In: Castaldi, C., Bishop, P.J., Hoerner, E.F., eds. Safety in ice hockey: second volume, ASTM STP 1212, C.R., Philadelphia: American Society for Testing and Materials; 1993.

28. Coventry, M. Winter sports injuries. The Lancet 85:66-70; 1965.

29. Daly, P.; Foster, T.; Zarins, B. Injuries in ice hockey. In: Renstrom, P., ed. Clinical practice of sports injury prevention and care. London: Blackwell Scientific Publications; 1994:375-391.

30. Daly, P.; Sim, F.; Simonet, W. Ice hockey injuries: a review. Sports Medicine 10(3):122-131; 1990.

31. Dick, R.W. Injuries in collegiate ice hockey. In: Castaldi, C., Bishop, P.J., Hoerner, E.F., eds. Safety in ice hockey: second volume, ASTM STP 1212, C.R., Philadelphia: American Society for Testing and Materials; 1993:21-30.

32. Downs, J. Incidence of facial trauma in intercollegiate and junior hockey. Physician Sportsmed. 7(2):88-92; 1979.

33. Fekete, J. Severe brain injury and death following minor hockey accidents: the effectiveness of the "safety helmets" of amateur hockey players. CMAJ. 99:1234-1239; 1968.

34. Feriencik, K. Trends in ice hockey injuries: 1965 to 1967. Physician Sportsmed. 7(2):81-82; 1979.

35. Finke, R.; Goodwin-Gerberich, S.; Madden, M.; Funk, S.; et al. Shoulder injuries in ice hockey. J. Ortho. Sports Phys. Therapy 10(2):54-58; 1988.

36. Fox, E.; Bowers, R.; Foss, M. The physiological basis for exercise and sport, 5th edition. Madison, WI: Brown and Benchmark; 1993.

37. Gibbs, R. Unsafe headgear faulted in critical hockey injuries. Physician Sportsmed. 2(2):39-42; 1974.

38. Goodwin-Gerberich, S.; Finke, R.; Madden, M.; Priest, J.; Aamoth, G.; Murray, K. An epidemiological study of high school ice hockey injuries. Child's Nervous System 3:59-64; 1987.

39. Green, H.; Bishop, P.; Houston, M.; McKillop, R.; Norman, R.; Stothart, P. Time-motion and physiological assessments of ice hockey performance. J. Applied Physiology 40(2):159-163; 1976.

40. Hastings, D.; Cameron, J.; Parker, S.; Evans, J. A study of hockey injuries in Ontario. Ont. Medical Review 41:686-692; 1974.

41. Hayes, D. An injury profile for hockey. Can. J. Applied Sport Sciences 3:61-64; 1978.

43. Hayes, D. Risk factors in sport. Human Factors 16(5):454-458; 1974.

44. Hayes, D. An injury profile for hockey. In: Landry, F., Orban, W., eds. Ice hockey: research, development and new concepts. Miami, FL: Symposia Specialists, Inc; 1978:89-95.

45. Hayes, D. College ice hockey injuries frequent but mostly minor. Hospital Tribune 23: Jan. 21; 1974.

46. Hayes, D. Hockey injuries: how, why, where, and when? Physician Sportsmed. 3(1):61-65; 1975.

47. Hayes, D. The nature, incidence, location, and causes of injury in intercollegiate ice hockey. In: Taylor, A. Application of science and medicine to sport. Springfield, IL: Charles C Thomas; 1975: 292-300.

48. Hayes, D. Reducing risks in hockey: analysis of equipment and injuries. Physician Sportsmed. 6(1):67-70; 1978.

49. Hornof, Z.; Napravnik, C. Analysis of various accident rate factors in ice hockey. Med. and Science in Sports 5(4):283-286; 1973.

50. Horns, R. Blinding hockey injuries. Minnesota Medicine 59(4):255-258; 1976.

51. Houston, M.; Green, H. Physiological and anthropometric characteristics of elite Canadian ice hockey players. J. Sports Med. 16:123-128; 1976.

52. Hovelius, L. Shoulder dislocation in Swedish ice hockey players. Amer. J. Sports Med. 6(6):373-377; 1978.

53. Hoyt, W. Etiology of shoulder injuries in athletes. J. Bone Joint Surg. 49:755-766; 1967.

54. Hulley, S.; Cummings, S. Designing clinical research. Baltimore, MD: Williams and Wilkins; 1988.

55. Hunter, R. Chapter 30: Hockey. In: Reider, B., ed. Sports medicine: the school-age athlete. Philadelphia, PA: W.B. Saunders; 1991:590-600.

56. Hunter, J. Hockey takes a heavy injury toll. Globe and Mail 141:42:Nov. 3:S1, S5; 1984.

57. Janes, J. Ice-hockey injuries. Clin. Orthopaedics 23:67-74; 1962.

58. Jorgensen, U.; Schmidt-Olsen, S. The epidemiology of ice hockey injuries. Brit. J. Sports Med. 20(1):7-9; 1986.

59. Kraus, J.; Anderson, B.; Meuller, C. The effectiveness of a special ice hockey helmet to reduce head injuries in college intramural hockey. Med. Sci. Sports 2(3):162-164, 1979.

60. Kropp, D.; Marchant, L.; Warshawski, J. An analysis of head injuries in hockey and lacrosse. Sport Safety Research Report, Fitness and Amateur Sport Branch, Department of National Health and Welfare, 1974-1975.

61. L'Abbé, Detsky, O'Rourke. Meta-analysis in clinical research. Amer. J. of Internal Med. 107:224-233; 1987.

62. Legault, P. Personal Communication. Registrants in the Canadian Amateur Hockey Association; data released for 1992-93 season; 1993.

63. Lorentzon, R.; Werden, H.; Pietila, T.; Gustavsson, B. Injuries in international ice hockey: a prospective, comparative study of injury incidence and injury types in international and Swedish elite ice hockey. Amer. J. Sports Med. 16(4):389-391; 1988a.

64. Lorentzon, R.; Werden, H.; Pietila, T. Incidence, nature, and causes of ice hockey injuries: a three-year prospective study of a Swedish elite ice hockey team. Amer. J. Sports Med. 16(4):392-396; 1988b.

65. Lysens, R.; de Weerdt, W.; Nieuwboer, A. Factors associated with injury proneness. Sports Medicine 12(5):281-289; 1991.

66. MacIntosh, S.; Shephard, R. Athletic injuries at the University of Toronto. Medicine and Science in Sports 3(4):194-199; 1971.

67. Mack, R. Ice hockey injuries. Sports Medicine Digest 3(1):1-2; 1981.

68. Muller, P.; Biener, K. Eishockeysportunfälle. Munch med Wschr. 115(13):564-567; 1973.

69. Von Napravnik, C. Kopfverletzungen beim Eishockey. Medizin und Sport 12:45-47; 1972.

70. Neron, G. La violence au hockey. Haut-Commissariat a la jeunesse, aux loisirs et au sports. Gouvernement du Québec; 1977.

71. Nordin, M. Biomechanics of ligaments. In: Törnquist, C., ed. Proceedings of the 3rd international conference on the coaching aspects of ice hockey. Gothenburg, Sweden: The Swedish Ice Hockey Association; 1981.

72. Norfray, J.; Tremaine, M.; Homer, C.; Groves, M.; Bachman, M. The clavicle in hockey. Amer. J. Sports Med. 5(6):275-280; 1977.

73. Noyes, F.; Albright, J. Sports injury research. J. of Sports Med. 16(Suppl. 1); 1988.

74. Park, R.; Castaldi, C. Injuries in junior ice hockey. Physician Sportsmed. 8(2):81-90; 1980.

75. Pashby, T.; Pashby, R.; Chisholm, L.; Crawford, J. Eye injuries in Canadian hockey. CMAJ. 113:663-666, 674; 1975.

76. Pashby, T. Eye injuries in Canadian hockey. Phase II. CMAJ. 117(6):670-678; 1977.

77. Pashby, T. Eye injuries in Canadian amateur hockey. Amer. J. Sports Med. 7(4):254-257; 1979.

78. Pashby, T. Eye injuries in hockey. Inter. Ophthalmology Clin. 21(4):59-81; 1981.

79. Pashby, T. Eye injuries in Canadian amateur hockey. Can. J. Ophthalmology 20(1):2-4; 1985.

80. Pashby, T. Eye injuries in Canadian amateur hockey: still a concern. Can. J. Ophthalmology 22(6):293-296; 1987.

81. Pashby, T. Eye injuries in sports. Journal of Ophthalmic Nursing & Technology 8(3):99-101; 1989.

82. Pelletier, R.; Montelpare, W.J.; Taylor, B.; Yakutchik, D. Injury profile in Canadian interuniversity hockey. Can. J. Sport Sciences. 15(4):abstracts; 1990.

83. Pelletier, R.; Montelpare, W.; Stark, R. Intercollegiate ice hockey injuries: a case for uniform definitions and reports. American Journal of Sport Medicine 21(1):78-82; 1993.

84. Pforringer, W.; Smasal, V. Aspects of traumatology in ice hockey. J. Sport Sciences 5(3):327-336; 1987.

85. Reeves, J.; Mendryk, S. A study of the incidence, nature and cause of hockey injuries in the greater Edmonton metropolitan area. In: Taylor, A., ed. Application of science and medicine to sport. Springfield, IL: Charles C Thomas; 1975:301-308.

86. Rielly, M. The nature and causes of hockey injuries: a five year study. Athletic Training 17(2):88-90; 1982.

87. Rovere, G.; Gristina, A.; Nicastro, J. Medical problems of a professional hockey team: a three-season experience. Physician Sportsmed. 6(1):58-63; 1978.

88. Roy, A.; Bernard, D.; Roy, B.; Marcotte, G. Body checking in pee-wee hockey. The Physician and Sport Medicine 17(3):119-126; 1989.

89. Sane, J.; Ylipaavalniemi, P.; Leppanen, H. Maxillofacial and dental ice hockey injuries. Med. Sci. Sports Exercise 20(2):202-207; 1988.

90. Sim, F.; Chao, E. Injury potential in modern ice hockey. Amer. J. Sports Medicine 6(6):378-384; 1978.

91. Sutherland, G. Fire on ice. Amer. J. Sports Med. 4(6):264-269; 1976.

92. Tator, C.; Edmonds, V. Acute spinal cord injury: analysis of epidemiologic factors. Can. J. Surg. 22(6):575-578; 1979.

93. Tator, C. Spinal injuries due to hockey. CMAJ. 127(11):1077; 1982.

94. Tator, C.; Edmonds, V. National survey of spinal injuries in hockey players. CMAJ. 130(7):875-880; 1984.

95. Tator, C. Neck injuries in ice hockey: a recent, unsolved problem with many contributing factors. Clin. Sports Med. 6(1):101-114; 1987.

96. Tator, C.; Edmonds, V.; Lapczak, L. Spinal injuries in ice hockey: review of 182 North American cases and analysis of etiological factors. In: Castaldi, C., Bishop, P.J., Hoerner, E.F., eds. Safety in ice hockey: second volume, ASTM STP 1212, C.R., Philadelphia: American Society for Testing and Materials; 1993:11-20.

97. Toogood, T.; Love, W. Hockey injury survey. CAHPER 32(2):20-23; 1966.

98. Tredget, T.; Godberson, C.; Bose, B. Myositis ossificans due to hockey injury. CMAJ. 116(1):65-66; 1977.

99. Trudel, P.; Bernard, D.; Boileau, R.; Marcotte, G.; Audette, S. The study of performance and aggressive behaviors of ice hockey players. In: Castaldi, C., Bishop, P.J., Hoerner, E.F., eds. Safety in ice hockey: second volume, ASTM STP 1212, C.R., Philadelphia: American Society for Testing and Materials; 1993:95-102.

101. Vinger, P. Ocular injuries in hockey. Arch Opthalamol. 94(1):74-76; 1976.

102. Clarke, K.; Powell, J. Football helmets and neurotrauma—an epidemiological overview of three seasons. Med. and Science in Sports 11(2):138-145; 1979.

103. Wilson, K.; Cram, B.; Rontal, E.; Rontal, M. Facial injuries in hockey players. Minn. Med. 60:13-19; 1977.

104. Pollard. The nature and occurrence of injuries in ice hockey. In: Mathe, E., ed. Proceedings of Conference on Winter Sports Injuries, Madison, WI; 1967:156-167.

105. Daffner, R. Injuries in amateur ice hockey: A two year analysis. J. of Family Practice 4(2):225-227; 1977.

# 16

# Martial Arts

## Willy Pieter

## 1. Introduction

Oriental martial sports have become increasingly popular in the West, especially since WW II. National and international competitions are held in several of these sports and one of them, judo, has become an Olympic sport. Taekwondo was a demonstration sport at the 1988 and 1992 Olympic Games, and karate practitioners aspire to the Olympics. Tournaments are not only organized for adult participants, but also for young athletes. For instance, the U.S. Junior Olympic National Taekwondo Championships experienced a 124% increase in participation rate between 1989 and 1991. Despite this interest in martial sports, research on the epidemiology of martial sports injuries is scarce and in some cases nonexistent. On occasion, martial sports injuries were included as part of a larger survey on sports injuries (3, 22, 81, 95, 102), but in these cases, no separate injury rates were reported for the martial sports.

Judo competition and training always involve contact. Competition in karate and taekwondo may be full contact or noncontact. Injuries discussed in this chapter on the latter two martial sports will be predominantly on full contact taekwondo and noncontact karate because of lack of information in the other variations of the sports.

The purpose of this chapter is to present information related to injuries in judo, karate, and taekwondo because these three forms offer the majority of injury data. The literature search included all studies published in English, French, German, or Dutch as well as unpublished theses and dissertations. This choice of languages is partly related to the fact that more studies on injuries in the selected martial sports are published in one or more of these languages (especially French and German) as opposed to injury studies in Hungarian or Portuguese, for instance, and partly to this author's limited linguistic skills. No studies in Chinese, Japanese, and Korean are included, for the computer searches did not yield an appreciable number of publications in any of these languages. In addition, we have included no anecdotal or theoretical discussions of potential injuries in martial sports for review.

We accomplished data collection using the following procedures: (a) ancestry approach—retrieval of research cited in published research; (b) computer searches—the Sport Discus database (key words were martial arts injuries, judo injuries, karate injuries, taekwondo injuries), the Medline database (key words were martial arts injuries, taekwondo injuries, karate injuries, judo injuries), and Sportwissenschaft Datenbank Spolit (key words were martial arts injuries, budo injuries, judo injuries, karate injuries, taekwondo injuries); and (c) articles by the author that have been submitted for publication in 1994. The computer searches were conducted from 1960 through 1993 to incorporate as much information as possible.

Most of the information found on injuries in the martial sports are from case and case series studies. Although these studies will give a general indication of the occurrence of certain injury types in the martial sports, the limitations are prohibitive in gaining a better understanding of the occurrence of injuries in the general population of martial sports athletes and in identifying high risk groups as well as risk factors for injury (101). On the other hand, the retrospective and prospective studies included in this review have contributed much to what is presently known about injuries in martial sports, although they are limited by their inconsistencies in injury definition, data collection methods, and treatment of data.

# 2. Incidence of Injury

## 2.1 Injury Rates

A comparison of injury rates based on retrospective and prospective studies on martial sports injuries in men and women is shown in Tables 16.1 and 16.2, respectively. As expected, these injury rates were calculated differently across studies. In cases where injury rates per 100 participants were not reported, this author, based on the information provided in the respective studies, calculated the rates by dividing the total number of injuries by the number of participants, the quotient of which

was then multiplied by 100. The obvious weakness of this approach is that not every participant is equally exposed to the risk of sustaining an injury (101). If exposure data were provided in the literature searched, injury rates per 1,000 athlete-exposures (A-E) were calculated by this author by dividing the number of injuries by the number of A-E and multiplying by 1,000.

Perusal of Tables 16.1 and 16.2 suggests that more injuries were incurred in male noncontact karate without the use of protective padding than in the other martial sports reviewed, perhaps because more data are available on injuries in male than in female martial sports athletes. Part of this

**Table 16.1  A Comparison of Injury Rates in Men's Martial Sports**

| Sport/study | Design | Data collection | Duration | # injuries | Sample # part. | Rate per 100 part. | Rate 1,000 A-E | Rate per 1,000 pract. hours |
|---|---|---|---|---|---|---|---|---|
| Judo | | | | | | | | |
| Azuma, 1971 | Prospect | Questionnaire | 5 years | 1,735 | 1,672 | 103.8 | — | — |
| Barrault et al., 1983 | Prospect. | Questionnaire | 1 year | 3,941 | 16,496 | 23.9 | 122.6 | — |
| Ransom & Ransom, 1989 | Prospect. | Questionnaire | 3 tournaments | 485 | 181[a] | 268.0[a] | — | — |
| Rabenseifer, 1984 | Prospect. | Questionnaire | 1 year | 542 | 100 | 542.0 | — | — |
| Non-contact karate (with padding) | | | | | | | | |
| Buckley, 1990 | Prospect. | Questionnaire | 9 tournaments | 108 | — | — | 46.0 | — |
| Johannsen & Noerregaard, 1988 | Prospect. | Questionnaire | 4 tournaments | 74 | 270 | 27.4 | 127.6 | — |
| McLatchie & Morris, 1977 | Prospect. | Questionnaire | 3 tournaments | 49 | — | — | 22.2 | — |
| Non-contact karate (without padding) | | | | | | | | |
| Hirata, 1971 | Propsect. | Not reported | 1 year | 221 | 666 | 31.2 | — | — |
| Johannsen & Noerregaard, 1988 | Prospect. | Questionnaire | 3 tournaments | 153 | 403 | 38.0 | 123.4 | — |
| Kurland, 1980b | Prospect. | Questionnaire | Not reported | 11 | 32 | 34.4 | — | 18.4 |
| McLatchie, 1976 | Prospect. | Questionnaire | 1 tournament | 80 | — | — | 135.6 | — |
| McLatchie & Morris, 1977 | Prospect. | Questionnaire | 5 tournaments | 147 | — | — | 98.8 | — |
| Poirier, 1990 | Prospect. | Questionnaire | 6 years | 548[a,b] | — | — | 154.3 | — |
| Stricevic et al., 1983 | Prospect. | Questionnaire | 6 tournaments | 82 | 284 | 28.9 | 132.7 | — |
| Full-contact karate | | | | | | | | |
| McLatchie et al., 1980 | Prospect. | Questionnaire | 1 tournament | 37 | 70 | 52.9 | — | — |
| Full-contact taekwondo | | | | | | | | |
| Oler et al., 1991 | Prospect. | Questionnaire | 1 tournament | 52[a] | 700[a,b] | 7.4[d] | — | — |
| Oler et al., 1991 | Prospect. | Questionnaire | 1 tournament | 102[a,c] | 700[a,c,d] | 3.4[d] | — | — |
| Pieter & Lufting, 1994 | Prospect. | Questionnaire | 1 tournament | 12[e] | 273 | 4.4[e] | 22.9[e] | — |
| Pieter et al., 1994 | Prospect. | Questionnaire | 1 tournament | 36 | 67 | 53.7 | 139.5 | — |
| Pieter & Zemper, 1994a | Prospect. | Questionnaire | 4 years | 324 | 1,665 | 19.5 | 95.1 | — |
| Pieter & Zemper, 1994b | Prospect. | Questionnaire | 3 years | 353[c] | 3,274[c] | 10.8 | 58.2 | — |
| Zemper & Pieter, 1989 | Prospect. | Questionnaire | 1 tournament | 27 | 48 | 56.3 | 127.4 | — |

[a]Includes males and females.

[b]Includes juniors and seniors.

[c]Junior (6-16 years) taekwondo athletes.

[d]Estimated based on data provided by authors.

[e]Number of significant injuries (significant=at least one week absence from participation).

**Table 16.2    A Comparison of Injury Rates in Women's Martial Sports**

| Sport/study | Design | Data collection | Duration | # injuries | Sample # part. | Rate per 100 part. | Rate 1,000 A-E | Rate per 1,000 pract. hours |
|---|---|---|---|---|---|---|---|---|
| Judo | | | | | | | | |
| Barrault et al., 1983 | Prospect. | Questionnaire | 1 year | 350 | 1,099 | 31.9 | 130.6 | — |
| Non-contact karate (without padding) | | | | | | | | |
| Kurland, 1980b | Prospect. | Questionnaire | Not reported | 7 | 17 | 41.2 | — | 21.0 |
| Full-contact taekwondo | | | | | | | | |
| Pieter & Lufting, 1994 | Prospect. | Questionnaire | 1 tournament | 3[e] | 160 | 1.9[e] | 9.7[e] | — |
| Pieter et al., 1994 | Prospect. | Questionnaire | 1 tournament | 11 | 30 | 36.7 | 96.5 | — |
| Pieter & Zemper, 1994a | Prospect. | Questionnaire | 4 years | 174 | 742 | 23.5 | 105.5 | — |
| Pieter & Zemper, 1994b | Prospect. | Questionnaire | 3 years | 87[c] | 865[c] | 10.1 | 56.6 | — |
| Zemper & Pieter, 1989 | Prospect. | Questionnaire | 1 tournament | 20 | 48 | 41.7 | 90.1 | — |

[a]Includes males and females.

[b]Includes juniors and seniors.

[c]Junior (6-16 years) taekwondo athletes.

[d]Estimated based on data provided by authors.

[e]Number of significant injuries (significant=at least one week absence from participation).

lack of injury data for female martial sports athletes may be related to the following:

- Lower number of female martial sport participants (3, 95).
- Until recently, females were excluded from competition (91).
- Some researchers reported injuries and injury rates for a combined sample of adult men and women or of young males and females (6, 40, 63, 64, 75, 77, 83, 108).

Combining the injuries for males and females may be based on the notion that they incur the same type and degree of injury in the same body part (7). The injury type may be the same in males and females, but certainly the degree of injury may be different.

## 3. Injury Characteristics

### 3.1 Injury Onset

It should come as no surprise, because of the contact aspect of martial sports, that injuries reported in the literature are predominantly sudden onset (see Table 16.3).

### 3.2 Injury Types

Tables 16.4 and 16.5 represent the percent comparison of injury types incurred in men's and women's

martial sports, respectively. Because of lack of information in most studies, the data are based on most, but not all, of the prospective studies displayed in Tables 16.1 and 16.2. A review of Tables 16.4 and 16.5 suggests the following observations:

- Certain injury types were reported in some but not all samples (e.g., nerve injury).
- Some injury types were combined in most studies (e.g., sprains and strains).
- Studies used different names for some injury types (e.g., hemorrhage instead of epistaxis).

Information on injury types in women is available for only full contact taekwondo athletes. Tables 16.4 and 16.5 suggest that contusions and sprains are injury types common to all three martial sports reviewed.

### 3.2.1 Judo

Among male judo athletes, sprains and contusions emerge as the most frequently occurring injuries in the prospective data. However, the number of subjects in the two prospective studies differs so greatly that further discussion of the data would be meaningless.

### 3.2.2 Karate

The most frequently occurring injury type in non-contact karate without padding is the contusion (range 3.8-72.0%), followed by the laceration

**Table 16.3   A Percent Comparison of Nature of Injury Onset in Men's and Women's Martial Sports**

| Sport/study | Design | # of participants | Injury onset Sudden | Gradual |
|---|---|---|---|---|
| **Men karate** | | | | |
| Kurland, 1980b | Prospect. | 32 | 77.8 | 22.2 |
| **Taekwondo** | | | | |
| Pieter & Zemper, 1994a | Prospect. | 1,665 | 99.1 | 0.9 |
| Pieter & Zemper, 1994b[a] | Prospect. | 3,274 | 98.6 | 1.4 |
| Zemper & Pieter, 1989 | Prospect. | 48 | 100.0 | 0.0 |
| **Women taekwondo** | | | | |
| Pieter & Zemper, 1994a | Prospect. | 742 | 98.8 | 1.2 |
| Pieter & Zemper, 1994b[a] | Prospect. | 865 | 96.6 | 3.4 |
| Zemper & Pieter, 1989 | Prospect. | 48 | 95.0 | 5.0 |

[a]Percentages refer to Junior Olympic athletes.

(range 10.0-24.4%). Contusions also appear to be very frequent in noncontact karate when padding is used. The one prospective study presently available on full contact karate reported the most frequently occurring injury type as nonspecific (35.1%), followed by the hematoma (24.3%) (55).

As in judo, bone fractures in karate may occur to the lower (10, 82) as well as the upper extremities (20, 60). Dental fractures also have been reported in both martial sports (46). Hand techniques are used more often in karate, as opposed to taekwondo in which leg techniques are dominant, so it should come as no surprise that bone fractures to the hands of karate athletes have appeared in case reports and series data (3, 20, 36, 43, 44, 107).

The injury rate for fractures in noncontact karate for adult males was found to be 8.09/1,000 A-E, and that for full contact taekwondo was 6.07/1,000 A-E (70). Regardless of whether protective equipment was used in noncontact karate, the result should be of interest, since no contact was supposed to have occurred. Padding may have decreased the chances of fractures in noncontact karate, however (34).

### 3.2.3 Taekwondo

A large percentage of contusions are common in both karate (range 40.2-68.3% if the maverick value of 3.8% is deleted) and taekwondo (range 41.0-63.0% for males, 36.8-90.0% for females). One would not expect such a similarity between a noncontact and a full contact event. One explanation may be that martial sports athletes seem to punch and kick harder when wearing protective equipment (85, 89). This may explain the relatively frequent occurrence of the epistaxis in noncontact karate with padding.

In full contact taekwondo, 54.5% of injuries reported to a local hospital during a large international tournament consisted of fractures (87). Punches and kicks to the head may lead to brain injury in karate and taekwondo. No case reports or case series studies were found on brain injury in karate and taekwondo. However, prospective studies (91, 108) have shown rather alarming injury rates for cerebral concussions. The injury rate for cerebral concussions in noncontact male karate athletes was 1.62/1,000 A-E and in full contact taekwondo, 7.34/1,000 A-E. The injury rate for cerebral concussions for adult female taekwondo athletes is 3.03/1,000 A-E (72), but no comparative data for female karate athletes are available.

The rates for cerebral concussions sustained at single tournaments vary in karate and taekwondo:

- For male noncontact karate athletes, 11.86 concussions per 1,000 A-E were reported (51).
- For taekwondo athletes, the rates are 15.27/1,000 A-E (males) and 3.23/1,000 A-E (females) (68), and 15.50/1,000 A-E (males) and 8.77/1,000 A-E (females) (71).
- For young male and female taekwondo athletes, the rates are 5.4/1,000 A-E and 4.6/1,000 A-E, respectively (73).

## 3.3 Injury Location

Tables 16.6, 16.7, and 16.8 show a percent comparison of body parts injured in men's judo and men's and women's full contact taekwondo. The information is based on the prospective studies displayed in Tables 16.1 and 16.2. Clearly, the body parts injured are not consistently reported across

**Table 16.4   A Percent Comparison of Injury Types in Men's Martial Sports**

| Sport/study | Design | # of part. | # of inj. | Abras. | Conc. | Contus. | Disloc. | Epist. | Fract. | Lacer. | Nonspec. | Sprain | Strain | Other |
|---|---|---|---|---|---|---|---|---|---|---|---|---|---|---|
| **Judo** | | | | | | | | | | | | | | |
| Azuma, 1971 | Prospect. | 1,672 | 1,735 | — | — | 13.3 | 14.3 | — | 10.0 | — | — | 56.6 | — | — |
| Koiwai, 1965 | Retrosp. | — | 70 | — | 5.7 | 5.7 | 38.6 | — | 30.0 | — | — | 10.0 | — | 2.9 |
| Rabenseifer, 1984 | Prospect. | 100 | 542 | — | 0.7 | 56.8 | — | — | 1.5 | — | — | 38.9 | — | 2.0 |
| **Non-contact karate (with padding)** | | | | | | | | | | | | | | |
| Johannsen & Noerregaard, 1988 | Prospect. | 270 | 74 | — | 10.0 | 66.0 | — | 10.0 | 1.4 | 12.0 | — | — | — | — |
| McLatchie & Morris, 1977 | Prospect. | — | 49 | — | 4.5 | — | 6.4 | 10.5 | — | 12.0 | — | — | — | — |
| **Non-contact karate (without padding)** | | | | | | | | | | | | | | |
| Hirata, 1971 | Prospect. | 666 | 221 | — | — | 68.3 | — | — | 8.2 | 10.0[a] | — | 9.1 | — | 0.5 |
| Johannsen & Noerregaard, 1988 | Prospect. | 403 | 153 | — | 11.0 | 44.0 | — | 12.0 | 9.0 | 24.0 | — | — | — | — |
| McLatchie, 1976 | Prospect. | — | 80 | — | — | 3.8 | 5.0 | 11.3 | — | 21.3 | 37.5 | 8.8 | — | — |
| McLatchie & Morris, 1977 | Prospect. | — | 147 | — | 6.0 | — | 6.7 | 16.4 | — | 12.0 | 3.2 | — | — | — |
| Poirier, 1990[b] | Prospect. | — | 548 | — | — | 72.0 | 9.0[c] | 33.0 | — | — | — | — | — | — |
| Schmid & Schwarz, 1977 | Retrosp. | 60 | 210 | — | 1.0 | — | — | — | 19.5 | 21.0 | — | 44.8 | — | 13.8 |
| Stricevic et al., 1983 | Prospect. | 284 | 82 | 4.9 | 1.2 | 40.2 | — | 13.4 | 6.1 | 24.4 | — | 7.3 | 1.2 | 1.2 |
| **Full-contact karate** | | | | | | | | | | | | | | |
| McLatchie et al., 1980 | Prospect. | 70 | 37 | — | 5.4 | — | 5.4 | 13.5 | 2.7 | 8.1 | 35.1 | — | 5.4 | — |
| **Full-contact taekwondo** | | | | | | | | | | | | | | |
| Pieter et al., 1994 | Prospect. | 67 | 36 | — | 11.1 | 50.0 | — | 5.6 | 11.1 | 8.3 | — | 11.1 | — | 2.8 |
| Pieter & Zemper, 1994a | Prospect. | 1,665 | 324 | — | 7.7 | 46.9 | 0.6 | — | 5.9 | 11.1 | — | 11.4 | 1.5 | 2.5 |
| Pieter & Zemper, 1994b[d] | Prospect. | 3,274 | 353 | 1.7 | 9.3 | 43.9 | 0.6 | — | 2.6 | 6.0 | 6.5 | 21.3 | 4.5 | — |
| Zemper & Pieter, 1989 | Prospect. | 48 | 27 | 3.7 | 3.7 | 63.0 | — | — | 14.8 | 3.7 | — | 3.7 | 3.7 | — |
| Zandbergen, n.d. | Prospect. | — | 85 | — | 2.4 | 41.0 | — | — | 5.9 | 17.7 | 3.5 | 17.7 | — | 10.6 |

[a]Combination of lacerations and abrasions.
[b]Male and female young and adult athletes.
[c]Combination of dislocations and fractures.
[d]Junior (6-16 years) taekwondo athletes.

**Table 16.5   A Percent Comparison of Injury Types in Women's Martial Sports**

| Sport/study | Design | # of part. | # of inj. | Abras. | Conc. | Contus. | Disloc. | Epist. | Fract. | Lacer. | Nonspec. | Sprain | Strain | Other |
|---|---|---|---|---|---|---|---|---|---|---|---|---|---|---|
| **Full-contact taekwondo** | | | | | | | | | | | | | | |
| Pieter et al., 1994 | Prospect. | 30 | 11 | — | 9.1 | 90.0 | — | — | — | — | — | — | — | — |
| Pieter & Zemper, 1994a | Prospect. | 742 | 174 | 2.3 | 2.3 | 53.5 | 0.6 | — | 5.8 | 8.6 | — | 8.6 | 3.5 | 3.5 |
| Pieter & Zemper, 1994b[a] | Prospect. | 865 | 87 | — | 8.1 | 36.8 | — | — | 5.8 | 2.3 | 9.2 | 27.6 | 6.9 | 3.5 |
| Zemper & Pieter, 1989 | Prospect. | 48 | 20 | — | 5.0 | 75.0 | 5.0 | — | — | — | — | 5.0 | 5.0 | 5.0 |

[a]Junior (6-16 years) taekwondo athletes.

**Table 16.6   A Percent Comparison of Injury Location in Men's Judo**

| Location | Barrault et al., 1983 (n=16,496) (# inj.=3,941) Prospect. | Koiwai, 1965 (n=?) (# inj.=70) Retrosp. | Rabenseifer, 1984 (n=100) (# inj.=542) Prospect. | Ransom & Ransom, 1989 (n=181) (# inj.=485) Prospect. |
|---|---|---|---|---|
| Head/spine/trunk | 25.1 | 12.8 | 4.8 | 18.6 |
| Skull | — | — | — | 2.3 |
| Face | — | — | — | — |
| Eye | — | — | — | 0.8 |
| Ear | — | — | — | 2.5 |
| Nose | — | — | — | 4.1 |
| Jaw | — | — | — | 0.4 |
| Mouth/teeth | — | — | — | 2.7 |
| Chest | — | — | — | — |
| Groin | — | 1.4 | — | 1.7 |
| Rib | — | — | — | 3.7 |
| Stomach | — | — | — | 0.4 |
| Upper extremity | 44.3 | 58.6 | 39.7 | 47.0 |
| Shoulder | 16.7 | 1.4 | — | 16.1 |
| Clavicle | — | — | — | 5.0 |
| Arm | — | — | — | 1.0 |
| Elbow | 15.6 | 1.4 | — | 8.0 |
| Forearm | — | — | — | — |
| Wrist | 2.1 | — | — | 6.2 |
| Hand/finger | 9.9 | — | — | 10.7 |
| Lower extremity | 30.5 | 15.7 | 50.7 | 36.6 |
| Pelvis/hip | 1.0 | — | — | — |
| Thigh | — | — | — | — |
| Knee | 10.6 | 2.9 | — | 9.1 |
| Leg | — | — | — | 1.7 |
| Ankle | 7.4 | — | — | 7.4 |
| Heel | — | — | — | — |
| Foot/toe | 10.4 | — | — | 18.4 |

studies. Similar to injury types, injury locations were combined in some studies (e.g., upper and lower extremities), which makes it difficult to reveal the actual injury potential of these body regions. Perusal of the tables suggests the following observations:

- In judo, the upper extremity (range 39.7-47.0%) appears to be the most frequently injured anatomic region according to prospective data, followed by the lower extremity (range 30.5-50.7%) and the head/spine/trunk (range 4.8-25.1%).
- In full contact taekwondo, the head/spine/trunk (range 8.0-69.0%) were most frequently injured in the males, followed by the lower extremity (range 13.0-70.0%).
- In the women, on the other hand, the lower extremity (range 41.4-75.0%) was most frequently injured, followed by the head/spine/trunk (range 20.0-35.9%).

Data from karate injuries are not plentiful. Nonetheless, indications from prospective data are that in noncontact karate (34, 51, 57, 75, 91), as well as full contact karate (55), regardless of whether padding was worn, the head/spine/trunk seems to be most frequently injured.

### 3.3.1 Head/Spine/Trunk

Brain injury and its potentially debilitating consequences deserve special attention. Strangulation in judo may lead to subdural hematoma (61), reduced regional cerebral blood flow (78) with memory disturbance for verbal material as a result of a left temporal lobe lesion (28). It is recommended to exercise caution when applying strangulation in judo, especially because it may lead to fatal injuries (39).

Unfortunately, there are only a limited number of case reports, case series, and cross-sectional studies that can provide insight into body areas

**Table 16.7    A Percent Comparison of Injury Location in Men's Full-Contact Taekwondo**

| Location | Oler et al., 1991[a] (n=700) (# inj.=52) Prospect. | Pieter et al., 1994 (n=67) (# inj.=36) Prospect. | Zandbergen, no date (n=?) (# inj. = 85) Prospect. | Zemper & Pieter, 1989 (n=48) (# inj.=27) Prospect. | Oler et al., 1991[b] (n=700) # inj.=102) Prospect. | Pieter & Zemper, 1994a (n=1,665) (# inj.=324) Prospect. | Pieter & Zemper, 1994b (n=3,274) (# inj. 353) Prospect. |
|---|---|---|---|---|---|---|---|
| Head/spine/trunk | 55.0 | 39.0 | 8.0 | 33.3 | 69.0 | 45.9 | 45.7 |
| Skull | — | 5.6 | — | 3.7 | — | 7.4 | 10.5 |
| Face | — | — | — | 3.7 | — | 7.4 | 5.1 |
| Eye | — | — | — | 3.7 | — | 1.9 | 3.4 |
| Ear | — | — | — | — | — | — | — |
| Nose | — | 11.1 | — | 3.7 | — | 3.7 | 5.7 |
| Jaw | — | 11.1 | — | — | — | 2.2 | 3.4 |
| Mouth/teeth | — | 5.6 | 4.0 | 7.4 | — | 5.9 | 5.1 |
| Chest | — | — | — | 3.7 | — | 0.6 | — |
| Groin | 4.0 | 2.8 | — | — | 8.0 | 2.2 | 4.8 |
| Rib | — | — | — | 7.4 | — | 2.8 | 1.7 |
| Stomach | — | 2.8 | — | — | — | 0.6 | 2.3 |
| Upper extremity | 21.0 | 8.3 | 18.0 | 22.2 | 14.0 | 12.8 | 13.9 |
| Shoulder | — | — | — | — | — | — | 1.1 |
| Clavicle | — | — | — | 3.7 | — | 0.9 | — |
| Arm | — | — | — | — | — | 0.6 | 0.9 |
| Elbow | — | — | — | — | — | 0.3 | 0.6 |
| Forearm | — | — | — | — | — | 0.9 | — |
| Wrist | — | — | — | — | — | 1.5 | 2.8 |
| Hand/finger | — | 8.3 | — | 18.5 | — | 8.6 | 8.5 |
| Lower extremity | 23.0 | 52.8 | 70.0 | 44.4 | 13.0 | 48.2 | 38.3 |
| Pelvis/hip | — | 2.8 | — | — | — | 2.8 | 1.7 |
| Thigh | — | — | — | 3.7 | — | 2.5 | 4.0 |
| Knee | — | — | — | 11.1 | — | 9.3 | 5.1 |
| Leg | — | 16.7 | — | 11.1 | — | 4.6 | 5.1 |
| Ankle | — | — | — | — | — | 9.9 | 6.2 |
| Heel | — | — | — | — | — | 0.3 | 0.6 |
| Foot/toe | — | 33.3 | — | 18.5 | — | 18.8 | 15.6 |

[a]Combined sample of male and female adult athletes.

[b]Combined sample of male and female Junior Olympic athletes.

particularly at risk of injury, and too few of these address injuries in female martial sport athletes. The few studies on martial sports injuries to the head/spine/trunk reveal the following observations:

- Most reported maxillofacial injuries were bone and dental fractures (24, 43, 46, 87).
- Subacute thyroiditis (11), injuries to the cervical spine (6, 29) and dorso-lumbar areas (6) occur in judo.
- Liver laceration, perforated liver, perirenal hematoma, hematuria, lung and cerebral hemorrhage as well as pancreatic transection were found in karate (15, 26, 59, 99).
- Injury to the trachea, facial lacerations, cerebral concussion, and dental fractures were found in taekwondo (87).

Blows to the head and neck in karate are implicated in such injuries as cerebral concussions, and spinning kicks are related to cervical spine injuries (52). The head striking the floor has been observed to lead to brain damage, and hand blows or kicks to the trunk region have caused visceral injuries (52, 84). It is not surprising that punches were the leading injury mechanism in karate (91), because punches are most frequently used in karate compared with taekwondo, in which kicks dominate. A case in point is the study by Siana et al. (87), who reported that all head and neck injuries in full contact taekwondo were due to kicks. In karate, McLatchie (53) suggested outlawing the round and spinning back kicks because they were implicated in such serious injuries as depressed skull fractures, orbital blowout fractures, and cervical dislocations.

**Table 16.8    A Percent Comparison of Injury Location in Women's Full-Contact Taekwondo**

| Location | Pieter et al., 1994 (n=30) (# inj.=11) Prospect. | Pieter & Zemper, 1994a (n=742) (# inj.=174) Prospect. | Pieter & Zemper, 1994b (n=865) (# inj.=87) Prospect. | Zemper & Pieter, 1989 (n=48) (# inj.=20) Prospect. |
|---|---|---|---|---|
| Head/spine/trunk | 27.3 | 34.2 | 35.9 | 20.0 |
| Skull | — | 2.9 | 8.1 | 5.0 |
| Face | — | 4.6 | 3.5 | 5.0 |
| Eye | — | 2.9 | 3.5 | 5.0 |
| Ear | — | — | — | — |
| Nose | — | 7.5 | 3.5 | — |
| Jaw | 9.1 | 1.7 | 4.6 | 5.0 |
| Mouth/teeth | — | 4.0 | 2.3 | — |
| Chest | — | — | 1.2 | — |
| Groin | 18.2 | 1.2 | — | — |
| Rib | — | 1.2 | 2.3 | — |
| Stomach | — | 1.2 | 2.3 | — |
| Upper Extremity | 9.1 | 16.3 | 20.8 | — |
| Shoulder | — | — | 1.2 | — |
| Clavicle | — | — | — | — |
| Arm | — | 0.6 | — | — |
| Elbow | — | 1.2 | 1.2 | — |
| Forearm | 9.1 | 1.2 | — | — |
| Wrist | — | 1.2 | 1.2 | — |
| Hand/finger | — | 12.1 | 17.2 | — |
| Lower extremity | 63.7 | 51.6 | 41.4 | 75.0 |
| Pelvis/hip | — | — | 1.2 | — |
| Thigh | 27.3 | 3.5 | 4.6 | 15.0 |
| Knee | — | 5.2 | 6.9 | 15.0 |
| Leg | 27.3 | 10.9 | 6.9 | 5.0 |
| Ankle | — | 10.3 | 12.6 | — |
| Heel | — | — | — | — |
| Foot/toe | 9.1 | 21.8 | 9.2 | 40.0 |

### 3.3.2 Upper Extremity

**3.3.2.1 Judo.** The upper extremities appear to sustain most fractures in judo (2, 37), mostly due to improper falling techniques (23, 29, 31, 56, 65). A hideous fracture of the olecranon process and of the radial neck with posterior dislocation of the elbow joint was reported by McLatchie et al. (56). The injury was a result of a breakfall attempt, and its prognosis in adults is considered poor, which consequently led to the athlete's leaving the sport. In 66% of the karate athletes mentioned by Danek in his cross-sectional study of 20 athletes (21), detrimental change was found in the dominant wrist. This included loss of wrist extension and in some also loss of flexion; 48% showed decreased blood flow to the ulnar region of the hand. Only one study was located on upper extremity injuries in female judo athletes (33). The authors reported an anterior dislocation of the shoulder in a 19-year-old female judo athlete with concomitant damage to the long thoracic and dorsal scapular nerves and with extensive anterior labrum defect.

Being thrown on the shoulder and poorly executed breakfalls seem to be among the mechanisms of injury to the upper extremity (33, 56, 79). Grappling techniques have been implicated in injuries to the fingers (25).

**3.3.2.2 Karate.** Upper extremity injuries in karate include dislocations, fractures, hypertrophic infiltrative tendinitis, nerve injury, hemoglobinuria after trauma of the hands, occlusion of arteries, and muscular captation (1, 20, 27, 36, 43, 44, 55, 60, 90, 93, 97, 107).

### 3.3.3 Lower Extremity

**3.3.3.1 Judo.** Studies on judo injuries in male athletes have focused on fungal contamination (4). The most frequently identified source of contamination was the shower room, followed by the judo mat and on the morphology of the feet (12, 88). Only one study was found on lower extremity injuries in female judo athletes (19), and it described a fibular head dislocation.

***3.3.3.2 Karate.*** The feet were the topic of reviews of injuries in karate, aikido, and judo, but no empirical data were presented (98, 105). Several years ago, it was thought that feet of karate athletes were seldom injured (5), which may still be the case (see Tables 16.6 and 16.7). Danek (21) found that injuries to the feet occur eight times more frequently during competition than during training. However, because of the small sample size (20 athletes) and the nature of the study (cross-sectional), this result should be viewed with caution. In addition to the feet, other body parts injured in the lower extremity are the femur (82) and the pelvis (10).

***3.3.3.3 Taekwondo.*** It is estimated that 18% of all injuries in noncontact taekwondo are to the feet (9), for leg techniques in taekwondo are more prevalent than in karate. One would expect to find many reports of injuries to the lower extremity of taekwondo athletes. Yet, only one case has been reported in the literature, an 11-year-old female athlete with Sever's disease (104).

# 4. Injury Severity

## 4.1 Time Loss

Only in noncontact karate has a study been conducted that reported time loss (5). Sixty percent of the combined sample of male and female karate athletes studied sustained 49 foot injuries. This resulted in time loss from participation of one week (81.6%), with 9 of these 49 injuries (18.4%) leading to time loss of one month (5).

In their survey of a combined sample of martial sports, Birrer and Birrer (8) reported a time-loss injury rate of 0.19% for injuries that resulted in more than 4 weeks away from practice. However, no information is provided about injuries that would result in time off from practice of less than 4 weeks.

## 4.2 Catastrophic Injuries

There are fatalities in judo (31, 38, 39, 62), karate (30, 84), and taekwondo (64, 84). Hand blows or kicks to the trunk region in both karate and taekwondo lead to fatal injuries (84). A rotational kick, the spinning hook kick, was the underlying mechanism that led to a fatal injury in full contact taekwondo competition (64).

Only one nonfatal catastrophic injury has been reported (56).

# 5. Injury Risk Factors

In the literature on martial sports injuries, no analytical information is available identifying risk factors that would predispose an athlete to injury. However, pending future research, several potential risk factors may be gleaned from the descriptive research carried out to date and reported in sections 1 through 4.

## 5.1 Intrinsic Factors

### 5.1.1 Physical Characteristics

Although research has been conducted to assess physical characteristics of martial sports athletes (18, 49, 66), no studies are available to relate injuries to these characteristics. Similarly, strength profiles of martial sports athletes have been determined (49, 69, 94), but again no relationship between the occurrence of injuries and the athlete's strength has been established. Hence, it is not known whether individuals with a low level of strength, for instance, will be at a higher risk of incurring an injury.

***5.1.1.1 Age.*** In Pieter and Zemper's (73) study, age was positively related to injury prevalence rate of young athletes, That is, the older the participant, the higher the prevalence rate.

***5.1.1.2 Body Weight.*** An increase in body weight may predispose taekwondo competitors to injury. Two prospective studies reported this tendency in young males (73, 74), whereas in young female athletes and tournament adults there was no tendency (73, 74).

### 5.1.2 Motor/Functional Characteristics

***5.1.2.1 Skill Level.*** Such factors as skill level and flexibility have been implicated in 80% of ruptures and 67% of sprains in Zandbergen's prospective study (106). Skill level is related to experience and may be distinguished from technical mastery per se.

The total number and prevalence rate of injuries were found to increase with increased skill level in some studies (6, 83, 86) and to decrease with increased skill level in other studies (8, 47, 76, 91). The differences in study designs, injury definition, populations, and martial sports disciplines account for these contrasting results. The studies simply cannot be compared in a meaningful way.

*5.1.2.2 Technique.* Prospective and series data suggest that a lack of refined technique may contribute to injury (32, 64, 71, 73, 100). Poor fist technique may be related to hand fractures in karate (43), and competing with open hands in taekwondo will likely invite fractures or other injuries to the fingers (108). However, as mentioned before, in the absence of control groups in these studies with proper identification of the population at risk, no definitive conclusions can be drawn.

## 5.2 Extrinsic Factors

### 5.2.1 Exposure

Although no data exist that substantiate this, the number of bouts fought (16, 50) and repetitive subconcussive blows to the head (42) may be more related to brain damage than knockouts per se.

### 5.2.2 Environment

*5.2.2.1 Opponent.*  Prospective data indicate that receiving a blow is among the major injury mechanisms in full contact taekwondo (71, 73, 109). Zandbergen (106) found that 86% of all contusions in full contact taekwondo were due to extrinsic factors (all those factors that are nonathlete-related, such as opponent and equipment). The major extrinsic factor that led to injuries was hypothesized to be the opponent. However, the results should be viewed with caution, because no control group was used consisting of those who were not injured. In judo, improper throwing techniques by the opponent were among the major injury mechanisms in Koiwai's retrospective study (37).

### 5.2.3 Equipment

Some research on martial sports equipment seems to indicate potential risk factors. For instance, Kurland (40) prospectively found that 55% of all recorded aikido injuries during training were mat related, such as getting caught between two mats. The rate for mat-related injuries in judo has been found to be 70.3/1000 A-E, which includes all mat-related injuries in young and adult male and female judo athletes of local, regional, and national levels (6).

In noncontact karate, Johannsen and Noerregaard (34) noted the total number of injuries and total number of injuries per 100 participants were fewer when fist pads were used, but this is deceiving. In terms of athlete-exposures, the injury rate is actually higher when protection was used (see Table 16.1). They also found significantly more contusions when pads were used and significantly more lacerations and fractures when pads were not used. No differences were apparent between using fist protection and not using protection in terms of epistaxis and TKO's. Although protective equipment may not reduce the chances of brain damage, it will certainly decrease the occurrence of other injuries.

Unfortunately, the lifespan of fist or foot padding is limited (89, 92), which would require regular testing of the protective gear. For instance, fist padding was found to have lost its protective function after only the fifth impact (89). Percentage attenuation for the top, heel, and side of foot pads ranged from 23-55%, 36-70%, and 24-41%, respectively (92). The lifespan of this foot protective gear varied between 300 and 3,000 impacts; that is, the first ruptures of the material started to become apparent after those impacts. However, this does not answer the question of when the footwear started to decrease in its protective qualities. It is entirely feasible that impacts before the first ruptures manifested themselves are within the zone of concussion.

No research has been conducted on the helmet and chest protector worn in full contact taekwondo. However, some evidence exists that suggests that the chest protector may do a better job in absorbing energy from rotational kicks, such as the round kick compared to thrust kicks, such as the side kick (17).

## 6. Suggestions for Injury Prevention

Joos (35) has distinguished two types of preventive measures in martial sports. Primary prevention refers to prevention of injuries that may occur, and secondary prevention refers to prevention of reinjuries. In fact, reinjuries may be considered yet another (intrinsic) risk factor. Meeuwisse (58) suggests that if several risk factors are known to lead to injury, modification of these factors may help reduce the occurrence of the injury. Because the occurrence of injuries in martial sports will most likely be related to several risk factors, an interdisciplinary approach seems logical. Therefore, close collaboration between coach, referee, sports science, and sports medicine personnel will have a better chance of contributing to the reduction of some injuries seen in martial sports competitions.

Unfortunately, as indicated in the Introduction to this chapter as well as the preceding section on Risk Factors, the limitations of some martial sports studies are prohibitive relative to the formulation of sound preventive measures. In addition, no intervention studies have been conducted. Although it is recognized that recommendations for injury prevention in the martial sports should be based on more reliable data than the studies offer, the literature provides a starting point from which to address preventive measures (see Table 16.9). Suggestions for injury prevention are grouped

**Table 16.9  Suggestions for Injury Prevention**

| Preventive measure | Examples/suggestions | Study / *level of evidence* |
| --- | --- | --- |
| **The martial sport athlete** | | |
| Education of martial sports athletes | Athletes in martial sports should be educated relative to injury risks and should be taught not to enter competition prematurely. | Oler et al., 1991 / *Prospective* |
| | Athletes should learn early that improper attitude may be related to injury: the "macho" participant will likely receive and deliver avoidable injuries. | Birrer, 1984 / *Review*<br>Jaffe & Minkoff, 1988 / *Review* |
| **Martial sports** | | |
| Modification of rules | It is strongly recommended that beginning karate or taekwondo athletes should not be allowed to engage in the free exchange of blows. | Oler et al., 1991 / *Prospective* |
| | Modification of the present rules in karate and taekwondo, which allow blows to the face/head, may help reduce serious injuries to this body part, such as cerebral concussions. | Cantu, 1992<br>Oler et al., 1991<br>Zemper & Pieter, 1991 / *Prospective* |
| | Caution during strangulation in judo may help prevent fatalities. | Koiwai, 1987 / *Case series* |
| Modification of technique | It is suggested to compete with closed fists instead of open hands in karate and taekwondo to help reduce fractures to the hands and fingers. | Zemper & Pieter, 1991 / *Prospective* |
| **External environment** | | |
| Use of mats | Mandatory use of mats should be enforced at all levels of competition in karate and taekwondo | McLatchie et al., 1979 / *Case report* |
| | Preferably, the mats should be of one piece with no folds in the cover, so that no body parts will get caught between mats, which could lead to injury. | Koiwai, 1965 / *Retrospective* |
| | The mats should be all around the ring with plenty of room *beyond* the borders of the ring. They should not be too soft, for this may lead to toe injuries as well as ankle or knee injuries. DO NOT use carpets or similar substitutes. | Lekszas, 1973 / *Review* |
| Padding | Less skilled practitioners in karate should wear padding. | McLatchie, 1976 / *Prospective*<br>Scarponi et al., 1986 / *Case report* |
| | In non-contact karate, fist padding may reduce injuries to hands and fingers. | Johannsen & Noerregaard, 1988 / *Prospective* |
| | Kurland suggests that about 72% of injuries in practice could have been prevented if hand, foot, and chest protectors had been used. | Kurland, 1980b / *Prospective* |
| Experienced referees | Referees should have competition experience, preferably at the national level as a minimum requirement to better assess the nature of blows being exchanged in the ring and other relevant aspects of a bout. | McLatchie et al., 1992 / *Prospective* |
| | Illegal moves should be penalized immediately and competition interrupted if injuries are imminent. | McLatchie, 1981 / *Review* |

| Preventive measure | Examples/suggestions | Study / *level of evidence* |
| --- | --- | --- |
| Instructor/coach training | Guidelines are needed for minimum coursework requirements for prospective instructors and coaches. | Birrer, 1984 / *Review* Koiwai, 1987 / *Case series* Jaffe & Minkoff, 1988 / *Review* Pieter & Heijmans, 1994 / *Prospective* |
| Health support system Preparticipation examination | The preparticipation examination is recommended for all those who have plans to enter competition. This PPE should be conducted once a year thereafter and also should be done to assess whether the athlete is fit to return to competition after serious injury. For young martial sports athletes, the PPE should include maturity assessment. | |
| Education/certification of coaches | Coaches should be required to take first aid and be familiar with basic injury care and prevention. Continuing education in these areas also should be implemented. | McLatchie et al., 1992 / *Prospective* |
| Improved medical evaluation | Medical examiners should eliminate athletes from further competition if any of the following conditions exist: pain in the cervical spine radiating to the shoulders; loss of motion in the neck; tingling in the upper extremities; loss of consciousness (real or imagined) secondary to trauma that is not caused by a choke. | Koiwai, 1987 / *Case series* |
| | On-site medical personnel should be trained to recognize and treat head and neck injuries, and to evaluate if/when the athlete can safely return to participation. | Cantu, 1992 / *Case report* Oler et al., 1991 / *Prospective* |

according to the following subheadings: martial sport athlete, martial sports, external environment, and the health support system. It is acknowledged that the preventive value of these suggested preventive measures awaits further study.

# 7. Suggestions for Further Research

As alluded to in section 6, injury prevention programs in martial sports should be based on reliable research data. To this end, investigators are encouraged to agree on the same definition of injury. This author would like to suggest that injury be defined as any condition resulting from practice or competition for which treatment is sought by the attending physician, no matter how minor its nature. Time loss could then be defined as the athlete's having to miss the rest of the day of competition because of an injury and one or more days thereafter from participation in the activity. In this way, all martial sports injuries incurred during practice or competition will be recorded so that a more complete injury profile may be obtained. As

well, the population of study should be extended to include athletes at the club, elementary and high school, collegiate, and elite levels. In addition, more females should be included as subjects. Finally, large-scale prospective studies should be carried out on both injured and noninjured athletes by multidisciplinary research teams, using both questionnaires and interview techniques.

Research in martial sports in general and martial sports injuries in particular is lacking. Early studies are characterized by anecdotal or theoretical discussions of potential injuries in martial sports (62). Empirical investigations have only recently been attempted. Considering the diversity of the martial sports in several respects, it is not advisable to treat them as one group as far as occurrence of injuries is concerned. Ideally, injuries should be reported by individual martial sports even if several of them are being investigated at the same time. Suggestions for future research derived from the present review of the literature are shown in Table 16.10. They follow the format of the chapter relative to the sections upon which they are based.

**Table 16.10    Suggestions for Further Research**

| Research component | Research directions/questions |
| --- | --- |
| **Incidence of injury** | |
| Injury rates | Injury rates should preferably be reported relative to athlete-exposures or time of exposure and not only as prevalence rates. Expressed this way, what are the injury rates at various levels of skill and competition (local, regional, national, continental, world)? What are the injury rates in practice versus competition? How do injury rates of young athletes compare to those of their adult counterparts? |
| Reinjury rates | Reinjury rates should be determined according to uniform definition for reinjury and uniform criteria for recording by body part, body side, injury type, nature of onset, and history of injury the previous season. |
| **Injury characteristics** | |
| Injury onset | Future research should investigate both acute and gradual onset of injuries including the injury mechanism(s) for each. How do acute and gradual onset injuries differ by level of competition, training, gender, age, and maturity status? Injury mechanism should also include the exact technique (e.g., round kick in taekwondo) that led to the injury. |
| Injury types | Injury types need to be uniformly reported across studies on martial sports injuries. |
| Injury location | What is or are the location(s) most frequently injured by type of injury? How does this differ between gender, level of competition, training, age, and skill level? |
|  | More research is needed to assess the nature, extent, and mechanism of injuries to the head and neck region in karate and taekwondo, particularly the effects of repetitive head trauma. Head and neck injuries in these martial sports comprise a high percentage of total injuries relative to body part. |
|  | In karate and taekwondo, future research should assess the injuries to the hand and fingers (including thumb) in practice (e.g., hand conditioning) and competition (e.g., fractures) and their mechanisms. |
|  | The foot deserves special attention in future research on taekwondo injuries. It is the body part most frequently injured because the feet are the ones in contact with the opponent during kicking in taekwondo competition. |
| **Injury severity** | |
| Time loss | Time loss in relation to injury type, location, and duration needs to be calculated in future research. Are there any differences by gender, skill level, competition level, age, or body weight? |
| **Injury risk factors** | |
| Intrinsic factors | No information is available on the relationship between such factors as somatotype, strength levels, body weight, maturity status, and psychological profile as they relate to injuries in martial sports. |
|  | Age of young taekwondo athletes may be related to the occurrence of injuries (Pieter & Zemper, 1994b), but sound evidence is presently lacking. This relationship should be investigated in young athletes in other martial sports. In addition, is the same relationship apparent in adult athletes? |
|  | Future research should express skill level in terms of years of experience in competition or years of training rather than belt rank, for the latter is less reliable because of differing criteria for promotion to a higher rank between martial sports schools and organizations, even within the same sport. |
| Extrinsic factors | Research needs to be carried out investigating the relationship between exposure (number of bouts) and the occurrence of injuries. |
|  | Research on karate injuries seems to suggest that padded flooring was instrumental in reducing the injury prevalence rate (McLatchie et al., 1992). Research is needed to study this relationship in taekwondo. Furthermore, in judo, studies are needed to investigate what is the best way to reduce mat-related injuries. |
|  | More systematic research should address the relationship between the occurrence of injuries in martial sports and such variables as the opponent, instructor/coach, and referee. |
|  | More systematic research is needed to study the relationship between the use of protective equipment and the occurrence of injuries in martial sports. As well, the lifespan and attenuation rates of protective equipment should be investigated. |
| Injury prevention | There is a need for longitudinal studies that evaluate injury prevention measures with regards to their effectiveness in reducing injury rate in martial sports (Van Mechelen, Hlobil & Kemper, 1992). |

# References

1. Arriaza, R.; Del Cerro, M.; Vaquero, J. Dislocation of the four ulnar carpometacarpal joints in a karate player. J. Sport Traum. Rel. Res. 12:255-259; 1990.

2. Azuma, T. Judo. In: Larson, L.A., ed. Encyclopedia of sport sciences and medicine. New York: MacMillan; 1971:546-548.

3. Backx, F.J.G. Sports injuries in youth. Etiology and prevention, Rijksuniversiteit Utrecht: Janus Jongbloed Research Centrum; 1991.

4. Badillet, G.; Puissant, A.; Jourdan-Lemoine; Barrault, D. Pratique du judo et risque de contamination fongique (Judo practice and the risk of fungal contamination). Ann. Dermatol. Venereol. 109:661-664; 1982.

5. Barnes, L. Karate kicks seldom injure feet. Phys. Sports Med. 6:20; 1978.

6. Barrault, D.; Achou, B.; Sorel, R. Accidents et incidents survenus au cours des compétitions de judo (Accidents and incidents incurred during judo competitions). Symb. 15:144-152; 1983.

7. Birrer, R.B. Martial arts injuries: Their spectrum and management. Sports Med. Digest. 6:1-3; 1984.

8. Birrer, R.B.; Birrer, C.D. Martial arts injuries. Phys. Sports Med. 10:103-104, 107-108; 1982.

9. Birrer, R.; Birrer, C.; Son, D.S.; Stone, D. Injuries in taekwondo. Phys. Sports Med. 9:97-103; 1981.

10. Birrer, R.B.; Robinson, T. Pelvic fracture following karate kick. NY State J. Med. 91:503; 1991.

11. Blum, M.; Schloss, M.F. Martial-arts thyroiditis. New Eng. J. Med. 311:199-200; 1984.

12. Boudjemaa, B.; Potier, K. Profil podologique d'un club de judo (Podiatric profile of a judo club). Méd. Sport. 66:17-18; 1992.

13. Buckley, T. Karate injuries. A compilation of 1,000 kumite matches. Unpublished report, Everett, WA: U.S.A. Karate Federation of Washington; 1990.

14. Cantu, R.C. Cerebral concussion in sport. Sports Med. 14:64-74; 1992.

15. Cantwell, J.D.; King, J.T. Karate chops and liver lacerations. JAMA 224:1424; 1973.

16. Casson, I.R.; Sham, R.; Campbell, E.A.; Tarlau, M.; Didomenico, A. Neurological and CT evaluation of knocked-out boxers. J. Neur. Neur. Sur. Psych. 45:170-174; 1982.

17. Chuang, T.Y.; Lieu, D.K. A parametric study of the thoracic injury potential of basic taekwondo kicks. In: Min, K., ed. Taekwondo. USTU Instructors Handbook. Berkeley, CA: United States Taekwondo Union Instructors (sic) Certification Committee; 1991:118-126.

18. Claessens, A.; Beunen, G.; Lefevre, J.; Mertens, G.; Wellens, R. Body structure, somatotype, and motor fitness of top-class Belgian judoists and karateka. A comparative study. In: Reilly, T.; Watkins, J.; Borms, J., eds. Kinanthropometry III. London: E. & F.N. Spon; 1986:53-57.

19. Cossa, J-F.; Evrard, C.; Poilleux, F. Un des inconvénients du judo: luxation isolée de l'articulation péronéo-tibiale supérieure (One of the inconveniences of judo: isolated luxation of the superior peroneal-tibial articulation). Rev. Chir. Orthop. Répar. App. Mot. 54:211-214; 1968.

20. Crosby, A.C. The hands of karate experts. Clinical and radiological findings. Brit. J. Sports Med. 19:41-42; 1985.

21. Danek, E. Martial arts: the sound of one hand chopping. Phys. Sports Med. 7:140, 144; 1979.

22. De Loës, M.; Goldie, I. Incidence rates of injuries during sport activity and physical exercise in a rural Swedish municipality: Incidence rates in 17 sports. Int. J. Sports Med. 9:461-467; 1988.

23. De Meersman, R.E.; Wilkerson, J.E. Judo nephropathy: trauma versus non-trauma. J. Trauma. 22:150-152; 1982.

24. Dupeyrat, G. Traumatismes maxillo-faciaux pour certains sports de combats. Risques encourus et prévention (Maxillar-facial trauma in selected combative sports. Incurred risks and prevention). Cinés. 24:453-458; 1985.

25. Frey, A.; Müller, W. Heberden-Arthrosen bei Judo-Sportlern (Heberden arthrosis in judo athletes). Schweiz. Med. Wochenschr. 114:40-47; 1984.

26. Fujita, S.; Kusunoki, M.; Yamamura, T.; Utsunomiya, J. Perirenal hematoma following judo training. NY State J. Med. 88:33-34; 1988.

27. Gardner, R.C. Hypertrophic infiltrative tendinitis (HIT) syndrome of the long extensor. JAMA 211:1009-1010; 1970.

28. Glynn Owens, R.; Ghadiali, E.J. Judo as a possible cause of anoxic brain damage. J. Sports Med. Phys. Fit. 31:627-628; 1991.

29. Godt, P.; Vogelsang, H. Seltene Verletzungen beim Judo. Unfallh. 82:215-218; 1979.

30. Hirata, K.I. Karate. In: Larson, L.A., ed. Encyclopedia of sport sciences and medicine. New York: MacMillan; 1971:548-549.

31. Jackson, F.; Earle, K.M.; Beamer, Y.; Clark, R. Blunt head injuries incurred by marine recruits in hand-to-hand combat (judo training). Mil. Med. 132:803-808; 1967.

32. Jaffe, L.; Minkoff, J. Martial arts: a perspective on their evolution, injuries, and training formats. Orthop. Rev. XVII:208-209, 213-215, 220-221; 1988.

33. Jerosch, J.; Castro, W.H.M.; Geske, B. Damage of the long thoracic and dorsal scapular nerve after traumatic shoulder dislocation: case report and review of the literature. Act. Orthop. Belgica. 56:625-627; 1990.

34. Johannsen, H.V.; Noerregaard, F.O.H. Prevention of injury in karate. Brit. J. Sports Med. 22:113-115; 1988.

35. Joos, E. Preventie van letsels bij gevechtssporten (Prevention of injuries in martial sports). Vlaams Tijdschr. Sportgen. Sportwet. 14:73-85; 1993.

36. Kelly, D.W.; Pitt, M.J.; Mayer, D.M. Index metacarpal fractures in karate. Phys. Sports Med. 8:103-105; 1980.

37. Koiwai, E.K. Major accidents and injuries in judo. Ariz. Med.: J. Ariz. State Med. Ass. 22:957-962; 1965.

38. Koiwai, E. K. Fatalities associated with judo. Phys. Sports Med. 9: 61-66; 1981.

39. Koiwai, E.K. Deaths allegedly caused by the use of "choke holds" (shime waza). J. For. Sci. 32:419-432; 1987.

40. Kurland, H. A comparison of judo and aikido injuries. Phys. Sports Med. 8:71-74; 1980a.

41. Kurland, H. Injuries in karate. Phys. Sports Med. 8:80-85; 1980b.

42. Lampert, P.W.; Hardman, J.M. Morphological changes in brains of boxers. JAMA 251:2676-2679; 1984.

43. Larose, J.H.; Kim, D.S. Knuckle fracture. A mechanism of injury. JAMA 206:893-894; 1968.

44. Larose, J.H.; Kim, D.S. Karate hand-conditioning. Med. Sci. Sp. 1:95-98; 1969.

45. Legrand, M.; Lamendin, H. Traumatologie bucco-dentaire des judoka (Oral-dental trauma in judo athletes). Symb. 15:173-178; 1983.

46. Legrand, M.; Lemoine, J.J.; Wouters, F.; Lamendin, H. Traumatismes bucco-dentaires dans la pratique des sports martiaux Japonais (Oral-dental injuries in Japanese martial sports). Méd. Sp. 54:18-23; 1980.

47. Lekszas. G. Sportartspezifische Verletzungen im Judo-Kampfsport, Unfallmechanismen und Hinweise zur Prophylaxe (Sport-specific injuries in judo, mechanisms and recommendations for prevention). Med. Sport. 13:79-84; 1973.

48. Lissner, H.R.; Lebow, M.; Evans, F.G. Experimental studies on the relation between acceleration and intracranial pressure changes in man. Surg. Gyn. Obstet. 111:329-338; 1960.

49. Little, N.G. Physical performance attributes of junior and senior women, juvenile, junior and senior men judokas. J. Sports Med. Phys. Fit. 31:510-519; 1991.

50. McCunney, R.J.; Russo, P.K. Brain injuries in boxers. Phys. Sports Med. 12:52-67; 1984.

51. McLatchie, G.R. Analysis of karate injuries sustained in 295 contests. Injury: Brit. J. Accident Surg. 8:132-134; 1976.

52. McLatchie, G.R. Injuries in combat sports. In: Reilly, T., ed. Sports fitness and sports injuries. London: Faber & Faber; 1981:168-174.

53. McLatchie, G. Karate and karate injuries. Brit. J. Sports Med. 15:84-86; 1981.

54. McLatchie, G.R.; Commandre, F.A.; Zakarian, H.; Vanuxem, P.; Lamendin, H.; Barrault, D.; Chau, P.Q. Injuries in the martial arts. In: Renström, P.A.F.H., ed. Clinical practice of sports injury prevention and care. Volume V of the Encyclopaedia of Sports Medicine. Oxford: Blackwell Scientific Publications; 1992:609-623.

55. McLatchie, G.R.; Davies, J.E.; Caulley, J.H. Injuries in karate—a case for medical control. J. Trauma. 20: 956-958; 1980.

56. McLatchie, G.R.; Miller, J.H.; Morris, E.W. Combined force injury of the elbow joint—the mechanism clarified. Brit. J. Sports Med. 13:176-179; 1979.

57. McLatchie, G.R.; Morris, E.W. Prevention of karate injuries—a progress report. Brit. J. Sports Med. 11:78-82; 1977.

58. Meeuwisse, W.H. Predictability of sports injuries. What is the epidemiological evidence? Sp. Med. 12:8-15; 1991.

59. Nielsen, T.H.; Jensen, L.S. Pancreatic transection during karate training. Brit. J. Sports Med. 20:82-83; 1986.

60. Nieman, E.A.; Swann, P.G. Karate injuries. Br. Med. J. 1:233; 1971.

61. Nishimura, K.; Fujii, K.; Maeyama, R.; Saiki, I.; Sakata, S.; Kitamura, K. Acute subdural hematoma in judo practitioners. Report of four cases. Neurol. Med. Chir. (Tokyo). 28:991-993; 1988.

62. Norton, M.L.; Cutler, P. Injuries related to the study and practice of judo. J. Sports Med. 5:149-151; 1965.

63. Nyst, M.; Laundly, P. Injuries incurred in the practice of karate. Sp. Health. 5:7-10; 1987.

64. Oler, M.; Tomson, W.; Pepe, H.; Yoon, D.; Branoff, R.; Branch, J. Morbidity and mortality in the martial arts: A warning. J. Trauma. 31:251-253; 1991.

65. Orava, S.; Virtanen, K.; Holopainen, Y.V.O. Post-traumatic osteolysis of the distal ens (sic) of the clavicle. Ann. Chir. Gyn. 73:83-86; 1984.

66. Pieter, W. Performance characteristics of elite taekwondo athletes. Kor. J. Sport Sci. 3:94-117; 1991.

67. Pieter, W; Heijmans, J. Taekwondo. Training, Tecknik und Selbstverteidigung (Taekwondo. Training, technique and self-defense). Aachen: Meyer & Meyer Verlag; 1994.

68. Pieter, W.; Lufting, R. Injuries at the 1991 taekwondo world championships. J. Sport Traum. Rel. Res. (in press); 1994.

69. Pieter, W.; Taaffe, D. Peak torque and strength ratios of elite taekwondo athletes. In: Commonwealth and international conference proceedings. Volume 3. Sport Science. Part 1. Auckland, New Zealand: NZAHPER; 1990:67-79.

70. Pieter, W.; Van Ryssegem, G. Serious injuries in karate and taekwondo. J. Asian Mart. Arts (accepted); 1994.

71. Pieter, W.; Van Ryssegem, G.; Lufting, R.; Heijmans, J. Injury situation and injury mechanism at the 1993 European Taekwondo Cup. (submitted for publication); 1994.

72. Pieter, W.; Zemper, E.D. Competition injuries in adult taekwondo athletes. (submitted for publication); 1994a.

73. Pieter, W.; Zemper, E.D. Injury rates in children participating in taekwondo competition. (submitted for publication); 1994b.

74. Pieter, W.; Zemper, E.D.; Heijmans, J. Taekwondo blessures (Taekwondo injuries). Geneesk. Sport. 23:222-228; 1990.

75. Poirier, E. Traumatologie du karaté en competition (Traumatology of karate competition). Unpublished M.D. thesis. Paris: Université Paris Val-De-Marne; 1990.

76. Rabenseifer, L. Sportverletzungen und Sportschäden im Judosport (Sports injuries and sports damage in judo). Unfallh. 87:512-516; 1984.

77. Ransom, S.B.; Ransom, E.R. The epidemiology of judo injuries. J. Osteop. Sports Med. 3:12-14; 1989.

78. Rodriguez, G.; Francione, S.; Gardella, M.; Marenco, S.; Nobili, F.; Novellone, G.; Reggiani, E.; Rosadini, G. Judo and choking: EEG and regional cerebral blood flow findings. J. Sports Med. Phys. Fit. 31:605-610; 1991.

79. Russo, M.T.; Maffulli, N. Dorsal dislocation of the distal end of the ulna in a judo player. Acta Orthop. Belgica. 57:442-446; 1991.

80. Ryan, A.J. Eliminate boxing gloves. Phys. Sports Med. 11:49; 1983.

81. Sahlin, Y. Sport accidents in childhood. Br. J. Sports Med. 24:40-44; 1990.

82. Scarponi, R.; Bianchetti, M.; Cadlolo, R.; Carnelli, F.; Maggioni, E.; Guazzetti, R. Bone injuries in karate. Int. J. Sp. Traum. 4:259-262; 1986.

83. Schmid, P.; Schwarz, R. Karate und Trauma (Karate and injuries). Öster. J. Sport Med. 7:29-32; 1977.

84. Schmidt, R.J. Fatal anterior chest trauma in karate trainers. Med. Sci. Sports. 7:59-61; 1975.

85. Schwartz, M.L.; Hudson, A.R.; Fernie, G.R.; Hayashi, K.; Coleclough, A.A. Biomechanical study of full contact karate contrasted with boxing. J. Neur. Surg. 64:248-252; 1986.

86. Sherrill, P.M. Martial-art injuries at a major Midwest tournament. Results of a cumulative two-year study and a comparison with other recent studies. J. Osteop. Sports Med. 3:8-11; 1989.

87. Siana, J.E.; Borum, P.; Kryger, H. Injuries in taekwondo. Brit. J. Sports Med. 20:165-166; 1986.

88. Sion, M.; Rooze, M.; Klein, P. Comparaison podoscopique entre des judokas et des sujets témoins (Podiatric comparison of judo athletes and control subjects). Méd. Sport. 62:140-145; 1988.

89. Smith, P.K.; Hamill, J. Karate and boxing glove impact characteristics as functions of velocity and repeated impact. In: Terauds, J.; Barham, J.N., eds. Biomechanics in Sport II. Proceedings of ISBS 1985. Del Mar, CA: Academic Publishers; 1985:123-133.

90. Streeton, J.A. Traumatic haemoglobinuria caused by karate exercises. Lancet. II:191-192; 1967.

91. Stricevic, M.V.; Patel, M.R.; Okazaki, T.; Swain, B.K. Karate: historical perspective and injuries sustained in national and international tournament competitions. Am. J. Sports Med. 11:320-324; 1983.

92. Thomas, M.; Prince, P. Capacité d'atténuation d'impact et durée de vie des protecteurs de pied utilisés dans la pratique de sports de combat (Impact attenuation and lifespan of foot padding used in combative sports). Can. J. Sport Sci. 12:136-143; 1987.

93. Tondeur, M.; Haentjens, M.; Piepsz, A.; Ham, H.R. Muscular injury in a child diagnosed by $^{99m}$Tc-MDP bone scan. Eur. J. Nucl. Med. 15:328-329; 1989.

94. Tumilty, D.; Hahn, A.; Telford, R.D. A physiological profile of well-trained male judo players, with proposals for training. Excel. 2:12-14; 1986.

95. Van Galen, W.; Diederiks, J. Sportblessures (Sports injuries). Haarlem: Uitgeverij De Vrieseborch; 1990.

96. Van Mechelen, W.; Hlobil, H.; Kemper, H.C.G. Incidence, severity, aetiology and prevention of sports injuries. A review of concepts. Sports Med. 14:82-99; 1992.

97. Vayssairat, M.; Priollet, P.; Capron, L.; Hagege, A.; Housset, E. Does karate injure blood vessels of the hand? Lancet II:529; 1984.

98. Villiaumey, J.; Brondani, J.C. Pathologie du pied au cours des arts martiaux japonais (Pathology of the feet in Japanese martial arts). Méd. Sport. 54:15-17; 1980.

99. Von Brettel, H.F. Verletzungen durch Karateschläge (Injuries following karate strikes). Beitr. Ger. Med. 39:87-90; 1981.

100. Von Brüggemann, G. Sportverletzungen und Sportschäden beim Judo (Sports injuries and sports damage in judo). Orthop. Praxis. 14:396-398; 1978.

101. Walter, S.D.; Sutton, J.R.; McIntosh, J.M.; Connolly, C. The aetiology of sports injuries. A review of methodologies. Sp. Med. 2:47-58; 1985.

102. Weightman, D.; Browne, R.C. Injuries in eleven selected sports. Brit. J. Sports Med. 9:136-141; 1975.

103. Whiting, W.C.; Gregor, R.J.; Finerman, G.A. Kinematic analysis of human upper extremity movements in boxing. Am. J. Sports Med. 16:130-136; 1988.

104. Wirtz, P.D.; Vito, G.R.; Long, D.H. Calcaneal apophysitis (Sever's disease) associated with taekwondo injuries. J. Am. Pod. Med. Assoc. 78:474-475; 1988.

105. Zakarian, H.; Commandré, F.; Bourgat, M.; Fabre, J.; Azario, J. Le pied du karatéka ((The feet of karate athletes). Méd. Sport. 66:14-16; 1992.

106. Zandbergen, A. Taekwondo Blessures en Fysiotherapie (Taekwondo injuries and physical therapy). Unpublished Thesis. Enschede: Twentse Akademie voor Fysiotherapie; no date.

107. Zeichner, D.M.; Hoehn, J.G. Karate-induced hand injuries. Orthop. Rev. 10:127-131; 1981.

108. Zemper, E.D.; Pieter, W. A two-year prospective study of taekwondo injuries at national competitions, presented at the International Congress and Exposition on Sports Medicine and Human Performance, Vancouver, BC, Canada, April 16-20; 1991.

109. Zemper, E.D.; Pieter, W. Injury rates during the 1988 US Olympic Team Trials for taekwondo. Brit. J. Sports Med. 23:161-164; 1989.

110. Zigun, J.R.; Schneider, S.M. "Effort" thrombosis (Paget-Schroetter's syndrome) secondary to martial arts training. Am. J. Sports Med. 16:189-190; 1988.

# 17

## Ocean Sports

### G. Harley Hartung and Deborah A. Goebert

## 1. Introduction

In the United States, sports and recreational injuries are considered a major source of disabilities and deaths. This includes most of the drownings, 14% of spinal injuries, 10% of brain injuries, and 13% of facial injuries (5, 34, 55, 56, 95, 104). The prevention of injury related to most types of ocean recreation remains nearly unresearched (70).

Aquatic sports in ocean waters are restricted to a relatively few areas in the world by geographic, oceanographic, and climatic limitations. Similar to many sports, there has been a rapid increase in the popularity of ocean sports in the past 20 to 25 years. With increased numbers of participants and contestants, the number of injuries associated with these activities has also increased dramatically. Unlike most other sports, aquatic sports are doubly hazardous in that serious injury also predisposes the participant to submersion and drowning.

Ocean aquatic sports and recreational activities, except a relatively few isolated competitive events such as surfing, windsurfing, paddling, and ocean swimming, are of a recreational nature as opposed to a competitive orientation. Such activities are almost entirely individual; there are some teams, but they are generally sports clubs and not scholastic related. Few have competent coaches. The only professional or semiprofessional participants are in the high-profile events such as board surfing and windsurfing.

Many participants are inexperienced in activities they engage in only periodically. For example, millions of persons have obtained scuba certification, but relatively few dive often enough to become truly experienced. Unlike many other sports, injuries occurring during ocean activities often have alcohol or drug use involved as a contributing factor.

The research data on ocean-related sports and recreational injuries are inadequate and fraught with limitations. Surveillance and study efforts to date have sporadically concentrated on mortality and morbidity data. There is virtually no information on some activities and few systematic studies. Ocean sports and recreational activities account for a relatively large number of serious or potentially serious injuries in certain locations around the world, but few of the existing studies have documented the true extent of the problem.

Almost all the studies to date have focused attention on specific activities, such as diving, scuba, or surfing, or on specific injuries, such as drowning or spinal cord injury (SCI). Certainly, these data are needed in order to provide a basis for injury prevention and safety efforts, but such studies tend to neglect the risks of less serious injuries, or less popular or less dangerous activities.

This is the first inclusive review of articles published that address injuries in all types of ocean sports and recreational activities. The objective of this review was to retrieve and report all studies from 1975, published in English, which relate to ocean sports injuries. Some studies published earlier have been included when there were few recent studies, or when it was thought that they provided important background data.

We accomplished data collection for this review using the following procedures: (a) the ancestry approach (retrieval of papers cited in recently published research reports and literature reviews); (b) computer searches (the Medline database using key words diving, surfing, drowning, aquatic, ocean, and injuries; the UnCover database using the same keywords); (c) published and unpublished abstracts and reports that are not cited in the computer databases used; and (d) unpublished data of the authors and colleagues.

In some studies reviewed we included data on fresh water sports combined with that of ocean injuries (i.e., diving and swimming). We have attempted to focus on the salt water injuries, but in some reports it was impossible to determine the exact numbers of cases in each category. Reports were found from around the world, including Australia, Canada, Israel, and South Africa in addition to the states of California, Maryland, North Carolina, Florida, Texas, and Hawaii in the U.S.A.

# 2. Incidence of Injury

## 2.1 Injury Rates

Accurate estimates of overall injury incidence of ocean sports and recreational activities are difficult, because most studies report data on specific activities or types of injuries. Another problem is the difficulty in accurately determining the number of persons at risk for such injuries because most occur during recreational activities. Some studies have used de facto or resident population as the denominator, but this can be misleading because only a percentage of most populations is truly at risk.

The data in Table 17.1 are from various studies in Hawaii. These are the only studies that were found that provide injury rates for all types of ocean sports and recreational activities. These studies may not provide good cross-study comparisons because of differences in methodology but may give estimates of possible rates of injury. Note that the two studies using emergency treatment data provide similar rates, which are higher than the rate of hospitalizations.

Hawaii has high morbidity and mortality from ocean recreation and sports. The hospitalization rate for ocean-related sports and recreational injuries is 10.2 per 100,000 de facto population with rates for individual islands ranging from 7.1 (Oahu) to 29.8 (Maui) (23, 37). Hawaii's mortality rate for ocean sports injuries in the state is 5.2 per 100,000 de facto population (23, 48). Rates are lower for Oahu (3.8) than for Hawaii, Maui, and Kauai counties (7.9, 8.7, and 13.9, respectively). Mortality rates for the nonresident population is even higher at 15.1 per 100,000.

## 2.2 Reinjury Rates

Published data on repeat injuries incurred during ocean sports are not available. The authors' experience is that there are injury-prone individuals who participate in ocean sports. Given that the majority of participants and those injured during surfing are young males, often teenagers (3, 51, 60), risk-taking behavior is not surprising. Our anecdotal experience through medical record review of ocean-related recreational injuries confirms these findings, particularly for surfing activities (43). For example, one teenager required emergency room treatment three times in one week for different surf-boarding incidents.

# 3. Injury Characteristics

## 3.1 Injury Onset

### 3.1.1 Chronic Injuries

There are very few data related to the incidence of chronic injuries resulting from ocean sports and recreational activities (see Table 17.2). Conditions that could be common to many ocean activities are the following:

**Table 17.1   Comparison of Injury Rates in Ocean Sports**

| Study | Design | Data collection | Duration of study | # injuries | Population at risk | Rate: # injuries /100,000 |
|---|---|---|---|---|---|---|
| Dept. of Health, 1989 | R | RR[a] | 3 yr | 185 | De facto | 5.2 |
| Hartung et al., 1990 | P | I, RR | 10 mo | 276[b] | De facto | 31.2 |
| Yamamoto et al., 1992 | P | I, RR | 1 yr | 108[c] | Resident | 38.5 |
| Goebert, 1993 | R | RR | 5 yr | 485[d] | De facto | 10.2 |

*Note.* P = prospective; R = retrospective; I = interview; RR = record review.

[a]Death certificates.

[b]Emergency room visits.

[c]Pediatric emergency room visits.

[d]Hospitalized injuries.

**Table 17.2    Case Studies and Case Series of Chronic Injuries in Ocean Sports**

| Study | Design | # Ss | Age | Sex | Findings |
|---|---|---|---|---|---|
| Swift, 1965<br>California | Case study | 1[a] | ? | Male | Surfer's knots, knees, and feet |
| Gelfand, 1966<br>California | Case series | 8 | ? | Male | Surfer's knots, bone changes |
| Erickson & von Gemmingen, 1967<br>California | Case series | 30 | 13-22 yr | Male | Surfer's knots, skin ulcers |
| Blankenship, 1971<br>California | Incident report | | | | Ear, eye, nose, neck, shoulder, skin, knee, foot |
| Tashima, 1973<br>Hawaii | Case study | 1 | 47 | Male | Surfer's knot, chest |
| McDanal & Anderson, 1977<br>Hawaii | Case study | 1 | 30 | Male | Surfer's elbow |

[a]Exact N not given.

- Chronic musculoskeletal injuries involving the shoulder and neck (10, 98, 102)
- Chronic ear conditions resulting in vertigo and possible disorientation when submerged (9, 10)
- Chronic sinusitis from prolonged exposure to the elements (10)
- Chronic eye problems from excessive exposure to sun, wind, and salt water (10, 49, 87)
- Skin problems such as premature aging, nonmalignant cancers, and melanoma from excessive exposure to ultraviolet radiation (10, 33)

### 3.1.2 Acute Injuries

Almost all other injuries accompanying ocean sports activities are of sudden onset and include lacerations, fractures, dislocations, concussions, and submersions. Dunkelman et al. (27) describe an unusual case of pectoral major muscle rupture in windsurfing. Although rare, shark attacks may lead to loss of blood or drowning.

### 3.2 Injury Type

Only two Hawaii studies (37, 43) have examined injury type for all ocean sports and recreational activities. See Table 17.3 for a percent comparison of injury type in these studies.

### 3.2.1 Swimming, Snorkeling, Scuba

There are few studies reporting the incidence of injury specific to ocean swimming. However, the majority of submersion injuries occur while swimming, and consistent with expectation, the most common injury diagnosis from swimming in the ocean is submersion injury (drowning or near drowning) (37, 43, 74). Swimming injuries are presented in Table 17.4. Three studies in Hawaii, focusing on differing severity, have documented ocean submersion injuries based on data from death records, hospital records, and emergency room records.

Death certificates (23, 24, 48):

- Forty-six deaths occurred during swimming, snorkeling, and scuba (2.8 per 100,000).
- Swimming accounted for 75% of all water-related deaths.
- Majority of swimming-related deaths are from submersion.

Hospital admissions (37):

- Submersion accounted for 78% of injuries while swimming.
- Fractures accounted for 19% of injuries while swimming.
- Submersion injury was the most frequent diagnosis.

Emergency room visits (43):

- Swimming accounted for 30% of ocean injuries.
- A wide variety of diagnoses related to swimming.
- Swimming associated with 50% of near drownings.
- More than 75% of the stings occurred during swimming.

**Table 17.3    Percent Comparison of Injury Types in Ocean Sports**

| Study | Design | Total # injuries | Abrasion/ contusion | Concussion | Decomp. Sick. | Dislocation | Drown & near | Fracture | Laceration /tear | Sprain /strain | Sting | Other |
|---|---|---|---|---|---|---|---|---|---|---|---|---|
| Hartung, 1990 | P | 268[a] | 5.6 | 1.5 | 7.5 | 4.1 | 6.0 | 6.0 | 28.6 | 6.3 | 24.3 | 10.1 |
| Goebert, 1993 | R | 485[b] | 2.3 | 4.3 | 6.6 | 2.1 | 46.2 | 30.1 | 2.3 | 0.2 | 0 | 5.9 |

*Note.* P = prospective; R = retrospective.

[a]Emergency room visits.

[b]Hospitalized injuries.

**Table 17.4    Percent Comparison of Injury Types by Ocean Sport Activity**

| Study | Design | Total # injuries | Abrasion/ contusion | Concussion | Decomp. Sick. | Dislocation | Drown & near | Fracture | Laceration /tear | Sprain /strain | Sting | Other |
|---|---|---|---|---|---|---|---|---|---|---|---|---|
| Swimming/scuba | | | | | | | | | | | | |
| Hartung, 1990 | P | 115[a] | 3.5 | 0 | 17.5 | 2.6 | 8.7 | 2.6 | 12.2 | 4.4 | 39.5 | 11.6 |
| Goebert, 1993 | R | 199[b] | 1.5 | 1.5 | 16.0 | 0.5 | 71.3 | 7.0 | 0.5 | 0 | 0 | 1.7 |
| Surfing | | | | | | | | | | | | |
| Barry, 1982 | P | 348 | 1.7 | — | — | ? | 3.5 | 2.9[c] | 56.9 | 6.9 | 20.4 | 7.7 |
| Lowdon, 1983 | R | 337 | 3.3 | — | — | ? | 0 | 14.8 | 40.9 | 35.3[c] | — | 5.6 |
| Hartung, 1990 | P | 119[a] | 6.1 | 3.5 | 0 | 5.2 | 2.6 | 9.6 | 48.2 | 9.6 | 8.8 | 6.4 |
| Goebert, 1993 | R | 158[b] | 4.4 | 5.7 | 0 | 3.8 | 15.2 | 52.5 | 5.7 | 0.6 | 0 | 12.0 |
| Diving into ocean | | | | | | | | | | | | |
| Hartung, 1990 | P | 6[a] | 16.7 | 0 | 0 | 0 | 0 | 16.7 | 50.0 | 16.7 | 0 | 0 |
| Goebert, 1993 | R | 28[b] | 0 | 7.1 | 0 | 0 | 3.6 | 85.7 | 0 | 0 | 0 | 3.6 |

*Note.* P = prospective; R = retrospective.

[a]Emergency room visits.

[b]Hospitalized injuries.

[c]Includes dislocations.

Snorkeling is often classified in the same category as swimming. Similar to swimming, the most common diagnosis for hospitalized snorkeling activities is submersion injury, accounting for nearly 90% of cases (37). Hartung et al. (43) found that snorkeling was involved in only 2.2% of emergency room visits for ocean-related activities, but Goebert (37) found that snorkeling accounted for ~10% of hospitalized ocean sports injuries.

Free diving can be considered a special class of snorkeling. Shallow water blackout is a condition that can occur from breath holding. It results in the loss of consciousness because of diminished hyperbaric urge to breathe. To increase bottom time, some free divers hyperventilate. Hyperventilation lowers the concentration of carbon dioxide, which indicates to the body the need to breathe. This condition is rarely reported in medical records and only anecdotal accounts are available (37; Lin,

U.C. personal communication, May 1993). The diagnosis for someone suffering shallow water blackout is submersion injury. Lin suspects that most near drownings occurring to free divers may be a result of shallow water blackout.

Scuba-diving injuries are most frequently the result of submersion injury, barotrauma, and decompression sickness. Drowning is the cause of death in greater than 69% of scuba diving fatalities (12). Conditions such as nitrogen narcosis, hypoxia, equipment failure, disorientation, panic, and barotrauma can all result in drowning or near drowning.

In a Hawaii study of hospitalized injury, near drowning accounted for 33% of the scuba injuries (37). The second most common reason for admission was barotrauma. "Barotrauma" refers to damage inflicted on tissues and organs by uncompensated ambient pressure change during ascent or descent. From an analysis of 155 dysbarism cases treated by the United States Navy hyperbaric chambers at Pearl Harbor, Hawaii, more than a third of all cases had at least initial spinal cord involvement (54). Hartung et al. (43) reported similar findings.

### 3.2.2 Diving

A number of reports of SCI related to diving into various bodies of water have been found in the literature. Kurtzke (57), reviewing SCI data from all over the world, found that diving was the cause of injury in 2.2 to 14% of total SCI cases in various studies done prior to 1975. Subsequent studies in North America have reported that diving was the cause in 10.6 to 18% of total cases of SCI (2, 52, 93, 94).

The largest diving study has been reported by Bailes et al. (4) who found that 9% of 2,435 cases of SCI treated in the Chicago area resulted from diving injury, but only 13 of these were ocean injuries. Kewalramani and Kraus (53) have determined an annual incidence for diving-related spinal injuries of 0.28/100,000 de facto population in northern California, but this also included only a few salt water cases.

In Hawaii, ~6% of 485 hospitalized ocean-related injuries were caused by diving into the water (see Table 17.4), and 25 of the 28 injuries were spinal fractures and/or SCI (37).

The large majority of the spinal injuries related to diving have been cervical fractures with or without SCI (45). Many other injuries resulting from diving go largely unreported in the literature. Skull fractures, concussions with or without loss of consciousness, drownings or near drownings, and lacerations are other consequences of diving injury that could result in hospitalization or medical treatment (37, 43).

### 3.2.3 Surfing

Studies of overall acute surfing injury types are presented in Table 17.4 and include board surfing, body surfing, body boarding, and wind surfing or sailboarding. The studies are limited to injuries serious enough to justify at least paramedical treatment, with many less serious injuries self-treated and unreported. It is difficult to determine the actual incidence of surfing injuries in most of the studies, but an early study from San Diego reported an injury rate of 68 per 10,000 surfers (9). An Australian mail survey (60) found a rate of 3.5 per 1,000 surfing days for all reported acute injuries. In Hawaii, a lower rate of hospitalized

injuries of 1 in 17,500 surfing days was reported from one hospital at an area of Oahu which has relatively mild surf conditions (3). The persons injured in these studies are typically young males.

Shields et al. (88) found that surfing was the activity involved in 19% of 152 sports-related SCI in southern California. In Texas, however, only ~1% of 218 sports SCI were related to (body) surfing (16). An Australian study showed that 10.5% of 200 SCI occurring during aquatic sports involved surfing (13).

Body surfing spinal injuries occur when a person riding a wave hits the sand at an angle that allows the head to snap forward or backward. Both a Maryland study on body surfing injuries at Ocean City area beaches and a Waikiki area hospital study found the vast majority of those individuals hospitalized had residual permanent injuries (3, 21, 69). At a hospital serving a larger area of Oahu, another study of hospitalizations related to body surfing found the majority of cases were spinal injuries (20).

In spite of numerous studies reporting spinal injury related to surfing, the actual number of cases involved is small. There are enough data, however, to show that body surfing is much more likely to be related to serious spinal injury (fracture or dislocation with SCI) than are other types of surfing activities (26, 38, 91). Douglas and Douglas (26) reported that 73% of surfing-related SCI over an 11-year period in Hawaii were a result of body surfing.

Cheng et al. (21) reported that middle-aged men were especially susceptible to SCI related to body surfing because of preexisting spinal canal narrowing or degenerative spondylosis. In Hawaii, the mean age of hospitalized body surfers was 35.7 years and that of boogie boarders was 34.8, with older participants having more serious injuries (37). Board surfers and wind surfers who were hospitalized were much younger, averaging 24.7 and 28.9 years, respectively. Earlier studies also reported that body surfing spinal injuries occurred primarily in men who were older than injured board surfers (3, 20, 91).

### 3.2.4 Paddling

There are no epidemiologic or even comprehensive case studies dealing with injury type in ocean paddling activities.

### 3.3 Injury Location

Except recent Hawaii data (37), there are no studies of injury location in overall ocean sports (see Table 17.5).

There are skull fractures, intracranial injuries, spinal injuries, limb fractures, dislocations, and open wounds associated with surfing activities (see Table 17.6). Limb fractures, internal injuries, drowning, air embolism, and barotrauma may be associated with other ocean activities. Lacerations, contusions, abrasions, and marine animal stings can all occur to any part of the body in association with any ocean sport activity.

### 3.3.1 Head/Spine/Trunk

Injuries to the head and neck, including fractures, concussions, lacerations, and drowning or near drowning appear to account for the majority of serious ocean sport injuries. In Hawaii, 5.9% of hospitalized injuries were skull fractures (37). A prospective study from a small hospital emergency room near the north shore area of Oahu, Hawaii, found that 83% of surfing injuries treated were lacerations, 50% of those to the head (65).

In paddlers, the chest and back muscles are subject to frequent strain, primarily because they serve as the power generators. These injuries are usually acute, with the exception of chronic lower back pain and disc herniation. Low-back pain is most

**Table 17.5    Percent Comparison of Injury Location by Activity for Hospitalized Participants in Ocean Sports in Hawaii**

| Location | Swim/ snorkel /scuba | Surfing | Diving | Paddling | Total |
|---|---|---|---|---|---|
| Head | 1.3 | 8.6 | 0.5 | 0 | 10.4 |
| Spine/trunk | 2.9 | 16.4 | 6.3 | 0 | 25.6 |
| Upper extremity | 1.0 | 4.7 | 0.5 | 0 | 6.2 |
| Lower extremity | 1.6 | 3.4 | 0 | 0 | 5.0 |
| Physiologic/internal | 44.5 | 8.3 | 0 | 0 | 52.8 |
| Total | 51.3 | 41.4 | 7.3 | 0 | 100.0 |

*Note.* Retrospective data.

**Table 17.6    Percent Comparison of Injury Location in Surfing**

| Location | Blankenship, 1971 (n = 150) Incident report | Kennedy, 1975 (n = 584) Prospective | Kennedy, 1976 (n = 786) Prospective | Barry, 1982 (n = 384) Prospective | Lowdon, 1983 (n = 337) Retrospective | Goebert, 1993[a] (n = 159) Retrospective |
|---|---|---|---|---|---|---|
| Head | (67.6) | (69.9)[b] | (63.5)[b] | (22.6) | (31.2) | (11.8) |
| Skull | 31.0 | | | | 10.4 | 11.8 |
| Face | 25.9 | | | 2.6 | 18.4 | |
| Teeth | 10.7 | | | | 2.4 | |
| Spine/trunk | (6.9) | — | — | (17.5) | (18.1) | (35.4) |
| Neck | 1.9 | | | | 4.2 | |
| Back | 0.6 | | | 8.9 | 6.8 | |
| Rib | 2.5 | | | | 4.7 | |
| Chest | 0.6 | | | 8.6 | — | |
| Abdomen | 1.3 | | | | 2.4 | |
| Upper extremity | (10.2) | (6.7) | (7.6) | (21.5) | (9.2) | (10.1) |
| Shoulder | 3.2 | | | | 6.2 | |
| Arm | 1.9 | | | | 3.0[c] | |
| Elbow/wrist | 1.9 | | | | 0 | |
| Hand/finger | 3.2 | | | | — | |
| Lower extremity | (9.5) | (7.5) | (13.5) | (36.4) | (29.1) | (7.3) |
| Pelvis/hip | 3.2 | | | | 2.4 | |
| Thigh | 0 | | | | 3.0 | |
| Knee | 1.9 | | | | 5.3 | |
| Leg | 2.5 | | | | 5.3 | |
| Ankle | 0 | | | | 4.2 | |
| Foot | 1.9 | | | | 8.9 | |
| Internal or physiologic | (4.0) | — | (0.1) | (0.3) | (5.6) | (17.9) |

[a]Hospitalized injuries only.

[b]Includes neck.

[c]Includes hand.

common during heavy training and among older paddlers (98).

A number of sport and recreational activities including diving, body surfing, and scuba diving contribute to aquatic spinal injury (see Tables 17.4-17.6). Diving into the water accounts for 60 to 65% of all recreational SCI, with approximately 1,000 diving-related SCI occurring in the U.S. each year.

### 3.3.2 Upper Extremity

Attempts to generate power from the arms and wrists result in overuse of these relatively small muscles in paddlers. Stress on the wrist and forearm is the most common cause of pain and swelling to this area, usually a result of the paddler maintaining a tight grip on the paddle. Paddlers often develop tendinitis of the wrist. It can be due to increased training, colder weather, or improper stroking. Carpal tunnel syndrome is another chronic condition to the wrist area caused by overuse (98).

There are generally two categories of shoulder injury. The first category is the common muscle strain and is due to overuse or sudden unaccustomed movement. The second is restrictive activity including recurrent shoulder dislocation, rotator cuff and subacromial impingement syndromes. These injuries occur during the stroke when the body is far from the plant of the blade (98).

### 3.3.3 Lower Extremity

Chronic hamstring muscle injuries usually originate in the buttocks of paddlers, probably caused by prolonged sitting and rotation in the kayak or canoe. Although uncommon, strain and small tears in these tendons can take time to heal. Inflammation of the prepatellar bursa occurs frequently among paddlers who kneel. Paddlers who kneel should examine their knees for signs of inflammation (98).

### 3.3.4 Physiologic and Systemic Injury

The incidence of drowning in the world is difficult to estimate because not all countries report information. However, the probable incidence is 6.0 deaths per 100,000 persons (77). Some reported rates that contain information on drowning in natural bodies of water from various countries are presented in Table 17.7. These include Australia with 2.6 to 4.7 drownings per 100,000 persons; Japan with 9 drownings per 100,000 persons; United Kingdom with 9 drownings per 100,000

persons, and the United States with 1.4 to 15.6 drownings per 100,000 persons (5, 75, 79).

Most drownings occur in natural bodies of water, including creeks, rivers, lakes, dams, canals, bays, and oceans (5, 17, 18, 25, 41, 44, 64, 72, 76, 77, 84, 101) while swimming, wading, or boating (25, 41, 83). Many of these studies involve coastal states, and many deaths are associated with ocean activities (see Table 17.7).

Although Hawaii's reported mortality rate from drowning (2.8 per 100,000 persons) is similar to that of other states (23, 24, 48), current statistics are not representative of the actual situation because only residents are included. In a 3-year study of death certificates completed by the Hawaii State Department of Health (48), there were 121 drownings (ocean, pool, other) of which 48, or 40%, were nonresidents. When the results were delimited to ocean-related drownings, the percentage of drownings occurring to nonresidents increased to 50%.

Near drowning, occurring when an individual is submerged long enough to suffer the consequences of oxygen deprivation (97), is seldom reported in injury and disability data (89). The landmark volume, *Cost of Injury* (83) estimated the rate of hospitalization from near drownings to be 2.3 per 100,000 persons and estimated the rate of non-hospitalized near drownings to be 11 per 100,000 persons. More than two thirds (67%) of persons hospitalized from near drownings suffer apraxia (29). The number of potential drownings in which persons are rescued without identified medical consequences is unknown but believed to be substantial (89, 96).

Research data from Hawaii (37, 43) indicate the primary reason for hospitalization from ocean-related injuries was near drowning, accounting for 44%. Of those hospitalized, nearly 75% were male.

Stings from marine animals are perhaps the most commonly occurring injury associated with ocean sports activities. The stings from jellyfish, men-o-war, and similar coelenterates are usually not serious, but certain individuals may react to the venom and the result may be temporarily serious. Stingrays can and do cause serious injury and even death, especially if the stinger penetrates to the abdominal cavity (22). Cases of cardiac disrhythmias following stingray envenomation have been reported (47) as have regional vascular insufficiencies after jellyfish stings (99).

In Australia, 20% of 348 surfing-related injuries were reported to be marine animal stings (6). Similarly, in Hawaii 24% of 276 ocean sports injuries

**Table 17.7    Comparison of Submersion Injury Rates in Ocean and Other Natural Bodies of Water**

| Study | Design | Data collection | Duration of study | # of injuries | Population at risk | Rate: # of injuries/100,000/yr |
|---|---|---|---|---|---|---|
| Dietz & Baker, 1974 | R | RR (medical examiner records) | 1972 (1 yr) | 2 | Resident population | 0.04 |
| Fandel & Bancalari, 1976 | R | RR (hospital charts) | 1968-1974 (5 yr) | 2 | Children under 14 admitted to hospital | — |
| Pearn & Thompson, 1977 | R | RR (death certificates and hospital charts) | 1971-1975 (5 yr) | 40 | Resident population | 1.66 (natural bodies of water) |
| Rowe et al., 1977 | R | RR (medical examiner records) | 1964-1974 (10 yr) | 294 | De facto population | 1.73 |
| Pearn et al., 1979 | R | RR (hospital records) | 1973-1977 (5 yr) | 140 | Resident population (children only) | 12.2 (1-4 yr) 4.0 (5-9 yr) 3.7 (10-14 yr) |
| CDC, 1982 | R | RR (death certificates) | 1980 (1 yr) | 150 | — | — |
| CDC, 1986 | R | RR (death certificates) | 1980-1984 (5 yr) | 1,052 | — | — |
| Wintemute et al., 1987 | R | RR (death certificates) | 1974-1984 (10 yr) | 80 | Resident population | 2.29 (natural bodies of water) |
| Gulaid & Sattin, 1988 | R | RR (death certificates) | 1978-1984 (7 yr) | 6,503/yr | — | — |
| Manolios & Mackie, 1988 | P | RR (lifeguard reports) | 1973-1983 (10 yr) | 262 | — | — |
| O'Carroll et al., 1988 | R | RR (death certificates) | 1976-1984 (8 yr) | 270 | Resident population | 0.71 |
| Patetta & Biddinger, 1988 | R | RR (death certificates) | 1980-1984 (5 yr) | 101 | Resident population | 0.38 |
| Department of Health, 1989 | R | RR (death certificates) | 1986-1988 (3 yr) | 46 | De facto population | 2.8 |
| Markrich, 1989 | R/P | RR/I (life guard reports and death certificates) | 1988 (1 yr) | 41 | 65,750 beach attendance/day | 0.61/beach day |
| Hartung et al., 1990 | P | RR/I (emergency room) | 1988-1989 (10 mo) | 15 | De facto population | 0.33 |
| Hedberg et al., 1990 | R | RR (death certificates and Dept. of Natural Resources records) | 1980-1985 (5 yr) | 216 | Resident population | 2.1 (natural bodies of water) |
| Goebert, 1993 | R | RR (hospital charts) | 1985-1988 (4 yr) | 142 | De facto population | 2.99 |

*Note.* P = prospective; R = retrospective; RR = record review; I = interview.

seen in hospital emergency rooms were the result of mostly coelenterate stings (43).

## 4. Injury Severity

### 4.1 Time Loss (Hospitalization/Length of Stay)

A measure of injury severity and time loss is length of hospital stay. Unfortunately, this information was not available in most of the literature on ocean-related injuries. Information presented in this section is from an ongoing study in Hawaii which has

not yet been published (37). Table 17.8 presents the following data related to length of hospital stay.

Hospitalized ocean-related injuries in Hawaii had an average length of stay of 6.5 days (s.d. 15.7), ranging from less than 24 hours to 205 days. Persons sustaining submersion injuries had the longest length of stay (5.5 days, s.d. 16.6), ranging from less than 1 to 205 days, and persons sustaining fractures had the longest average length of stay (9.9 days, s.d. 19.1), ranging from less than 1 to 131 days. Persons with central spinal cord syndrome were admitted for an average of 6.4 days (s.d. 2.7), ranging from 3 to 11 days. Persons involved in incidents resulting in decompression

**Table 17.8   Severity of Injury by Ocean-Related Sport Activity Based on Length of Hospital Stay in Hawaii**

| Activity | Mean (days) | Std. dev. | Range (days) | Cases |
|---|---|---|---|---|
| Surfing | | | | |
|   Body surfing | 9.6 | 19.5 | < 1-131 | 77 |
|   Boogie boarding | 5.5 | 10.3 | < 1-54 | 26 |
|   Board surfing | 4.0 | 3.5 | < 1-17 | 40 |
|   Wind surfing | 2.3 | 1.2 | < 1-5 | 13 |
|   Skim boarding | 1.5 | 0.7 | 1-2 | 2 |
| Swimming | | | | |
|   Swimming | 6.9 | 23.6 | < 1-205 | 95 |
|   Scuba | 5.2 | 6.2 | < 1-31 | 43 |
|   Snorkeling | 3.1 | 2.2 | < 1-9 | 45 |
| Diving into ocean | 15.8 | 22.3 | 1-114 | 28 |
| Paddling | 0 | 0 | — | 0 |

sickness or air embolism were hospitalized for 5.4 days (s.d. 4.6) and 5.0 days (s.d. 4.4), respectively. These injuries resulted in hospitalization periods between less than 1 and 16 days.

The activity resulting in the longest average length of stay was diving into the ocean (37). The hospitalization period averaged more than 2 weeks (15.8 days), ranging from 1 to 114 days. However, swimming and body surfing resulted in the longest individual periods of hospitalization with 205 days and 131 days, respectively. Body surfing resulted in an average hospital stay of more than one week while swimming resulted in average hospitalization stay approaching one week.

## 4.2 Catastrophic Injuries

The incidence of drowning in studies from around the world have been presented in Table 17.7. Table 17.9 outlines other known instances of catastrophic injury in relation to ocean sports activities.

An early study by Blankenship (9) listed 18 deaths related to surfing in California and Hawaii, most of them caused by drowning. Among 276 emergency room visits, Hartung, et al. (43) found 5 deaths (3 from drowning) caused by ocean sports and recreational activities in Hawaii. One death from drowning was reported in each of two Australian studies of surfing injuries (6, 51).

Because most recreation-related SCI result in permanent paralysis (91, 96), they have been labeled "fates worse than death" (83). The majority of approximately 700 aquatic spinal injuries resulted in permanent paralysis (17), and it is known

that a large number of diving and body surfing injuries result in quadriplegia (3, 16, 21, 26, 40, 91). The impact of these sudden injuries can be devastating to the victims, their families, and society as a whole.

The incidence of residual brain injury associated with ocean sports activities is unknown. The large number of head injuries (skull fractures, lacerations, concussions, etc.) associated with board surfing make it possible that many participants receive substantial blows to the head and may have associated brain injury (56). This requires further study.

Scuba divers with neurologic decompression sickness usually have spinal cord involvement (39, 59). Fifteen to twenty percent of divers with SCI will have permanent residual damage and abnormal neurologic function (12, 37). Brain injury has not been found to be a consequence of routine diving. However, an air embolism to the brain will result in permanent injury (71). Studies in commercial divers with repeated incidents of decompression sickness indicate permanent brain injury may occur (12).

## 5. Injury Risk Factors

### 5.1 Intrinsic Factors

#### 5.1.1 Alcohol and Drug Use

The Centers for Disease Control and Prevention (CDC) estimates that 25 to 50% of adult and adolescent drowning victims had consumed alcohol near the time of death. A Massachusetts study found that 36% of men and 11% of women had consumed alcohol on their last aquatic recreational outing (19). Other studies confirm that more than 25% of fatal submersions in persons 15 years of age and older have alcohol as a possible contributing factor (61, 78).

A study by Plueckhahn (80) of drownings in the Geelong area of Australia found that 35% of all men and 56% of those aged 30 to 64 years had blood alcohol concentrations (BAC) of > .08%. Of the 35 drownings involving ocean swimming and surfing, 73% of men in the 30- to 64-year age group had alcohol in the blood, and 45% had a BAC > .15%.

Many studies of diving and surfing injuries report that the use of alcohol and/or drugs may be significantly related to injuries during these activities (15, 37, 68, 86, 91). Alcohol and drugs may slow reaction time, affect judgment, and reduce inhibitions, all of which could increase the risk of injury during ocean activities.

**Table 17.9  Catastrophic Injuries Occurring in Ocean Sports**

| Study | Design | Subjects | Injuries | Findings |
|---|---|---|---|---|
| **Swimming/scuba** | | | | |
| Frankel, 1977 | Case reports | 8 | SCI | Paraplegia; includes some professional divers |
| Melamed & Ohry, 1980 | Retrospective | 35 | Neuro. | 5 with residual complications |
| Kizer, 1980 | Case series | 9 | Neuro. | Minimal recovery |
| Girard, 1980 | Case reports | 2 | SCI | Complete paraplegia |
| Hartung et al., 1990 | Prospective | 3 | 1 drown, 2 SCI | SCI due to scuba; 1 permanent quadriplegia |
| Goebert, 1993 | Retrospective | 10 | Drown | 6 swimming, 4 snorkeling |
| **Surfing** | | | | |
| Blankenship, 1971 | Retrospective Prospective | 18 | 17 drown, 1 SCI | Fatal |
| Kennedy & Vanderfield, 1976 | Prospective Retrospective | 1 | Drown | Fatal |
| Allen et al., 1977 | Case series | 8 | 7 SCI, eye rupture | 1 quadriplegia, 1 enucleation |
| Shields et al., 1978 | Retrospective | 29 | SCI | 74% C5-6 quadriplegia |
| Good & Nickel, 1980 | Retrospective | 23[a] | SCI | Nonfatal; all cervical |
| Griffiths, 1980 | Retrospective | 2 | SCI | All cervical |
| Chang & McDanal, 1980 | Retrospective | 10 | SCI | 1 permanent paralysis |
| Buchta, 1981 | Case | 1 | Internal | Ruptured spleen |
| Scher, 1981 | Retrospective | 1 | SCI | |
| Barry et al., 1982 | Prospective | 12 | Drown | 1 fatal, 11 near drown |
| Lowdon et al., 1983 | Retrospective | 4 | SCI | Spinal fracture |
| Brophy & Merry, 1985 | Retrospective | 21 | SCI | 19 body, 2 board surfing |
| Hartung et al., 1990 | Prospective | 5 | 2 drown, 3 SCI | 1 permanent quadriplegia |
| Douglas & Douglas, 1991 | Retrospective | 83 | SCI | > 80% cervical; 29 complete, 16 incomplete quadriplegia |
| Goebert et al., 1991 | Retrospective | 1 | SCI | |
| Cheng et al., 1992 | Case series | 14 | SCI | Body surfing; 10 permanent quadriplegia or paraplegia |
| Goebert, 1993 | Retrospective | 38 | SCI | Body surfing |
| **Diving into ocean** | | | | |
| Burke, 1972 | Retrospective | 16 | SCI | 10% fatal, 50% tetraplegia |
| Carter, 1977 | Retrospective | 12 | SCI | 98% quadriplegia |
| Kewalramani & Kraus, 1977 | Retrospective | 3 | SCI | Tetraplegia |
| Scher, 1978 | Retrospective | 18[a] | SCI | |
| Shields et al., 1978 | Retrospective | 82[a] | SCI | |
| Hall & Burke, 1978 | Retrospective | 100[a] | SCI | 14 fatal; 47 complete quadriplegia |
| Good & Nickel, 1980 | Retrospective | 57[a] | SCI | Nonfatal; all cervical |
| Griffiths, 1980 | Retrospective | 65[a] | SCI | All cervical |
| Gaspar & Silva, 1980 | Retrospective | 4 | SCI | C-5 tetraplegia |
| Scher, 1981 | Retrospective | 46[a] | SCI | 40 fracture; 6 fracture/dislocation |
| Mennen, 1981 | Retrospective | 21[a] | SCI | 80.5% C4-6; mostly permanent tetraplegia |
| Ohry & Rozin, 1982 | Retrospective | 8 | SCI | Complete and incomplete quadriplegia |
| Brophy & Merry, 1985 | Retrospective | 159[a] | SCI | 99% cervical |
| Bailes et al., 1990 | Retrospective | 13 | SCI | All cervical |
| Goebert et al., 1991 | Retrospective | 1 | SCI | |
| Cheng et al., 1992 | Case series | 28 | SCI | |
| Goebert, 1993 | Retrospective | 24 | SCI | |

[a]Exact number of ocean injuries not given.

## 5.2 Extrinsic Factors

### 5.2.1 Exposure

Lowdon et al. (60) determined surfing exposure in a questionnaire survey of 346 Australian surfers. Although years of participation, surfing days, and hours of surfing per day were determined, the only relation with injury was that surfing experience correlated significantly with incidence of head lacerations, skull fractures, and other fractures. These relationships were thought to be caused solely by exposure, because the more competent the surfer, the more frequently he or she will be surfing and in more challenging conditions.

### 5.2.2 Environment

Our studies in Hawaii have indicated certain risk conditions, locations, and other factors that could be used in predicting when, where, to whom, and what type of injuries might be expected to occur. Almost 43% of these injuries occurred on the weekend and 62% occurred between the hours of 6:00 a.m. and 2:00 p.m. (43).

Other environmental factors that have been mentioned as risks in our and other studies include the following:

- Waves and currents
- Wind
- Impact with stationary objects
- Impact with floating objects
- Impact with other persons

Our research data for Hawaii (37, 43) reveal specific sites and target groups for spinal injuries. For example, on Oahu there were 42 cases of neck and spinal injury in the 4-year study period. Sandy Beach, locally called the "neck-breaking capital of the world," and Makapuu Beach ranked the highest of the locations where injuries occurred, accounting for 55% of the spinal and neck injuries. On Maui, there were 47 cases of spinal injury. Ka'anapali, Makena, Fleming, and Wailea beaches ranked the highest of the locations where injuries occurred, accounting for 70% of the injuries. The other islands had relatively few spinal injuries. Statewide, over 80% of all those injured were male. The injuries occurred while body surfing (51%), diving into shallow water (19%), and boogie boarding and swimming (8% each).

### 5.2.3 Equipment

Most modern surfboards have pointed noses and tails, protruding fins, and sharp skegs, all of which can and do inflict serious injury (65, 91).

## 6. Suggestions for Injury Prevention

Just as the occurrence of injury requires the interaction of several factors, the prevention of injury may require a number of interventions. One of the earliest systems to address injury prevention was developed by Haddon beginning in 1962 (96) and described in chapter one of that work. A more recently developed model, PRECEDE, is also useful for considering and planning prevention strategies (96). The PRECEDE model focuses on determinants of behavioral change. It suggests that three types of variables should be targeted to influence health behaviors. Predisposing variables are precursors to the injury and include relevant knowledge, beliefs, attitudes, and values. Enabling variables are those required to perform the activity leading to the injury. They also include availability and accessibility of personnel and community resources. Reinforcing variables are factors subsequent to the injury that provide incentives or disincentives for the continuation of the activity the individual was engaged in prior to the injury. The use of the Haddon strategies and the PRECEDE model are helpful in designing and selecting injury prevention interventions for ocean-related sports and recreation.

Drowning has frequently been the focus of recreational injury prevention, primarily because it is a major contributor to injury mortality. Although the majority of morbidity and mortality from drowning occur in natural bodies of water, prevention efforts have targeted barriers to swimming pools, adult supervision of young children, life preservers, telephone availability, and resuscitation. Little attention has been given to the prevention of ocean-related sports and recreational injuries. Prevention projects have not addressed the dangers of natural aquatic environments such as currents, waves, and various lake, river, and ocean bottoms (17, 25, 44, 72, 75, 84, 89) nor have they targeted transient groups of participants. Multiple prevention strategies are needed that address the variety of participants, the different ocean sports activities, the environment, and the health support system. Relevant suggestions are shown in Table 17.10.

### 6.1 Participants

#### 6.1.1 Education

In addition to prevention strategies presented in Table 17.10, a few relevant education projects are highlighted below. "Project Wipeout" is a campaign designed by Hoag Memorial Hospital in California, and is dedicated to educating young people about water safety and prevention of surfing injuries. The project was a response to the growing number of SCI occurring at the local beaches. The project is conducted in cooperation with physicians, lifeguards, spinal cord injured persons, and many others. Another model project being used at a number of locations is "Think First"

**Table 17.10  Suggestions for Injury Prevention in Ocean Sports**

| Preventive measure | Examples/suggestions | Study/level of evidence |
| --- | --- | --- |
| **The participant** | | |
| Alcohol and drug abuse education | Because the use of alcohol and/or drugs may be significantly related to injuries during ocean sports activities, participants should be educated about the consequences. | Burke, 1972/retrospective<br>CDC, 1990/retrospective<br>Goebert, 1993/retrospective<br>Mackie, 1978/literature review<br>Mennen, 1981/retrospective<br>Plueckhahn, 1975/retrospective<br>Plueckhahn, 1982/retrospective<br>Scher, 1981/retrospective<br>Taniguchi et al., 1985/case reports |
| Water safety education | Existing programs aimed at prevention of diving-related injuries include basic education for those at risk, projects to reinforce this message in the community, and promotion of legislative measures to prevent injuries. | NCIPC, 1989/literature review<br>UAB, 1990/N.A. |
| **The sport/activity** | | |
| Modification of vessel design | Surfboards: The sharp pointed nose and tail of the board should be rounded or made of a material that is softer than fiberglass. The fin and skegs could be made less pointed and the training edge less sharp without significant decrements in performance. | Lowdon et al., 1983/retrospective<br>McCrerey, 1979/case reports<br>Taniguchi et al., 1985/case reports |
| | Kayaks: Manufacturers need to create a "safety" boat design. | Ray, 1989/anecdotal evidence |
| | Adding foam padding to the shell increases lower body control but could impede exit if too tight. | Bechdel, 1990/anecdotal evidence |
| Use of helmets | Since most board surfing injuries are lacerations of the head and skull and nose fractures, helmets and nose guards could reduce the incidence of these injuries. | Lowdon et al., 1983/retrospective<br>McCrerey, 1979/case reports<br>Taniguchi, 1985/case report |
| | Helmets should be worn when kayaking near shallow reefs. | Bechdel, 1990/anecdotal evidence |
| Use of PFDs or life jackets | Paddlers should wear personal flotation devices (PFD) or life jackets that are approved by the Coast Guard. | Bechdel, 1990/anecdotal evidence |
| Training and conditioning | Neck strengthening exercises by body surfers may protect them from some types of cervical spine injuries. | Cheng et al., 1992/case series<br>Douglas & Douglas, 1991/retrospective |
| | General rough water swimming training may increase endurance. | Laird, 1989/case series |
| Rescue training | Basic rescue skills, such as the ability to assist swimmers and perform CPR, should be required for all competitive paddlers and surfers and recommended for everyone. | Bechdel, 1990/anecdotal evidence |
| **External environment** | | |
| Signage | Posting of warning signs with water safety symbols near hazardous areas and educating users of those areas through brochures can make a difference in injury control. | Hawaii Dept. of Health, 1992/comparative study (prospective) |
| Lifeguards | Ocean beaches patrolled by lifeguards have substantially fewer fatal submersion incidents than other beaches. | Mackie, 1979/literature review |
| Segregation of beach use by activity | To avoid user conflict over surf breaks, caused by over-crowding and increased popularity of various kinds of surfing, beaches should be designated for a particular kind of activity at given times. Also, restricting power vessels from near-shore waters has been effective. | Birnie, 1983/anecdotal evidence<br>Blattau, 1981/prospective; case series<br>McCrerey, 1979/case report<br>Taniguchi et al., 1985/case report |
| **Health support system** | | |
| Hyperbaric chambers | The immediate availability of hyperbaric chambers and rehabilitation facilities can make a difference in the severity of scuba injuries. The sooner a person with decompression sickness or arterial gas embolism can reach a recompression facility, the better the chance of complete recovery. | Pratt, 1986/prospective<br>Bove, 1989/case reports |
| First responder training | Beach lifeguards should acquire first responder training like that of paramedics, police, and firefighters in addition to lifeguard, first aid, and CPR certification. | Hiller et al., 1987/case series<br>Laird, 1989/case series<br>Howe, 1993/personal communication |

developed at the West Florida Regional Medical Center. This program stresses all activities in which young people participate, including swimming and diving, and emphasizes safe behavior. A film, *Consequences*, was produced by the University of Washington and focuses on risk-taking behaviors and their possible consequences. It includes activities such as surfing and diving and provides prevention alternatives for these situations. The message is "Be a free spirit . . . do it, but do it safely."

## 6.2 The Sport/Activity

### 6.2.1 Safety Equipment

There has been a great deal of emphasis on high technology equipment with little training for its use. When new equipment is introduced, instructional sessions, articles, and so forth need to focus on training. Similarly, hazards are often identified, but no programs to train participants to avoid them exist (82). Safety information and techniques need to be made more available, and international standards need to be developed for all ocean sports activities (1). Manufacturers are inhibited from making safety equipment, designing and manufacturing products for safety for fear of liability. It appears that once they recognize the "risk" and attempt to reduce it, they become legally responsible (1).

Table 17.10 presents suggestions on equipment modification. In addition, the use of helmets while surfing is gradually becoming accepted by board surfers, especially by those who have had head injuries and those who ride the large, dangerous waves on the north shore of Oahu. Helmets specially made for use in salt water are now being sold in surf and diving shops in Hawaii. Recent pictures in surfing publications showing surfers competing while wearing helmets and the availability of special surfing helmets may make their use more common (see *Surfer*, Jan. & Mar. 1993). It is essential that they be made more visible in the media to encourage teenagers and young adult males to wear them. Because most surfers are in these two age groups, they would not consider wearing a helmet for fear it may be inconsistent with their macho image (91).

The use of a leash, tether, or leg rope as they have been called in Australia is of controversial benefit in injury prevention and safety (6, 50, 91). These cords, which attach the surfboard to the leg of the surfer, may help reduce incidence of injury from loose boards impacting others in the water and help the surfer stay with his board, which can

be used as a flotation device in case of injury. On the other hand, these leashes appear to increase the risk of injury from the surfer's own board, encourage poor swimmers who rely on the board for flotation to surf under dangerous conditions, and encourage surfing in areas where other ocean activities are being conducted (6, 50, 91). In paddling activities, however, tethering the paddle to the canoe or kayak is an important safety measure and is required for novice competitors (personal communication, Adams, 1993).

### 6.2.2 Training and Conditioning

Some, but not the most serious, injuries related to ocean sports might be prevented or minimized by better physical conditioning or training. Lowdon et al. (60) found no significant correlation between strains and sprains in board surfers and frequency of mobility (stretching) exercise workouts. They found that 57% of their sample reported never or rarely doing such exercises, and only 25% did these exercises twice a week or more often. They also found that more experienced and mature surfers recommended that stretching and warm-up activities be used before surfing.

Dehydration is one of the most common health hazards encountered by paddlers in Hawaii (personal communication, Adams, 1993). Boats can be rigged to carry a water bottle. Plastic tubing can be used so that the paddler can drink on demand. Additionally, boats should be equipped with a first aid kit.

### 6.2.3 Competitive Requirements

There are few competitive requirements for ocean activities mainly because there are relatively few competitive events. Surfing and windsurfing have professional competitions open only to members of the pro tour. Most other activities do not have any restrictions based on skill or experience level.

## 6.3 External Environment

### 6.3.1 Signage

Signage has been used to warn individuals of the hazards of ocean activities related to a particular geographical area. Litigation has played a major role in initiating the "signage" movement. There has been almost no research to demonstrate the effectiveness of signage. In a study conducted in Texas, signage parameters (size, color, lettering, and symbols) were examined (personal communication, Howe, J., Nov. 1992, Feb. 1993). The use of symbols, particularly pictorial representation, was shown to be most effective. International water safety symbols have been developed, and continue to be developed, by the International Lifeguard Association.

The Honolulu Aquatic Safety Intervention Project studied the exposure to educational materials, including international water safety symbols (personal communication, Hawaii Dept. of Health, 1992). Intervention strategies involved the following: (a) the posting of warning signs with water safety symbols near hazardous areas at a particular beach frequented by tourists and (b) promoting recognition of these warning symbols. The study demonstrated that targeted educational interventions, like signage and a brochure to promote recognition of those signs, can make a difference in injury control. The study found that exposure to the displays significantly increased knowledge of the beach hazards and that rescued persons were less likely to have seen the large display.

### 6.3.2 Lifeguard Availability

Intuitively, the presence of lifeguards is an effective measure of preventing ocean sports injuries; however, this has not been thoroughly studied. Beaches are more often attended and more people participate in ocean-related recreational activities when lifeguards are available. Still, it is likely that rates of injury are less on lifeguarded beaches (personal communication, Howe, J., Feb. 1993).

### 6.3.3 Specific Usage Areas

Injuries occasionally result from multiple activity use and user conflicts in certain ocean shore areas. In order to promote safety of persons and protection of property as related to the use of the ocean, it is sometimes necessary to designate areas in which certain activities are restricted (8).

## 6.4 Health Support System

In order to effectively minimize injury and disability, an adequate health support system is necessary. Components of this system include not only first responders (lifeguards, police, firefighters, and paramedics) and an effective emergency response time to reach an emergency treatment facility, but also the availability of hyperbaric chambers and rehabilitation facilities. The risk of drowning in all ocean sports and recreation requires immediate medical or paramedical assistance (81).

## 7. Suggestions for Further Research

Studies already suggest that ocean-related sports and recreational injuries represent an important problem in coastal states and countries. The serious injuries appear to be drownings, near drownings, SCI, and decompression sickness. Additionally, there are fractures, lacerations, musculoskeletal injuries, and contusions and abrasions. These injuries are the result of varied activities. This information has been useful for the formulation of priorities, new research directions, and intervention strategies.

- An effective ocean-related sports and recreational injury prevention program depends on detailed epidemiological studies that identify the following specifics: (a) activities, (b) risk factors, and (c) target groups (70, 72, 95).
- Ways to more accurately determine exposure rates for various ocean activities need to be developed. Such data are extremely difficult to estimate, especially for recreational activities, but are essential in calculating injury rates and comparing activities.
- Efforts should be made to initiate longitudinal ocean sports injury surveillance or reporting in areas where such activities are popular (Hawaii, California, Florida, Australia, South Africa).
- More data are needed on risk factors for injury, such as environmental conditions, injury mechanisms, and alcohol and drug use.
- More research is needed on rehabilitation outcomes and the incidence of residual disabilities in the severely injured cases.
- Also needed are studies of the effects of new injury prevention programs and other interventions on the incidence of injuries of certain types or in specific areas.

Although the information from currently available studies demonstrates and contributes to the development of solutions, further study would provide a much broader picture of all degrees of ocean-related sports and recreational injury. The acquisition of such data is essential for program evaluation of targeted interventions.

## References

1. Anonymous. Playing it safe. Canoe. May:16; 1990.
2. Albrand, O.W.; Corkill, G. Broken necks from diving accidents: a summer epidemic in young men. Am. J. Sports Med. 4:107-110; 1976.

3. Allen, R.H.; Eiseman, B.; Straehley, C.J.; Orloff, B.G. Surfing injuries at Waikiki. J.A.M.A. 237:668-670; 1977.

4. Bailes, J.E.; Herman, J.M.; Quigley, M.R.; Cerullo, L.J.; Meyer, P.R. Diving injuries of the cervical spine. Surg. Neurol. 34:155-158, 1990.

5. Baker, S.P.; O'Neill, B.O.; Ginsburg, M.J.; Li, G. The injury fact book. New York: Oxford Univ. Press; 1992.

6. Barry, S.W.; Kleinig, B.J.; Brophy, T. Surfing injuries. Austral. J. Sports Med. 14:49-51; 1982.

7. Bechdel, L. Start with safety: the essentials of whitewater safety. Canoe. May:43-48; 1990.

8. Birnie, I. User conflict in studies on marine policy and law. Proceedings of the Seminar on Water Safety: Ho'ike i ke kai. Pfund, R.T., ed. UNIHI-SeaGrant MP 84-01. Honolulu: 1983:25-29

9. Blankenship, J.R. Board surfing (acute and subacute injury). In: American College of Sports Medicine, ed. Encyclopedia of Sport Sciences and Medicine. New York: MacMillan; 1971:501-507.

10. Blankenship, J.R. Board surfing (chronic injury). In: American College of Sports Medicine, ed. Encyclopedia of Sport Sciences and Medicine. New York: MacMillan; 1971:598-599.

11. Blattau, J. Sportsmanship and surfing: 1958-1981. Hawai'i Surf Sea. 3:27; 1981.

12. Bove, A.A. Diving medicine: the long term effects of diving. Skin Diver. August:28-31; 1989.

13. Brophy, T.O.; Merry, G.I. Spinal injuries in aquatic sports. Presented at the 2nd World Congress on Emergency and Disaster Medicine, Pittsburg, PA, 1981. Cited in: ref 91 (Taniguchi, R.M.; Blattau, J.; Hammon, W.M. Surfing. In: Schneider, R.C.; Kennedy, J.C.; Plant, M.L., eds. Sports injuries: Mechanisms, prevention, and treatment. Baltimore: Williams & Wilkins; 1985:271-289.)

14. Buchta, R.M. A ruptured spleen due to body surfing. J. Adolesc. Health Care. 1:317-318; 1981.

15. Burke, D.C. Spinal cord injuries from water sports. Med. J. Austral. 2:1190-1194; 1972.

16. Carter, R.E. Etiology of traumatic spinal cord injury: statistics of more than 1,100 cases. Tex. Med. 73(6):61-65; 1977.

17. Centers for Disease Control. Aquatic deaths and injuries—United States. MMWR. 31:417-419; 1982.

18. Centers for Disease Control. North Carolina drowning, 1980-1984. MMWR. 35(40):635-639; 1986.

19. Centers for Disease Control. Alcohol use and aquatic activities—Massachusetts, 1988. MMWR. 39:332-334; 1990.

20. Chang, L.A.; McDanal, C.E. Board-surfing and body-surfing injuries requiring hospitalization in Honolulu. Hawaii Med. J. 39:117; 1980.

21. Cheng, C.L.Y.; Aizik, L.W.; Mirvis S.; Robinson W.L. Bodysurfing accidents resulting in cervical spinal injuries. Spine. 17:257-260; 1992

22. Cross, T.B. An unusual stingray injury—the skin-diver at risk. Med. J. Austral. 2:947-948; 1976.

23. Department of Business and Economic Development, Research & Statistics Office. Hawai'i Data Book, 1988. Honolulu, HI: DBED; 1989.

24. Department of Health, Research & Statistics Office. Statistical report, Department of Health, State of Hawai'i, 1988. Honolulu, HI: Department of Health; 1989.

25. Dietz, P.; Baker, S. Drowning: epidemiology and prevention. Am. J. Public Health 64:303-312; 1974.

26. Douglas, G.L.; Douglas, M.T. Spinal column injuries in surfing. Unpublished report, Honolulu, HI: 1991.

27. Dunkelman, N.R.; Marini, S.G.; Ladin, K.S.; Nagler, W.; Brennan, M.J. Pectoral major muscle rupture in windsurfing. Arch. Phys. Med. Rehabil. 71:774-775; 1990 (abstract).

28. Erickson, J.G.; von Gemmingen, G.R. Surfer's nodules and other complications of surfboards. J.A.M.A. 201:134-136; 1967.

29. Fandel, I.; Bancalari, E. Near drowning in children: clinical aspects. Pediatrics. 58:573-579; 1976.

30. Frankel, H.L. Paraplegia due to decompression sickness. Paraplegia. 14:306-311, 1977.

31. Gaspar, V.G.; Silva, R.M.E. Spinal cord lesions due to water sports and occupations: our experience in 20 years. Paraplegia. 18:106-108; 1980.

32. Gelfand, D.W. Surfer's knots: associated bone changes and medical problems. J.A.M.A. 197:149-150; 1966.

33. Gentile, D.A.; Auerbach, P.S. The sun and water sports. Clin. Sports Med. 6:669-684; 1987.

34. Gerberich, S. Sports injuries: implications for prevention. Public Health Rep. 100:670-671; 1985.

35. Girard, R. Paraplegia during skin-diving (13 cases). Paraplegia. 18:123-126; 1980.

36. Goebert, D.A.; Ng, M.Y.; Varney, J.M.; Sheetz, D.A. Traumatic spinal cord injury in Hawai'i. Hawaii Med. J. 50:44-50; 1991.

37. Goebert, D.A. Unpublished data, Honolulu, HI; 1993.

38. Good, R.P.; Nickel, V.L. Cervical spine injuries resulting from water sports. Spine. 5:502-506; 1980.

39. Greer, H.D.; Massey, E.W. Neurological injury from undersea diving. Neurol. Trauma. 10:1032-1045; 1992.

40. Griffiths, E.R. Spinal injuries from swimming and diving treated in the spinal department of Royal Perth Rehabilitation Hospital: 1956-1978. Paraplegia. 18:109-117; 1980.

41. Gulaid, J.A.; Sattin, R.W. Drownings in the United States, 1978-1984. MMWR. 37:27-33; 1988.

42. Hall, J.C.; Burke, D.C. Diving injury resulting in tetraplegia. Med. J. Austral. 1:171; 1978.

43. Hartung, G.H.; Goebert, D.A.; Taniguchi, R.M.; Okamoto, G.A. Epidemiology of ocean sports-related injuries in Hawaii: akahele o ke kai. Hawaii Med. J. 49:52-56; 1990.

44. Hedberg, K.; Gunderson, P.D.; Vargas, C.; Osterholm, M.T.; MacDonald, K.L. Drownings in Minnesota, 1980-1985: a population-based study. Am. J. Public Health. 80:1071-1074; 1990.

45. Herman, J.M.; Sonntag, V.K.H. Diving accidents: mechanisms of injury and treatment of the patient. Crit. Care Nurs. Clin. N. Am. 3:331-337; 1991.

46. Hiller, W.D.B.; O'Toole M.L.; Fortess, E.E.; Laird, R.H.; Imbert, P.C.; Sisk, T.D. Medical and physiological considerations in triathlons. Am. J. Sports Med. 15:164-167; 1987.

47. Ikeda, T. Supraventricular bigeminy following a stingray envenomation: a case report. Hawaii Med. J. 48:162-164; 1989.

48. Injury Prevention and Control Office, Hawai'i Department of Health. Unpublished data; 1990.

49. Josephson, J.E.; Caffery, B.E. Contact lens considerations in surface and subsurface aqueous environments. Optom. Vis. Sci. 68:2-11; 1991.

50. Kennedy, M.; Vanderfield, G.; Huntley, R. Surfcraft injuries. Austral. J. Sports Med. 7:53-54; 1975.

51. Kennedy, M.; Vanderfield, G. Medical aspects of surfcraft usage. Med. J. Austral. 2:707-709; 1976.

52. Kewalramani, L.S.; Orth, M.S.; Taylor, R.G. Injuries to the cervical spine from diving accidents. J. Trauma. 15:130-142; 1975.

53. Kewalramani, L.S.; Kraus, J.F. Acute spinal-cord lesions from diving—epidemiological and clinical features. West J. Med. 126:353-361; 1977.

54. Kizer, K.W. Dysbarism in paradise. Hawaii Med. J. 39:109-116; 1980.

55. Kraus, J.F.; Branti, C.E.; Riggins, R.S.; Richards, D.; Borhani, N.O. Incidence of traumatic spinal cord lesions. J. Chronic Disease. 28:471-492; 1975.

56. Kraus, J.F.; Black, M.A.; Hessol, N.; Ley, P.; Rokaw, W.; Sullivan, C.; Bowers, S.; Knowlton, S.; Marshall, L. The incidence of acute brain injury and serious impairment in a defined population. Am. J. Epidemiol. 119:186-201; 1984.

57. Kurtzke, J.F. Epidemiology of spinal cord injury. Exp. Neurol. 48:163-236; 1975.

58. Laird, R.H. Medical care at ultraendurance triathlons. Med. Sci. Sports Exerc. 21:S222-S225; 1989.

59. Lehman L.B. Scuba and other sports diving: nervous system complications. Postgrad. Med. 80(2): 68-71; 1986.

60. Lowdon, B.J.; Pateman, N.A.; Pitman, A.J. Surfboard-riding injuries. Med. J. Austral. 2:613-616; 1983.

61. Mackie, I. Alcohol and aquatic disasters. Med. J. Austral. 1:652-653; 1978.

62. Mackie, I. Death in the water—world talks. AMA Gazette. Feb. 1:16; 1979.

63. Manolios, N.; Mackie, I. Drowning and near-drowning on Australian beaches patrolled by lifesavers: a 10-year study, 1973-1983. Med. J. Austral. 148:165-171; 1988.

64. Markrich, M. Hawaii's beaches are not safe enough—there are too many drownings, too many accidents. Honolulu. (October): 57-85; 1989.

65. McCrerey, L. North shore injuries. Surfer. 20:38-45; 1979.

66. McDanal, C.E.; Anderson, B. Surfer's elbow. Hawaii Med. J. 36:108-109; 1977.

67. Melamed, Y.; Ohry, A. The treatment and the neurological aspects of diving accidents in Israel. Paraplegia. 18:127-132; 1980.

68. Mennen, U. A survey of spinal injuries from diving. S. Afr. Med. J. 59:588-590; 1981.

69. Miller, S. Body-surfing called hazardous to 40-and-over males. Newsletter of the National Head and Spinal Cord Injury Prevention Program. 1(3):31; 1989.

70. National Research Council and Institute of Medicine. Injury in America. Washington, DC: National Academy Press; 1985.

71. Neuman, T.S.; Bove, A.A. Combined arterial gas embolism and decompression sickness following no-stop dives. Undersea Biomed. Res. 17:429-436; 1990.

72. O'Carroll, P.W.; Alkon, E.; Weiss, B. Drowning mortality in Los Angeles County, 1976 to 1984. J.A.M.A. 260:380-383; 1988.

73. Ohry, A.; Rozin, R. Spinal cord injuries resulting from sport. The Israeli experience. Paraplegia. 20:334-338; 1982.

74. Patetta, M.J.; Biddinger, P.W. Characteristics of drowning deaths in North Carolina. Pub. Health Rep. 103:406-411; 1988.

75. Pearn, J.; Thompson, J. Drowning and near-drowning in the Australian Capital Territory: a five-year total population study of immersion accidents. Med. J. Austral. 1:130-133; 1977.

76. Pearn, J.H.; Wong, R.Y.K.; Brown, J., III; Ching, Y.-C.; Bart, R., Jr.; Hammar, S. Drowning and near-drowning involving children: a five-year total population study from the city and county of Honolulu. Am. J. Public Health. 69:450-454; 1979.

77. Plueckhahn, V.D. The aetiology of 134 deaths due to "drowning" in Geelong during the years 1957 to 1971. Med. J. Austral. 62(2):1183-1187; 1972.

78. Plueckhahn, V.D. Death by drowning? Geelong 1959-1974. Med. J. Austral. 2:904-906; 1975.

79. Plueckhahn, V.D. Drowning: community aspects. Med. J. Austral. 2:226-228; 1979.

80. Plueckhahn, V.D. Alcohol consumption and death by drowning in adults. J. Stud. Alcohol. 43:445-452; 1982.

81. Pratt, F.D.; Haynes, B.E. Incidence of "secondary drowning" after saltwater submersion. Ann. Emerg. Med. 15:1084-1087; 1986.

82. Ray, S. International safety symposium held in England. Canoe. May:11-12; 1989.

83. Rice, D.P.; MacKenzie, E.J.; & Associates. Cost of injury in the United States: A report to congress. San Francisco, CA: Institute for Health & Aging, University of California and Injury Prevention Center, Johns Hopkins University; 1989.

84. Rowe, M.; Arango, A.; Allington, G. Profile of pediatric drowning victims in a water-oriented society. J. Trauma. 17:587-591; 1977.

85. Scher, A.T. Spinal cord injuries due to diving accidents. J. Sports Med. 18:67-70; 1978.

86. Scher, A.T. Diving injuries to the cervical spinal cord. S. Afr. Med. J. 59:603-605; 1981.

87. Seiff, S.R. Ophthalmic complications of water sports. Clin. Sports Med. 6:685-693; 1987.

88. Shields, C.L.; Fox, J.M.; Stauffer, E.S. Cervical cord injuries in sports. Phys. Sportsmed. 6(9)71-76; 1978.

89. Spyker, D. Submersion injury: epidemiology, prevention, and management. Pediatr. Clin. N. Am. 32:113-125; 1985.

90. Swift, S. Surfers' "Knots." J.A.M.A. 192:223-224; 1965.

91. Taniguchi, R.M.; Blattau, J.; Hammon, W.M. Surfing. In: Schneider, R.C.; Kennedy, J.C.; Plant, M.L., eds. Sports Injuries: Mechanisms, Prevention, and Treatment. Baltimore: Williams & Wilkins; 1985: 271-289.

92. Tashima, C.K. Surfer's chest knots. J.A.M.A. 226:468; 1973.

93. Tator, C.H.; Edmonds, V.E. Acute spinal cord injury: analysis of epidemiologic factors. Can. J. Surg. 22:575-578; 1979.

94. Tator, C.H.; Edmonds, V.E.; New, M.L. Diving; a frequent and potentially preventable cause of spinal cord injury. Can. Med. Assoc. J. 124:1323-1324; 1981.

95. Tator, C.; Edmonds, V. Sports and recreation are a rising cause of spinal cord injury. Physician Sportsmed. 14:157-167; 1986.

96. The National Committee for Injury Prevention and Control. Injury prevention: Meeting the challenge. New York: Oxford University Press; 1989.

97. UAB Department of Rehabilitation Medicine, Spain Rehabilitation Center. Resources: a national directory of spinal cord injury prevention programs. Birmingham, AL: University of Alabama at Birmingham; 1990.

98. Walsh, M. Sports medicine for paddlers: the cause, care and treatment of paddler's injuries. Canoe. May:36-38+; 1989.

99. Williamson, J.A.; Burnett, J.W; Fenner, P.J.; Hach-Wunderle, V.; Hoe, L.Y.; Adiga, K.M. Acute regional vascular insufficiency after jellyfish envenomation. Med. J. Austral. 149:698-701; 1988.

100. Wintemute, G.J.; Kraus, J.F.; Teret, S.P.; Wright, M. Drowning in childhood and adolescence: a population-based study. Am. J. Public Health. 77: 830-832; 1987.

101. Wintemute, G.J.; Kraus, J.F.; Teret, S.P.; Wright, M.A. The epidemiology of drowning in adulthood: implications for prevention. Am. J. Prev. Med. 4:343-348; 1988.

102. Withers, P.M. Paddlers and risk. Canoe. May:73-89; 1988.

103. Yamamoto, L.G.; Yee, A.B.; Matthews, W.J., Jr.; Wiebe, R.A. A one-year series of pediatric ED water-related injuries: the Hawaii EMS-C project. Pediatr. Emerg. Care. 8:129-133; 1992.

104. Young, J.S.; Burns, P.E.; Bowen, A.M.; McCutchen, R. Spinal cord injury statistics: Experience of the regional spinal cord injury systems. Phoenix: Good Samaritan Medical Center; 1982.

# 18

# Racquet Sports

*Nick Mohtadi and Alex Poole*

## 1. Introduction

Racquet sport injuries are becoming a matter of increasing concern in the world of sports medicine. The number of participants is rising, and these sports are played by an older population compared with contact sports. The equipment and environmental factors make for unique circumstances in which injury may occur. The public exposure of professional athletes and the vast amount of money involved, particularly in tennis, impact upon the young, aspiring racquet sport enthusiasts. This leads to greater pressure to practice, higher expectations of performance, and increasing demands on the human body. It is intuitive that these factors would combine to result in a greater susceptibility to injury. However, it is important to establish the baseline information on the incidence, type, severity, mechanisms, and risk factors of the injuries. This information can provide the basis to delineate strategies for injury prevention.

This chapter will present an overview of the literature pertaining to the racquet sports badminton, racquetball, squash, and tennis. There are obvious similarities in the injuries seen in each sport, but there are also specific problems that are unique to one activity or the other.

This overview involved searching Medline for the years 1975-1993 inclusively. We performed the search using the following key words: injury, tennis, squash, badminton, racquetball, and racquet sports. The articles obtained were then cross referenced to identify additional articles or texts. All articles were included, irrespective of their methodological strength or research design. This all-inclusive policy was required because the literature is entirely descriptive with case series and case reports predominating.

## 2. Incidence of Injury

### 2.1 Injury Rates

The true understanding of racquet sport injury requires information on the epidemiology or distribution of these injuries. Although much is written about these sports, the incidence and prevalence of injury are not clearly described. Injury definition, characterization of the population at risk, and systematic data collection have been identified as the three major methodological problems in this area of sport injury epidemiology (74). With these three concerns in mind the most important information with respect to sport-related injury is the incidence rate. This describes the number of new cases over a specified period of time as compared with the population at risk (74).

There are only a few studies in badminton in which this information is readily available (46, 76). In 1990, Kroner et al. reported on a population-based study that showed an incidence of 208 injuries out of a population of 10,032 badminton players, or roughly 20 per 1,000 players (58). These injuries were reported from the emergency rooms of the two community hospitals. Compared with other sports, badminton injuries represented 4.1% of the total (58). Other studies have shown frequencies of badminton injury at 1% (4) and 3.1% (68) compared with other sports. The disparity in the literature can be explained by the differences in population and sporting participation.

In racquetball there are no population-based studies available. One study reported 70 new cases of injury in a 15-month period (98) at a university student health service. Another study collected 157 racquetball injuries over two time periods and at two institutions. This information does not allow determination of incidence figures (104).

In squash the information available is not population based. Most studies have brought attention to eye injuries (6, 8, 30, 35) and sudden death (66, 89). A retrospective telephone survey attempted to identify squash-related injuries from an epidemiological perspective (11). The overall injury rate of the 155 surveyed squash players was 44.5%. This represented those individuals who responded, out of a group of 200 players selected at random from two separate squash clubs. This information cannot be classified as incidence or prevalence data because all injuries over the course of their playing history were evaluated (11).

In tennis most of the reported information has been devoted to tennis elbow (19, 37, 62, 70, 81, 87). The incidence of tennis elbow was estimated at 9.1% in a self-reported questionnaire from individuals at a private tennis club (39). The prevalence over this 2-month study period was 14.1%, and a total of 39.7% reported that they had at one time been afflicted by this problem (39). Other estimates are that up to 50% of tennis players will have problems with their elbows (3, 43). The incidence of other injuries is not established. It has been stated that the majority of adolescents playing tennis will have their playing temporarily interrupted by an injury, with lower extremity problems predominating. These estimates are not based on documented evidence (37).

There is very little information on the comparison of injury rates sustained in racquet sports versus other sporting activities. Tennis accounted for only 0.3% and badminton for 0.1% of the total of 1,576 injuries in a population of school-aged children (111). When these sports were compared as injury rates per 1,000 participant hours, tennis had 0.01 and badminton essentially 0 injuries per 1,000 hours (111). These compare with 5.68 in track and field and 1.05 in football per 1,000 participant hours (111). Similar low injury rates were found in Irish children, where the injury rate in tennis was less than 1% of the total number of injuries (109). A 2-year prospective study in high school sports compared the total injury rate between a number of sports (33). This was calculated by dividing the number of injuries by the number of participants based upon sex. Tennis had an injury rate of 0.03 and 0.07 for females and males respectively, and in badminton the rate was 0.06 for females (33).

A recent population-based study in England and Wales surveyed a random sampling of the population to identify sport and recreation injury, (84). The population sample was based upon a postal survey of 16- to 45-year-old individuals throughout a one year period. The incidence of injury was compared per 1,000 occasions of participation by each activity. Overall the substantive new injury rate was higher in squash (5 per 1,000), followed by badminton (3 per 1,000),and then tennis (2 per 1,000). These figures are dramatically less than the highest risk sport of rugby (50 per 1,000) (84).

## 2.2 Reinjury Rates

Information regarding reinjury rates is available only for tennis elbow. Injury recurred in 24% of tennis players (39). This information is based upon self-reported questionnaires and suffers from recall bias.

## 2.3 Injury Rates in Competitive vs. Recreational Players

Information comparing competitive and recreational players is not readily available. It is estimated that lateral epicondylar pain is 10 times more frequent than medial in beginner or average players, whereas medial tennis elbow is three times more frequent in expert players (59). Injury rate was evaluated in elite junior tennis players aged 13 to 19 from the United States, Sweden, and England (55). An injury was defined as a condition lasting 5 or more days, that arose from playing tennis, caused alteration in playing level or performance, or caused cessation of playing. Over 60% of these elite players had at least one injury fulfilling these criteria over the previous 2 years. These juniors were playing 11 to 24 hours per week (55). Another reference to competitive players stated 24% of 270 competitive juniors reported shoulder pain, the figure rising to 50% in an older population (63). This information was not substantiated by any specific details as to the definition of injury or diagnoses.

## 3. Injury Characteristics

Any discussion of injury characteristics invokes the necessary description of the definition of the injury. Indeed it has been stated that there is no basic scientific distinction between injury and disease (41). The most difficult problem in comparing the injuries between sports is that each article uses a different definition. Anatomical definitions are used, such as the type of tissue involved (muscle, tendon, bone, etc.), or the anatomical region (upper extremity, lower extremity or ankle, knee, head, and neck, etc.), and an etiological definition of whether the injury occurred as a result of acute trauma or overuse. There is also a selection bias introduced in many of the studies. Reports from emergency departments (58, 104) will selectively identify acute traumatic injuries. Overuse injuries will be more common in a sports injury clinic (20, 98), and information collected from a population of participants (11), will likely be a combination of both, but specific to the sport involved. Caution must be used when comparing the variety of injuries and their respective locations.

## 3.1 Injury Onset

Most of the common problems related to racquet sports are due to repetitive use (see Table 18.1). The overuse mechanism is particularily likely to involve the upper extremity (37, 63). Rotator cuff tendinopathy, tennis elbow, and wrist problems have been associated with overuse injury (87, 93). Similarly in the lower limb, problems in the knees and feet are related to the constant pounding that occurs during play (34, 61). The spine and abdomen are also susceptible to repetitive injury (5, 31, 64, 72).

Many musculoskeletal injuries occur from acute overload of the involved tissue, whether it is musculotendinous, ligamentous, or bony (20). The musculotendinous injuries such as "tennis leg" (32) or rupture of the medial head of the gastrocnemius (75) occur because of excessive eccentric overload. The same mechanism is implicated in acute rotator cuff tears, although a fall on the outstretched arm or a direct axial load could lead to a direct tear. Badminton injuries typically result from an intrinsic mechanism in which the player stumbles or falls while making an attempt to play a shot. Extrinsic injuries caused by collisions, being hit by the racquet or shuttlecock, are much less likely (46, 58). This mechanism did account for the

eye injuries sustained. When squash and racquetball are compared with tennis and badminton, it is evident that there are a greater number of acute or sudden onset injuries in the former (20). The great majority of facial and head injuries including ocular trauma are a result of direct trauma from the racquet or ball (6, 8, 11, 20, 21, 25, 98, 104, 106).

## 3.2 Injury Type

It is estimated that the vast majority of racquet sport injuries involve the musculoskeletal system. This can be gleaned from the number of articles devoted to musculoskeletal injuries and in particular those that consider the sport overall (11, 58, 59, 98). The majority of information available is based upon case reports and generic reviews of injuries that are related to the racquet sports (61). As Table 18.2 would suggest, there is little specific epidemiologic evidence to comment upon. A variety of injuries have been reported, including acute musculotendinous injuries (34, 36, 52, 99) and acute ligamentous sprains, particularly involving the ankle as the most common site (11). Overuse syndromes involving tendons (7, 19, 39, 47, 62, 70, 81, 86, 87, 105) are very prevalent, especially in the elbow. In younger players injuries related to the growth plates can occur. Shoulder subluxation, labral tears, "Osgood-Schlatter disease of the shoulder," and slipped capital humeral epiphysis are implicated without specific documentation (37). Osteochondritis desiccans of the humeral head in a 44-year-old tennis player (48), fractures

Table 18.1  Injury Onset by Sport

| Injury onset | Tennis (Chard, 1987, N = 131) | Badminton (Jorgensen, 1990, N = 229) | Squash (Chard, 1987, N = 372) | Racquetball (Rose, 1979, N = 70) |
|---|---|---|---|---|
| Overuse | 30% | 74% | 20% | 10% |
| Acute trauma | 70% | 26% | 80% | 90% |

Table 18.2  Injury Type by Sport

| Injury type | Tennis (Chard, 1987, N = 131) | Badminton (Kroner, 1990, N = 217) | Squash (Berson, 1981, N = 69) | Racquetball (Soderstrom, 1982, N = 157) |
|---|---|---|---|---|
| Joint/ligament /sprain | 64% | 58.5% | 20.3% | 34% |
| Muscle | 10% | 19.8% | 18.8% | Not incl. |
| Tendon | 18% | 8.8% | 7.2% | 1.3% |
| Skin[a] | Not incl. | 5.1% | 36.2%[b] | 46.5%[c] |
| Bone | Not incl. | 5.1% | 2.9% | 7.6% |
| Eye | Not incl. | 2.3% | | 5.7% |
| Inflammation | Not incl. | Not incl. | 14.5% | 1.9% |
| Nasal/dental | Not incl. | Not incl. | | 3.1% |
| Other | 8% | 0.5% | See above | Not incl. |

[a]Including lacerations and contusions.

[b]Other injuries also included.

[c]43.4% being facial.

and dislocations of the wrist (112), and injuries to the hook of the hamate (40) have been reported. Case reports of stress fractures (9, 67, 79, 96) are also present in the literature.

Ophthalmologic, neurologic, cardiovascular, and miscellaneous injuries including lacerations to the face, hematomas involving the scalp, nasal hematomas and fractures, and dental injuries make up the remaining injury types (74). Neurologic injuries are uncommonly reported and include peripheral neuropathies (15, 42, 97, 100) but only rarely head injuries (21). The peripheral nerve injuries are related both to overuse and the anatomical peculiarities of the radial, long thoracic, and suprascapular nerve. There is no information on the incidence of these injuries, but the senior author has seen three suprascapular nerve neuropathies in tennis players. Two of these individuals were highly successful professional players despite this problem.

Heat-related illness caused by the environmental conditions of temperature and humidity are well recognized in tennis (80) and squash (44). The spectrum of heat-related problems can range from heat cramps to heat stroke, a medical emergency (80). Ophthalmologic and cardiovascular concerns will be discussed in section 4.2 on catastrophic injury.

## 3.3 Injury Location

Information on injury location is roughly divided into the areas of the axial structures, the upper and lower extremities (see Table 18.3).

### 3.3.1 Head/Spine/Trunk

The majority of injuries occurring in racquet sports in the head and neck region are related to direct trauma through contact with the racquet or ball.

**Table 18.3   Injury Location by Sport**

| Injury location | Tennis (Chard, 1987, N = 131) | Badminton (Kroner, 1990, N = 217) | Squash (Berson, 1981, N = 69) | Racquetball (Soderstrom, 1982, N = 157) |
|---|---|---|---|---|
| Head/neck | Not incl. | 4.1% | 18.8%* | 52.9% |
| Upper extremity | 35% | 11.1% | 23% | 12.1% |
| Trunk/spine | 45% | 1.8% | 10.1% | 3.2% |
| Lower extremity | 20% | 82.9% | 48.1% | 31.8% |

*Estimated.

Racquetball and squash participants are particularly susceptible to these injuries because they involve close contact between players in an enclosed court. In two series of racquetball injuries, the facial and head injuries accounted for more than 50% of all trauma reported (98, 104). Similar injuries in squash have been reported with an incidence estimated at 18.8% (11).

Abdominal and groin injuries have also been described in tennis players (5). Most thoraco-abdominal injuries are due to indirect trauma (64), although this information is not supported with good evidence.

With respect to the spine, most of the specific injuries are presentations of low-back pain. These include lumbar disc disease, mechanical low-back pain, and acute traumatic injury (72). A survey of professional men's tennis players revealed an overall incidence of back pain of 38% (72). Of 143 players surveyed, 43 had chronic pain, and 38 suffered more acute injuries. The authors stated that 11 had injuries of the lumbo sacral spine. In a series of badminton injuries, only 1.8% involved the back (58). Racquetball had an even lower incidence of back sprain at 2 out of 75 (104). Specific diagnostic details are not available in these reports. Anecdotal reports of other injuries, such as inferior vena cava thrombosis, demonstrate the variety of problems encountered in racquet sports (102).

### 3.3.2 Upper Extremity

The upper extremity is particularily susceptible to injury in racquet sports because of the use of the racquet and its effect on the dominant limb. Yet it is not involved in injury as much as the lower limb (11, 58). Most upper extremity problems are related to musculotendinous injury (58) around the shoulder (83) and elbow. Wrist problems are less frequently found, especially in tennis. This is believed to be due to the mechanism of the tennis stroke (93).

The shoulder has been implicated in tennis players as an area of concern. "Tennis shoulder" was originally described as a deformity in 1976 (94, 95). It characteristically involves a downward droop or depression of the dominant shoulder with an apparent scoliosis. This was present in more than 50% of 84 expert tennis players. The correlation between tennis shoulder and symptoms of shoulder pain as a constant relationship could not be made. The implication, however, was that this posture could lead to impingement and irritation of the rotator cuff and even to thoracic outlet syndrome (94, 95). The epidemiology of shoulder impingement was addressed comparing a number of sports. The tennis players had a higher rate of shoulder pain and impingement at 50%, with badminton at 37%, and squash at 25% (65). Rotator cuff tears have also been discussed, including their treatment with surgical repair. These tears occurred in tennis players at an average age of 58 (13).

The remainder of the literature is devoted to tennis elbow (19, 39, 47, 62, 70, 81, 86, 87, 105). It has been estimated that at one time or another, 50% of tennis players will suffer from tennis elbow (3). This can occur both medially and laterally, and occasionally in the triceps insertion posteriorly.

### 3.3.3 Lower Extremity

Lower extremity injury occurs consistently more frequently than other injury in racquet sports (11, 58, 104). The knee accounted for the majority of lower limb injuries. Ligament or meniscal injuries were more common in squash and badminton than in tennis, in which patellar problems predominated (20). In another series of racquet sport injuries, 222 of 404 were related to the knee. Thirty percent of the total required arthroscopy, with a diagnosis of meniscal lesions in the majority of patients (71). In squash (11) and badminton (58) the ankle is more likely to be involved in injury. "Tennis leg," otherwise known as rupture of the medial head of the gastrocnemius (34, 36, 99), osteitis pubis (31), which has been reported in both tennis and squash, and iliotibial band syndrome are predominantly associated with tennis (7). Achilles tendon rupture is present in all racquet sports but seems to be more prevalent in badminton (52). In this series of ruptures, 40% occurred in badminton compared with only 18% in soccer, even though it is estimated that far more people participate in soccer (52).

Achilles tendonitis and other hindfoot problems are also reported in all racquet sports. Less commonly reported cases include, flexor hallucis longus tendon injury, resulting in the so-called trigger foot (78), posterior tibial tendon rupture (110), acute superficial posterior compartment syndrome (2), and an even more bizarre occurrence in which a squash player was impaled through the leg by a piece of the wooden floor (23).

## 4. Injury Severity

### 4.1 Time Loss

The literature does not lend itself to determining the time loss of injury. Injury severity is reported in different ways. In squash 47% of the reported injuries were considered to be disabling, resulting in a time loss of greater than two weeks (11). In badminton severity has been measured by patient disposition. In one study, although most injuries were minor, 31% required further treatment and 6.8% were hospitalized. In racquetball there is no specific information regarding severity, although injuries such as Achilles tendon ruptures and serious eye injuries have required hospitalization and surgery. Similarly in tennis, the information is not clear with respect to injury severity (59).

## 4.2 Catastrophic Injury

Catastrophic injury in racquet sports refers to ocular trauma and sudden death. For the purposes of this chapter catastrophic injury is defined as that which cannot be overcome with treatment and rehabilitation.

### 4.2.1 Ocular Trauma

Most accounts of ocular injuries are included in generic eye injury reports, rather than those related to racquet sports. One retrospective study in Australia identified 5% of racquet-related eye trauma resulting in long-term sequelae. This study focussed on a population of squash players and identified an injury rate of 1.75 per 1,000 hours played (35). There were two permanent eye injuries involving impairment of vision but no cases of blindness.

Most of the available information is presented as case reports or series of eye injuries with no information as to the population at risk (21, 24, 25, 35, 46, 49, 53, 66, 82, 101). Squash appears to be the most dangerous of the racquet sports, based upon these reports, but there is no direct evidence comparing the various racquet sports. A general study of ocular trauma revealed that out of 202 injuries, 11.4% were due to racquetball and 7.4% due to tennis (60). These figures compare with 28.7% in basketball. The denominator or population at risk, however, is indeterminate and therefore comparisons are misleading. Squash and tennis were not represented.

These and other methodologic concerns are present in the literature. Most of the articles looked at ocular injury only. It is not possible to compare the incidence of these injuries with other racquet sport injuries. In badminton, the incidence of eye injury was 2.3%, the details of which were not disclosed (58). In racquetball, eye injuries accounted for 9 out of 157 total injuries in one study

(104). Permanent visual impairment (21, 25, 35, 49, 53, 101) and blindness (24, 46, 49, 82) were found to occur in all racquet sports; however, there were no figures detailing the incidence of loss of an eye.

### 4.2.2 Sudden Death

Despite a number of references to sudden death occurring during racquet sport participation, there is no reliable evidence of the incidence of this problem because of the lack of denominator data (27). Most articles have looked at the underlying causes, which include hypertrophic cardiomyopathy, congenital abnormalities of the coronary arteries, aortic valve rupture in younger patients (73), coronary artery disease in older participants (54), and less frequently myocarditis (88). It has been shown that racquet sports can significantly increase the heart rate response, with badminton and squash (91) reaching 80 to 85% of predicted maximum and tennis roughly 70% (22).

Specific articles relating sudden death to racquet sports include those that occurred during squash and tennis (88-90, 92). No reports of sudden death in badminton or racquetball were found. The probable cause of death in most of these individuals was an episode of arrhythmia (107) because of increased catecholamine levels in a susceptible heart (103). Blood pressure changes have also been implicated, but the evidence does not support this etiology (17).

## 4.3 Injury Outcome

### 4.3.1 Dropping Out

There is no information of any significance on whether racquet sport players stop playing the sport because of injury. Even with serious eye injuries, the information is poor with respect to return to the sport (101). In one instance of complete eye removal, the tennis player returned to competitive play (24). In squash many injuries resulted in the players being out of their sport for more than 2 weeks, but only rarely were the injuries considered disabling (11).

### 4.3.2 Clinical Outcome

The clinical outcomes of most injuries sustained during racquet sport play are good (62). Common problems such as tennis elbow have a reported recurrence rate of 25%, with successful treatment in the remainder (39). Even tennis players with full thickness rotator cuff tears undergoing surgical treatment have had a successful clinical outcome (13).

# 5. Injury Risk Factors

## 5.1 Intrinsic Factors

### 5.1.1 Physical Characteristics

It is very difficult to extract the necessary information to identify specific risk factors. Most of the information is based upon patients presenting with problems rather than prospective data looking at the population at risk.

Most of the studies reveal a male preponderance of injury (20, 46, 51, 58, 98) even if time and exposure are accounted for. Warm-up and stretching have been advocated to prevent injury, but there is no evidence that lack of warm-up or inflexibility are risk factors (11, 98). Age is considered a risk factor for most overuse or degenerative conditions, particularly rotator cuff problems in the shoulder and tennis elbow (11).

Another consideration involves general fitness, which has been addressed in a number of publications (10, 38, 55, 69, 77). The racquet sports are characterized by periods of intense activity with intermittent periods of rest. This profile demands both aerobic and anaerobic training. Poor fitness is a risk factor for cardiac problems (69) and may even contribute to overuse and acute injuries, although this is speculative.

### 5.1.2 Psychological and Psychosocial Characteristics

There is no information relating these concerns with injuries in racquet sports. The only inference is with respect to the male preponderance of injury caused by more aggressive, reckless play (98). This is particularly the case in racquetball when men play what is known as "cut throat." This involves three players on the court at one time, and there is always a two-on-one situation with a greater potential for injury.

## 5.2 Extrinsic Factors

### 5.2.1 Exposure

When one considers exposure as a risk factor in racquet sports, it is difficult to make any clear statements other than the intuitive comment that a greater amount of play would result in more injuries. This is implied because elite badminton players suffer more injuries per season, but when exposure is taken into account there are no differences between recreational and elite players (50). In tennis, the exposure to match play seems to have a greater effect on injury than simply the number of hours played (55). This information is gleaned from a comparison of junior competitive players from England, Sweden, and from two programs in the United States. The Swedish players are involved in match play almost one third of the time and twice as much as the other programs. All but one of the Swedish juniors (92%) reported an injury whereas the other groups reported injuries in 55 to 66% of their members (55). It is evident that match play is not the only reason for the difference but the evidence is contributory. The evidence in badminton is in the opposite direction with more injuries occurring during training rather than in match play (50).

### 5.2.2 Training Conditions

There is little information to implicate any specific type of training with injury. The junior tennis player information (55) suggests that improved flexibility will reduce the level of injury, but this has yet to be validated.

### 5.2.3 Environment

Again there is little information specifically dealing with the environmental factors surrounding racquet sports (85). It is surprising because a sport like tennis is played on at least three types of surfaces in both indoor and outdoor environments. There have been some references to these issues but not in the English literature (12, 16, 57, 108). A slippery surface accounted for 21% of injuries in one study (12), and in others the hardness of the surface was implicated (16, 59, 108). In Nigg's study, the type of surface clearly showed a difference, with the harder surfaces showing a greater frequency of injury. This was a self-reported study of pain and injury without a clear description or injury definition. They also included upper extremity injury, which is likely to occur irrespective of the playing surface (85).

The environment certainly plays a role when one compares racquetball and squash with tennis and badminton. The enclosed court inevitably leads to contact between the player and the walls, the other player, and the racquet and ball (98). It is this difference between the sports that accounts for the majority of nonorthopaedic injuries (11). The type of surface for the indoor court sports is also of importance, particularly in squash and racquetball where the buildup of moisture can affect the frictional characteristics of the shoe-court interface (18).

### 5.2.4 Equipment

The institution of regulations enforcing appropriate eye protection in the form of closed eye guards have essentially eliminated eye injuries from ball impact in squash and racquetball. These eye guard standards have been set by testing different types of eye wear (14, 29). Standards have now been set, and many organizations have instituted rules mandating their use (26). There are still many injuries that occur because of contact with the racquet and the opposing player, but the eye is relatively well protected. The variety of tennis racquets and materials used in their construction have been implicated in the prevention of injury, but there is no scientific evidence to support this.

## 6. Suggestions for Injury Prevention

There are many aspects of racquet sport injuries that can be looked at in terms of prevention. The important factors include the individual players, the sport itself, the environment, and the health support system (1). Further reduction in injury may be afforded through improved education of the players to avoid dangerous situations (104). The catastrophic injuries related to the eye (26) and sudden death are the obvious ones to consider (27).

With respect to sudden death, there are no specific tests other than a careful medical check up for those at risk. This involves an assessment of the players and their level of conditioning. A common-sense approach, by matching the sport to the individual and cautioning people with cardiac risk factors, is recommended (27). Eye injuries in squash and racquetball have been significantly reduced by including eye protection as part of the sport (26).

Tennis elbow has received attention through biomechanical studies aimed at prevention (45). The use of grip bands to reduce vibration has been considered. The clinical relevance of this biomechanical information has yet to be demonstrated. Another study recommended using smaller grip forces and using racquets that minimize off-center impacts to reduce the risk of tennis elbow (56). With these injuries, the focus has been on the equipment and technique aspects of the sport. Here again, clinical confirmation is required.

An intrinsic approach through individual strengthening has been advocated to prevent shoulder tendinitis and associated rotator cuff problems (28).

In consideration of problems such as heat stroke, prevention requires adequate hydration (80) and an understanding of the environmental conditions.

Many other aspects of prevention could be illustrated for racquet sports. These measures, such as an ankle brace to prevent sprains, an adequate warm-up and stretching to prevent muscle tears, and avoidance of overuse situations, are generic to most sports.

# 7. Suggestions for Further Research

One of the prevalent problems with the current literature on racquet sport injuries is the lack of consistent injury definition. The literature confuses readers with injuries related to location, injury type, and severity. There needs to be more specific information to identify the acuity, location, type, and severity of each injury, rather than only one or two of these parameters. Furthermore, the selection bias that is introduced when the population at risk is not identified makes any or all conclusions about the injury incidence impossible. Further research should concentrate on prospective data collection, based upon clearly defined inclusion and exclusion criteria. It should focus on populations of racquet sport participants rather than those who present with injuries. This requires accurate information on the baseline exposure of the population under study. Once the exposure is defined, injury rates can be calculated on the basis of hours of play rather than just a percentage of the people involved. Injury prevention is a speculative task until this kind of information becomes available.

More specifically, racquet sports are unique in that they require the participant to utilize a racquet, usually in the dominant hand, and contact a ball of different sizes or a shuttlecock. Each sport has its own adaptive physical and mental aspects. The tennis player develops the so-called tennis shoulder, which in itself is not an injury but an adaptive physical posture very similar to a volleyball player or a baseball pitcher. The badminton player develops a combination of wrist flexibility and dynamic strength in order to clear a shuttlecock from one backhand corner to the other. The squash and racquetball players are constantly bending low to the ground with adaptive lower extremity muscle strength and fitness. The key to further research involves the delineation of what is an adaptive change to improve performance versus a maladaptation that predisposes to injury. This requires a great deal of investigation on normal racquet sport participants rather than just those who are presenting with an injury. The case series or reports serve to establish hypotheses but cannot answer any questions about causation or suggest plausible directions for prevention.

The focus should be on the younger junior players. It is in this category that the most likely benefit will be achieved. Based upon current trends these juniors are playing 20 to 30 hours per week and at younger and younger ages. The physical stresses on these growing individuals are tremendous, not to mention the psychological effects of training at these levels.

Another focus should be the use of education to investigate its effect on injury. This would be particularly useful in the area of catastrophic injury. Logical questions would be: Can education regarding use of eye protection increase the compliance with its use and lower the incidence of eye injuries? Can education lower the occurrence of sudden death? A greater understanding of the risks to people predisposed to heart problems may lead to a lowering incidence of sudden death caused by cardiovascular disease.

The area of biomechanical research designed to identify the factors surrounding injury, although vital, needs to be based upon sound epidemiological information. A detailed understanding of the uninjured player is necessary before inferences can be made about the injured athlete.

In order to carry out this type of investigation into racquet sport injury, many resources are required, particularly personnel. The research assistant is central to this process. They can provide ongoing contact with the participating groups, clubs, or organizations. They would be directly involved in data collection through questionnaires or with the support of trainers associated with teams, who can document both exposure and injury information.

The impact of injury in racquet sports is not as obvious as in a contact sport in which disabling injuries are commonplace. Nevertheless, the number of participants recreationally and the intensity of competition at the elite level magnify the need for a much clearer understanding of injury in racquet sports.

# References

1. Adrian, M. Action model to evaluate and reduce risk of catastrophic injuries. In: Adams, S.H., Adrian, M.J., Bayless, M.A., ed. Catastrophic injuries in sports: Avoidance strategies. 2nd ed. Indianapolis: Benchmark Press; 1987:243-249.
2. Allen, M.J.; Barnes, M.R. Unusual cause of acute superficial posterior compartment syndrome. Injury. 23(3):202-203; 1992.

3. Allman, F.L. Tennis elbow: Etiology, prevention and treatment. Clin. Orthop. 3:308; 1975.

4. Axelsson, R.; Renstrom, P.; Svensson, H. Akuta idrottsskador pa et centrallaserett. Lakartidningen. 77:3615-3617; 1980.

5. Balduini, F.C. Abdominal and groin injuries in tennis. Clin. Sports Med. 7(2):349-357; 1988.

6. Bankes, J.L.K. Squash rackets: A survey of eye injuries in England. Brit. Med. J. 291:1539; 1985.

7. Barber, F.A.; Sutker, A.N. Iliotibial band syndrome. Sports Med. 14(2):144-148; 1992.

8. Barrell, G.V.; Cooper, P.J.; Elkington, A.R.; MacFadyen, J.M.; Powell, R.G.; Tormey, P. Squash ball to eye ball: The likelihood of squash players incurring an eye injury. Brit. Med. J. 283:893-895; 1981.

9. Bell, R.H.; Hawkins, R.J. Stress fracture of the distal ulna. Clin. Orthop. 209:169-171; 1986.

10. Bergeron, M.F.; Maresh, C.M.; Kraemer, W.J.; Abraham, A.; Conroy, B.; Gabaree, C. Tennis: A physiological profile during match play. Int. J. Sports Med. 12:474-479; 1991.

11. Berson, B.L.; Rolnick, A.M.; Ramos, C.G.; Thornton, J. An epidemiologic study of squash injuries. Am. J. Sports Med. 9(2):103-106; 1981.

12. Biener, K.; Caluori, P. Tennissportunfaelle (Tennis injuries). Medizinische Klinik. 72:754-757; 1977.

13. Bigliani, L.U.; Kimmel, J.; McCann, P.D.; Wolfe, I. Repair of rotator cuff tears in tennis players. Am. J. Sports Med. 20 (2):112-117; 1992.

14. Bishop, P.J.; Kozey, J.; Caldwell, G. Performance of eye protectors for squash and racquetball. Phys. Sports Med. 10:63-69; 1982.

15. Black, K.P.; Lombardo, J.A. Suprascapular nerve injuries with isolated paralysis of the infraspinatus. Am. J. Sports Med. 18:225-228; 1990.

16. Bochi, L; Fontanesi, G; Orso, C.A.; Camurri, G.B. La patologia del piede nel tennis in rapporto al terreno di gioco (The pathology of the foot in tennis in connection with playing surfaces). Int. J. Sport Traumatology. 6:325-332; 1984.

17. Bridgeon, G.S.; Hughes, L.O.; Broadhurst, P.; Raftery, E.B. Blood pressure changes during the game of squash. Europ. Heart J. 13:1084-1087; 1992.

18. Chapman, A.E.; Leyland, A.J.; Ross, S.M.; Ryall, M. Effect of floor conditions upon frictional characteristics of squash court shoes. J. Sports Sci. 9:33-41; 1991.

19. Chard, M.D.; Hazleman, B.L. Tennis elbow—A reappraisal. Brit. J. Rheum. 28(3):186-190; 1989.

20. Chard, M.D.; Lachman, S.M. Racquet sports patterns of injury presenting to a sports injury clinic. Brit. J. Sports Med. 27(4):150-153; 1987.

21. Clemett, R.S.; Fairhurst, S.M. Head injuries from squash: A prospective study. NZ Med J. 92:1; 1980.

22. Docherty, D. A comparison of heart rate responses in racquet games. Brit. J. Sports Med. 16(2):96-100; 1982.

23. Dudley, M.J. An unusual squash injury. Br. J. Sport Med. 25(3):138; 1991.

24. Duke, M. Tennis players and eye injuries. JAMA. 236(20):2287; 1976.

25. Easterbrook, M. Eye injuries in racquet sports: A continuing problem. Can. Med. Assoc. J. 123:269; 1980.

26. Easterbrook, M. Eye protection in racquet sports. Clin. Sports Med. 7(2):253-265; 1988.

27. Eichner, E.R. Sudden death in racquet sports. Clin. Sports Med. 7(2):245-251; 1988.

28. Ellenbecker, T.S.; Davies, G.J.; Rowinski, M.J. Concentric versus eccentric isokinetic strengthening of the rotator cuff. Am. J. Sports Med. 16(1):64-69; 1988.

29. Feigelman, M.; Sugar, J.; Jednock, N.; Read, J.S.; Johnson, P.L. Assessment of ocular protection for racquetball. JAMA. 250:3305-3309; 1984.

30. Fowler, B.J.; Seelenfreund, M.; Newton, J.C. Ocular injuries sustained playing squash. Am. J. Sports Med. 8(2):126-128; 1980.

31. Fricker, P.A.; Taunton, J.E.; Ammann, W. Osteitis pubis in athletes. Sports Med. 12(4):266-279; 1991.

32. Froimson, A.I. Tennis leg. JAMA. 209:415-416; 1969.

33. Garrick, J.G.; Requa, R.K. Injuries in high school sports. Pediatrics. 61:465-469; 1978.

34. Gecha, S.R.; Torg, E. Knee injuries in tennis. Clin. Sports Med. 7(2):435-452; 1988.

35. Genovese, M.T.; Lenzo, N.P.; Lim, R.K.; Morkel, D.R.; Jamrozik, K.D. Eye injuries among pennant squash players and their attitudes towards protective eyewear. Med. J. Aust. 153:655-658; 1990.

36. Gilbert, T.; Ansari, A. A tennis player with a swollen calf. Hosp. Practice. November 15, 1991:209-212; 1991.

37. Gregg, J.R.; Torg, E. Upper extremity injuries in adolescent tennis players. Clin. Sports Med. 7(2): 371-385; 1988.

38. Groppel, J.L.; Roetert, E.P. Applied physiology of tennis. Sports Med. 14(4):260-268; 1992.

39. Gruchow, H.W.; Pelletier, B.S. An epidemiologic study of tennis elbow. Am. J. Sports Med. 7(4):234-238; 1979.

40. Gupta, A.; Risitano, G.; Crawford, R.; Burke, F. Fractures of the hook of the hamate. Injury. 20(5): 284-286; 1989.

41. Haddon, W., Jr.; Baker, S.P.; Injury control. In: Clark, D.W.; MacMahon, B., eds. Preventative and community medicine. 2nd ed. Boston: Little, Brown; 1981:109-140.

42. Hama, H.; Ueba, Y.; Morinaga, T.; Suzuki, K.; Kuroki, H.; Yamamuro, T. A new strategy for the treatment of suprascapular entrapment in athletes: Shaving of the base of the scapular spine. J. Shoulder Elbow Surg. 1(5):253-260; 1992.

43. Hang, Y.; Peng, S. An epidemiologic study of upper extremity injury in tennis players. J. Formosan Med. Assoc. 83:307; 1984.

44. Hansen, R.D.; Brotherhood, J.R. Prevention of heat-induced illness in squash players. Med. J. Aust. 148:100; 1988.

45. Hatze, H. The effectiveness of grip bands in reducing racquet vibration transfer and slipping. Med Sci Sports Exercise. 24(2):226-230; 1992.

46. Hensley, L.D.; Paup, D.C. A survey of badminton injuries. Brit. J. Sport Med. 13:156-160; 1979.

47. Ilfeld, F.W. Can stroke modification relieve tennis elbow? Clin. Orthop. 276:182-186; 1992.

48. Ishikawa, H.; Ueba, Y.; Yonezawa, T.; Kurosaka, M; Ohno, O.; Hirohata, K. Osteochondritis dissecans of the shoulder in a tennis player. Am. J. Sports Med. 16(5):547-550; 1988.

49. Jones, N.P. Eye injuries in sport. Brit. J. Sports Med. 21(4):169-170; 1987.

50. Jorgensen, U.; Winge, S. Epidemiology of badminton injuries. Int. J. Sports Med. 8:379-382; 1987.

51. Jorgensen, U.; Winge, S. Injuries in badminton. Sports Med. 10(1):59-64; 1990.

52. Kaalund, S.; Lass, P.; Hogsaa, B.; Nohr, M. Achilles tendon rupture in badminton. Br. J. Sports Med. 23(2):102-104; 1989.

53. Kelly, S.P. Serious eye injuries in badminton players. Brit. J. Ophth. 71:746-747; 1987.

54. Kenny, A.; Shapiro, L.M. Sudden cardiac death in athletes. Brit. Med. Bull. 48(3):534-545; 1992.

55. Kibler, W.B.; McQueen, C.; Uhl, T. Fitness evaluations and fitness findings in competitive junior tennis players. Clin. Sports Med. 7(2):403-406; 1988.

56. Knudson, D.V. Factors affecting force loading on the hand in the tennis forehand. J. Sports Med. Phys. Fitness. 31(4):527-531; 1991.

57. Kraemer, J.; Schmitz-Benting, J. Ueberlastungsschaeden am bewegungsapparat bei tennisspielern (Damage on the locomotor system of tennis players due to overload). Deutsche Zeitschrift fuer Sportmedizin. 2:44-46; 1979.

58. Kroner, K.; Schmidt, S.A.; Nielsen, A.B.; et al. Badminton injuries. Brit. J. Sport Med. 24(3):169-172; 1990.

59. Kuland, D.N.; McCue, F.C.; Rockwell, D.A.; Gieck, J.H. Tennis injuries: Prevention and treatment. Am. J. Sports Med. 7(4):249-253; 1979.

60. Larrison, W.I.; Hersh, P.S.; Kunzweiler, T.; Shingleton, B.J. Sports-related ocular trauma. Ophthalmology. 97(10):1265-1269; 1990.

61. Leach, R.E. Leg and foot injuries in racquet sports. Clin. Sports Med. 7(2):359-370; 1988.

62. Leach, R.E.; Miller, J.K. Lateral and medial epicondylitis of the elbow. Clin. Sports Med. 6(2):259-272; 1988.

63. Lehman, R.C. Shoulder pain in the competitive tennis player. Clin. Sports Med. 7(2):309-327; 1988.

64. Lehman, R.C. Thoracoabdominal musculoskeletal injuries in racquet sports. Clin. Sports Med. 7(2):267-276; 1988.

65. Lo, Y.P.C.; Hsu, Y.C.S.; Chan, K.M. Epidemiology of shoulder impingement in upper arm sports events. Brit. J. Sports Med. 24(3):173-177; 1990.

66. Locke, A.S. Squash rackets: A review—Deadly or safe? Med. J. Aust. 143:565-567; 1985.

67. Loosli, A.R.; Leslie, M. Stress fracture of the distal radius. Am. J. Sports Med. 19(5):523-524; 1991.

68. Lorentzen, R.; Johansson, C.; Bjonstig, U. Fotbollen orsaker flest skador men badmintonskaden ar dyrast. Lakartigningen. 81:340-434; 1984.

69. Lynch, T.; Kinirons, M.T.; O'Callaghan, D.; Ismail, S.; Brady, H.R.; Horgan, J.H. Metabolic changes during serial squash matches in older men. Can. J. Sport Sci. 17(2):110-113; 1992.

70. Maffulli, N.; Regine, R.; Carrillo, F.; Capasso, G.; Minelli, S. Tennis elbow: An ultrasonographic study in tennis players. Brit. J. Sports Med. 24(3): 151-155; 1990.

71. Marans, H.J.; Kennedy, D.K.; Kavanagh, T.G.; Wright, T.A. A review of intra-articular knee injuries in racquet sports diagnosed by arthroscopy. Can. J. Surg. 1(3):199-201; 1988.

72. Marks, M.R.; Haas, S.S.; Wiesel, S.W. Low back pain in the competitive tennis player. Clin. Sports Med. 7(2):277-287; 1988.

73. Maron, B.J.; Roberts, W.C.; McAllister, H.A.; Rosing, D.R.; Epstein, S.E. Sudden death in young athletes. Circulation. 62(2):218-229; 1980.

74. Maylock, F.H. Epidemiology of tennis, squash and racquetball injuries. Clin. Sports Med. 7(2):233-243; 1988.

75. Miller, W.A. Rupture of the musculotendinous junction of the medial head of the gastrocnemius muscle. Am. J. Sports Med. 5:191-193; 1977.

76. Mills, D.M.S.. Injuries in badminton. Brit. J. Sports Med. 11:51-53; 1977.

77. Montpetit, R.R. Applied physiology of squash. Sports Med. 10(1):31-41; 1990.

78. Moorman, C.T.; Monto, R.R.; Bassett, F.H. So-called trigger ankle due to an aberrant flexor hallucis longus muscle in a tennis player. J. Bone Joint Surg. 74-A(2):294-295; 1992.

79. Murakami, Y. Stress fracture of the metacarpal in an adolescent tennis player. Am. J. Sports Med. 16(4):419-420; 1988.

80. Murphy, R.J. Heat problems in the tennis player. Clin. Sports Med. 7(2):429-433; 1988.

81. Murtagh, J.E. Tennis elbow. Aust. Fam. Phys. 17(2): 90-95; 1988.

82. Nanavati, B.A. Eye injuries in racquet sports. Brit. Med. J. 302:1599; 1991.

83. Neer, C.S., II; Welsh, R.P. The shoulder in sports. Orthop. Clin. North Am. 8(3):583-591; 1977.

84. Nicholl, J.P.; Coleman, P.; Williams, B.T. Injuries in sport and exercise. The Medical Care Research Unit, University of Sheffield; Commissioned by The Sports Council of England and Wales; 1991: 1-8.

85. Nigg, B.M.; Segesser, B. The influence of playing surfaces on the load on the locomotor system and on football and tennis injuries. Sports Med. 5:375-385; 1988.

86. Nirschl, R.P. Soft-tissue injuries about the elbow. Clin. Sports Med. 5(4):637-652; 1986.

87. Nirschl, R.P. Prevention and treatment of elbow and shoulder injuries in the tennis player. Clin. Sports Med. 7(2):289-308; 1988.

88. Northcote, R.J.; Ballentyne, D. Sudden cardiac death in sport. Brit. Med. J. 287:1357-1359; 1983.

89. Northcote, R.J.; Evans, A.D.B.; Ballentyne, D. Sudden death in squash players. Lancet. (1):148-151; 1984.

90. Northcote, R.J.; Flannigan, C.; Ballantyne, D. Sudden death and vigorous exercise—A study of 60 deaths associated with squash. Brit. Heart J. 55:198-203; 1986.

91. Northcote, R.J.; Macfarlane, P.; Ballantyne, D. Ambulatory electrocardiography in squash players. Brit. Heart J. 50:372-377; 1983.

92. Opie, L.H. Sudden death and sport. Lancet. 1:263-266; 1975.

93. Osterman, A.L.; Moskow, L.; Low, D.W. Soft-tissue injuries of the hand and wrist in racquet sports. Clin. Sports Med. 7(2):329-348; 1988.

94. Priest, J.D. The shoulder of the tennis player. Clin. Sports Med. 7(2):387-402; 1988.

95. Priest, J.D.; Nagel, D.A. Tennis shoulder. Am. J. Sports Med. 4(1):28-42; 1976.

96. Rettig, A.C.; Beltz, H.F. Stress fracture in the humerus in an adolescent tennis player. Am. J. Sports Med. 13:55-58; 1985.

97. Roles, N.C.; Maudsley, R.H. Radial tunnel syndrome: Resistant tennis elbow as a nerve entrapment. J. Bone Joint Surg. 54-B:499-508; 1972.

98. Rose, C.P.; Morse, J.O. Racquetball injuries. Phys. Sports Med. (January):73-78; 1979.

99. Sando, B. Calf strain. Aust. Fam. Phys. 17(12):1060-1061; 1988.

100. Schultz, J.S.; Leonard, J.A. Long thoracic neuropathy from athletic activity. Arch Phys. Med. Rehabil. 73:87-90; 1992.

101. Seelenfreund, M.H.; Freilich, D.B. Rushing the net and retinal detachment. JAMA. 235(25):2723-2726; 1976.

102. Sheehan, N.J.; Rainsbury, R.M. Inferior vena cava thrombosis following a game of squash. Royal Soc. Med. 52; 1987.

103. Shepherd, R.H. Death on the squash court? Can. J. Sport Sci. 17(2):152; 1992.

104. Soderstrom, C.A.; Doxanas, M.T. Racquetball: A game with preventable injuries. Am. J. Sports Med. 10(3):180-183; 1982.

105. Stratford, P.W.; Norman, G.R.; McIntosh, J.M. Generalizability of grip strength measurements in patients with tennis elbow. Phys. Ther. 69(4):276-281; 1989.

106. Verow, P. Sports injuries: Squash. Practitioner. 233:876-879; 1989.

107. Visser, F.C.; Mihciokur, M.; van Dijk, C.N.; den Engelsman, J.; Roos, J.P. Arrythmias in athletes: Comparison of stress test, 24h Holter and Holter monitoring during the game in squash players. Europ. Heart J. 8(Supplement D):29-32; 1987.

108. von Salis-Sogli, G. Sportverletzungen und sportschaeden beim tennis (Sport injuries in tennis) Deutsche. Zeitschrift Fuer Sportmedizin. 8:244-247; 1979.

109. Watson, A.W.S. Sports injuries during one academic year in 6,799 Irish school children. Am. J. Sports Med. 12(1):65-71; 1984.

110. Woods, L.; Leach, R.E. Posterior tibial tendon rupture in athletic people. Am. J. Sports Med. 19(5):495-498; 1991.

111. Zaricznyj, B.; Shattuck, L.J.M.; Mast, T.A.; Robertson, R.V.; D'Elia, G. Sports-related injuries in school-aged children. Am. J. Sports Med. 8(5):318-323; 1980.

112. Zemel, N.P.; Stark, H.H. Fractures and dislocations of the carpal bones. Clin. Sports Med. 5(4):709-724; 1986.

# 19

# Resistance Training

*V. Patteson Lombardi*

## 1. Introduction

This chapter compares the injuries associated with five distinct resistance training modes: (a) recreational weight training, (b) Olympic lifting, (c) power lifting, (d) body building, and (e) strength training for other sports (e.g., American football). Details concerning each of these different forms of resistance training can be found in other sources (17, 37).

Only a small percentage of those who use weights participate in competitive weight lifting and results from the few weight lifting injury studies cannot be applied to the general public. Therefore, a goal of this chapter is to describe weight-training-associated injuries and deaths for an entire population. Three valuable incident data files obtained from the United States Consumer Product Safety Commission (US CPSC) were analyzed for recreational weight training injuries and deaths: (a) the National Electronic Injury Surveillance System (NEISS), which monitors 91 hospital emergency rooms in the U.S. and Puerto Rico, (b) the current Injury and Potential Injury Incident file (IPII), a collection of news articles, medical examiner reports, inquiries, and complaints; and (c) the Death Certificate file, investigation synopses or verbatim details of fatalities as noted in coroner reports. Except where specific examples are given, US CPSC data files on weight training injuries for 3 years, 1982, 1991, and 1992, were partitioned, analyzed, then averaged to provide an accurate representation of trends over the decade, but with a bias toward recent years.

Together with an analysis of US CPSC recreational weight training data, the chapter reviews the limited U.S. and international, prospective and retrospective studies from 1970 to present on competitive, resistance-trained athletes. The methods used to find these studies included (a) Medline searches (University of Washington Information Navigator System) with the keywords weight training, weight lifting, Olympic lifting, power lifting, body building, injury, and sports injuries, (b) cross-referencing, and (c) direct communication with authors. Since 1970, only one true prospective study examining college football players (77), and three retrospective studies, examining adolescent power lifters (8), Olympic lifters (34), and high school football players (53), have been published in the U.S. Only two international, retrospective investigations, one studying body builders and power lifters (21), and the other, Olympic lifters (31), have been published more recently. It is these six, U.S. and international, prospective and retrospective studies that form the basis of the analysis for competitive resistance training.

Since 1970, there have been more than 150 case or series reports of injuries in recreational weight trainers and resistance-trained athletes. These were found by the same methods indicated previously. Case report and series designs are numerator based and often difficult to interpret (73), so only those that seemed to support the prospective and retrospective data were detailed. Other selected, interesting case or series reports were condensed for review in the form of a table.

The precise definition of *injury* is an important consideration in evaluating injuries associated with any sport or activity. The variety of definitions used make it difficult to compare studies. Some researchers tabulate injuries only when they cause a participant to miss a week or more of training, which leads to a disproportionate representation of severe cases. Some injuries have been reported by athletes, whereas others have been evaluated by sports medicine physicians. Although athletes may properly evaluate the anatomical location of injuries, their personal diagnoses are often unreliable (73). Additionally, even when physicians evaluate injuries, the methods they use may bias the results. For example, orthopedic physicians using clinical exams and X rays are more likely to find bone, muscle, and joint injuries, whereas internists or cardiovascular specialists may isolate an entirely different set of abnormalities. All of these problems appear to be common to most injury studies regardless of the sport or activity.

There are many more obstacles associated with resistance-training injury research. It can be argued that relative to any other sport or activity, resistance training has the widest diversity of participants with a multitude of goals and experiences. Yet in most cases, researchers have not categorized their subjects appropriately as recreational weight trainers or Olympic lifters, power lifters, body builders, or other strength-trained athletes. When scientists have documented injuries, they have implied often that these are the direct result of resistance training, even though they have not evaluated individual characteristics, including medical history and genetic predisposition for injury.

Resistance training has the potential for almost endless combinations of exercise *mode, intensity, duration, frequency*, and *distribution* of training sessions, yet these have been documented in research only rarely. [Descriptions of each of these exercise variables can be found in other sources (3, 17, 37).] Injury rates for resistance training (and other activities and sports) may depend less upon exercise mode and more upon injury predisposition, general fitness level, previous training experience, and total work output (exercise intensity × duration × frequency).

The unique characteristics of the individual, the exercise, and the environment must all be considered to derive meaningful conclusions about injuries associated with resistance training or any form of exercise (Table 19.1). When each of these crucial factors is isolated, the true causes of activity- or sport-associated injuries will be revealed rather than obscured by the lack of ability to control variables.

## 2. Incidence of Injury

### 2.1 Injury Rates

All techniques used to characterize injuries in groups of subjects have advantages and disadvantages. A true *injury rate*, which implies some element of exposure time or training duration, gives more precise information, but may require units of

**Table 19.1   Selected Variables That Must Be Controlled to Derive Meaningful Conclusions From Sport and Activity Injury Research**

| Variable | Specific example |
|---|---|
| Exercise | Weight training |
|   Mode (What kind?) | Isotonic free weight training; barbell and dumbbell systems; military press exercise |
|   Intensity (How hard?) | Muscular strength training; influenced by specific training phase, time of year; periodization, light, medium, heavy workouts; ≥ 75% 1-RM |
|   Duration (How long?) | Actual training time vs. total training time per year, month, week, day, or session; influenced by number and speed of repetitions, number of sets, rest interval time; 10.5 min |
|   Frequency (How many?) | Number of training sessions per week or day, number of sets or repetitions per exercise; 3 sets of 8 repetitions, 3 days/wk |
|   Distribution of training sessions (How often and when?) | Influenced by program design including aerobics and cross training; periodization: base, load, peak, competitive, recovery phases; major-minor muscle group, split alternate plan; aerobics on light weight training days |
| Environmental characteristics | Environmental temperature, humidity and ventilation (indoor vs. outdoor facility); availability: facility and equipment, belts, other supportive devices, training partners, coaches; water and other nutrients; ergogenic aids and other factors |
| Individual characteristics | Genetic and environmental influences; age, general physiological and psychological status; nutritional and sleep status; gender; predisposition for injury; not cleared, conditionally cleared, or cleared for weight training; training goals: for rehabilitation, recreation, fitness, improvement in another sport, or competitive Olympic lifter, power lifter or body builder; use of drugs or ergogenic aids; exercise technique |

expression that are essentially incomprehensible, incomparable, or perhaps even meaningless. True injury rates could be estimated only for three studies, which examined adolescent power lifters (8), junior high and high school football players (53), and college football players (77). An attempt was made to explain these injury rates in a meaningful, practical way. Injury rates could not be estimated for any other resistance training studies because exercise regimen information was insufficient or unavailable. It was surprising that most studies did not quantify the retroactive nature of questionnaires or interviews, making it unclear whether current, recent, past, or all injuries were reported.

Some have chosen to report the *cumulative incidence* of injuries, or the percentage of those injured relative to the total number of participants. Although perhaps more practical from a coaching standpoint, this method essentially omits multiple injuries to the same individual and may underestimate substantially the actual frequency of injuries. Also, it is difficult to derive this calculation from most studies because specifics about multiple or repeat injuries to the same individual are often excluded. More details about cumulative incidence and alternative ways to represent injury rates can be found in other sources (40, 45, 52).

The *injury probability*, obtained simply by dividing the total number of injuries by the total number of participants, was calculated for all of the studies presented in Table 19.2. This ratio represents the probability of finding injuries in a specific group and may provide a general sense of the risk associated with a specific resistance training *mode* along with an easy way to compare the results of several studies. However, these numbers must be interpreted with caution because they do not contain an element of time, and are most certainly influenced by the study design (e.g., retrospective vs. prospective nature) and the author's definition of injury (e.g., 1 or more days of missed training vs. ≥ 8 days of disability vs. hospitalization). Furthermore, the injury probability may reflect many variables other than resistance mode, which are isolated or described rarely, including individual, exercise, and environmental characteristics presented previously (Table 19.1).

### 2.1.1 Weight Training

Only by combining two independent sources of information for the same year, 1985 data from NEISS (68) and American Sports Data (36), can an injury probability for recreational weight training be derived. For 1985 (the only year for which participation data is available), an estimated 36 million adults trained with weights, roughly 3 million more than those who engaged in running and jogging during that same year (36). Given an estimated total of 50,876 hospital-reported injuries and 36 million participants (68), a crude injury probability of 0.0014 for the entire U.S. population can be calculated. This implies that during 1985, for every 1,000 participants in weight training, 1.4 were injured and reported to a hospital (Table 19.2). This crude injury probability may be overestimated by about 20%, since American Sports

Data (36) predicted the number of U.S. adult participants, while the NEISS (68) estimated hospital-reported injuries for all age groups (of which children made up about 20%).

### 2.1.2 Olympic Lifting

Eighty junior Olympic lifters were asked about their previous injuries and overuse problems and were filmed during a contest (34). Although the subjects' mean age was not reported, the group averaged 5 years training experience and included adolescents and young adults. These athletes reported 111 injuries for an absolute injury probability of 1.39 injuries per participant (Table 19.2).

A total of 202 injuries was reported by 121 Olympic lifters (31) including experienced, world-class athletes. This equates to an injury probability of 1.67. Thus, data from two retrospective studies including younger (34) and more experienced athletes (31), predict that an Olympic lifter would report an average of 1 to 2 injuries at some random time prior to a competitive event. Since Olympic lifting research has not documented exposure time, true injury rates cannot be calculated.

### 2.1.3 Power Lifting

Seventy-one young male power lifters, with about 1 1/2 years training experience, sustained 98 injuries (8). This confers an injury probability of 1.38 injuries per lifter (Table 19.2). All of these young athletes were unsupervised over half of their training time, while remarkably, 19-year-olds were unsupervised nearly all (99%) of the time. As seen in Table 19.2, the injury probabilities for young, male, power lifters (8) and Olympic lifters (34) are nearly identical.

The study of adolescent, male, power lifters by Brown and Kimball (1983) is one of the few for which a true injury rate can be calculated. The 71 adolescents trained for an average of 99.2 minutes, 4.1 times per week for 17.1 months, and sustained 98 injuries (8). This is equivalent to 0.3 injuries per 100 hours of training or about 1 injury per participant year (~340-350 hours of training) (8, 74). In other words, if 100 adolescent power lifters trained using a similar regimen, we would expect one injury to occur about every 6 to 7 hours of training (about every 4 training sessions) or each athlete to be injured an average of once per year. Assuming that a year encompasses about three typical athletic seasons, this rate of 1 injury per participant year is comparable to the 0.25 to 0.35 injuries per participant season for high school basketball, soccer, and track and lower than that

**Table 19.2   Overview of Retrospective and Prospective Injury Studies on Recreational Weight Trainers, Competitive Olympic Lifters, Power Lifters, Body Builders, and Strength-Trained American Football Players**

| Author (year) (ref. #) | Study type (recorder) | Study duration | Sample, ♂ / ♀ (n, age) | Training experience | Total # injuries | Injury probability (injuries/ participants) |
|---|---|---|---|---|---|---|
| American Sports Data & US CPSC, NEISS combined (1985) (36, 68) | Prospective MD hospital emergency room report (hospital clerk) & estimates | 12 months | Weight trainers recreational ♂ & ♀ adults ASD estimate (n = 36,000,000, unknown) | Unknown | 50,876[a] US CPSC | 0.0014 |
| Kulund et al. (1978) (34) | Retrospective interview (orthopod, MD) | Unknown | Olympic lifters ♂ adolescents? (n = 80, unknown) | 60.8 months | 111[b] | 1.39 |
| König & Biener (1990) (31) | Retrospective questionnaire (participants with MD) | Unknown | Olympic lifters ♂ adults including world class athletes (n = 121, unknown) | Unknown | 202[c] | 1.67 |
| Brown & Kimball (1983) (8) | Retrospective questionnaire (participants) | Unknown | Power lifters ♂ adolescents (n = 71, unknown, but est. 16.7 yr) | 17.1 months | 98[d] | 1.38 |
| Goertzen et al. (1989) (21) | Retrospective questionnaire (participants) & orthop. exam (MD) | 18 months | Power lifters ♂ young adults (n = 39, 28.3 yr) | 82.8 months | 120[e] | 3.08 |
| Goertzen et al. (1989) (21) | Retrospective questionnaire (participants) & orthop. exam (MD) | 18 months | Power lifters ♀ young adults (n = 21, 29.4 yr) | 64.8 months | 40[e] | 1.90 |
| Goertzen et al. (1989) (21) | Retrospective questionnaire (participants) & orthop. exam (MD) | 18 months | Body builders ♂ young adults (n = 240, 25.9 yr) | 43.2 months | 235[e] | 0.98 |
| Goertzen et al. (1989) (21) | Retrospective questionnaire (participants) & orthop. exam (MD) | 18 months | Body builders ♀ young adults (n = 118, 30.4 yr) | 34.8 months | 53[e] | 0.45 |
| Risser et al. (1991) (52, 53) | Retrospective questionnaire (participants) & physical exam (MD & ATC) | 1 month | Football players ♂ jr. high & high school (n = 354, 15.4 yr) | 11.2 months | 27[f] | 0.08 |
| Zemper (1990) (77) | Prospective questionnaire (ATC) | 4 seasons | Football players ♂ college (n = 10,908, unknown, but est. 20 yr) | Unknown | 38[g] | 0.0035 |

*Note.* The injury probabilities were calculated by dividing the total number of injuries by the total number of participants. These numbers should be evaluated with care, since experimental designs, injury definitions, and individual, exercise, and environmental factors varied.

[a]Total projected from 1985 hospital-reported injuries recorded in 64 hospital emergency rooms in the U.S. and its territories. Compared to NEISS estimates before 1990, those after 1990 have been 18% higher due to a new sampling procedure. A correction factor of 1.18 was applied to the original number of injuries projected for 1985 to account for underestimation.

[b]Olympic lifters reported injuries and overuse problems that lasted from 1 day to more than 2 years.

[c]Olympic lifters reported injuries that resulted in an inability to participate from 0-7 days up to over 28 days.

[d]Power lifters reported the occurrence and level of pain when lifting, immediately after, and between workouts, and injuries that caused them to discontinue training for at least 1 day.

[e]Power lifters or body builders reported acute pain and overuse injuries (injury time was not noted) in a questionnaire. Some were examined later by an orthopedic physician. Depending on the athlete's experience, X rays were taken of the shoulder, elbow, knee, and vertebral column. Total number of injuries is likely underestimated by ~9%, since only the most prevalent injuries (~91% of the total) were reported by the authors.

[f]Football players completed a questionnaire during preparticipation physical exams by an MD. Injuries that caused ≥ 8 days of missed participation were recorded for the previous year and verified by an athletic trainer.

[g]Head athletic trainers recorded weight room injuries that kept players from participating in football for 1 day or more. Football players engaged in pre-season and in-season resistance training.

reported for high school football, women's gymnastics, and wrestling (20, 74).

Goertzen and colleagues (1989) should be commended for being the only researchers to have studied males and females across competitive resistance training modes. Their unique study (21) essentially combined a retrospective medical questionnaire with prospective X rays and orthopedic exams as a follow-up in selected athletes. The male and female power lifters surveyed were similarly aged, but the males had 1 1/2 years more training experience. The authors detailed 120 injuries in 39 males, and 40 in 21 females. [Only the most prevalent injuries (91% of the total) were reported, which means that the total number analyzed was underestimated by about 9%.] Despite underreporting of data, the injury probabilities can be estimated as 3.08 for males and 1.90 for females. Only about 5% of the mostly professional power lifters indicated that they trained under "educated supervision" and just over 50% engaged in any other sports (e.g., jogging, racquetball, squash). While gender may have played a significant role, the lower injury probability for females may have been influenced by their fewer years of experience, safer exercise selection, lower absolute training intensity, superior exercise technique, enhanced spotting, or underreporting of injuries. Despite the lack of control for many individual, exercise, and environmental variables, these data (21) imply that athletes with considerable experience, regardless of their gender, can expect about 2 to 3 injuries when training for a power lifting meet. It is unfortunate that exposure time and the survey's retroactive nature were not documented.

### 2.1.4 Body Building

Goertzen and associates also administered an injury questionnaire to 240 male and 118 female, young, adult body builders (21). Both groups had similar training experience. Only a small percentage of these athletes (e.g., < 2% of the males) always trained under "educated supervision." Two-hundred-and-thirty-five injuries were described in the males for an estimated injury probability of 0.98. Fifty-three injuries were noted in the females for an estimated injury probability of 0.45 (Table 19.2).

The slight difference in training experience (~1/2 yr) could not have accounted for the injury probability differences between females and males, yet training intensity, duration, and other variables noted previously may have played a role. Nevertheless, it is interesting that as for power

lifters, the injury probability for female body builders is considerably lower than that for males. It can be predicted from Goertzen's data (21) that compared with experienced females, experienced male body builders (or power lifters) have about a 1 1/2- to 2-fold greater likelihood of reporting injuries. One could speculate that these differences do not arise from genetic or biological origin, but simply depend on the females' tendency to stress exercise technique more than resistance.

### 2.1.5 Football

Risser, Risser, and Preston (1990) studied weight training injuries in 354 junior high and high school football players (53). The players, who averaged about 15 years of age, had just over 11 months of training experience. Only 27 injuries were reported for a relative injury probability of 0.08 (Table 19.2). This equates to approximately 1 injury for every 13 players. This is significantly lower than the injury probability reported for young, male, Olympic lifters (34) and power lifters (8) (Table 19.2). It is also significantly lower than that reported for football participation (1 in 4 athletes injured) in similar, age group males (49, 53).

Risser and colleagues (1990) also provided enough information to allow for a true injury rate calculation. The 354 high school football players trained an average of 3.2 sessions per week, 52.2 minutes per session, for 11.2 months, and sustained 27 injuries (52, 53). This equates to 0.06 injuries per 100 hours of training or 0.08 injuries per participant year. In other words, if 100 junior high and high school football players were highly supervised and trained according to this same regimen, we would expect one athlete to be injured about every 17 hours of training or about every 19 training sessions. Junior high players had the highest injury rate (0.11 injuries/participant year), while high school varsity players had the lowest (0.05 injuries/participant year). When athletes are well-coached and supervised by knowledgeable professionals who are concerned for their safety, their likelihood of being injured in the weight room is far lower than when playing football. A study in college football players yielded similar results.

Zemper (1990) analyzed weight room injuries in a national sample of 10,908 college football players over four football seasons (77). This rare prospective study relied on certified head athletic trainers at each university or college to complete weekly exposure and injury data report forms, about 99% of which were submitted. Surprisingly, only 38 time-loss, weight-room-related injuries were reported (out of a total of 5,158 football-associated injuries). This represents an injury probability of near 0.0035 per player or an injury rate of 0.35 injuries per 100 players (about the size of an average team) per season (Table 19.2). Zemper also described this as 0.13 injuries per 1,000 athlete-exposures, with an exposure defined as one athlete participating in one practice or competition with the potential of being injured. In other words, in 3 years, the average college football team can expect about one time-loss injury from strength training. Zemper concluded that although football players may spend a considerable amount of time in the weight room, they do not appear to incur an inordinate number of injuries there (especially relative to playing football). It is important to note that compared with out-of-season strength training, in-season training is often conducted at a considerably lower intensity with a de-emphasis on maximum lifting. To fully separate the influence of resistance training from football on the incidence of weight room injuries, out-of-season injury data should be collected.

Zemper (77), Risser and associates (53), and Brown and Kimball (8) have taken important steps in improving the ability to isolate variables in resistance-training injury studies.

# 3. Injury Characteristics

## 3.1 Injury Onset

As in other sports and activities, the acute or chronic nature of a resistive-training injury depends on a multitude of individual, environmental, and exercise characteristics (Table 19.1). While most resistive-training studies have documented acute injuries, there have been some reports of chronic injuries involving the low back, shoulder, and knee.

### 3.1.1 Weight Training

The acute versus chronic nature of injuries has not been examined in recreational weight trainers. Only the acute, hospital-reported injury data tabulated prospectively by the NEISS of the US CPSC is available (65, 66, 67, 68, 70). Research is needed in this area.

### 3.1.2 Olympic Lifting

Over 90% of young, Olympic lifters examined in a case series study (32) complained of low-back pain sometimes (50%) or always (> 40%), while less than 10% expressed no episodes of low-back

pain. Acute bouts of low-back pain were experienced during the transition phase of the clean and jerk or just before and after pressing weights overhead. The vertebral segment of L-5/S-1 is particularly vulnerable to high forces during overhead lifting (1). X rays verified that about one third of the Olympic lifters had spondylolysis, which was noted as being about six times higher than the expected incidence (5-7%) in normal adults of the general population (32). The highest incidence of spondylolysis was in competitors with 4 years experience, while spondylolysis accompanied by low-back pain was most prevalent in the lighter weight classes. It may have been premature for the authors to conclude that spondylolysis occurs more frequently in lighter weight classes, because over 75% of the lifters were in classes less than or equal to middle weight. Additional studies with an even distribution of competitors in each weight class would help to clarify this presumption.

A high incidence of spondylolysis in Olympic weight lifters was confirmed by X rays and review of clinical records of 3,132 Italian Olympic athletes over 26 years (54). Twenty-two of 97 (23%) Olympic lifters had spondylolysis, which was noted as being considerably higher than the rate found in the normal population (~4-6%). Thus, two case series studies (32, 54) indicate that Olympic weight lifting may exacerbate spondylolysis, but likely in genetically predisposed individuals. A more recent, retrospective study implies that chronic knee, shoulder, and other low-back problems may be associated with Olympic lifting.

Although recognizing the difficulty in distinguishing between acute and chronic injuries at the time of diagnosis, König and Biener (1990) found multiple overuse injuries of ligaments, tendons, and joint capsules in experienced Olympic lifters (31). Knee injuries, which accounted for 25% of the total, were seldom the result of acute trauma, but rather involved degenerative processes. There were multiple cases of shoulder arthritis noted as being unresponsive to therapy. One third of the athletes stated that they had back problems at least once in their lifetime, yet apparently this does not exceed the incidence in the general population (22). Back problems accounted for just over 20% of all Olympic lifting injuries, but often occurred without obvious reason. One lifter's low-back pain disappeared completely when he was finally diagnosed with pelvic torsion and successfully treated with orthotics. Further research will help to differentiate chronic injuries induced solely by Olympic lifting from those precipitated by genetic predisposition, inadequate conditioning, poor technique, continued training in spite of joint pain, or failure to seek proper medical advice.

Although acute incidents of blackout have been reported in Olympic lifters during competition (12), the long-term effects of these isolated events on the cardiovascular and cerebrovascular systems are unknown. Blackouts are induced by the performance of Valsalva's maneuver, involving breath holding or forcing against a closed glottis, which is nearly reflexive with lifts greater than 50% of one-repetition maximum (1-RM). Olympic lifters are most vulnerable to blackout, when the bar compresses vessels in the neck, just prior to pressing the weight overhead during heavy clean and jerks. Valsalva's maneuver may be advantageous for supporting the spine during heavy lifting (26, 35). However, the mechanical advantages of using Valsalva's maneuver may be offset by the undesirable effects on the heart and vessels, lungs, brain, spinal cord, and cerebrospinal fluid (12, 37).

### 3.1.3 Power Lifting

A study of young power lifters may imply that power lifting is associated with chronic injuries (8). Approximately two thirds of adolescent power lifters experienced low-back pain during, after, and between workouts, while about one fifth had low-back pain approaching severe. Just over half noted mild to severe pain in the shoulder region with one third reporting this pain sometimes or always. About one fifth to one third noted knee pain sometimes to always, with over one third noting the pain was mild to severe (8). Less than one quarter of all injuries that caused these athletes to stop training were treated by a physician, athletic trainer, or other sports medicine professional. These results imply that power lifting may lead to chronic low-back, shoulder, and knee joint pain. However, the apparent chronic nature of these injuries may have been averted, if athletes had (a) been adequately conditioned, (b) used superior technique, and (c) discontinued training and sought proper medical treatment when joint pain occurred. Yet, another study of more experienced, young, adult male and female power lifters reveals the actual presence of degenerative joint changes.

Joint degeneration was documented by orthopedic exams and X rays in experienced male and female power lifters by Goertzen and associates (21). Although, it was not clear whether bilateral joint degeneration was counted once or twice in a given athlete, there were 22 cases of shoulder arthritis documented in 39 males (injury probability = 0.56) and 3 cases in 21 females (injury probability = 0.14). Repetitive, high-intensity bench presses, dips, and push-ups may induce shoulder-

girdle bone microtrauma and osteolysis (bone breakdown) of the distal clavicle (9), which may be similar to a premature aging process.

Goertzen and associates (21) also reported 38 cases of degenerative/irregular patellar cartilage in males (injury probability = 0.97) and 11 cases in females (injury probability = 0.52). Although vertebral column injuries were prevalent in both male and female athletes, these power lifters had an incidence of spondylolysis or spondylolisthesis similar to that of the general population (~5-8%). Nevertheless, these cases do confirm the presence of degenerative joint disease in relatively young (age = 28-29 yr), yet experienced (training = ~5-7 yr) adult male and female power lifters. Longitudinal research is needed to compare the incidence of degenerative joint changes in wide age-ranged groups of resistance- and nonresistance-trained females and males.

### 3.1.4 Body Building

Goertzen's group (1989) documented the presence of joint degeneration in male and female body builders. There were 69 cases of shoulder arthritis in 240 male (injury probability = 0.29), and 9 cases in 118 female body builders (injury probability = 0.08). Knee cartilage pathology was found also in athletes of both genders (21). These cases do confirm the presence of degenerative joint disease in relatively young, moderately experienced, male and female body builders, but more comparative work is needed with the general population.

Although individual (e.g., genetic predisposition, training despite joint pain, use of steroids), exercise (e.g., selection, technique, intensity), and environmental (e.g., knee wraps, spotting) characteristics may have confounded the results, cumulative data from Goertzen and associates (21) imply that compared to power lifters, body builders have a lower probability of joint degeneration.

Blood pressures as high as 480/350 mmHg in body builders doing a series of double leg presses and 232/154 mmHg in subjects using only 50% of 1-RM have been recorded intra-arterially (19, 38). Although, higher than anticipated pressures may have occurred because an inverted leg press was used (by body builders who may have taken steroids), it certainly seems prudent to have those with serious, preexisting cardiovascular complications avoid heavy resistance training. High pressures during heavy lifting can severely limit or even temporarily abolish the output of the heart, decrease the blood supply to the brain, and induce blackout (12, 37). While some have speculated that heavy resistance training demonstrates the plasticity or dynamic nature of the cardiovascular system, no well-designed studies using 24-hour ambulatory recordings have examined the long-term effects of resistance training on blood pressure. One study has demonstrated that systolic blood pressure can remain elevated for up to 15 minutes after high-intensity (80% 1-RM) resistance training, in contrast to what occurs following aerobic exercise (47). Longitudinal research using 24-hour monitors is needed to determine if acute blood pressure changes may induce chronic hypertension in genetically predisposed individuals.

### 3.1.5 Football

Two season-ending injuries (a leg fracture and an L-4 disc rupture) were reported in a prospective study of strength-trained, college football players (77). While these weight room injuries, along with three cases of heat exhaustion and one concussion, may have resulted in extended problems, the long-term effects of strength-training for football have not been examined. This is a difficult area for research since football participation may influence a player's susceptibility to weight room injuries and subsequent chronic problems.

## 3.2 Injury Type

Table 19.3 is a comparison of injuries partitioned according to diagnosis and resistive-training mode. These percentages should be viewed with care since they may have been skewed by differences in basic study design, definition of injury, and individual, environmental, and exercise variables.

### 3.2.1 Weight Training

The percentages presented in Table 19.3 for recreational weight training are averages of 3,836 hospital-reported cases monitored by the NEISS of the US CPSC during 1982, 1991, and 1992 (65, 66, 67). These injuries involved males and females of all age groups (0-65+ yr). However, the data is biased toward males, who accounted for about 80%, and adolescents and young adults (15-24 yr), who accounted for about 45% of all injuries during the 3 years (65, 66, 67). Additional data partitioning and analyses are needed to define gender and age group differences.

The most prevalent injuries in recreational weight trainers are muscle strains and ligament sprains, accounting for almost 40%, and contusions and abrasions, accounting for slightly more than 20% of the total (65, 66, 67). Thus, about 60% of all hospital-reported injuries are due to overtaxed muscles and ligaments and bruises and scrapes. Also note in Table 19.3, that relative to other forms of resistance training, recreational weight training has the highest percentage of fractures. In fact, the percentage of fractures in the general population is four-fold greater than any other resistance-training category, except for strength-trained, adolescent football players. While other resistance-training modes may slightly skew the hospital-reported data (e.g., a fracture in a high school football player may have been treated at the hospital), because of the diverse hospital-reporting system (currently, 91 hospitals in the U.S. and Puerto Rico) and large NEISS data sampling, this influence is probably minimal (69). These data imply that in the general population, injury mechanisms involve inadequate specific warm-up, poor exercise technique, premature use and mishandling of heavy weights, and lack of spotting.

### 3.2.2 Olympic Lifting

König and Biener (1990) and Kulund and colleagues (1978) did not partition injuries specifically by diagnosis, but rather emphasized a listing of injuries by anatomical site. The text of these two retrospective studies (31, 34) was carefully analyzed so each injury noted by the authors was tabulated. During this process, logical assumptions were made about diagnoses that are most common to specific joints. For example, if it was not noted by the authors, it was assumed that wrist injuries involved ligament sprains or tendon inflammations rather than muscular strains or bony fractures. From this careful review with basic assumptions, diagnosis categories and percentage approximations were formulated. Since these approximations are by no means perfect, they must be viewed with caution. However, they do provide a foundation, which was previously nonexistent, for partitioning Olympic lifting injuries by diagnosis.

Ligament sprains account for the greatest percentage of injuries in younger (34) and older (31) Olympic lifters, some 35-40% of the total (Table 19.3). Muscle strains are the next most prevalent category, contributing approximately 30%. Despite performing far more technically difficult, repetitive, high-intensity, overhead lifts, Olympic lifters have a low percentage of total injuries as fractures (0-2%), especially relative to recreational weight trainers (Table 19.3). The low fracture percentage may be attributed to the outstanding musculature

**Table 19.3　A Comparison of Resistive-Training Injuries Partitioned According to Diagnosis**

| US CPSC (NEISS)[a] (1982, 1991, 1992) (65, 66, 67) Weight training ♂ & ♀ prospective | Kulund et al.[c] (1978) (34) Olympic lifting ♂ retrospective | König & Biener[c] (1990) (31) Olympic lifting ♂ retrospective | Brown & Kimball (1983) (8) Power lifting ♂ retrospective | Goertzen et al.[d] (1989) (21) Power lifting ♂ retrospective | Goertzen et al.[d] (1989) (21) Power lifting ♀ retrospective | Goertzen et al.[d] (1989) (21) Body building ♂ retrospective | Goertzen et al.[d] (1989) (21) Body building ♀ retrospective | Risser et al. (1991) (52, 53) HS football ♂ retrospective | Zemper[e] (1990) (77) College football ♂ prospective |
|---|---|---|---|---|---|---|---|---|---|
| Strain/sprain[b] (39%) | Ligament sprain (~36%) | Ligament sprain (~39%) | Muscle strain (61%) | Arthritis (29%) | Tendinitis (25%) | Cartilage degen. (32%) | Tendinitis (33%) | Muscle strain (74%) | Muscle strain (40%) |
| Contusion/ abrasion (22%) | Muscle strain (~32%) | Muscle strain (~29%) | Tendinitis (12%) | Tendinitis (28%) | Arthritis (17%) | Tendinitis (23%) | Cartilage degen. (28%) | Ligament sprain (11%) | Ligament sprain (18%) |
| Fracture (13%) | Other (~24%) | Other (~25%) | Muscle spasm (10%) | Cartilage degen. (17%) | Ligament sprain (17%) | Arthritis (18%) | Ligament sprain (13%) | Fracture (7%) | Subluxation/ separation (11%) |
| Laceration (13%) | Tendinitis (~6%) | Cartilage injury (~3%) | Ligament sprain (4%) | Nerve injury (10%) | Muscle strain (11%) | Nerve injury (10%) | Arthritis (8%) | Tendinitis (4%) | Heat exhaustion (8%) |
| Other (5%) | Dislocation (~1%) | Muscle spasm (~1%) | Abrasion (4%) | Muscle strain (6%) | Bone degeneration (11%) | Muscle strain (7%) | Muscle strain (8%) | Nerve injury (4%) | Tendinitis (5%) |
| Dislocation (2%) | Hernia (~1%) | Fracture (~2%) | Nerve injury (3%) | Ligament sprain (6%) | Cartilage degen. (9%) | Ligament sprain (6%) | Nerve injury (8%) | | Disc injury (5%) |
| Hematoma (1%) | Fracture (~0%) | Contusion/ abrasion (~1%) | Fracture (2%) | Bone degeneration (2%) | Nerve injury (8%) | Bone degeneration (3%) | Bone degeneration (3%) | | Fracture (3%) |
| Crushing (1%) | | Amputation (< 1%) | Other (2%) | Disc injury (1%) | Disc injury (2%) | Disc injury (2%) | Disc injury (3%) | | Abrasion/ contusion (3%) |

*Note.* As many as eight injury diagnosis categories are presented in descending order of prevalence for each study. The percentage contribution of each diagnosis to the total is listed in parentheses. Care should be used when evaluating percentages, since experimental designs and injury definitions, and individual, environmental, and exercise characteristics varied.

[a]Percentages presented are an average of hospital-reported injuries for 3 years over the most recent decade.

[b]Separate categories were not used for muscular strains and ligament sprains. To classify hospital-reported injuries, the US CPSC, like other organizations, relies on the International Classification of Diseases. It can be argued that this grouping may be more realistic, because different diagnoses may occur simultaneously and/or be difficult to distinguish (e.g., about the shoulder joint). Thus, separate categories may create a false partitioning.

[c]The authors did not partition injuries specifically by diagnosis. Diagnosis categories and percentage approximations were formulated by carefully reviewing the authors' text, by tabulating each specific injury reported, and by making logical assumptions about diagnoses that are most common to specific joints. For example, if not noted, it was assumed that wrist injuries were ligament sprains or tendon inflammations, rather than muscular strains or bony fractures.

[d]The authors detailed only the most prevalent injuries (91.4% of the total). Diagnosis categories and percentage approximations were formulated from this impartial listing.

[e]The author and reporting athletic trainer detailed each injury specifically. The merging of several categories would induce higher values for the most prevalent diagnoses, yet create additional problems with overlap or redundancy. For example, a low-back disc injury may involve a combination of cartilaginous, ligamentous, muscular, and bony insults.

and refined techniques developed by Olympic lifters, which may in essence cushion or protect their bones. Also, compared with controls, Olympic lifters have a significantly higher bone mass at every site except the head (30). Yet, compared with junior lifters (34), older, more experienced lifters, including World Champions (31), have a slightly higher percentage of total injuries attributed to fractures (Table 19.3). However, two cases of wrist fractures may have been equipment related, that is, induced by poorly rotating Olympic bars (31).

### 3.2.3 Power Lifting

Muscle strains account for about 60% of the total injuries in adolescent male power lifters (8), but only 6% in experienced, adult male (21) and only 11% in experienced, adult female (21) power lifters (Table 19.3). There have been no reports of arthritis in young power lifters (8), but arthritis is the first or second most prominent diagnosis for experienced male and female power lifters (21). Tendinitis diagnoses appear to be less than half as common in younger versus older power lifters (Table 19.3). Cartilage degeneration follows a similar pattern, accounting for a greater percentage of total injuries in experienced athletes. These results imply that older power lifters, regardless of their gender, are susceptible to chronic overuse injuries and degenerative joint disease. Yet, the orthopedic exams and X rays used along with surveys, to evaluate the more experienced athletes (21), made it easier to detect arthritis and other chronic problems. Certainly, further research is needed, particularly in young female power lifters, to isolate a multitude of variables. It is impossible to conclude that power lifting (or any other type of resistance exercise) induces long-term injuries, which may be caused by those who are skeletally malaligned training despite joint pain and avoiding medical treatment.

### 3.2.4 Body Building

Experienced male and female body builders (21) have a high percentage of overuse and degenerative injuries (Table 19.3). Tendinitis is the primary diagnosis in females, accounting for one third of the total. Cartilage degeneration/abnormality and arthritis also account for a large percentage of injuries in females. Similarly, male body builders have a large fraction of chronic overuse injuries, including cartilage degeneration/abnormality, tendinitis, and arthritis.

Although any number of individual, environmental, and exercise characteristics may play a role, whether body building or power lifting, females appear to have (or at least report) a greater percentage of their injuries as tendinitis and sprains, and a lower percentage as arthritis, compared to males engaging in these same competitive events.

### 3.2.5 Football

Muscle strains are most common in strength-trained, junior high and high school football players (52, 53), accounting for nearly 75% of all injuries (Table 19.3). Ligament sprains are next most prevalent, contributing just above 10% to the total. Note from Table 19.3, that compared to all groups except recreational weight trainers, the adolescent football players have a higher percentage of fractures.

Risser and colleagues (53) noted that two junior high school athletes sustained fractures: one of the distal radial and ulnar epiphyses during a military press and the other of two proximal phalanges during an unidentified exercise. [The finger fractures were probably caused by weight mishandling or poor spotting technique.] Since Risser actually describes four fractures in two athletes, it may have been more appropriate to note that fractures accounted for about 14% (9/29) of all injuries. This percentage more closely approximates that of the general population.

Radial and ulnar fractures have been reported during overhead lifts, particularly the clean and jerk and military press in adolescents (24, 55). Youngsters during peak growth periods may be susceptible when they handle resistance in excess of their body weight (5, 28). However, three recent prospective studies indicate that prepubescents who engage in short-term training with overhead and Olympic lifts have a low injury rate and no clinically evident skeletal damage, provided they are supervised closely by trained sports medicine professionals (51, 58, 59).

As in younger football players, those in college experience most (40% of total) weight room injuries as muscle strains (77). The next most prevalent diagnosis in strength-trained college players is the ligament sprain. These results and others from Table 19.3 imply that once muscles become well-developed, they appear to be protected somewhat from injuries, which are diffused to other body parts. For every resistance training mode, the youngest athletes have the highest percentage of muscle strains. This seems logical since those who are older have had considerably more time to perfect neuromuscular patterning. Despite this fine tuning, when exercise intensity increases (the goal of competitive weight lifting), other body tissues must bear the brunt of the weight. Table 19.3 implies the presence of an injury hierarchy from muscles to tendons to ligaments to bones.

### 3.3 Injury Location (Anatomical Site)

Injuries partitioned by anatomical site are illustrated in Table 19.4. These data, obtained from the retrospective and prospective studies cited previously, are examined according to each resistance training mode. An overview of selected case reports and series is presented in Table 19.5. Primary sites of injury are noted together with exercises implicated.

#### 3.3.1 Weight Training

The finger is the most common site of hospital-reported weight training injuries, accounting for an average of 14% of the total for 1982, 1991, and 1992 (65, 66, 67). The lower trunk is a close second contributing 13%, while the upper trunk, shoulder, and toe each contribute about 10% to the total (Table 19.4). Most injuries in children are to the finger, toe, head, and face, while those in adolescents and adults involve the lower trunk, upper trunk, and shoulder (65, 66, 67). Additional data partitioning and analyses are needed to characterize more fully age group and gender differences.

In adolescents and adults, finger injuries imply mishandling of free weight barbells, plates, or dumbbells, or entangling of fingers in circuit machine cables or plates. In young children, finger injuries are likely induced by a lack of supervision and unsecured equipment. Recent US CPSC reported incident data files and individual injury listings (70, 71, 72) document many serious finger trauma cases in adults who dropped weights and in children who were free to explore unsecured weight training, cycle ergometer, treadmill, and stair-climbing devices.

In addition to US CPSC reports, several case studies implicate specific exercises with unique sites of injury (Table 19.5). Over two thirds of pectoralis major ruptures during recreational activities are associated with bench presses and chest flies (33, 50). Ruptures are most common near the humeral insertion and are induced by direct trauma or an extra force being applied when the muscle is at full tension. Most suspected partial tears reveal complete rupture upon surgery. As long as it occurs soon after injury, surgery followed by rehabilitation is highly successful in relieving

patients of pain, and restoring strength and normal chest contour (33).

A deconditioned musculotendinous unit, or one that is irritated from previous injury, is most susceptible to rupture. McMaster's early animal research (1933) demonstrated that a tendon will not rupture unless it is injured, and rather than the tendon itself, the tendon insertion or the musculotendinous junction will tear when exposed to extreme loads (42, 50). Muscles and tendons are likely most vulnerable during the transition phase of an exercise, midway between the eccentric and concentric components. Pectoral ruptures may be precipitated during failed maximal attempts, when a subject thrusts the head, neck, and trunk upward toward an immovable bar. Kretzler and Richardson (1989) stress that although pectoral muscle ruptures are uncommon, they are not rare (33).

Upper extremity compartment syndromes have been described in male and female weight trainers, interestingly, both of whom were 30 years of age (6, 57) (Table 19.5). Excessive, high-repetition arm and forearm exercises may have precipitated these injuries, but genetically small arm and forearm compartments or other factors may have played a role.

#### 3.3.2 Olympic Lifting

Olympic lifters most commonly injure the knee and the shoulder, which together account for nearly 50% of their total injuries (31, 34) (Table 19.4). About 35 to 40% of the remaining injuries occur in the wrist, back, and elbow. The clean and jerk and snatch are associated with shoulder and elbow injuries, the deep squat with knee injuries, and the dead lift with lower back injuries (34). While the clean and jerk may account for nearly 50% of all injuries (34), it may be unjust to characterize it as the most hazardous Olympic training lift prior to equating its frequency with other exercises. The deep squat contributes about 25%, the snatch 20%, and other pressing movements or the dead lift less than 10% to the total (34). It is not possible to predict which phase of the Olympic or ancillary training lifts might contribute to lower versus upper back injuries, because both retrospective, Olympic lifting studies (31, 34) grouped these distinct regions into a single *back* category.

Kulund and associates (1978) comment that Olympic lifters have a low incidence of back injuries (less than 10% of the total), which they attribute to enhanced paravertebral muscle strength, spinal flexibility, and straight-backed lifting style (34). However, a relatively low incidence of acute

**Table 19.4  A Comparison of Resistive-Training Injuries Partitioned According to Anatomical Site**

| US CPSC (NEISS)[a] (1982, 1991, 1992) (65, 66, 67) Weight training ♂ & ♀ prospective | Kulund et al. (1978) (34) Olympic lifting ♂ retrospective | König & Biener (1990) (31) Olympic lifting ♂ retrospective | Brown & Kimball (1983) (8) Power lifting ♂ retrospective | Goertzen et al. (1989) (21) Power lifting ♂ retrospective | Goertzen et al. (1989) (21) Power lifting ♀ retrospective | Goertzen et al. (1989) (21) Body building ♂ retrospective | Goertzen et al. (1989) (21) Body building ♀ retrospective | Risser et al. (1991) (52, 53) HS football ♂ retrospective | Zemper (1990) (77) College football ♂ prospective |
|---|---|---|---|---|---|---|---|---|---|
| Finger (14%) | Shoulder (23%) | Knee (25%) | Lower back (50%) | Vertebral column[e] (33%) | Knee (28%) | Shoulder (34%) | Knee (31%) | Lower back (48%) | Lower back (42%) |
| Lower trunk[b] (13%) | Knee (23%) | Shoulder girdle[d] (22%) | Knee (8%) | Shoulder (32%) | Vertebral column[e] (24%) | Elbow (21%) | Shoulder (29%) | Shoulder (15%) | Shoulder (11%) |
| Upper trunk[b] (10%) | Wrist (18%) | Back[c] (21%) | Thigh (7%) | Elbow (13%) | Shoulder (22%) | Knee (17%) | Vertebral column[e] (14%) | Upper back (11%) | Knee (11%) |
| Shoulder (10%) | Elbow (10%) | Wrist (12%) | Chest (7%) | Knee (10%) | Elbow (10%) | Hand (16%) | Hand (12%) | Hand (7%) | Neck (8%) |
| Toe (9%) | Back[c] (7%) | Elbow (6%) | Shoulder (6%) | Hand (6%) | Hand (10%) | Vertebral column[e] (10%) | Elbow (10%) | Knee (7%) | Heat exhaustion[f] (8%) |
| Foot (7%) | Thigh (5%) | Thigh (4%) | Elbow (6%) | Foot (6%) | Foot (4%) | Hip (2%) | Foot (2%) | Neck (4%) | Upper back (5%) |
| Face (6%) | Hand (5%) | Hand (2%) | Upper back (4%) | | Hip (2%) | Foot (1%) | Hip (2%) | Wrist (4%) | Head (3%) |
| Head (5%) | Neck (3%) | Head (2%) | Hand (4%) | | | | | Ankle (4%) | Chest (3%) |

*Note.* As many as eight anatomical sites are presented in descending order of prevalence for each study. The percentage contribution of each site to the total is listed in parentheses. Care should be used when evaluating percentages, since experimental designs and injury definitions, and individual, environmental, and exercise characteristics varied.

[a]Percentages presented are an average of hospital-reported injuries for 3 years over the most recent decade.

[b]This classification system was based on the 9th revision of the International Classification of Diseases. Separate categories were not used for anterior or posterior divisions, making it impossible to differentiate between lower back and abdominal injuries or upper back and chest injuries.

[c]The authors did not partition injuries into upper and lower back categories.

[d]Includes bony injuries to the scapula and clavicle and sprains of associated ligaments.

[e]Likely denotes all bony, ligamentous, muscular, and tendinous injuries associated with vertebrae, including the cervical vertebrae through the coccyx. Similar to combining neck, upper back, and lower back categories.

[f]Heat exhaustion is a complex problem caused by water or salt depletion and may involve abnormally functioning nervous, endocrine, cardiovascular, renal, and/or digestive systems.

**Table 19.5   Overview of Selected Case Reports/Series of Injuries in Recreational Weight Trainers and Competitive Resistance-Trained Athletes**

| Author (year) (ref. #) | Subject category (number of cases) | Subject gender (age) | Training experience | Primary site of injury | Injury diagnosis | Exercise implicated |
|---|---|---|---|---|---|---|
| Kotani et al. (1971) (32) | Olympic lifter (26) | Males (18-24 yr) | Unknown, but national caliber lifters | Lower back | Spondylolysis, lumbar spine deformity, spina bifida occulta | Snatch & clean & jerk, but genetic predisposition important |
| Kulund et al. (1978) (34) | Olympic lifter, adolescent? (1) | Male (unknown) | Unknown, but American Jr. National Champion | Chest | Rib fracture, with serratus anterior m. tear | Clean & jerk maximum attempt during contest |
| Kulund et al. (1978) (34) | Olympic lifter, adolescent? (1) | Male (unknown) | Unknown | Elbow | Elbow dislocation | Snatch, heavy resistance |
| Dangles & Bilos (1980) (13) | Power lifter, adult (1) | Male (39 yr) | ≥ 20 years, 110-kg class World Champion | Elbow & hand | Ulnar nerve neuritis | Dead lift, bench press & squat, heavy resistance, but genetic predisposition & elbow trauma important |
| Brady, Cahill, & Bodnar (1982) (7) | High school athletes, adolescents (29) | Males & females (15.8 yr, range: 13-19 yr) | Unknown | Lower back | Lumbosacral syndrome, ligamentous & disc injuries, spondylolisthesis | Leaper exercise machine, dead lift, circuit weight machine |
| Brady, Cahill, & Bodnar (1982) (7) | High school athletes, adolescents (6) | Males, females? (13-19 yr?) | Unknown | Hip | Avulsion of anterior superior iliac spine | Leaper exercise machine, dead lift, back hyperextension |
| Brady, Cahill, & Bodnar (1982) (7) | High school athletes, adolescents (4) | Males, females? (13-19 yr?) | Unknown | Knee | Meniscal laceration | Leg curl, dead lift |
| Brady, Cahill, & Bodnar (1982) (7) | High school athletes, adolescents (4) | Males, females? (13-19 yr?) | Unknown | Neck | Acute cervical ligament sprain | Leaper exercise machine |
| Cahill (1982) (9) | Power lifters, football players, body builders, & other athletes, adults (45) | Males (23.3 yr, range: 18-34 yr) | Unknown, but all extensively trained athletes | Shoulder | Distal clavicle osteolysis | Bench press, dip, & push-up |
| Gumbs et al. (1982) (24) | Olympic lifters or recreational weight trainers? adolescents (2) | Males (12 yr, 14 yr) | Unknown | Forearm | Bilateral distal radial & ulnar fractures | Military press 149 lb, clean & jerk 88 lb, both ≥ body weight |
| Bird & McCoy (1983) (6) | Recreational weight trainer, adult (1) | Female (30 yr) | Unknown, but licensed physical therapist | Forearm | Unilateral volar (forearm) compartment syndrome | Arm & forearm exercises & genetic predisposition |
| Mannis (1983) (39) | Football player, adolescent (1) | Male (17 yr) | Unknown, but likely ≥ 4 yr | Ankle | Transchondral fracture dome of talus | Squat 300 lb, eccentric phase, high repetitions |
| Shea (1986) (60) | Recreational weight trainer (1) | Female (26 yr) | Unknown, but health club instructor | Spinal cord | Quadriplegia C4-C6 spinal cord fusiform swelling | Lat pull? but perhaps induced by wrestling or oral contraceptives |
| Holder & Michael (1988) (27) | Football player, adult (1) | Male (23 yr) | Unknown, but ≥ 5 yr | Spinal column | Osteoid osteoma, benign spongy bone tumor | Likely unrelated to specific exercise, genetic predisposition important |

| Study | Population | Sex (Age) | Experience | Body region | Injury | Exercise/Cause |
|---|---|---|---|---|---|---|
| Mochizuki & Richter (1988) (44) | Body builder, adult (1) | Male (32 yr) | ≥ 16 years | Brain, heart, & vessels | Cerebrovascular accidents (2) & cardiomyopathy | Likely unrelated to specific exercises, but induced by ~16 yr self-administration of ~15 steroids |
| Segan et al. (1988) (57) | Recreational weight trainer or competitive weight lifter? (1) | Male (30 yr) | Unknown | Arm & forearm | Bilateral upper extremity compartment syndrome | Arm & forearm exercises high repetitions heavy resistance, overtraining, & genetic predisposition |
| Kretzler & Richardson (1989) (33) | Recreational weight trainers? & others (11) | Males? (32.5 yr, range: 20-59 yr?) | Unknown | Chest | Complete rupture of pectoralis major m. | Bench press & chest fly |
| Francobandiera et al. (1990) (18) | Body builder (1) | Female (23 yr) | Unknown | Wrist | Distal radio-ulnar joint dislocation | Barbell lifted with single-hand supinated grip; unusual accident induced by accidental push from partner |
| Jordan et al. (1990) (29) | Power lifter, adult (1) | Male (44 yr) | Unknown, but likely ≥ 20 years | Neck | Acute radiculopathy, cervical neural foramina impingement @ C4-5 and C5-6 | Unknown, but likely bench press, squat, &/or dead lift |
| Jordan et al. (1990) (29) | Recreational weight trainer? adult (1) | Male (37 yr) | Unknown | Neck | Acute radiculopathy, herniated nucleus pulposus @ C6-7 w/ spinal cord compression | Dead lift, 310-lb lift |
| Jordan et al. (1990) (29) | Recreational weight trainer, adult (1) | Male (36 yr) | Unknown | Neck | Acute radiculopathy, small herniated nucleus pulposus @ C5-6 | Upright row, 80-lb lift |
| Rossi & Dragoni (1990) (54) | Olympic lifters (22) | Male (20.6 yr; range: 15-27 yr?) | Unknown, but Olympic athletes | Lower back | Spondylolysis | Repetitive, forced hyperextension exercises, clean & jerk & snatch |
| Casamassima et al. (1991) (11) | Recreational weight trainer, adolescent (1) | Male (16 yr) | Unknown | Chest internal injury | Pneumopericardium: air in pericardial cavity | Bench press ~120 lb with powerful Valsalva's maneuver; but genetic predis. important |
| Reut et al. (1991) (50) | Body builder, adult (1) | Male (31 yr) | Unknown | Chest | Complete pectoralis major rupture | Bench press, 275-lb lift, eccentric phase |
| Gross et al. (1993) (23) | Recreational weight trainers & athletes, adolescents & adults (20; 16 males & 4 females) | Males & females (28 yr, range: 15-43 yr) | Unknown | Shoulder | Anterior shoulder instability | Bench press (wide grip), chest fly, pull over, lat pull, behind-the-neck press |

*Note.* In a few instances, data was extracted from prospective and retrospective studies to highlight the occurrence of a unique injury. For each case, by carefully reviewing the author's text, an attempt was made to isolate the exercise or exercises implicated. Although these data may indicate that specific injuries are associated with resistance training, it is impossible to make definitive conclusions without more information about genetic and environmental predispositions for injury.

injuries does not imply the absence of chronic problems. In section *3.1.2 Injury Onset, Olympic Lifting*, it was noted that Olympic lifters have a prevalence of spondylolysis higher than the normal population. It would be interesting to evaluate long-term, back injuries in the athletes studied by Kulund.

Compared to younger Olympic lifters (34), those more experienced (31) have over a three-fold higher percentage of injuries to the back (Table 19.4). Over 90% of Olympic lifters experience low-back pain sometimes or always (32). These data imply the progressive onset of chronic back problems. Further research will help distinguish chronic injuries induced solely by Olympic lifting from those precipitated by genetic predisposition, inadequate conditioning, poor technique, training in spite of joint pain, or failure to seek proper medical advice.

### 3.3.3 Power Lifting

Half of the injuries in adolescent power lifters (8) are to the lower back (Table 19.4). More experienced, male, power lifters also have a high percentage of vertebral column injuries (one third of the total), but nearly one third of their injuries are to the shoulder, with degenerative changes being most prominent (21).

It is interesting that adult female power lifters of similar age as males, but with 1 1/2 years less training experience, demonstrate a markedly different pattern of injuries according to anatomical site (21). While the knee accounts for only one tenth of the injuries in males, it is the most prominent site in females, contributing nearly one third to the total. The vertebral column is the second most prevalent site injured in female power lifters, accounting for nearly one quarter of all injuries. While other individual, environmental, and exercise characteristics certainly may be instrumental (e.g., differences in absolute exercise intensity), the unique distinctions between male and female bony pelves, femurs, and articular surfaces of long bones may contribute to these differences. For example, the more extreme hip and thigh joint angles, and smaller articular ends of long bones in females, may predispose them to knee problems during heavy squats of power lifting. The generally lighter and less dense upper extremity bones of females may make them less susceptible than males to shoulder joint arthritis.

### 3.3.4 Body Building

Female body builders have a high percentage of knee injuries, nearly double that of male body builders (21). This trend, also found in female power lifters, supports the contention that anatomical differences may predispose females to knee injuries, particularly when they train with heavy weights. About one third of the injuries in both male and female body builders are in the shoulder region, yet males have more than double the relative percentage of elbow injuries. Although more heavy and dense bones may predispose male body builders to shoulder and elbow injuries, their performance of heavy bench presses, despite chronic shoulder and elbow joint pain, probably plays a more important role.

### 3.3.5 Football

Nearly 50% of the injuries in strength-trained junior high and high school football players (53) are to the lower back (Table 19.4). Over 75% of injuries to freshman and junior varsity athletes involve the back (53). During these years, high-speed, ballistic (power clean, clean and jerk, and snatch) and more static, maximum lifts (dead lift and squat) are introduced. Despite enhanced supervision and coaching at the high school level, the inclusion of ballistic and static maximum lifts increases the likelihood of lower back injuries.

Knee meniscus tears have been associated with the leg curl and dead lift exercises in strength-trained, high school athletes including football players (7). These exercises and others, when performed with extreme, forced knee flexion, make subjects susceptible to injury. Back hyperextensions, dead lifts, and the *Leaper* machine (designed to improve jumping ability through violent extension contractions), have been associated with avulsions of the sartorius tendon from the anterior superior iliac spine (7). Poor exercise technique with excessive resistance and ballistic extensions through extreme ranges of motion make young athletes vulnerable to this painful, debilitating injury.

In college football players (77), the lower back is also the most injury-prone region, accounting for over 40% of all injuries (Table 19.4). Defensive and offensive lineman account for nearly one half of all injuries. These two groups of players, more so than others, are subjected repeatedly to sudden, violent extension contractions combined with twisting movements that are most often associated with low-back injuries (10).

Compared to high school football players, college players tend to include more Olympic lifts in their training. Although there is substantial variability, college regimens are usually a broad mix of both Olympic and power lifts, while high school programs include mainly power lifts. Note from Table 19.4, that college football players (77) have a high percentage of lower back injuries similar to adolescent power lifters (8) and high school football players (52, 53), but also relatively high percentages of shoulder and knee injuries, roughly half those of Olympic lifters (31, 34).

# 4. Injury Severity

## 4.1 Time Loss

### 4.1.1 Weight Training

Over 95% of the hospital-reported weight training injuries during 1982, 1991, and 1992 involved patients who were treated and released (65, 66, 67). About 3% involved treatment with referrals, 1% hospitalizations, and 0.009% deaths. A peak of one dozen, weight training-associated deaths occurred between March of 1991 and April of 1992 as confirmed by a review of US CPSC Death Certificate, Accident Investigation, and Reported Incident Files (63, 64, 72). These fatalities are reviewed in section 4.2 on *Catastrophic Injury*.

Along with treatment and referral categories, injuries evaluated at NEISS hospital emergency rooms are assigned a number between 1 and 8, with higher numbers indicating increased severity (69, 75). Over 80% of the hospital-reported injuries during 1981, 1991, and 1992 were less than class four, implying that most weight training injuries were mild to moderate.

### 4.1.2 Olympic Lifting

Junior Olympic lifters reported that nearly 30% of their injuries result in "no impairment" (34), which implies that they ignored their injuries or at least viewed them as being insignificant. Olympic lifters often train and compete with painful, hand calluses, and torn blisters, yet these are rarely reported since they are considered a part of training. Of the more significant injuries noted by young Olympic lifters, just over 30% lasted 2 weeks to 2 months, while less than 10% extended 2 months to 2 years. Athletes reported only about 5% of their injuries as being chronic/recurrent or lasting more than 2 years (34).

Nearly 75% of wrist, shoulder, elbow, or knee injuries caused experienced Olympic lifters to miss 0-7 days participation (31). Only 10% of knee injuries caused lifters to miss more than 8 days, while less than 5% resulted in an inability to work with

an average time loss of 0.7 days. In contrast, about 50% of back injuries caused athletes to miss 0-7 days, while over 45% resulted in more than 8 days of missed activity. Seven percent of back injuries caused experienced lifters to miss work for an average of 1.2 days. These results imply that in Olympic lifters, back injuries are more debilitating than injuries to other sites.

### 4.1.3 Power Lifting

Seventy-one adolescent power lifters missed a total of 1,126 training days due to 98 injuries (8). This equates to an average of 11.5 days missed per injury. The lower back accounted for just over 40%, while muscle pulls accounted for over 50% of total time lost (8).

### 4.1.4 Body Building

Time loss data for body builders has not been published.

### 4.1.5 Football

Only significant injuries, those inducing a disability of $\geq 8$ days, were tabulated in a study of strength-trained adolescent football players (52, 53). Almost 90% of the injuries in these young athletes were considered moderate (8-21 days disability) and just over 10% major (> 21 days impairment). About 40% of the injuries were treated by a physician, but none were classified as severe or permanently disabling.

Only 38 time-loss, weight room injuries were recorded over four seasons in 10,908 college football players (77). These resistance-training injuries represented less than 1% of the total in-season injuries related to football. Only 2 of these injuries (5% of the total) were season ending. Of the remaining 36 injuries, the time loss ranged from 1 to 42 days with an average of 7.4 days.

## 4.2 Catastrophic Injury

### 4.2.1 Weight Training

There were one dozen deaths associated with weight training equipment within 378 days between March of 1991 and April of 1992 (62, 64, 72) (Table 19.6). This equates to approximately one death every 32 days during this period. Eleven of 12 cases involved males at home dying of asphyxia and anoxia due to neck or chest compression by a barbell (62, 64, 72). A 4-year-old child died when his chest was pinned between a barbell and a bench press (64). Along with this case, a recent disturbing

**Table 19.6  Deaths Associated With Resistance Exercise Equipment From March, 1991, Through April, 1992**

| Date | City, state | Age | Gender | Body part | Diagnosis | Location | Product/exercise implicated |
|------|-------------|-----|--------|-----------|-----------|----------|-----------------------------|
| 03-19-91 | Conroe, TX | 25 | Male | Neck | Asphyxia | Home | Bench press |
| 05-27-91 | Burke, VA | 14 | Male | Neck | Asphyxia | Home | CWT machine cable |
| 06-23-91 | Middletown, NJ | 28 | Male | Neck | Asphyxia | Home | Bench press |
| 06-27-91 | Palmer, AK | 4 | Male | Chest | Asphyxia | Home | Bench press |
| 06-28-91 | College, PA | 17 | Male | Neck/chest | Asphyxia | Other | Bench press |
| 07-15-91 | Oyster Bay, NY | 27 | Male | Neck | Asphyxia | Home | Bench press |
| 08-14-91 | Saginaw, MI | 23 | Male | Neck | Asphyxia | Home | Bench press |
| 11-05-91 | Hazle, PA | 38 | Male | Neck | Asphyxia | Home | Bench press |
| 11-11-91 | Lattimer Mines, PA | 38 | Male | Neck | Asphyxia | Home | Bench press |
| 01-20-92 | Rochester, NY | 40 | Male | Neck | Asphyxia | Home | Bench press |
| 02-25-92 | Orlando, FL | 28 | Male | Neck | Asphyxia | Home | Bench press |
| 04-01-92 | Buffalo, NY | 37 | Male | Neck | Asphyxia | Home | Bench press |

*Note.* Data was compiled from US CPSC Death Report and Injury and Potential Injury Incident (IPII) files (63, 64, 67). All of these needless fatalities may have been prevented if spotters had been present, partners had been training nearby, or parents had secured equipment and supervised their children. The bench press is implicated as the most high-risk resistance exercise, particularly when performed without a spotter in the home. Widespread adult and adolescent education, as well as mandatory product warning information are the keys to preventing resistance training deaths.

incident of a boy dying after falling from a bunk bed and hitting his head on nearby weights (72) emphasizes that parents must recognize that all weights and exercise equipment are potentially fatal and must be secured to ensure inaccessibility to unsupervised children. There is no question that the performance of the bench press in the home without a spotter is a high-risk, potentially deadly activity.

One death of a 14-year-old male in May of 1991 was extremely unusual in that it apparently involved an accidental hanging (64) (Table 19.6). Since it was not clear what exercise may have been associated with the death, an additional accident investigation report was obtained and reviewed (63). This synopsis indicated that the male became entrapped in a weight machine in the basement of his home and died from a metal cord tightening around his neck. It was confirmed later in a US CPSC Reported Incident file and a newspaper article that the boy was performing a neck exercise improperly (72). This single death associated with a circuit weight machine may have been prevented with proper instruction.

The following case report of an accident investigation of possible equipment malfunction was provided by the US CPSC (62). A 15-year-old male was completing a repetition using an 80-pound barbell on an inclined bench press. During this repetition, the base of the bench collapsed beneath him causing the barbell to fall onto his chest. Fortunately, his father grasped and secured the weight immediately and the boy escaped with a minor

chest bruise. This single case indicates that the presence of a spotter can make the difference between minor and severe injury or even life and death.

Additional catastrophic injuries, ones that induce permanent changes in lifestyle, have been associated with weight training. Six severe injuries that required hospitalization were found in the 1991 and 1992 US CPSC data files (62, 63, 72) (Table 19.7). At least half of these involved female participants, five of six included severe finger injuries, and four of six involved amputations.

Shea (1986) described a tragic case of quadriplegia that occurred in an apparently fit, 26-year-old, female, health club instructor who had just completed a normal, light workout (Table 19.5). It is tempting to speculate that direct cervical spine trauma during lat pulls (the last exercise of the workout) provoked spinal cord swelling and permanent paralysis. However, the young instructor did not report poor technique (60), which usually involves hitting the neck with the bar in the C7 to C8 region, substantially lower than where the (C4 through C6) spinal cord swelling occurred. The subject's use of oral contraceptives, previous day wrestling, and most importantly, genetic susceptibility to spinal cord infarct may have precipitated this tragic event.

Thus, most deaths involved males performing heavy, free-weight bench presses in the home. Catastrophic, nonfatal injuries included females using circuit weight devices, especially combination leg extension/leg curl machines with cables or chains.

**Table 19.7   Representative Catastrophic Injuries Other Than Deaths Associated With Resistance Exercise Equipment During 1991 and 1992**

| Date | City, state | Age | Gender | Body part | Diagnosis | Location | Product/exercise implicated |
|---|---|---|---|---|---|---|---|
| 06-27-91 | Austin, TX | 4 | Female | Head | Concussion | Home | Bench press |
| 01-12-92 | Phoenix, AZ | 13 | Male | Finger | Amputation | UNK | CWT machine cable |
| 01-22-92 | Manheim, PA | 23 | Male | Finger | Amputation | UNK | Comb. bench/leg extension |
| 03-16-92 | Tyrone, GA | 36 | Female | Finger | Amputation | Home | Comb. bench/leg curl |
| 07-00-92 | Prairie Village, KS | UNK | Female | Finger | Amputation | UNK | UNK |
| 12-28-92 | Lyons, NY | UNK | UNK | Finger | Laceration Crushing | UNK | Comb. bench/leg extension |

*Note.* Cases were documented in US CPSC, IPII, Reported Incident or Accident Investigation files (62, 63, 72). Some were verified by newspaper accounts. UNK or 00 indicates that the variable was unknown or impossible to determine conclusively from US CPSC reports or newspaper articles.

### 4.2.2 Olympic Lifting

There have been no reports of fatalities or catastrophic head injuries associated with Olympic lifting. There have been isolated reports of severe injuries that may have induced permanent lifestyle changes. One world-class athlete had part of his finger amputated when it was pinned between the bar and the rack after a squat exercise (31). Perhaps, inappropriate spotting and a poorly designed squat rack played a role in this injury, but it is more likely that the lifter was exhausted after completing a heavy set and simply misjudged the position of the bar supports. Previously cited chronic shoulder arthritis and back problems (31) and the high incidence of spondylolysis (32, 54) in Olympic lifters could also be viewed as lifelong injuries.

### 4.2.3 Power Lifting

No reports of fatalities or catastrophic injuries have been associated with power lifting without the implication of steroid use. Half of the injuries in adolescent power lifters involved the lower back (8), which could induce chronic, disabling problems (8). Goertzen and associates (21) found a high percentage of vertebral column injuries, shoulder arthritis, and knee cartilage pathologies in experienced male and female power lifters. Male and female power lifters also reported several cases of carpal tunnel syndrome. Potentially, these injuries could be hindering for a lifetime.

### 4.2.4 Body Building

No reports of fatalities or permanent disabilities have been associated with body building without the implication of steroid use. For example, dual cerebrovascular accidents and cardiac myopathy were diagnosed in a 32-year-old, male body builder (44). Although heavy lifting with Valsalva's maneuver may have been involved, the thromboembolic nature of the cerebral events and the subject's reduction in myocardial ejection fraction implicate his use of at least 15 different steroids over the past 16 years as the primary cause.

A high percentage of injuries in male and female body builders involve shoulder arthritis, knee cartilage degeneration, and tendinitis, which may induce permanent disability (21).

### 4.2.5 Football

Two epiphyseal fractures were reported in 354 strength-trained, adolescent football players (53). One disc rupture, one leg fracture, one concussion, and three cases of heat exhaustion were documented in 10,908 strength-trained, college football players (77). Although these acute injuries involved only a few athletes, they certainly could develop into lifelong problems.

## 5. Injury Risk Factors

There are a multitude of individual, exercise, and environmental factors that increase the likelihood of injury during resistance training. Age, genetic predisposition for injury, medical history, nutritional status and use of ergogenic aids, previous training, current physical and psychological condition, use of general and specific warm-up, exercise characteristics (mode, intensity, duration, frequency, and distribution of training sessions), training equipment, supervision, and spotting are some of the variables that must be considered. While it is certainly impossible to isolate each of these, previous research has focused on implicating exercise factors, without really considering individual and environmental variables. Until this is done, it will be virtually impossible to compare the effects of different resistance training modes (or other sports or activities) on the frequency and characteristics of acute and long-term injuries.

Despite the relative lack of control of confounding variables in resistance training and most sports injury research, some risk factors have been implicated repeatedly. US CPSC data proves that using heavy weights without a spotter in the home can be deadly (63, 64, 72). It also indicates that using a machine without adequate instruction or awareness of potential hazards can be fatal or induce severe injury (62, 63, 64). When equipment is not secured, young unsupervised children and adolescents are particularly vulnerable. Poor technique and faulty equipment have been implicated in some injuries (31), yet despite outstanding technique and superbly designed devices, injuries do occur in experienced, world-class, competitive Olympic lifters (31), power lifters, and body builders (21). This implies that repetitive, heavy resistance movements induce injuries, which may be chronic when body signals like joint pain and follow-up medical evaluations are ignored.

Some exercises and equipment appear to be associated with a high risk of injury. The free weight bench press is the most deadly piece of equipment, particularly when used by a novice in the home without a spotter. Leg curl/leg extension machines have been implicated in nonfatal, but severe injuries such as amputations. The bench press, squat, and dead lift have been associated with acute and chronic shoulder, knee, and lower back problems. Despite the doubling of supervision in adolescents, a greater performance of power cleans and clean and jerks is associated with a four-fold increase in back injuries (53). Other exercises or specific techniques have been associated with injuries.

Gross and associates (1993) found instability in 23 shoulders of 20 recreational weight trainers and athletes (23) (Table 19.5). All subjects indicated that resistance training was their sole or primary recreational activity and experienced posterior shoulder pain in the "at-risk" position, when the shoulder was forcibly abducted and externally rotated. Exercises that caused the most pain included the wide-grip bench press, supine or inclined chest fly, bent-arm pull over, lat pull, and behind-the-neck press. Using appropriately selected conservative or surgical treatments, together with extensive rehabilitation and exercise technique modification, the authors were highly successful in treating their patients. Many who train with weights have well-developed, large, upper extremity muscles, but frequently demonstrate asynchronous, weak rotator cuff and scapular stabilizers (23). The key to successful return to activity following conservative treatment or surgery was rehabilitation of deep shoulder muscles and modification of each subject's technique to avoid the "at-risk" position. The authors should be commended for their thoughtful presentation of such practical research.

Despite Kulund and associates' (34) claim that inflexibility and improper technique cause most lifting injuries, even highly trained American and World Champions, considered to have extensive muscular development and superbly refined exercise technique, have been injured seriously. Injuries are likely induced by multiple factors, including the use of repetitive, high-resistance, ballistic, extension contractions through extreme ranges of motion; genetic propensity for injury; and training history and previous injuries.

High-level, competitive athletes may tax the outer limits of muscle, bone, and joint integrity during their frequent, intensive training sessions and competitions. Despite the appearance of superficial muscular development, weak links may be present in deep rotational and stabilizing muscles of the spine and shoulder (23). When competitive lifters exceed their muscular limits, other tissues are stressed. The structural injury hierarchy seems to proceed initially from overtaxed, superficial muscles to deeper intrinsic muscles, tendons, and ligaments. Note in Table 19.3, that compared to college football players (77) and experienced Olympic lifters (31), adolescent power lifters (8) and young football players (53) have a higher percentage of muscle injuries. These younger athletes have not reached their full muscular potential and thus incur more muscular injuries. In contrast, a phasic shift of injuries from muscles to tendons to ligaments seems to have occurred in the older college football players and Olympic lifters.

When competitive principles emphasizing maximum lifting are applied inappropriately to children and the general population, injury frequency and severity are amplified. This is especially true when novices use improper technique and train maximally without supervision.

Research seems to indicate that lack of proper instruction and supervision (environmental variables), poor exercise technique (an exercise variable), and premature use of excessive resistance (exercise and individual variables) play major roles in precipitating injuries. Although much research is needed to isolate more fully these and other variables, exercise intensity appears to be the most important risk factor.

Since this chapter deals with injuries, its inherent tone is negative. We must keep in mind that despite acute and chronic injuries associated with unsupervised, heavy, resistance training, we have much to gain by training with weights. Recently, the American College of Sports Medicine recommended that moderate resistance training be included as an integral component of an optimal fitness program (3). No other form of exercise has the potential for enhancing as many components of health-related fitness (muscular strength/ endurance, flexibility, neuromuscular relaxation, cardiorespiratory endurance, % body fat) (37). Properly applied weight training can improve cardiovascular fitness (25), strengthen muscles and bones (30, 43, 46), reduce arthritis (41) and depression (48), and counteract muscle weakness and physical frailty (46), even in those over 90 years of age (15, 16).

## 6. Suggestions for Injury Prevention

It is clear with the increasing popularity of weight training that comprehensive efforts must be directed toward injury prevention. Models to enhance safety and to minimize injuries and deaths associated with resistance training are illustrated as hierarchical pyramids, including preliminary guidelines for participation (Figure 19.1) and exercise training guidelines (Figure 19.2).

Medical clearance by a sports medicine physician is the key starting point for injury reduction (Figure 19.1). Subjects are classified as not cleared, fully cleared, or conditionally cleared for weight training based on genetic predisposition and previous injuries. Those with severe hypertension may not be cleared until their blood pressure is normalized. Conditionally-cleared individuals may include children who should always be supervised and avoid maximum lifting, or those predisposed to spondylolysis for whom certain exercises can be modified. After medical clearance, adequate sleep and diet help to ensure energy nutrient availability and foster concentration during workouts. Appropriate dress, including hard-toe shoes with non-slick soles and light cotton absorptive clothing, can minimize lower extremity injuries and decrease the likelihood of heat illness.

Next to medical screening, the most important preliminary guideline is instruction by a qualified, sports medicine professional (Figure 19.1). Instructors, coaches, and trainers should seek certification by the American College of Sports Medicine (ACSM), the National Strength and Conditioning Association (NSCA), and the National Athletic

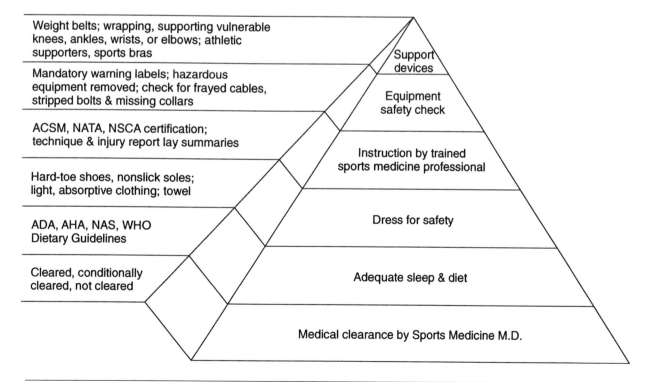

**Figure 19.1** Safety pyramid of preliminary guidelines for participation in resistance training. The foundation for minimizing injuries is a medical evaluation of each candidate by a physician trained in sports medicine.

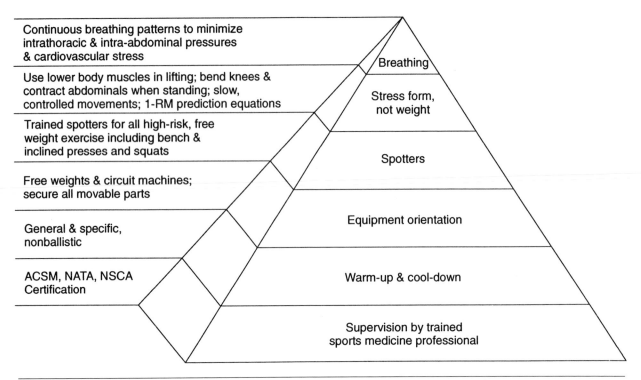

**Figure 19.2** Safety pyramid of training guidelines for resistance training. The key to reducing training injuries is supervision by trained sports medicine professionals, certified by organizations like the American College of Sports Medicine, the National Athletic Training Association, and the National Strength and Conditioning Association.

Training Association (NATA). Teaching the importance of technique and spotting for exercises like the bench press can make the difference between life and death. All participants should be encouraged to report even minor injuries and to seek treatment from qualified sports medical personnel to minimize the development of chronic problems. When direct, one-on-one instruction is not possible, lay summaries and peer-reviewed texts (2, 3, 4, 17, 37) should be made easily accessible.

To minimize heat injuries, the sports medicine staff should ensure that weight room ventilation is optimal, water is readily available, and resistance training intensity and distribution are adjusted based on sports practices in hot and humid conditions.

Equipment must be designed with safety in mind. Parents must be warned about the potential deadly nature of weight training and all exercise equipment. Product warning labels on bench presses, cable leg extension/leg curl and neck machines should be required to minimize deaths and amputations associated with these home training devices.

Once adequate instruction and equipment checks have taken place, support devices such as

belts and knee wraps may be helpful, particularly for those with vulnerable joints (14, 26, 35).

The most important training guideline, supervision by trained sports medicine professionals, is a key extension of instruction (Figure 19.2). Subjects who warm up and cool down provide for a rehearsal of the activity that is about to take place, minimize the chances of muscle pulls and delayed muscle soreness, and enhance the likelihood of lifelong participation (37). Although genetic predisposition and injury history must be considered, knee and thigh injuries may be reduced by thorough, light, specific warm-up and adductor stretches before moderate to heavy lifting. Chest, shoulder, and elbow injuries may be triggered by lack of specific warm-up on bench and inclined bench presses and the premature use of excessive resistance. Pectoral tears and chronic shoulder injuries may be prevented if athletes learn to avoid the "at-risk position" and seek medical attention at an early stage during the onset of an injury (23, 74).

Even though participants may have had adequate basic instruction, they must be familiarized with techniques prior to using new equipment. The use of a spotter for free weight bench presses and all other high-risk exercises cannot be over-emphasized (Figure 19.2).

It is important that instructors and coaches strongly consider the goals of each individual when prescribing resistance training programs. Certainly, for competitive Olympic and power lifters, a primary goal is to lift as much weight as possible. But for other athletes or even more so for the general population, encouraging maximum attempts can lead to a high injury rate, particularly when exercise technique is ignored. There is no question that improvements in strength for performance in sports and for overall fitness can be achieved without near-maximum or maximum lifting. Children, beginners, deconditioned lifters, and those who are pregnant or elderly should be encouraged to stress the form, not the weight (Figure 19.2). Slow, smooth, and methodical movements should be used to decrease joint shear and compression forces (37).

Some researchers advise that youngsters avoid maximum lifting until they have achieved Tanner Stage 5 developmental maturity, since they will have passed their maximal skeletal growth rate when epiphyses appear to be vulnerable to injury (2, 5, 61). Although there is much variation, this Stage is reached at approximately 15 years of age for both boys and girls. While it may be overly cautious to have youngsters and adolescents avoid overhead lifts, there is certainly a need for enhanced instruction and a de-emphasis on maximum attempts. One-repetition maximum prediction equations may provide an alternative motivational tool (37).

Data from Risser and colleagues (53) indicate that more supervision does not necessarily imply fewer injuries, but may depend also upon exercise selection. For example, even though they may be supervised, young athletes may incur a substantial number of low-back injuries, particularly when power cleans and clean and jerks are introduced prematurely (53). Preventative, prehabilitation exercises may be the key to minimizing injuries (74).

Athletes who participate in gymnastics, weight lifting, and football have the greatest risk of low-back injury (1). Most back injuries occur when an underdeveloped, unprepared, or overloaded spine is subjected to a sudden violent extension, especially when rotation is involved (10). Jesse suggests that athletes be required to complete a full year of forward and lateral flexion and rotation exercises before they are allowed to perform overhead extension movements or lifts greater than 40% of their body weight (28, 37). Multiplanar movements

that emphasize rotation, along with the body acting as its own stabilizer, may be quite helpful in preventing and rehabilitating back injuries (28, 37, 56).

Continuous breathing patterns should be emphasized to decrease intracavity pressures and minimize stresses on the cardiovascular system (37).

Each Safety Pyramid step should be tested rigorously to determine its independent effectiveness in reducing weight training injuries. Some suggestions for testing are provided in the next section.

# 7. Suggestions for Further Research

To make progress in research dealing with sports injuries, an important first task is to develop a standardized, universally applicable definition of *injury* and a practical and easy method for describing injury rates. These could be formulated and recommended by a panel of experts from an international sports epidemiology group. Additionally, since it occasionally uses confusing, nonspecific, anatomical terminology (e.g., lower trunk), and merges unique, diagnostic categories (e.g., strain/sprain), the commonly relied upon 9th revision of the International Classification of Diseases (75), although recently updated (76), should be carefully reevaluated and revised. It is crucial that a novel, standardized, universally accepted method for classifying injuries by specific anatomical location and diagnosis be developed. These fundamental steps will help immeasurably to ensure that comparisons across studies are meaningful and simplified.

Future research in resistance training should categorize subjects appropriately as recreational weight trainers, Olympic lifters, power lifters, body builders, or athletes who use weights to improve sports performance. Additionally, the training modes, intensities, durations, frequencies, and session distributions should be noted, and subject genetic predispositions for injury should be explored. These steps will help to establish injury rates specific to different subgroups of resistance trainers and determine the influence of key individual, exercise, and environmental variables.

The basic purpose of sports epidemiology research should continue to be questioned. Is the major goal of sports epidemiologists simply to describe injury rates in elite groups of athletes, or should more efforts be directed toward beginners and the general population? Is it important for epidemiologists to provide injury and safety guidelines for assisting parents and their children in choosing sports and fitness activities for a lifetime? Perhaps, our prior and current research directions should be reevaluated carefully, so that the results of future studies are more meaningful and applicable to the general public.

We should continue to ask some major questions. "What does this injury rate mean in practical terms?" "Where are most injuries taking place?" "How are they happening?" "Why is it important?" To help reduce the frequency and severity of injuries, sports injury specialists should suggest novel safety, evaluative, and rehabilitative programs rather than simply describe injury characteristics. After a universal system for injury description is formulated and implemented, there should be a strong effort to move beyond descriptive studies to the implementation of programs that can document injury reduction.

As noted in the introduction, it could be that exercise mode has relatively little to do with the frequency and severity of injuries reported by sports epidemiologists. Are exercise intensity, duration, and frequency more important? As has been proposed regarding the risk of cardiovascular disease, are injuries dependent more upon the total work performed rather than upon the type of work? Unless individual, exercise, and environmental variables are fully isolated, sports injury specialists will be limited to descriptive studies of highly specialized subjects that provide results that are difficult to interpret and generalize. By taking a more active role in designing stringently controlled research studies, and by using the results to implement well-designed preventative programs, sports epidemiologists can help to ensure that for all participants, resistance training is a safe, effective, and rewarding, lifelong experience.

## Acknowledgment

Special thanks to Patrick D. Shannon of the US Consumer Product Safety Commission (National Injury Information Clearinghouse, Washington, DC) for his help with technical information; Marc Kaltenhauser of the University of Oregon (Department of Exercise & Movement Science, Eugene, OR) for translating articles from German to English; and Dr. J. David Symons of Alliance Pharmaceutical Corporation (San Diego, CA) for his review of manuscripts.

## References

1. Alexander, M.J.L. Biomechanical aspects of lumbar spine injuries in athletes: a review. Can. J. Appl. Sci. 10(1):1-20; 1985.
2. American Academy of Pediatrics, Committee on Sports Medicine. Strength training, weight and power lifting, and body building by children and adolescents. Pediatrics. 86(5):801-803; 1990.
3. American College of Sports Medicine (ACSM). Position stand: the recommended quantity and quality of exercise for developing and maintaining cardio-respiratory and muscular fitness in healthy adults. Med. Sci. Sports Exerc. 22(2):265-274; 1990.
4. Baechle, T.R.; Groves, B.R. Weight training instruction: Steps to success. Champaign, IL: Human Kinetics Publishers; 1994.
5. Bailey, D.A.; Wedge, J.H.; McCulloch, R.G.; Martin, A.D.; Bernhardson, S.C. Epidemiology of fractures of the distal end of the radius in children as associated with growth. J. Bone Joint Surg. Am. 71(8):1225-1231; 1989.
6. Bird, C.B.; McCoy, J.W. Weight-lifting as a cause of compartment syndrome in the forearm. J. Bone Joint Surg. Am. 65:406; 1983.
7. Brady, T.A.; Cahill, B.R.; Bodnar, L.M. Weight training-related injuries in the high school athlete. Am. J. Sports Med. 10(1):1-5; 1982.
8. Brown, E.W.; Kimball, R.G. Medical history associated with adolescent powerlifting. Pediatrics. 72(5):636-644; 1983.
9. Cahill, B.R. Osteolysis of the distal part of the clavicle in male athletes. J. Bone Joint Surg. Am. 64-A(7):1053-1058; 1982.
10. Cantu, R.C. Lumbar spine injuries. In: Cantu, R.C., ed. The exercising adult. Lexington, MA: Collamore Press; 1980.
11. Casamassima, A.C.; Sternberg, T.; Weiss, F.H. Spontaneous pneumopericardium: a link with weight lifting? Physician Sports Med. 19(6):107-110; 1991.
12. Compton, D.; Hill, P.M.; Sinclair, J.D. Weight-lifters' blackout. Lancet. II(7840):1234-1237; 1973.
13. Dangles, C.J.; Bilos, Z.J. Ulnar nerve neuritis in a world champion weightlifter. Am. J. Sports Med. 8(6):443-445; 1980.
14. Duda, M. Weight-lifting belts may reduce injury risk. Physician Sports Med. 17(8):24-25; 1989.
15. Fiatarone, M.A.; Marks, E.C.; Ryan, N.D.; Meredith, C.N.; Lipsitz, L.A.; Evans, W.J. High-intensity strength training in nonagenarians: effects on skeletal muscle. JAMA. 263(22):3029-3034; 1990.
16. Fiatarone, M.A.; O'Neill, E.F.; Roberts, N.D.; Clements, K.M.; Solares, G.R.; Nelson, M.E.; Roberts, S.B.; Kehayias, J.J.; Lipsitz, L.A.; Evans, W.J. Exercise training and nutritional supplementation for physical frailty in very elderly people. N. Engl. J. Med. 330(25):1769-75; 1994.

17. Fleck, S.J.; Kraemer, W.J. Designing resistance training programs. Champaign, IL: Human Kinetics Publishers; 1987.

18. Francobandiera, C.; Maffulli, N.; LePore, L. Distal radio-ulnar joint dislocation, ulna volar in a female body builder. Med. Sci. Sports Exerc. 22(2):155-158; 1990.

19. Freedson, P.; Chang, B.; Katch, F.; Kroll, W.; Rippe, J.; Alpert, J.; Byrnes, W. Intra-arterial blood pressure during free weight and hydraulic resistive exercise (abstract). Med. Sci. Sports Exerc. 16(2): 131; 1984.

20. Garrick, J.G.; Requa, R. Medical care and injury surveillance in the high school setting. Physician Sports Med. 9:115-120; 1981.

21. Goertzen, V.; Schöppe, K.; Lange, G.; Schulitz, K.-P. Verletzungen und Überlastungsschäden beim Bodybuilding und Powerlifting. [Medical history associated with body building and power lifting.] Sportverletz. Sportschaden. 3:32-36; 1989.

22. Granhed, H.; Morelli, B. Low back pain among retired wrestlers and heavy weight lifters. Am. J. Sports Med. 16(5):530-533; 1988.

23. Gross, M.L.; Brenner, S.L.; Esformes, I.; Sonzogni, J.J. Anterior shoulder instability in weight lifters. Am. J. Sports Med. 21(4):599-603; 1993.

24. Gumbs, V.L.; Segal, D.; Halligan, J.B.; Lower, G. Bilateral distal radius and ulnar fractures in adolescent weight lifters. Am. J. Sports Med. 10(6):375-379; 1982.

25. Haennel, R.; Teo, K.K.; Quinney, A.; Kappagoda, T. Effects of hydraulic circuit training on cardiovascular function. Med. Sci. Sports Exerc. 21(5):605-612; 1989.

26. Harman, E.A.; Rosenstein, R.M.; Frykman, P.N.; Nigro, G.A. Effects of a belt on intra-abdominal pressure during weight lifting. Med. Sci. Sports Exerc. 21(2):186-190; 1989.

27. Holder, L.E.; Michael, R.H. Unexplained shoulder pain in a weight lifter. Physician Sports Med. 16(6):91-97; 1988.

28. Jesse, J.P. Olympic lifting movements endanger adolescents. Physician Sports Med. 5:60-67; 1977.

29. Jordan, B.D.; Istrico, R.; Zimmerman, R.D.; Tsairis, P.; Warren, R.F. Acute cervical radiculopathy in weight lifters. Physician Sports Med. 18(1):73-76; 1990.

30. Karlsson, M.K.; Johnell, O.; Obrant, K.J. Bone mineral density in weight lifters. Calcif. Tissue Int. 52(3):212-215; 1993.

31. König, M.; Biener, K. Sportartspezifische Verletzungen im Gewichtheben. [Sport-specific injuries in weight lifting.] Schweiz-Z. Sportmed. 38(1):25-30; 1990.

32. Kotani, P.T.; Ichikawa, N.; Wakabayashi, W.; Yoshii, T.; Koshimune, B.S.; Koshimune, M. Studies of spondylolysis found among weight lifters. Br. J. Sports Med. 6:4-7; 1971.

33. Kretzler, H.H.; Richardson, A.B. Rupture of the pectoralis major muscle. Am. J. Sports Med. 17(4):453-458; 1989.

34. Kulund, D.N.; Dewey, J.B.; Brubaker, C.E.; Roberts, J.R. Olympic weight-lifting injuries. Physician Sports Med. 6(11):111-119; 1978.

35. Lander, J.E.; Hundley, J.R.; Simonton, R.L. The effectiveness of weight-belts during multiple repetitions of the squat exercise. Med. Sci. Sports Exerc. 24(5):603-609; 1992.

36. Levine, A.; Wells, S.; Kopf, C. New rules of exercise. U.S. News World Rep. 101(6):52-56; 1986.

37. Lombardi, V.P. Beginning weight training: The safe and effective way. Dubuque, IA: Wm. C. Brown Company Publishers; 1989.

38. MacDougall, J.D.; Tuxen, D.; Sale, D.G.; Moroz, J.R.; Sutton, J.R. Arterial blood pressure response to heavy resistance exercise. J. Appl. Physiol. 58(3):785-790; 1985.

39. Mannis, C.I. Transchondral fracture of the dome of the talus sustained during weight training. Am. J. Sports Med. 11(5):354-356; 1983.

40. Mazur, L.J.; Yetman, R.J.; Risser, W.L. Weight-training injuries: common injuries and preventative methods. Sports Med. 16(1):57-63; 1993.

41. McCubbin, J.A. Resistance exercise training for persons with arthritis. Rheum. Dis. Clin. North Am. 16(4):931-943; 1990.

42. McMaster, P.E. Tendon and muscle ruptures: clinical and experimental studies on the courses and location of subcutaneous ruptures. J. Bone Joint Surg. Am. 15:705-722; 1933.

43. Menkes, A.; Mazel, S.; Redmond, R.A.; Koffler, K.; Libanati, C.R.; Gundberg, C.M.; Zizic, T.M.; Hagberg, J.M.; Pratley, R.E.; Hurley, B.F. Strength training increases regional bone mineral density and bone remodeling in middle-aged and older men. J. Appl. Physiol. 74(5):2478-2484; 1993.

44. Mochizuki, R.M.; Richter, K.J. Cardiomyopathy and cerebrovascular accident associated with anabolic-androgenic steroid use. Physician Sports Med. 16(1):108-114; 1988.

45. Mueller, F.O.; Ryan, A.J., editors. Prevention of athletic injuries: The role of the sports medicine team. Philadelphia: F.A. Davis; 1991.

46. Munnings, F. Strength training: not only for the young. Physician Sports Med. 21(4):133-140; 1993.

47. O'Connor, P.J.; Bryant, C.X.; Veltri, J.P.; Gebhardt, S.M. State anxiety and ambulatory blood pressure following resistance exercise in females. Med. Sci. Sports Exerc. 25(4):516-521; 1993.

48. Ossip-Klein, D.J.; Doyne, E.J.; Bowman, E.D.; Osborn, K.M.; McDougall-Wilson, I.B.; Neimeyer, R.A. Effects of running or weight lifting on self-concept in clinically depressed women. J. Consult. Clin. Psychol. 57(1):158-161; 1989.

49. Powell, J. Six-hundred, thirty-six thousand injuries annually in high school football. Athl. Train. 22:19-22; 1987.

50. Reut, R.C.; Bach, B.R.; Johnson, C. Pectoralis major rupture. Physician Sports Med. 19(3):89-96; 1991.

51. Rians, C.B.; Weltman, A.; Cahill, B.R.; Janney, C.A.; Tippett, S.R.; Katch, F.I. Strength training for pre-

pubescent males: is it safe? Am. J. Sports Med. 15(5):483-489; 1987.

52. Risser, W.L. Weight-training injuries in children and adolescents. Am. Fam. Physician. 44(6):2104-2108; 1991.

53. Risser, W.L.; Risser, J.M.H.; Preston, D. Weight-training injuries in adolescents. Am. J. Dis. Child. 144:1015-1017; 1990.

54. Rossi, F.; Dragoni, S. Lumbar spondylolysis: Occurrence in competitive athletes. J. Sports Med. Phys. Fitness. 30:450-452; 1990.

55. Ryan, J.R.; Salciccioli, G.G. Fractures of the distal radial epiphysis in adolescent weight lifters. Am. J. Sports Med. 4:26-27; 1976.

56. Saudek, C.E.; Palmer, K.A. Back pain revisited. J. of Orthop. Sports Phys. Ther. 8(12):556-566; 1987.

57. Segan, D.J.; Sladek, E.C.; Gomez, J.; McCoy, H.J.; Cairns, D.A. Weight lifting as a cause of bilateral upper extremity compartment syndrome. Physician Sports Med. 16(10):71-77; 1988.

58. Servedio, F.J.; Bartels, R.L.; Hamlin, R.L.; Teske, D.; Shaffer, T.; Servedio, A. The effects of weight training, using Olympic style lifts, on various physiological variables in pre-pubescent boys (abstract). Med. Sci. Sports Exerc. 17(2):288; 1985.

59. Sewall, L.; Micheli, L.J. Strength training for children. J. Pediatr. Orthop. 6(2):143-146; 1986.

60. Shea, J.M. Acute quadriplegia following the use of progressive resistance exercise machinery. Physician Sports Med. 14(4):120-124; 1986.

61. Tanner, S.M. Weighing the risks. Physician Sports Med. 21(6):105-116; 1993.

62. U.S. Consumer Product Safety Commission, Directorate for Epidemiology, National Injury Information Clearinghouse. Accident investigations: Exercise equipment (code 3277), January, 1992 - September, 1993. Washington, DC: US CPSC; 1994.

63. U.S. Consumer Product Safety Commission, Directorate for Epidemiology, National Injury Information Clearinghouse. Accident investigations: Weight lifting (code 3265), January, 1991 - September, 1993. Washington, DC: US CPSC; 1994.

64. U.S. Consumer Product Safety Commission, Directorate for Epidemiology, National Injury Information Clearinghouse. Death certificate file: Weight lifting (code 3265), January, 1991 - September, 1993. Washington, DC: US CPSC; 1994.

65. U.S. Consumer Product Safety Commission, Directorate for Epidemiology, National Injury Information Clearinghouse. Estimates & injury detail reports: National electronic injury surveillance system. Weight lifting, 1982 (codes 3264 & 3265). Washington, DC: US CPSC; 1983.

66. U.S. Consumer Product Safety Commission, Directorate for Epidemiology, National Injury Informa-

tion Clearinghouse. Estimates & injury detail reports: National electronic injury surveillance system. Weight lifting, 1991 (codes 3264 & 3265). Washington, DC: US CPSC; 1992.

67. U.S. Consumer Product Safety Commission, Directorate for Epidemiology, National Injury Information Clearinghouse. Estimates & injury detail reports: National electronic injury surveillance system. Weight lifting, 1992 (codes 3264 & 3265). Washington, DC: US CPSC; 1993.

68. U.S. Consumer Product Safety Commission, Directorate for Epidemiology, National Injury Information Clearinghouse. Estimates report: National electronic injury surveillance system. Weight lifting, 1985 (code 3265). Washington, DC: US CPSC; 1986.

69. U.S. Consumer Product Safety Commission, Directorate for Epidemiology, National Injury Information Clearinghouse. Explanation sheet for NEISS estimates report. Washington, DC: US CPSC; 1990.

70. U.S. Consumer Product Safety Commission, Directorate for Epidemiology, National Injury Information Clearinghouse. Individual injury listing: National electronic injury surveillance system. Exercise equipment (code 3277), June - September, 1993. Washington, DC: US CPSC; 1994.

71. U.S. Consumer Product Safety Commission, Directorate for Epidemiology, National Injury Information Clearinghouse. Individual injury listing: National electronic injury surveillance system. Weight lifting (code 3265), June, 1993. Washington, DC: US CPSC; 1994.

72. U.S. Consumer Product Safety Commission, Directorate for Epidemiology, National Injury Information Clearinghouse. Reported incident file: Weight lifting (code 3265), January, 1991 - September, 1993. Washington, DC: US CPSC; 1994.

73. Walter, S.D.; Hart, L.E. Application of epidemiological methodology to sports and exercise science research. In: Exercise and sport sciences reviews. Baltimore: Williams & Wilkins, 1990, Volume 18: 417-448.

74. Webb, D.R. Strength training in children and adolescents. Pediatr. Clin. North Am. 37(5):1187-1210; 1990.

75. World Health Organization (WHO). International classification of diseases: Basic tabulation list with alphabetical index, 9th revision (ICD 9). Geneva: WHO; 1978.

76. World Health Organization (WHO). International statistical classification of diseases and related health problems, 10th revision (ICD 10). Geneva: WHO; 1992.

77. Zemper, E.D. Four-year study of weightroom injuries in a national sample of college football teams. Nat. Str. Cond. Assoc. J. 12(3):32-34; 1990.

# 20

# Rock Climbing and Mountaineering

*David G. Addiss and Hubert A. Allen*

## 1. Introduction

Because of increasing popularity and diversity of rock climbing and mountaineering during the past two decades, the epidemiologic features of climbing-related injuries are heterogeneous and rapidly evolving. It is therefore difficult to characterize climbing-related injuries as a whole. The incidence, type, severity, and anatomic location of injuries, and the causes and risk factors associated with them depend on the specific type of climbing involved, the geographic features of the climbing area, and other factors. In addition, injury patterns appear to be changing as climbers increasingly participate in new types of climbing such as rapid alpine-style ascents of the world's highest mountains and competitive sport climbing on artificial walls.

We consider mountaineering, rock climbing, sport climbing, and vertical ice climbing as four distinct types of climbing. Mountaineering involves climbing on snow, rock, or ice to reach a peak or summit, usually at moderate or high altitude in remote areas. Rock climbing generally involves minimal exposure to snow or ice and usually occurs at relatively low or moderate elevations where altitude sickness is unlikely to be a complicating factor. Sport climbing includes organized rock-climbing competitions, climbing on indoor or outdoor training walls, rock climbing in areas used primarily for practice and training, and "bouldering" (i.e., climbing on large boulders close enough to the ground so climbers do not require ropes in the event of a fall). Vertical ice climbing, including climbing frozen waterfalls, has developed as a sport during the past two decades as new tools

and equipment have been developed. In part because this sport is so young, little information exists on ice-climbing injuries.

The purpose of this paper is to describe the epidemiologic features of rock-climbing and mountaineering injuries. We searched Medline, a computer database maintained by the National Library of Medicine, to identify articles in the medical literature published in all languages from 1970 to 1993 on mountaineering or rock-climbing injuries. This information was supplemented by published reports of the American Alpine Club and articles in climbing magazines. Although some references described injuries in inexperienced tourists or hikers who fell while trying to climb or descend cliffs, our review focuses on injuries in climbers (i.e., persons with more experience or preparation) who intended to complete a particular climb.

By and large, existing studies are descriptive rather than analytic. Sources of data include records of park rangers or search and rescue personnel; hospital or clinic charts or insurance claims; surveys of climbers; and other sources, including expedition records and compilations of accounts by injured climbers. Major weaknesses of existing data include lack of standard case definitions, the absence of comparison or control groups, difficulty in obtaining accurate denominator information, and the fact that few studies have been conducted prospectively. No intervention studies have been published. However, detailed clinical studies have described specific injuries associated with sport climbing.

## 2. Incidence of Injury

### 2.1 Injury Rates

Because accurate data on the number of climbers at risk ("denominator data") are difficult to obtain, only a few studies of climbing-related injuries have estimated injury rates, and even these have used imprecise denominators, such as the number of climbers registered in a particular climbing area (37, 44). Schussman and colleagues attempted to estimate the number of climber-hours of exposure by multiplying the number of climbers registered for a specific climb by the customary length of time it takes to complete each climb. Because climbing times vary widely, however, the accuracy of this estimate is uncertain. Oberli and colleagues used the number of person-nights of occupancy in mountain huts as a denominator (33), but this figure excludes one-day climbs and climbers who bivouac rather than stay in a hut. In only one investigation (a prospective study of students participating in the National Outdoor Leadership School [NOLS]), have injury rates been reported per 1,000 person-days of exposure (21). Unfortunately, most of the data from this study are presented in aggregate, and include activities other than climbing.

To facilitate comparison of injury rates among studies, shown in Table 20.1, we have used "person-climbs" as a common denominator wherever possible and have assumed that "person-

climbs" are roughly equivalent to "registered climbers" or "climbers." Given these assumptions, injury rates reported by various investigators appear to be influenced primarily by the type of climbing and the study design or method of detecting cases, which affect the sensitivity of the numerator. The most thorough injury case data and the highest rates have been observed in studies of mountaineers in which injuries were reported by the climbers themselves (44) or by persons reviewing insurance claim data (33). In contrast, studies of mountaineers in the Alps and Tetons that used hospital records or search and rescue data reported rates of 1.4 to 2.2 injuries per 1,000 person-climbs (19, 37). Such data lack sensitivity because they omit injuries that do not require hospitalization, evacuation, or search and rescue assistance.

Little information exists on the incidence of rock- or ice-climbing injuries. Even though case detection may be fairly complete in areas such as Yosemite Valley (12), accurate denominator data are unavailable because climber registration is seldom required in rock- or ice-climbing areas. However, in a prospective study of students at NOLS, the incidence of rock-climbing injuries was 1.6 per 1,000 person-days, compared with 2.2 for injuries

**Table 20.1   Incidence of Climbing-Related Injury Rates, by Location and Data Source**

| Reference | Setting | Data source and type of study[a] | No. climbers | No. injured climbers | Injury incidence |
|---|---|---|---|---|---|
| Wilson, 1978 | Denali, mountaineering | Retrospective survey and search and rescue records | 587 | 112 | 19.1/1,000 person-climbs |
| Schussman, 1982 | Tetons, rock climbing and mountaineering | Search and rescue records | 71,655 | 158 | 2.2/1,000 person-climbs |
| Schussman, 1990 | Tetons, rock climbing and mountaineering | Search and rescue records | 43,631 | 108[b] | 2.5/1,000 person-climbs[b] |
| Oberli, 1981 | Swiss Alps, mountaineering | Insurance claims | 100,000[c] | 4,000 | 14.3/1,000 hut-nights |
| Foray, 1982 | Mount Blanc, mountaineering | Hospital case series | 1,260,000[c] | 1,819 | 1.4/1,000 climbers |
| Gentile, 1992 | NOLS[d]-ice climbing | Prospective | **** | **** | 2.2/1,000 climber-days |
| Gentile, 1992 | NOLS[d]-snow mountaineering | Prospective | **** | **** | 1.4/1,000 climber-days |
| Gentile, 1992 | NOLS[d]-rock climbing | Prospective | **** | **** | 1.6/1,000 climber-days |

[a]Studies were retrospective unless otherwise indicated.

[b]Data are for "accidents" rather than number of injured climbers.

[c]Estimated number.

****Data not available for individual sports.

[d]NOLS = National Outdoor Leadership School.

involving snow mountaineering. The low rates of injuries on both rock and snow reported for these students is of particular interest, since case detection was probably more thorough than in other studies: an injury was reported if it restricted normal activities for 12 hours or longer. This study suggests that injury rates among climbers receiving well-organized instruction may be considerably lower than those among climbers in less structured settings.

Surveys of rock climbers suggest that the prevalence of climbing-related injury is high. Thirty-five (76.1%) of 46 rock climbers reported injury-related pain associated with climbing (39), and 455 (97.8%) of 460 self-identified climbers responding to a widely distributed survey in the United States reported having had ≥ 1 climbing-related injury (42). In clinical surveys of elite European rock climbers, 26% had signs of previous injury to the A2 pulley of the ring finger (9) and 35% had severe pain caused by tendinitis or tenosynovitis of the fingers (17).

## 2.2 Reinjury Rates

Little is known about the frequency of reinjury. Among Yosemite climbers seeking medical attention for a climbing-related injury, 31% reported having had a previous climbing-related injury more severe than minor abrasions (12), but it was unclear whether the current injury was related to the previous injury. Surveys suggest that many climbers, particularly those involved in competitive sport climbing, continue to climb even though injured (39); reinjury may be common in this group (10).

# 3. Injury Characteristics

## 3.1 Injury Onset

Nontraumatic overuse-type injuries, including inflammation of the brachialis tendon, flexion deformities of the fingers, and osteoarthritis, occur commonly among rock climbers and competitive sport climbers. Surveys of climbers suggest that "overuse" causes as many as 55% of injuries (42). However, most serious injuries in rock climbers and mountaineers are caused by acute trauma resulting from falls (1, 37, 38).

## 3.2 Injury Type

Different investigators have categorized climbing-related injuries in various ways, making it hard to compare the findings of these studies. In general, the types of injury reported depend on the type of climbing and the source of data, as shown in Table 20.2. In studies of mountaineers that used hospital records or search and rescue data, the most frequently reported injuries were fractures, 29% to 38% (1, 37, 38), and "trauma," 69% (19). In contrast, when investigators mailed questionnaires to mountaineers in Alaska after the 1976 climbing season, frostbite was the most frequently reported injury (52%), followed by acute mountain sickness (25%) (44). Altitude sickness, including acute cerebral and pulmonary edema, which may be fatal, is a particularly serious problem for mountaineers venturing to high altitudes, and may contribute directly or indirectly to trauma and other mountaineering-related injuries (32, 44). Mountaineers also suffer from sunburn (40), hypothermia (41), heat exhaustion (7), snowblindness (22), altitude retinopathy (14), and lightning strikes (2, 19).

A prospective clinic-based study suggests that fractures are the leading type of injury among rock climbers, shown in Table 20.2. Among 220 rock climbers who sought medical care in Yosemite Valley, 29% of injuries were fractures and 25% were abrasions (12). In contrast, in a survey of rock climbers, fractures comprised only 5.4% of 1,949 self-reported injuries, compared with 40.3% for tendinitis, sprains, and muscle strains (42).

## 3.3 Injury Location

The lack of a standardized system for categorizing the anatomical location of climbing-related injuries makes comparison of data from various studies difficult. Some investigators provide details on the location of the "most serious" injury, others describe all reported injuries separately, and others lump all climbers with more than one injury into a "multiple injury" category. Even with these limitations, however, it is apparent that the anatomical location of reported climbing-related injuries depends to a large extent on the type of climbing and method of case detection, as shown in Table 20.3.

Injuries to the skin and subcutaneous tissues are perhaps the most common climbing injuries. Among injured climbers in Yosemite Valley, 50% had injuries to the skin or subcutaneous tissue (12). In a large survey of climbers, abrasions, lacerations, and hematomas accounted for 32.6% of all self-reported injuries (42).

### 3.3.1 Head/Spine/Trunk

In retrospective studies of mountaineering injuries based on search and rescue data or hospital rec-

**Table 20.2   Most Commonly Reported Injuries, by Setting and Type of Study**

| Reference | Setting | Data source and type of study[a] | No. injuries | Injury type | Number (%) of injuries |
|---|---|---|---|---|---|
| Wilson, 1978 | Denali, mountaineering | Retrospective survey and search and rescue records | 112[b] | Frostbite<br>Acute mountain sickness<br>Fracture<br>Sprained ankle | 58 (52%)[c]<br>35 (31%)[c]<br>4 (4%)<br>4 (4%)[c] |
| Foray, 1982 | Mont Blanc, mountaineering | Hospital case series | 1,484[b] | Trauma<br>Frostbite<br>Acute mountain sickness<br>Hypothermia | 1,034 (69%)<br>254 (17%)<br>94 (6%)<br>73 (5%) |
| Schussman, 1982 | Tetons, rock climbing and mountaineering | Search and rescue records | 247 | Fracture<br>Laceration<br>Contusion<br>Abrasion<br>Sprain/strain<br>Dislocation (shoulder) | 83 (34%)<br>47 (19%)<br>40 (16%)<br>19 (8%)<br>11 (4%)<br>8 (3%) |
| Schussman, 1990 | Tetons, rock climbing and mountaineering | Search and rescue records | 149[b] | Fracture<br>Contusion or abrasion<br>Massive or multiple<br>Sprain/strain | 57 (38%)<br>30 (20%)<br>19 (13%)<br>18 (12%) |
| Addiss, 1989 | U.S. National Parks, rock climbing and mountaineering | Search and rescue records and injury reports | 115 | Multiple<br>Fracture<br>Sprain<br>Frostbite | 38 (33%)<br>33 (29%)<br>12 (10%)<br>6 (5%) |
| Bowie, 1988 | Yosemite, rock climbing | Prospective clinical case series | 451 | Fracture<br>Abrasion<br>Contusion<br>Laceration<br>Sprain/strain<br>Hypothermia<br>Dislocation | 130 (29%)<br>111 (25%)<br>66 (15%)<br>64 (14%)<br>47 (10%)<br>12 (3%)<br>9 (2%) |
| Tomczak, 1989 | United States, self-selected climbers | Self-administered questionnaire survey | 1,949 | Tendinitis<br>Abrasion<br>Sprain<br>Hematoma<br>Muscle strain<br>General pain<br>Fracture | 452 (23%)<br>423 (22%)<br>187 (10%)<br>163 (8%)<br>146 (8%)<br>109 (6%)<br>106 (5%) |
| Bollen, 1988 | Great Britain, competitive sport climbers | Self-administered questionnaire survey | 115 | PIP[d] joint tenoperiostitis<br>Rotator cuff tear, shoulder | 31 (27%)<br>16 (14%) |

[a]Studies were retrospective unless otherwise indicated.

[b]Number of injured climbers, rather than number of injuries.

[c]Estimated number.

[d]PIP = proximal interphalangeal joint.

ords, head injuries comprised 16% to 22% of all injuries (19, 37, 38). A necropsy study of fatally injured climbers and hikers in Scotland reported that 81% had suffered head injuries (35).

### 3.3.2 Upper Extremity

Among competitive sport climbers, injuries to the upper extremity predominate (9, 39). Cole (16) examined six rock climbers with injuries of the finger-

tips initially characterized by redness and serous exudate, followed by maceration and splitting of the skin, which healed following 1 to 2 weeks of rest. Bollen has described several injuries that occur primarily in competitive or high-level sport climbers. Anterior elbow pain, or "climber's elbow," is caused by tendinitis of the brachialis muscle, and is associated with climbing on overhanging surfaces for prolonged periods, during

**Table 20.3    Most Frequent Anatomical Locations of Injuries, by Setting and Type of Study**

| Reference | Setting | Data source and type of study[a] | No. injuries | Injury location | Number (%) of injuries |
|---|---|---|---|---|---|
| Foray, 1982[b] | Mont Blanc, mountaineering | Hospital case series | — | Skull<br>Spine<br>Chest<br>Trunk<br>Extremities | (16%)<br>(8%)<br>(3%)<br>(12%)<br>(56%) |
| Schussman, 1982 | Tetons, rock climbing and mountaineering | Search and rescue records | 247 | Head<br>Chest<br>Back<br>Arm<br>Lower extremity<br>Multiple | 54 (22%)<br>19 (7%)<br>13 (5%)<br>30 (12%)<br>73 (30%)<br>34 (14%) |
| Schussman, 1990 | Tetons, rock climbing and mountaineering | Search and rescue records | 149 | Head<br>Chest<br>Back<br>Upper extremity<br>Lower extremity<br>Multiple | 31 (21%)<br>9 (6%)<br>5 (3%)<br>16 (11%)<br>55 (37%)<br>25 (17%) |
| McLennan, 1983 | Sierras, rock climbing and mountaineering | Clinical case series | 215 | Axial skeleton<br>Upper extremity<br>Lower extremity | 23 (11%)<br>39 (18%)<br>153 (71%) |
| Biener, 1981 | Swiss Alps, Mountaineering | Questionnaire mailed to Swiss Alpine Club members | 85 | Head<br>Trunk<br>Upper extremity<br>Lower extremity | (8%)<br>(17%)<br>(20%)<br>(55%) |
| Bowie, 1988 | Yosemite, rock climbing | Prospective clinical case series | 451 | Skin/subcutaneous<br>Skull<br>Lower extremity<br>Upper extremity<br>Thorax | 227 (50%)<br>25 (6%)<br>127 (28%)<br>29 (6%)<br>11 (2%) |
| Tomczak, 1989 | United States, self-selected climbers | Self-administered questionnaire | 1,949 | Upper extremity<br>Lower extremity<br>Whole body | 1,144 (59%)<br>641 (33%)<br>164 (8%) |
| Bollen, 1988 | Great Britain, competitive sport climbers | Self-administered questionnaire | 115 | Hand - PIP joint<br>Hand - 1st MCP joint<br>Wrist<br>Elbow<br>Shoulder<br>Lower limb | 31 (27%)<br>12 (10%)<br>9 (8%)<br>20 (17%)<br>16 (14%)<br>12 (10%) |
| Della Santa, 1990 | | | | Finger<br>Elbow | 41 (59%)<br>18 (26%) |

[a]Studies were retrospective unless otherwise indicated.

[b]Does not include nontraumatic injuries.

which the forearm is flexed and pronated (11). Medial and lateral epicondylitis are found in 5% to 16% of competitive climbers (11). Injury of the A2 pulley, or "climber's finger," is associated with falls or sudden weight bearing on the fingers while using the "cling grip" or "crimping," in which climbers hold on to narrow ledges by flexing the proximal interphalangeal (PIP) joints and extending the distal interphalangeal (DIP) joints of the fingers. The ring finger is particularly susceptible to this injury. In one survey, 24% of competitive sport climbers had fixed flexion deformities of the PIP joints of 10 to 15 degrees (9). This injury may result from leaving the hand in the "position of rest" rather than performing range-of-motion exercises after sessions of hard climbing. Climbing-associated digital avulsion, tears of the collateral ligaments of the PIP joints, rupture of the flexor digitorum superficialis tendon, carpal tunnel syndrome, and osteoarthritis have also been described (8, 11, 39).

### 3.3.3 *Lower Extremity*

Among mountaineers and rock climbers seeking medical care and in surveys of climbers, the lower extremity is the site of 28% to 71% of injuries (6, 12, 32, 42). The ankle is involved in 25% to 53% of lower extremity injuries among mountaineers in the Tetons and Sierras (32, 37, 38) and in 64% of lower extremity injuries among rock climbers in Yosemite (12).

## 4. Injury Severity

### 4.1 Time Loss

Little information is available on the degree to which climbing injuries cause lost work or time away from climbing. In a case series of rock climbers who were injured at a training site in Czechoslovakia and admitted to a hospital, 4% had "permanent serious sequelae" (24). Among climbers surveyed in the United States, 58 to 62% reported having seen a physician for a climbing-related injury (39,42). In one survey of rock climbers, 58% were currently using anti-inflammatory medication for a climbing injury and half continued to climb while injured (39).

### 4.2 Catastrophic Injury

Two separate measures of the risk of climbing-related mortality appear in the literature: the case-fatality ratio and the incidence rate of fatal injury. The case-fatality ratio, the proportion of injuries that are fatal, is calculated by dividing the number of climbing deaths by the number of injured climbers and multiplying by 100. The case-fatality ratio is highly dependent on the completeness of injury case detection, making comparison between studies difficult. For example, when only search and rescue data are used to determine the number of injuries (i.e., the denominator), case-fatality ratios are high, ranging from 19.0 to 28.3% (Table 20.4). These values are artificially inflated because they omit injuries not requiring search and rescue assistance from the denominator. Studies with more thorough injury case detection, including most clinical case series (12, 32), climber surveys (44), and studies utilizing insurance claim data (33), report case-fatality ratios of 5.0 to 8.9%. One exception is a case-fatality ratio of 18.4% reported in a hospital case series of mountaineering injuries in the Alps (19); this high figure may be explained, in part, by the fact that all persons with nonfatal injuries were injured severely enough to be hospitalized. A very low case-fatality ratio, 0.9%, was reported in a clinical case series of climbers at a training area in Czechoslovakia (24), suggesting that climbing training may be associated with lower risk. The case-fatality ratio does not appear to be associated with type of climbing, perhaps

**Table 20.4   Climbing-Related Case-Fatality Ratios and Fatality Rates, by Type of Climbing and Data Source**

| Climbing type | Reference | Setting | Data source and type of study[a] | Case fatality ratio | Fatality rate |
|---|---|---|---|---|---|
| Expedition mountaineering | Wilson, 1978 | Denali | Retrospective survey and SAR[b] records | 8.9% | 12/1,000 person-climbs |
| | Pollard, 1988 | Himalaya | Expedition reports | — | 43/1,000 person-climbs |
| Mountaineering | Addiss, 1989 | United States National Parks | SAR[b] records, injury reports | 28.3% | — |
| | Schussman, 1982 | Tetons | SAR[b] records | 19.0% | 0.4/1,000 person-climbs |
| | Schussman, 1990 | Tetons | SAR[b] records | 23.1% | 0.6/1,000 person-climbs |
| | Oberli, 1981 | Swiss Alps | Insurance claims | 5.0% | 0.7/1,000 climber-nights |
| | McLennan, 1983 | Sierras | Clinical case series | 8.5% | — |
| | Foray, 1982 | Mont Blanc | Hospital case series | 18.4% | 0.27/1,000 climbers |
| Rock climbing | Bowie, 1988 | Yosemite | Prospective clinical case series | 5.9% | — |
| | Hubicka, 1977 | Czechoslovakia | Hospital case series | 0.9% | — |

[a]Studies are retrospective unless otherwise indicated.

[b]SAR = search and rescue.

because it is so dependent on the completeness of case detection.

The fatality rate, or incidence of fatal injury, is calculated as the number of fatal injuries divided by an appropriate measure of exposure, such as climber-hours of exposure. As is the case for climbing-related injury rates, precise data on exposure are lacking. Unlike case-fatality ratios, reported fatality rates are strongly associated with type of climbing.

The highest fatality rates, 43 and 12 deaths per 1,000 person-climbs, are reported for expeditionary mountaineers at high altitude in the Himalaya and in Alaska, respectively (34, 44). Fatality rates for alpine-style mountaineering, which include both rock and snow conditions, range from 0.27 to 0.6 deaths per 1,000 person-climbs, or 0.7 deaths per 1,000 climber-nights, shown in Table 20.4. Little is known about fatality rates among rock climbers or sport climbers, but these are probably lower.

Little information exists on the incidence of paralysis resulting from climbing-related injury, although 20 (4%) climbers in one survey reported paresthesia or nerve-related injury (42). At very high altitudes (more than 7,000 to 8,000 meters), climbers who do not use supplemental oxygen may develop long-term fine motor disturbances (26), deficits in concentration and memory (23), and abnormalities on magnetic resonance imaging of the brain indicative of cortical atrophy (20).

## 4.3 Clinical Outcome/Residual Symptoms

Fatal climbing injuries attract the most attention, but several investigators have commented on the minor nature of most climbing-related injuries, even among mountaineers (19, 36). Among competitive sport climbers, fatal injuries are extremely rare, but less severe injuries occur frequently; 69 (80.2%) of 86 competitive climbers in Europe reported having had climbing-related injuries that were symptomatic for 10 days or longer (8).

Injury severity scores (ISS) (4) have been calculated for injured climbers in two studies. Injuries with severity scores of < 5, 5 to 12, and 13 to 75 are generally considered "mild," "moderate," and "severe," respectively (12). Among rock climbers seeking medical attention in Yosemite, the median ISS was 4 (12). Among mountaineers in the Tetons who required search and rescue assistance but who were not fatally injured, the median ISS was 2 (38). Investigators in both studies commented on the mild nature of the vast majority of climbing-related injuries. Injury severity scores were higher for climbers who were leading at the time of injury (12) and for those whose injury involved an error in judgment (38). In Yosemite, injury severity scores also increased with distance of the climber above the ground, length of fall, occurrence of injury after 5 p.m., and climbing at Cathedral Rocks, a specific location within Yosemite Valley (12).

## 5. Injury Risk Factors

The various schemes developed by different investigators to describe the cause of climbing-related injuries are testament to the difficulty inherent in determining which factors are causally related to such events. Some authors focus on immediate causes (e.g., "foot slipped on rock") and secondary causes (e.g., "climbing above ability"), and others emphasize issues of "poor judgment" (32), "inexperience" (44) or "climber error" (37). Each year, injured climbers report thoughtful self-assessments in the informative annual report by the American Alpine Club, *Accidents in North American Mountaineering*. However, these observations are difficult to categorize for epidemiologic analysis.

Epidemiologic models of causal relationships often begin with an assessment of risk factors. Unfortunately, reliable data on risk factors for climbing injuries are lacking. Existing studies are primarily descriptive and do not include information on characteristics of uninjured climbers for comparison. Therefore, possible risk factors can be suggested, but not evaluated, from the information available. In some studies, characteristics of fatally injured climbers have been compared with those of nonfatal injuries, so that some information exists on risk factors for severe or fatal injury.

### 5.1 Intrinsic Factors

#### 5.1.1 Physical Characteristics

Because detailed denominator data are, for the most part, unavailable, it is not known whether age, gender, or other physical characteristics are associated with risk of climbing-related injury.

#### 5.1.2 Motor/Functional Characteristics

Although experience and skill are commonly thought to prevent climbing-related injury, the degree to which they actually decrease the risk of injury is unknown. Existing data, summarized in Table 20.5, are inconsistent.

**Table 20.5   Evidence for Hypotheses Regarding Potential Risk Factors for Climbing-Related Injuries**

| Hypothesis and evidence for or against the hypothesis | Reference | Data source and type of study |
|---|---|---|
| Hypothesis: Lack of experience is associated with greater risk of injuries. | | |
| *Evidence* | | |
| In the Tetons, "climbers with less experience were more frequently involved in accidents" (data not shown). | Schussman, 1990 | SAR[a] records |
| Of 201 climbers injured on Class V routes in the Sierras, only 43 (21.4%) had > 5 years experience on Class V routes. | McClennan, 1983 | Clinical case series |
| Climbing injury rates were 2.9 per 1,000 climber-days for NOLS instructors, compared with 1.4 per 1,000 climber-days for students. | Gentile, 1992 | Prospective |
| In Yosemite, 71% of injured climbers reported being able to lead climbs as difficult as 5.10 or higher; only 14% of falls occurred when victims were attempting climbs rated beyond their most recent standard. | Bowie, 1988 | Prospective clinical case series |
| "Most lead climbers who fell were attempting to make a 'move' that was above their ability level" (data not shown). | Schussman, 1990 | SAR[a] records |
| Hypothesis: The incidence of injury increases with altitude. | | |
| *Evidence* | | |
| On British expeditions to Himalayan peaks of ≥ 7,000 meters, 8 deaths occurred at < 6,500 meters, 15 deaths occurred at > 6,500 meters. | Pollard, 1988 | Expedition reports |
| Acute mountain sickness documented in 86 (42.8%) climbers injured in the Sierras. | McLennan, 1983 | Clinical case series |
| Hypothesis: The lead climber is more likely to be injured than the climber who follows. | | |
| *Evidence* | | |
| 92% of rock climbing accidents involved leaders falling while ascending. | Schussman, 1990 | SAR[a] records |
| 66% of injuries in Yosemite caused by leader falls. | Bowie, 1988 | Clinical case series |
| Hypothesis: Some routes, mountains, or climbing areas are more risky than others. | | |
| *Evidence* | | |
| 58% of injuries occurred in 4 U.S. national parks and 67% of fatalities occurred in 2 U.S. national parks. | Addiss, 1989 | SAR[a] records, injury reports |
| Several mountains in Tetons associated with higher incidence of accidents. | Schussman, 1990 | SAR[a] records |
| British fatality rate on K2 is 11%, compared with 5.8% on Everest. | Pollard, 1988 | Expedition reports |
| Hypothesis: More difficult climbs are associated with higher rates of injuries. | | |
| *Evidence* | | |
| Most climbers in the Tetons are injured on climbs of lesser difficulty (71% of injuries occurred on routes rated easier than 5.6). | Schussman, 1990 | SAR[a] records |
| 58% of accidents in Tetons occurred on "steep terrain," 36% occurred on "moderate terrain." | Schussman, 1982 | SAR[a] records |
| "No correlation between standard of difficulty of climbing and number or type of injury" among elite British climbers (data not shown). | Bollen, 1988 | Questionnaire survey |
| Hypothesis: Longer falls are more likely to be fatal. | | |
| *Evidence* | | |
| On snow or ice in the Tetons, average length of fall for fatal accidents was 1,205 feet, compared with 119 feet for nonfatal accidents; on rock, average length of fall for fatal accidents was 160 feet, compared to 33 feet for nonfatal accidents. | Schussman, 1990 | SAR[a] records |
| Median length of fall for fatal injuries in U.S. national parks was 91 meters, compared with 9 meters for nonfatal injuries. | Addiss, 1989 | SAR[a] records, injury reports |
| Hypothesis: Climbing on ice or snow is more risky and more likely to be fatal than rock climbing. | | |
| *Evidence* | | |
| 34% of accidents in the Tetons occurred on snow or ice, but most climbing is on rock; of 21 fatal accidents, 12 occurred during travel on snow and 9 occurred during travel on rock. | Schussman, 1990 | SAR[a] records |
| "Fatal accidents occurred more often while the climbers were traveling on snow" (data not shown). | Schussman, 1982 | SAR[a] records |
| Case-fatality ratio in U.S. national parks was 41% for injuries occurring on snow or ice, compared with 19% on rock. | Addiss, 1989 | SAR[a] records, injury reports |

[a]SAR = search and rescue.

### 5.1.3 Psychosocial Characteristics

Investigators have begun to explore the psychological, social, and hormonal aspects of climbing (18, 31, 43), but little work has focused on the relationship between these factors and climbing-related injury. One author has suggested that suicidal intent may be the cause of some fatal climbing injuries (27). Anecdotal information from injured climbers suggests that psychological factors may be important predictors of injury in the mountains. Climbers describe "the flow experience," during which the mind and body are intensely focused on climbing and performance is exceptionally high (31). In contrast, fear may "serve to disintegrate judgment and precipitate accidents" in the mountain environment (29).

## 5.2 Extrinsic Factors

### 5.2.1 Exposure

Available data, summarized in Table 20.5, suggest that climbing at high altitude increases risk of injury and that lead climbers are more likely to be injured than those who follow.

### 5.2.2 Training Conditions

Proper training techniques for high-level rock climbing have only recently been developed (8). Among sport climbers, pain in the fingers is common after training sessions. As many as one-third of rock climbers may be injured while using home training or muscle strengthening devices (39). Nearly half the injuries reported among elite British climbers occurred during training (8). It has been suggested that proper training and performing stretching exercises before climbing could reduce injuries to the lower extremity (32), but this seems unlikely because most of these injuries result from falls with a high transfer of energy to a small area of the body, regardless of strength (12). In a large survey of U.S. climbers, 73% of all climbers reported performing stretching exercises before climbing (42).

### 5.2.3 Environment

As one might expect, length of fall is associated with likelihood of fatal injury, as shown in Table 20.5. In addition, some climbs or climbing areas are more dangerous than others. Although the data are somewhat inconsistent, available evidence suggests that risk of injury is associated with the difficulty of the climb, and with climbing on snow or ice rather than on rock.

Evidence is inconclusive on whether injuries are more likely to occur during the ascent or the descent. In studies of mountaineers and rock climbers, 42 to 92% of injuries occurred while ascending (1, 32, 37, 38). However, in the Tetons, 81% of accidents on snow occurred during the descent (38), suggesting that risk of injury may be greater during descent on snow surfaces. Because the time spent descending a climb is often a fraction of that required for the ascent, the risk of injury during descent may be much higher than that during the ascent.

Higher numbers of injuries are reported during the peak climbing season in various locations (12, 24, 32), but few studies have examined the effect of time or season on injury rates. In Yosemite, 47% of injuries occur during the spring, suggesting that risk of injury may be higher in persons who have not been climbing recently (12). In addition, 43% of injuries in Yosemite occur on Saturday and Sunday; severe injuries are more likely to occur during the evening hours.

### 5.2.4 Equipment

Several retrospective studies of injured climbers suggest that equipment failure is unusual, causing approximately 6 to 7% of all climbing-related injuries (1, 32). None of the accidents in the Tetons were considered to have been caused by failure of equipment that was properly used (37, 38). However, in a prospective study of injured climbers seeking medical care in Yosemite, the climber's protection pulled out of the rock during 29% of leader falls that resulted in medically attended injury, suggesting that equipment misuse or failure may contribute to increased severity of some injuries (12).

# 6. Suggestions for Injury Prevention

Investigators have expressed a variety of ideas on how best to prevent climbing-related injuries. Unfortunately, there are no studies that demonstrate the effectiveness of recommended interventions. The sometimes complex causal web of injuries in the wilderness makes prevention difficult, as does the nature of climbing itself, which combines elements of personal challenge, physical skill, adventure, and risk. As a climber gains more experience and his or her abilities improve, so does the difficulty of climbs attempted. Traditionally, prevention efforts have focused on acquiring experience and good training, using proper equipment, and exercising good judgment. While these recommendations have undoubtedly prevented injury, their overall effectiveness is unclear (1).

This review has highlighted the influence both the type of climbing and the source of injury data have on the magnitude and characteristics of reported injury rates. These two factors are linked: studies of mountaineering use search and rescue data or hospital case series; studies of rock climbing rely largely on clinical case series; and studies of sport climbing have tended to use surveys. If we see climbing as a continuum with the two extremes represented by sport climbing on one end and expedition mountaineering on the other, we can distribute the epidemiologic characteristics of climbing-related injuries along this continuum, shown in Table 20.6. At the risk of oversimplification, as one moves from sport climbing through rock climbing and alpine mountaineering to expeditionary mountaineering, injury severity and fatality rates increase, and the injury pattern changes from tendinitis, tears, and sprains of the upper extremities caused by overtraining and overuse, to fractures of the lower extremities and trauma to the head caused primarily by falls and objective hazards of the mountaineering environment.

Preventive strategies must be developed that address the tremendous and growing diversity within the sport of climbing. Although some strategies may be applicable to all climbers, others must address specific issues about a single type of climbing. Thus, multiple prevention strategies are needed, and these should focus on the climbers, the sport itself, the climbing environment, and the health support system.

## 6.1 Climbers

Climbers can reduce mountaineering injuries associated with altitude sickness by ascending to high altitudes slowly, or if more rapid ascent is necessary, by taking acetazolamide prophylactically to reduce the likelihood of altitude sickness (13). Proper training and experience can undoubtedly reduce risk of serious injury, particularly in the mountaineering setting where, in critical situations, decisions or actions must be taken quickly and with profound consequences. Experiencing and dealing successfully with these moments of intensity is part of the lure of mountaineering. Thus, Foray et al. (19) suggest that the real issue in preventing traumatic mountaineering injuries is "prudence" rather than "prevention." It is widely accepted, although few data support this position, that proper training and experience will foster prudence, correct decision making, and sound judgment in critical mountaineering situations. Indeed, many injuries described by climbers in the annual report *Accidents in North American Mountaineering* are the result of ignorance or neglect of basic mountaineering principles. Each year, injured climbers report errors such as rapelling off the end of their ropes, wandering into avalanche zones, disregarding early signs of acute altitude sickness while ascending rapidly, and misuse of equipment (3). At the other end of the climbing spectrum, in the well-controlled setting of competitive sport climbing, judgment and decision making seem less important in preventing serious injury than are proper training and adequate periods of rest.

## 6.2 Climbing

Injury prevention has received increased attention among climbers and mountaineers in recent years,

---

Table 20.6    General Characteristics of Injuries Associated With Various Types of Climbing

| Characteristic | Sport climbing | Rock climbing | Alpine mountaineering | Expeditionary mountaineering |
| --- | --- | --- | --- | --- |
| Primary sources of data | Surveys, clinical surveys | Clinical case series, surveys | Search and rescue, clinical case series | Expedition reports, search and rescue records |
| Fatality rates | Approach zero | Low | 0.03-0.06% | 1.2-4.3% |
| Most common anatomical locations | Hands, forearms | Lower extremity | Lower extremity, head | Head, lower extremity, multiple |
| Injury type | Tendinitis, sprains | Fractures, abrasions, contusions | Fractures | Fractures, internal injuries |
| Severity | Mild | Moderate | Increasingly severe | Very severe |
| Primary causes | Overuse | Overuse, falls | Falls, other objective hazards | Falls, avalanche, altitude |

in part because access to major climbing areas has been threatened by concerns about the costs and dangers associated with search and rescue operations and by the desires of landowners to avoid potential liability in the event of climber injury. In the United States, mountain guides have established a professional association that specifies requirements for training and experience before a guide can be "certified." In what has become a highly competitive marketplace, manufacturers increasingly develop equipment that is ergonomically sound, highly durable, and functional. Synthetic materials have been used to produce lightweight, yet warm and comfortable clothing and footwear. Such technical developments can only improve the margin of safety in extreme mountaineering situations. Among sport climbers, educational materials have been developed to instruct climbers in proper training techniques, stretching exercises, and strength-building regimens.

### 6.3 External Environment

Since "meeting the mountain on its own terms" is the essence of mountaineering, major modification of the environment to decrease risk of injury is considered contrary to the spirit of climbing and is therefore undesirable. On popular rock-climbing routes, bolts can be placed in the rock to protect climbers from falls, but widespread bolting is controversial, and climbing "purists" have been known to remove bolts because they decreased the sense of adventure and risk associated with a climb, thereby degrading the climbing experience.

However, mountaineers consider it perfectly acceptable to modify their personal environment by wearing a helmet or using a rope for protection in the event of a fall. Thus, preventive strategies in the mountaineering or rock-climbing environments should focus not on environmental modification per se, but on measures that climbers can take to reduce risk of severe injury in a fall or other "accident." By contrast, since artificial climbing walls are man-made, environmental modification may be a feasible strategy for preventing injuries in competitive sport climbers. Injury patterns in indoor "climbing gyms" should be studied, climbing routes modified, and such interventions evaluated.

### 6.4 Health Support System

Access to emergency medical attention may be crucial for the survival of mountaineers and rock climbers with life-threatening injuries. However, it has been postulated that if climbers are aware of available search and rescue services, they may take unnecessary risks leading to injuries requiring emergency evacuation (25). The appropriate role of medical evacuation in the mountain setting, which is expensive and frequently endangers the lives of the rescue team, is a subject of much debate. In some areas, such as Denali, it is recommended that each climbing party carry a two-way radio in case of emergency.

In general, physicians are not well-informed about climbing-related injuries, particularly those sustained during training or competitive sport climbing (5, 8). In one study, only 24.4% of competitive British sport climbers sought medical attention for their climbing-related injuries, and "most were unimpressed at the treatment received, with an 'if you go climbing, what do you expect' attitude commonly encountered" (8). In contrast, knowledge appears to be greater among physicians practicing in areas where cold- and altitude-related mountaineering injuries are common, such as Alaska. Physicians in these areas have pioneered new techniques, contributed to scientific knowledge, and provided state-of-the art medical care for climbers with frostbite and hypothermia (30).

## 7. Suggestions for Further Research

Major weaknesses of existing data include lack of standard case definitions, the absence of comparison groups, difficulty in obtaining accurate denominator information, and the fact that few studies have been conducted prospectively.

To obtain better estimates of injury incidence, investigators should attempt to standardize case definitions. Injured climbers or injuries, rather than "accidents," should be the basic unit of analysis. The lack of accurate denominators limits our ability to interpret available data. Whenever possible, investigators should try to collect data that would allow for calculation of climber-hours of exposure. In sport climbing settings, this seems practical, and both numerator and denominator data should be collected separately for training and actual competition. In some National Parks, such as the Tetons, where denominator data are available because of enforced climber registration policies, climber-days may be calculated if climbers are required to register both before and after the climb. In other National Parks and in most local climbing areas, however, accurate denominators will continue to remain elusive. Even if policies in such areas are changed to require climber registration, compliance is likely to remain incomplete.

In the absence of large multicenter studies of climbing injuries, standard definitions are needed to compare injury type and location and to confirm apparent differences in injury patterns among different types of climbing and geographic locations. When possible, researchers should obtain the type and anatomical location of "multiple" injuries and should collect data in a disaggregated fashion to allow for recombination and later comparison. Reanalysis of existing data could be useful. For example, it may be possible to disaggregate the NOLS data on mountaineering and rock climbing from other activities to investigate the apparent discrepancy between low injury rates in the controlled instructional setting and higher rates under nontraining conditions.

Systematic assessment of injury severity is needed in studies of climbing-related injury. Injury severity should be assessed through use of injury severity scores (4, 12, 38) or, at a minimum, recording whether medical attention was sought, or hospitalization required, for the injury.

Identification of risk factors can often lead to preventive strategies, and case-control studies are needed that compare characteristics of injured and noninjured climbers. Longitudinal studies of cohorts of climbers would be preferable, but such studies are logistically more difficult, more time-consuming, and more expensive. Longitudinal data collection might be feasible, however, among competitive sport climbers.

Anecdotal evidence suggests that "climber error" and "lack of judgment" are major contributors to climbing-related injury (32, 37). Because the decision to climb is voluntary, and because all climbers in some way confront the notions of risk, challenge, and adventure, we need behavioral research to understand climber behavior, motivation, and judgment, and to identify, communicate, and implement practical preventive approaches. A few investigators have begun to address the psychological nature of climbing and have established a framework for discussion of these issues (29, 31).

Equipment manufacturers and others have already conducted considerable research on the physical forces experienced by the climber, the belayer, the rope, and other protective gear worn in the event of a fall (15, 28). This work has probably helped save many lives and reduce injury severity. Until recently, similar work had not been done on the tolerance of human tendons and ligaments to the stresses of high-level climbing. Although studies by Bollen and others have yielded insight into causes of injury among high-level competitive sport climbers, effective alternative climbing strategies (e.g., using different types of holds) have not yet been developed. Interestingly, however, competitive sport climbers themselves are aware of these injuries, and many have begun to tape the proximal phalanges before climbing in an effort to prevent A2 pulley tears, a measure that may have some effectiveness (10, 11). Evaluation of this and other strategies taken by climbers to reduce risk of injury would be of interest.

In summary, climbing is a diverse, rapidly growing sport. Injury patterns and risk factors are highly dependent on the location and type of climbing. Increasing diversity within the sport makes development, implementation, and evaluation of preventive strategies difficult. To date, most climbing-related research has been descriptive. Analytic studies are now needed to identify risk factors, test hypotheses, and develop interventions that prevent injury without threatening or degrading essential characteristics of the sport.

# References

1. Addiss, D.G.; Baker, S.P. Mountaineering and rock-climbing injuries in US national parks. Ann. Emerg. Med. 18:975-979; 1989.
2. Akahane, T.; Okishio, R. Lightning injury: report of two cases. Burns 10:45-48; 1983.
3. American Alpine Club; Alpine Club of Canada. Accidents in North American Mountaineering, Volume 6, Issue 45. New York: American Alpine Club; 1992.
4. Baker, S.P.; O'Neill, B.; Haddon, W., Jr.; et al. The injury severity score: A method for describing patients with multiple injuries and evaluating emergency care. J. Trauma 14:187-196; 1974.
5. Bannister, P.; Foster, P. Upper limb injuries associated with rock climbing. Brit. J. Sports Med. 20:55; 1986.
6. Biener, K.; Bosch, H. Sportsmedizinisches profil der alpinisten. Munch. Med Wschr. [German] 23:508-512; 1981.
7. Bloch, C. Heat exhaustion during a mountain climb [letter]. S. African Med. J. 61:342; 1982.
8. Bollen, S.R. Soft tissue injury in extreme rock climbers. Brit. J. Sports Med. 22:145-147; 1988.
9. Bollen, S.R.; Gunson, C.K. Hand injuries in competition climbers. Brit. J. Sports Med. 24:16-18; 1990.
10. Bollen, S.R. Injury to the A2 pulley in rock climbers. J. Hand Surg. 15:268-270; 1990a.
11. Bollen, S.R. Upper limb injuries in elite rock climbers. Brit. J. Sports Med. 25(Suppl):S18-S20; 1990b.

12. Bowie, W.S.; Hunt, T.K.; Allen, H.A., Jr. Rock-climbing injuries in Yosemite National Park. West. J. Med. 149:172-177; 1988.

13. Bradwell, A.R.; Wright, A.D.; Winterborn, M.; Imray, C. Acetazolamide and high altitude diseases. Int. J. Sports Med. 13:S63-S64; 1992.

14. Butler, F.K.; Harris, D.J.; Reynolds, R.D. Altitude retinopathy on Mount Everest. Ophthalmology 99: 739-746; 1989.

15. Butlin, P.A. Potential injury mechanisms to the climber's belayer. Brit. J. Sports Med. 19:188-191; 1985.

16. Cole, A.T. Fingertip injuries in rock climbers. Brit. J. Sports Med. 24:14; 1990.

17. Della Santa, D.R.; Kunz, A. Le syndrome de surcharge digitale lie a l'escalade sportive. Schweizerische Zeitschrift Fur Sportmedizin 38:5-9; 1990.

18. Ellis, S.R.; Walka, J.J. Biorhythmic patterns of victims of mountain climbing accidents. Psycholog. Rep. 53:612-614; 1983.

19. Foray, J.; Herry, J.P.; Vallet, J.H.; Lacoste, V.; Cote, D.; Cahen, C. Les accidents de montagne: Etude d'une statistique de 1819 observations. Chirurgie 108:724-733; 1982.

20. Garrido, E.; Castello, A.; Ventura, J.L.; Capdevila, A.; Rodriguez, F.A. Cortical atrophy and other brain magnetic resonance imaging (MRI) changes after extremely high-altitude climbs without oxygen. Int. J. Sports Med. 14:232-234; 1993.

21. Gentile, D.A.; Morris, J.A.; Schimelpfenig, T.; Bass, S.M.; Auerbach, P.S. Wilderness injuries and illnesses. Ann. Emerg. Med. 21:853-861; 1992.

22. Ghosh, A.; Ghosh, A. Ocular problems in mountaineering. J. Indian Med. Assoc. 80:98-100; 1983.

23. Hornbein, T.F. Long term effects of high altitude on brain function. Int. J. Sports Med. 13:S43-S45; 1992.

24. Hubicka, E. Rock climbing injuries sustained at the training centre in Cesky Raj [Cze]. Acta Chirurgiae Orthopaedicae Et Traumatologiae Cechoslovaca 44: 77-82; 1977.

25. Krakauer, J. Mean season on Denali. Outside August: 54-60, 121; 1992.

26. Kramer, A.F.; Coyne, J.T.; Strayer, D.L. Cognitive function at high altitude. Human factors 35:329-344; 1993.

27. Krueger, D.W.; Hutcherson, R. Suicide attempts by rock-climbing falls. Suicide and life-threatening behavior 8:41-45; 1978.

28. Magdefrau, H. Stress on the human body when falling into a rope harness and its sequelae. [German] Anthropologischer Anzeiger. 49:85-95; 1991.

29. Mason, G.W. Psychological aspects of mountain accidents. Northwest Medicine 1:35-38; 1969.

30. Mills, W.J., Jr. Frostbite: A discussion of the problem and a review of an Alaskan experience. Alaska Med. 15:27-59; 1973.

31. Mitchell, R.G. Mountain experience—The psychology and sociology of adventure. Chicago: University of Chicago Press; 1983.

32. McLennan, J.G.; Ungersma, J. Mountaineering accidents in the Sierra Nevada. American Journal of Sports Medicine 11:160-163; 1983.

33. Oberli, H. Der Burgunfall, alpines Rettungswesen. Z. Unfallmed Berufskr. 74:3-9; 1981.

34. Pollard, A.; Clarke, C. Deaths during mountaineering at extreme altitude [letter]. Lancet 1:1277; 1988.

35. Reid, W.A.; Doyle, D.; Richmond, H.G.; Galbraith, S.L. Necropsy study of mountaineering accidents in Scotland. J. Clin. Path. 39:1217-1220; 1986.

36. Richon, C.A. Notre experience chirurgicale en batiere de blesses de la montagne en 1978 et 1979. Zeitschrift fur Unfallmedizin und Berufskrankheitin 74:27-28; 1981.

37. Schussman, L.C.; Lutz, L.J. Mountaineering and rock climbing accidents. Physician and Sportsmedicine 10:53-61; 1982.

38. Schussman, L.C.; Lutz, L.J.; Shaw, R.R.; Bohnn, C.R. The epidemiology of mountaineering and rock climbing accidents. J. Wilderness Med. 1:235-248; 1990.

39. Shea, K.G.; Shea, O.F.; Meals, R.A. Manual demands and consequences of rock climbing. J. Hand Surg. 17A:200-205; 1992.

40. Singh, K.G.; Singh, R.G.; Girgla, H.S.; Usha, M.D. Incidence of sunburn during mountaineering expedition. J. Sports Med. 26:369-372; 1986.

41. Strang, P.J.H. Death due to exposure to cold in the New Zealand Mountains. N.Z. Med. J. 69:4-11; 1969.

42. Tomczak, R.L.; Wilshire, W.M.; Lane, J.W.; Jones, D.C. Injury patterns in rock climbers. J. Osteopath. Sports Med. 3:11-16; 1989.

43. Williams, E.S.; Taggart, P.; Carruthers, M. Rock climbing: Observations on heart rate and plasma catecholamine concentrations and the influence of oxprenolol. Brit. J. Sports Med. 12:125-128; 1978.

44. Wilson, R.; Mills, W.J., Jr.; Rodgers, D.R.; Propst, M.T. Death on Denali. West. J. Med. 128:471-476; 1978.

# 21

# Rodeo

*Robert Nebergall*

## 1. Introduction

Rodeo has experienced a growth spurt in popularity with fans, numbers of participants, and number of rodeos. It is a physically demanding sport in which the possibilities of injury loom constantly. This chapter, the first review of rodeo injury literature, will describe incidence, characteristics, location, severity, and risk factors of rodeo injuries as reported in the literature. Suggestions for injury prevention and further research will be presented. As rodeo continues to grow, more health care providers will be called upon to care for the rodeo athlete. The goal, then, for this chapter is to make available to the health care provider desperately needed information and to stimulate more contributions to the rodeo literature.

Rodeo as a competitive sport evolved from the working lifestyles of cowboys from the Old West. The cowboy developed roping and riding skills that they required to tend great herds of cattle on the open range. Competition developed between ranch hands (cowboys) and later between ranches to test who had the best cowboy skills. Although the working American cowboy flourished for a brief period from the mid-1860s to the mid-1880s, his friendly competitions have stayed with us in what we know as rodeo. Today, rodeo is an organized and highly competitive sport that experiences nationwide and limited international participation. Rodeos are organized at the high school, collegiate, and professional levels. Saddle bronc riding, bareback bronc riding, bull riding, team roping, calf roping, steer wrestling, and women's barrel racing are the events that comprise a rodeo. Women's rodeo is becoming very popular with their unique variations of the above events. The rodeo clowns perform bullfighting to protect the bull riders during and after dismount. Rodeo events are divided into two groups: rough stock and timed events. Judges score the ride at the successful completion of an 8-second ride. The 100 points are divided equally between the cowboy and the animal. Two judges each have 25 cowboy and 25 animal points available to them when scoring the ride. Timed events include team roping, calf roping, steer wrestling, and barrel racing. The time to complete the event is used as the score. Although bullfighters or rodeo clowns are not scored for their performances during rodeos, they are entrusted with the bull riders' lives.

We collected data from published articles and two articles in consideration for publication. These were identified using the ancestry approach and computer searches. We searched Medline database from 1983 to 1993 with rodeo, injury, and cowboy as the key words.

As demonstrated by the brief bibliography for this chapter, there is a severe paucity of literature on rodeo injuries. Of the studies published all are retrospective, with Nebergall and Meyers reporting injuries in relationship to exposures. The case reports and single injury studies will be described in the appropriate sections.

## 2. Incidence of Injury

### 2.1 Injury Rates

Injury rates in rodeo have been reported at the collegiate (8) and professional levels (3, 4, 11). They have been described as a percentage of contestants injured (Tables 21.1, 21.2), a ratio of exposure to injury (Table 21.3), and an injury per exposure percentage (Table 21.1), or more correctly described as injury exposure ratio.

**Table 21.1 Injury per Exposure Percentage of Rodeo Performers at the International Finals Rodeo, 1987 to 1992**

| Event | Number of participants | Number injured | Number of injuries | Percentage injured | Number of individual performances | Injury per exposure percentage[a] |
|---|---|---|---|---|---|---|
| Bull riding | 90 | 35 | 36 | 39 | 447 | 8.1 |
| Bareback bronc riding | 90 | 26 | 28 | 29 | 441 | 6.3 |
| Saddle bronc riding | 90 | 13 | 14 | 14 | 445 | 3.1 |
| Steer wrestling | 90 | 4 | 4 | 4 | 450 | 0.9 |
| Bullfighting (clowns) | 18 | 4 | 4 | 22 | 477 | 0.8 |
| Calf roping | 90 | 2 | 2 | 2.2 | 450 | 0.4 |
| Barrel racing | 90 | 2 | 2 | 2.2 | 450 | 0.4 |
| Team roping | 180 | 0 | 0 | 0 | 900 | 0 |
| Total | 738 | 86 | 90 | 11.7 | 4,060 | |

[a]This may be better described as injury exposure ratio.

**Table 21.2 Rodeo Injuries by Event**

| Event | Number of participants | Number injured | Percentage injured | Number of injuries | Percentage of total injuries |
|---|---|---|---|---|---|
| Bull riding | 40 | 18 | 45 | 20 | 32.8 |
| Saddle bronc riding | 40 | 12 | 30 | 13 | 21.3 |
| Bareback bronc riding | 40 | 12 | 30 | 13 | 21.3 |
| Steer wrestling | 40 | 5 | 12.5 | 5 | 8.2 |
| Calf roping | 40 | 4 | 10 | 5 | 8.2 |
| Bullfighting (clowns) | 8 | 3 | 37.5 | 4 | 6.6 |
| Team roping | 40 | 1 | 2.5 | 1 | 1.6 |
| Barrel racing | 40 | 0 | 0 | 0 | 0 |
| Total | 278[a] | 55 | — | 61 | 100.0 |

[a]Actual total was 278, as some participants competed in more than one event.

**Table 21.3 Collegiate Rodeo Injuries by Event**

| Event | Athlete exposures | Injuries | Percent of total injuries | Ratio of exposure to injury |
|---|---|---|---|---|
| Rough stock | 634 | 110 | 79.7 | 6:1 |
| Steer wrestling | 323 | 17 | 12.3 | 19:1 |
| Roping | 1,182 | 9 | 6.5 | 131:1 |
| Barrel racing | 1,153 | 2 | 1.5 | 577:1 |
| Total | 3,292 | 138 | 100.0 | 24:1 |

A rodeo may have one or several "go-rounds," or performances. A performance or go-round typically includes all seven rodeo events. During rodeos that include more than one go-round, a contestant may make several "rides" in one or more events. Describing the injury rate as a percentage of contestants injured at a rodeo does not give a clear picture of the incidence of injury if there is more than one go-round. Reporting injuries as an occurrence per exposure (one exposure equals one ride) develops data better suited for comparisons between events, rodeos, and other sports.

Injury rates appear dramatically higher for participants in the rough stock events than the timed events. Bullfighters experienced injury rates approaching rough stock contestant rates.

## 2.2 Reinjury Rates

Although no published data is available for reinjury in rodeo, it probably represents the most common type of injury. There is no injured reserve in professional rodeo. The cowboy historically has not sought medical attention for injuries, although this trend is slowly changing. The rodeo athlete typically spends a great deal of time traveling long distances to compete at numerous rodeos. They are not salaried, and their income is dependent on winning or placing at rodeos. These factors are incompatible with the appropriate treatment and rehabilitation of injuries. Injuries such as hyperextended elbows in bareback bronc riders and adductor strains in bull riders may become chronic or "nagging" and ultimately end the rodeo athlete's career. Meyers (8) reported that his results included acute as well as reinjury. He felt the chronic or repetitive injuries resulted from repetitive overload and time exposure to musculoskeletal microtrauma. Future research should include establishing injury and reinjury rates. Medical personnel present at rodeos should make themselves available for diagnosis and treatment of chronic as well as acute injuries.

## 2.3 Injury Rates in Practice vs. Competition

Injury rates in rodeo have only recently been reported (8, 11). No information on injury rates in practice is available and may represent an area for future research.

## 2.4 Specific Injury Types

Bauer has described a hand injury pattern that appears to be unique to the riding hand of bareback bronc riders (1). He reported an increase in palm diameter with enlargement of the first metacarpal phalangeal joint. The increase in hand size may be due to soft tissue hypertrophy with minimal bony involvement. This is due to the repetitive trauma caused by the hand in the bareback rigging and its compressive configuration.

# 3. Injury Characteristics

## 3.1 Injury Onset

The majority of rodeo injury literature reports acute injuries, and we will describe this in the sections on injury type and injury location. Although relatively unreported, chronic/overuse injuries are very common in rodeo. Meyers (9) may have best described this as "the lack of on site preventive care and education, leading to inadequate self treatment." Common overuse/chronic injuries include elbow hyperextension and groin pulls in the rough stock events. Steer wrestlers are commonly seen sporting knee braces for chronic laxity, patella

femoral pain, and meniscal injuries. Claussen (2) reported ulnar hypertrophy secondary to repetitive trauma in a bareback bronc rider. Nebergall described acute or chronic injuries involving a tibia fracture and an anterior cruciate deficient knee (11).

## 3.2 Injury Type

The information for Table 21.4 was compiled from data reported in rodeo injury studies by Griffin (4), Meyers (8), and Nebergall (11). Nebergall and Griffin described data gathered by on-site observation and examination, and Meyers reported data obtained "second hand."

Contusions, sprains, and strains were the three most commonly reported injuries at the professional and collegiate levels, with the majority of injuries occurring in the rough stock events. Of these injuries, 70% (11) occurred during the dismount, which may account for the frequency of sprains, strains, and contusions.

Collegiate rodeo athletes experienced concussions with the same frequency as sprains and strains. Fractures and dislocations each represented less than 10% of the total injuries reported in all studies.

Hand and finger injuries from team roping are common at both the competitive and recreational level but have been rarely reported. Team ropers injure or amputate fingers while "dallying," pinching the finger against the saddle horn with the rope. Tooth loss has been reported in bull riding (11). The extremely rare condition of burning hand syndrome has been described in a bareback bronc rider (12). The symptomatology was due to a herniated cervical disc.

Rodeo shares common mechanisms of injury with other collision sports but has several unique,

**Table 21.4   Percent Comparison of Injury Types**

| Injury | Collegiate Meyers | Professional | | |
|---|---|---|---|---|
| | | Griffin & Peterson | Nebergall | Range |
| Contusion | 42.0 | 36.0 | 21.0 | 21.0-36.0 |
| Sprain | 10.9 | 19.6 | 35.5 | 19.6-35.5 |
| Strain | 15.9 | 19.6 | 12.2 | 12.2-19.6 |
| Laceration | 3.6 | 6.5 | 5.5 | 5.5-6.5 |
| Fracture | 3.6 | 6.5 | 8.8 | 6.5-8.8 |
| Abrasion | 8.7 | 4.9 | — | |
| Concussion | 13.8 | 4.9 | 7.7 | 4.9-7.7 |
| Dislocation | 1.5 | 1.6 | 8.8 | 1.6-8.8 |

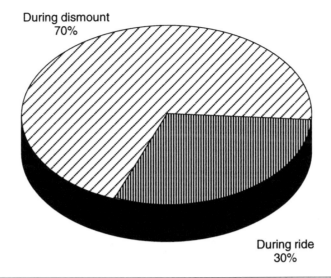

During dismount
70%

During ride
30%

**Figure 21.1**  Rough stock injuries.

sport specific mechanisms. Bareback bronc riders can "hang up" in the bareback rigging when the cowboy falls off "into his hand." In this situation the hand is acutely flexed over the top of the rigging handle, trapping the hand. When the cowboy is thrown "away" from his hand, the fingers and wrist are in extension allowing the hand to disengage from the rigging. Bull riders also hang up in their rigging, a rope wrapped around the bull's chest. At greatest risk for injury is the "hang up" bull rider who falls into the "well," the well being the center of the spin of a spinning bronc or bull. Saddle bronc riders may "blow a stirrup" (stirrup breaks) and lose their "seat" (bucked off). "Rigging and riding" describes other mechanisms of injury sustained during the ride because of equipment problems and/or trauma.

### 3.3 Injury Location

Information from retrospective rodeo injury studies was used to create the percent comparison of injury location seen in Table 21.5 (4, 8, 11).

The authors obtained data for the professional rodeo studies on-site as they observed the occurrence and then treated the injury. Information for the collegiate study was obtained from the athletes' postparticipation recollections and from records. Data obtained first hand will be most reliable because it avoids memory and interpretation of the records. In all studies the injury breakdown was evenly divided among the three categories of head/spine/trunk, upper extremity, and lower extremity. Head and neck injuries were the most common injury in the head/spine/trunk category.

**Table 21.5  Percent Comparison of Injury Location**

| Injury location | Collegiate Meyers | Professional Griffin & Peterson | Nebergall | Range |
|---|---|---|---|---|
| Head | (16.6) | (11.3) | (13.2) | |
|   Skull | 16.6 | 8.1 | 7.7 | 7.7-8.1 |
|   Face | — | 1.6 | 4.4 | 1.6-4.4 |
|   Teeth | — | 1.6 | 1.1 | 1.1-1.6 |
| Spine/trunk | (19.4) | (14.6) | (26.5) | |
|   Neck | — | 3.2 | 10.0 | 3.2-10.0 |
|   Upper back | — | — | 1.1 | |
|   Lower back | 5.0 | 4.9 | 6.6 | 4.9-6.6 |
|   Ribs | 14.4 | 6.5 | 7.7 | 6.5-7.7 |
|   Stomach | — | — | 1.1 | |
| Upper extremity | (30.2) | (44.0) | (33.1) | |
|   Shoulder | 10.1 | 8.1 | 7.7 | 7.7-8.1 |
|   Arm | — | 1.6 | 2.2 | 1.6-2.2 |
|   Elbow | 6.5 | 14.8 | 12.2 | 12.2-14.8 |
|   Forearm | 0.7 | 4.9 | — | |
|   Wrist | 2.8 | 3.2 | 3.3 | 3.2-3.3 |
|   Hand/finger | 10.1 | 11.4 | 7.7 | 7.7-11.4 |
| Lower extremity | (33.9) | (31.0) | (26.4) | |
|   Pelvis/hip | 5.8 | 9.8 | 3.3 | 3.3-9.8 |
|   Thigh | 3.6 | 4.9 | 1.1 | 1.1-4.9 |
|   Knee | 10.1 | 4.9 | 5.5 | 4.9-5.5 |
|   Leg | 8.0 | 6.5 | 2.2 | 2.2-6.5 |
|   Ankle | 5.7 | — | 11.0 | |
|   Heel/achilles | — | — | — | |
|   Foot/toe | 0.7 | 4.9 | 3.3 | 3.3-4.9 |

The most commonly injured body part in the upper extremity category was the shoulder in collegiate rodeo athletes and the elbow in the professionals. The knee was the most frequently injured in the lower extremity category.

### 3.3.1 Head/Spine/Trunk

Although most injuries occur during the dismount, this category represents injuries that typically occur during the ride in the rough stock events. Tremendous forces are generated through the head and spine as the animal jumps, twists, kicks, and turns trying to dislodge the cowboy. During the ride there can be violent whipping motions of the spine creating sprain, muscle spasm, and occasionally intervertebral disc rupture. The cumulative effect of this whiplash has motivated several bronc riders to wear neck braces during the ride for their chronic cervical strains. The dismount, whether premature or at the end of the 8-second ride, exposes the head and spine to injury. Concussions typically occur during the dismount, from a blow by the animal or landing on the head. The ribs and face are susceptible to contusions and lacerations from the animal and dismount.

### 3.3.2 Upper Extremity

Competitors in the rough stock events attempt to ride an animal for 8 seconds. The upper extremity is susceptible to injury because the athlete uses it to stay aboard. Injuries to the upper extremity are very common in the bull riding and bareback bronc events. Bull riders wrap their riding hand to the bull through the rigging, and bareback bronc riders wedge their riding hand into a handle on the rigging. Forces several times the rodeo athlete's body weight are generated across the upper extremity as the rider tries to stay on board. The combination of force and relatively rigid anchoring of the upper extremity to the animal sets the stage for injury in this event. In the professional ranks, Griffin and Nebergall (3, 4, 11) reported the elbow is the most commonly injured upper extremity part. Meyers (8) reported the shoulder and hand to be injured equally and most commonly in the upper extremity in collegiate rodeo athletes. The second and third most commonly injured areas of the upper extremity in professional rodeo athletes were the shoulder and hand. The wrist, forearm, and arm were a distant fourth, fifth, and sixth. Collegiate rodeo athletes experienced elbow injuries as the third most common upper extremity injury followed by wrist and forearm injuries.

### 3.3.3 Lower Extremity

Although most rodeo events require "riding" an animal, lower extremity injuries are quite common. Lower extremity injuries represented approximately one third of the injuries when evaluated by body location. The injury distribution was similar at the professional and collegiate levels. The lower extremity is injured during the dismount or when struck by an animal, the ground, a barrel, or the chutes. Groin pulls occur as the athlete strains the adductors attempting to remain on the animal. Pelvis/hips body location including groin pulls varied as a percentage of total injuries from study to study. Meyers reported 5.8% at the collegiate level; Griffin and Peterson reported 9.8% at the professional level; and Nebergall reported 3.3% at the elite professional level. The knee was frequently injured; however, at the professional level, the percentage of total injuries was half the collegiate level rate of 10.1%. Nebergall reported the ankle injuries at 11% at the elite professional level, and Griffin and Peterson reported no ankle injuries in their study of professional rodeo injuries.

## 4. Injury Severity

### 4.1 Time Loss

No studies are available describing the time lost from competition by rodeo athletes because of injury, and this represents an opportunity for further study.

### 4.2 Catastrophic Injuries

Although no catastrophic injuries have been reported in the literature during rodeo competition, deaths rarely occur. Bull riders have been killed, usually by being stepped on by the bull after being thrown.

### 4.3 Clinical Outcome/Residual Symptoms

Nebergall (11) reported that 8 of the 90 injuries treated from 1987 to 1992 at the International Finals Rodeo were severe enough for the athlete to end their competition at that Finals. A 9% injury rate that temporarily stopped competition is not an accurate reflection of the injury severity. What it does reflect is the extreme physical and mental toughness, commitment, and drive of the rodeo athlete (9). An example is the athlete who returns to competition against medical advice after reduction for a shoulder dislocation. In addition to this devotion by the rodeo athlete, two other factors contribute to why they continue to compete with severe injuries. One is the mentality of the rodeo athlete participating in a sport long on heritage and deep with tradition and unwritten protocol. The other is that there is no injured reserve list, worker's compensation, or unemployment benefits at the professional level. This is a hardcore example of the work ethic.

## 5. Injury Risk Factors

### 5.1 Intrinsic Factors

#### 5.1.1 Physical Characteristics

No reports are available describing physical characteristics of the rodeo athlete as they relate to injury risk factors. General somatotypes are found in each of the rodeo events (6). Bronc riders, calf ropers, and barrel racers are typically mesomorphs. Bull doggers are usually endomorphs, and ectomorph best describes bull riders, saddle bronc riders, and team ropers.

#### 5.1.2 Motor/Functional Characteristics

Again no literature was identified relating motor/functional characteristics to injury risk, and this too represents an area for future study.

#### 5.1.3 Psychosocial Characteristics

McGill (5) has studied the personality characteristics of professional rodeo cowboys. He described his subjects as "relatively alert, enthusiastic, and forthright individuals who tend to be reality based, self sufficient, and of a practical bent. There is a degree of drivenness and striving present." He described a relative elevation in internal attribution of health and associated this with successful rehabilitation after injury. Therefore, it becomes a factor in an athlete's ability to perform successfully in a sport where risk of injury is significant. Meyers (10) reported on psychological characterization of the collegiate rodeo athlete. He described intercollegiate rodeo participants as being "higher in vigor and lower in depression, fatigue, confusion, and total mood disturbance as determined through POMS when compared to the norms." Meyers (7) also reported "non-perceptualization of inherent injury reported by Endler among younger competitors may also extend to the collegiate age group as well, or observations may simply be specific to this type of sport athlete."

### 5.2 Extrinsic Factors

#### 5.2.1 Training Methods or Conditions

No studies have been reported on training as a factor in injury risk. Tuza (13) presented a program for flexibility and a general exercise prescription. He also discussed training for endurance, agility, and speed. This article should be standard reading for the health care provider involved with the rodeo athlete.

#### 5.2.2 Environment

The environment in which rodeo is conducted varies widely. Rodeos are held both indoors and outdoors. The arena floor varies considerably from hard to soft and dry to mud. It may also be well-worked dirt. Although not studied or reported, the playing surface represents a factor in injury risk. The chutes and arena fence are exposed metal on which the rodeo athlete may become injured.

#### 5.2.3 Equipment

Rodeo equipment and clothing are dictated to the rodeo athlete by rules and tradition. Protective pads and bracing have experienced limited exposure in rodeo.

## 6. Suggestions for Injury Prevention

Sports medicine education is paramount for injury prevention in rodeo. Unlike participants in team sports such as football, basketball, baseball, and so forth, many rodeo athletes have not been exposed through the training room, coaches, and team physicians to injury care and prevention.

Meyers (7) recommended developing event-specific training protocols. Year-round training in strength, flexibility, agility, speed, and endurance tailored to the lifestyle and competition requirements of rodeo will intuitively help with injury prevention and especially reinjury.

Meyers (8) has recommended increased use of orthotics for injury prevention. Elbow taping and bracing will help prevent elbow hyperextension injury and protect the joint from reinjury. Wrist taping should help prevent sprains in the rough stock events. Knee braces for steer wrestlers may help protect this joint from the chronic and acute injuries sustained in this event. Forearm pads and rib braces will protect these injury-susceptible areas from trauma. Nebergall (12) has described a cervical orthosis to prevent neck hyperextension in bareback bronc riding. A soft arena floor and appropriately padded chutes and arenas should soften the blow from falls and decrease the incidence of this mechanism of injury. "Flak" jackets are becoming very popular with bull riders. They utilize protective materials such as Kevlar and high density foam in a leather vest. This protects the thorax and abdomen from horns and hooves.

Access to health care providers for education and treatment in the rodeo arena and off-site should be a great help in injury prevention.

## 7. Suggestions for Further Research

After a review of the bibliography and the brevity of this chapter, it is apparent that opportunity for further research is wide open in rodeos.

I would encourage all health care providers covering a rodeo to keep records of the injuries that occurred. The following are recommendations for gathering and reporting rodeo injury data that is cross study comparable.

- Label the injury type using the standard nomenclature presented in this chapter and identify the body part location.
- Record the mechanism of injury and treatment rendered. It is important to determine the injury to exposure ratio and not simply document the percent of participants injured.
- Talk about and record the participant's old and chronic injuries. Find out how long they were out of competition, how the injury was treated, and what treatments did and did not work.
- Discuss with the rodeo athlete any brace, pad, warm-up routine, and so forth, and find out their rationale behind it and if it's effective. Save these discussions for postcompetition.
- Attend the same rodeo year after year to develop significant data.
- Injuries observed first hand provide better information than injuries reported second hand.

## References

1. Bauer, J.M.; Nebergall, R.W.; Eimen, R.M. Bareback Bronc Hand. In consideration for publication.
2. Claussen, B.F. Chronic hypertrophy of the ulna in the professional rodeo cowboy. Clin. Orthop. Related Research. 164:45-57; 1982.
3. Griffin, R.; Peterson, K.D.; Halseth, J.R. Injuries in professional rodeo. Phys. Sportsmed. 11(8):111-116; 1983.
4. Griffin, R.; Peterson, K.D.; Halseth, J.R. Injuries in professional rodeo: An update. Phys. Sportsmed. 15(2):104-115; 1987.
5. McGill, J.C.; Hall, J.R.; Ratlitt, W.R., et al. Personality of professional rodeo cowboys. J. Sports Behav. 9:143-151; 1986.
6. Medved, R. Body height and predisposition for certain sports. J. Sports Med. 6:89-91; 1966.
7. Meyers, M.C.; Elledge, J.R., et al. Exercise performance of collegiate rodeo athletes. Am. J. Sports Med. 20:410-415; 1992.
8. Meyers, M.C.; Elledge, J.R.; Sterling, J.C., et al. Injuries in intercollegiate rodeo athletes. Am. J. Sports Med. 18:87-91; 1990.
9. Meyers, M.C.; LeUnes, A.D.; Elledge, J.R., et al. Precompetitive mood state changes in collegiate rodeo athletes. J. Sport Behav. 13:114-121; 1990.
10. Meyers, M.C.; Sterling, J.C.; LeUnes, A.D. Psychological characterization of the collegiate rodeo athlete. J. Sport Behav. 11:59-65; 1988.
11. Nebergall, R.W.; Wilson, G. Burning hand syndrome in a bareback bronc rider. In consideration for publication.
12. Nebergall, R.W.; Bauer, J.M.; Eimen, R.M. Rough riders, how much risk in rodeo. Phys. Sportsmed. 20(10):85-92; 1992.
13. Tuza, G. Training considerations for rodeo. Natl. Strength Cond. Assoc. J. 6:38-41; 1985.
14. Wilkinson, J.G.; Meyers, M.C. Isokinetic leg strength and power in collegiate rodeo athletes. J. Strength Cond. Research 7(1):22-25; 1993.

# 22

# Running

## Kathleen Knutzen and Lawrence Hart

## 1. Introduction

Participation in running has increased over the past decade. As a result, there has also been an increase in the reported number of running-related injuries (36). In 1982, Koplan et al. (106) reported 17.1 million runners in the United States. They projected that one out of three would sustain an injury, and that one in ten would require medical attention per running year. Jacobs and associates in 1986 (94) estimated the number of runners to be 30 million, with 10 million projected to be running regularly, and 800,000 to 1 million participating in competitive races. It was projected in 1988 that 11% of the country's adults participated in running (209).

Because of the indirect link between the performance of running and a specific injury, running poses a special problem for medical professionals who treat or suggest preventive actions for the reduction of running injuries. The majority of injuries in running are attributable to overuse of the musculoskeletal system (232). A runner strikes the ground approximately 1,000 to 1,500 times per mile with forces of 2 to 3 times body weight (149, 232). Some runners tolerate this repeated cyclic loading of the body better than others. An injury can be caused by intrinsic or extrinsic factors that interfere with the runner's ability to withstand the repeated loading or that change the nature of the load itself (132).

This chapter presents the pertinent epidemiological literature on running injuries from 1975 to the present. Specifically, we reviewed the various studies to identify and summarize injury rates, injury type and location, and injury risk factors for running. Because running long distances has also been shown to interfere with certain bodily functions, we reviewed and summarized reports on

systemic alterations such as those seen in the gastrointestinal tract. Finally, we summarized suggestions for injury prevention and suggestions for future research using relevant sources from the literature.

We extracted the information utilized in this chapter from English articles found in journals, textbooks, proceedings, and published reports. We initially identified the articles through two computer searches for the years 1975 to the present. Two searches were conducted on the Sport Discus and Medline using the key words running and injury. Additional references were obtained from the articles themselves, review articles, and from textbook literature reviews.

The original reference list was extensive. Many articles on running injuries were written for the runner and contained practical information or general suggestions on running. We summarized articles in the present analysis if they contained injury data or statistics, or if they provided speculative information on risks associated with injury or ideas for the prevention of running injuries. We included a few review articles because of their reference to injury epidemiology.

The literature on running injuries presented in this chapter must be evaluated in light of the following strengths and weaknesses:

- Most articles on running injuries are case reports and case series. These studies may provide good information about the relative frequency of injury but they offer no robust information about specific factors (257). Such studies limit comparisons of running injuries within a group, because injury rates are calculated with reference to numbers of injured runners and do not account for all runners in a specific population. No absolute or relative risk can be calculated with these types of studies (257). Since preventive measures can only be prescribed if the etiology of the injury is identified, case series designs do not offer enough information for prevention prescription (246).

• The number of retrospective studies on running injuries are limited, and prospective studies are rare. The retrospective design offers good information on the relative risk of running injury and can be used to identify runners who are at a high risk of injury. However, the design does not allow for the computation of absolute risks (257) that can be obtained with a prospective study.

• Data collection is another weakness in running injury research. The most common data collection technique is the questionnaire, which is administered before or after a marathon or road race. The questionnaire is an instrument that is influenced by recall bias, motivational factors, and response rate. Injury rates are calculated retrospectively from self-report information extracted from the questionnaire.

• Few analytical studies on running attempt to identify and interpret different factors contributing to injury.

• The running injury literature, in most cases, does not distinguish between levels of running experience, and, as a result, information on elite, competitive, and recreational runners is usually combined.

• Running injury data on males and females are commonly combined, reducing the information on comparing injury characteristics between the sexes.

• It is difficult to compare studies and determine averages because of the inconsistencies in the techniques used in the various designs.

• A comparison of different injury types across studies is also limited by the lack of conformity in defining injuries. Hoeberigs (81) has identified several definitions of injury: ailment or pain, musculoskeletal, attributed to running, caused a reduction in running, or caused a visit to a health professional or use of medication. With no standardized definition of a running injury, it is difficult to make comparisons across studies.

• Most running injury studies are limited to very specific populations participating in marathons or road races. This limits the application of the results to a specific type of runner and does not address the risk of running across a larger population. There are no studies that have examined injury risk in the runner who runs but who does not compete in marathons or road races. Likewise, the case series designs only evaluate runners

who come to a physician or sports medicine clinic and do not consider runners who are injured and do not seek treatment. Consequently, running injury studies are negatively affected by sampling bias and nonrandom selection of participants.

• One strength of the running injury studies is the common involvement of physicians or other medical personnel in the assessment and reporting of running injuries. Medical personnel who work on a daily basis with injured runners write most case series and case reports. This has strengthened the diagnosis of running injuries.

## 2. Incidence of Injury

### 2.1 Injury Rates

Injury rates for specific running populations are presented in Tables 22.1, 22.2, and 22.3. These data have been extracted from both retrospective and prospective studies. Injury rates presented in these studies should be interpreted with the following limitations in mind:

• Injuries are typically reported for a specific time period using a questionnaire. Recall biases and the subjectivity of the participants' reports may influence this form of data collection.
• The number of participants in each study is reduced by the response rate of the participants, leaving a significant number of participants who do not respond and thereby, skew the injury statistics.
• Very few studies address the risks and incidence of running for entire populations. There was only one such study identified (46).
• Injury rates are presented for a specific time period with little reference to differences in exposure of an athlete to injury, for example, mileage run per week, days of running per week, types of training.

Because of the great variation in data collection techniques and protocol design, it is difficult to summarize injury rates. Given these restrictions, the data are presented within the framework of the different study designs.

• The annual incidence of injured runners ranged from 48 to 65% in the prospective studies and 24 to 60% in the retrospective ones. Additionally, there are very short term retrospective studies collected over the course of one marathon (38, 169, 243) that present incidences of injured runners in

**Table 22.1    A Comparison of Injury Rates in Running**

| Study | Design Pros/ret | Data collection Inter/ques | Duration inj. survey | # partic. | # of injured athletes | # of inj. athletes/N | Annual rate of inj. ath/N | # of injuries/N | Sex |
|---|---|---|---|---|---|---|---|---|---|
| Prospective studies | | | | | | | | | |
| Bovens et al., 1989 | P | I | 18-20 months | 115[a] | 62 | 0.54 | 0.29-.36 | 1.51 | — |
| Lysholm & Wiklander, 1987 | P | — | 1 year | 60[b] | 39 | 0.65 | 0.65 | 0.92 | M:44 F:16 |
| Macera et al., 1989 | P | | 1 year | 583 | 300 | 0.51 | 0.51 | — | M:485 F:98 |
| Ross & Schuster, 1983 | P | I | 5 years | 63 | 34 | 0.54 | 0.11 | 0.40 | — |
| Walter et al., 1989 | P | Q | 1 year | 1,288[c] | 620 | 0.48 | 0.48 | 0.56 | M:985 F:303 |
| *Range: Prospective studies* | | | | | | 0.48-0.65 | 0.11-0.65 | 0.40-1.51 | |
| Retrospective studies | | | | | | | | | |
| Blair et al., 1987 | R | Q | 1 year | 438 | 105 | 0.24 | 0.24 | 0.24 | M:76% F:24% |
| Eggold, 1981 | R | Q | — | 146[d] | — | — | — | 1.03 | |
| Estok & Rudy, 1986 | R | Q | past | 57[e] | — | — | — | 1.8 | F |
| Henderson, 1975 | R | Q | — | > 1,000[f] | — | 0.60 | — | — | — |
| Holmich et al., 1988 | R | Q | 1 year | 60[g] | 26 | 0.43 | 0.43 | — | M:60 |
| Holmich et al., 1989 | R | Q | 1 year | 1,426[e] | 442 | 0.31 | 0.31 | 0.92 | M:1,310 F:116 |
| Hughes et al., 1985 | R | Q | — | 1,266[e] | 725 prev. 360 present | 0.57 0.28 | | — — | M:1,078 F:188 |
| Jacobs & Bersen, 1986 | R | Q | 2 years | 451[h] | 210 | 0.47 | 0.24 | — | M:355 F:96 |
| Koplan et al., 1982[a] | R | Q | 1 year | 1,423[e] | 498 | 0.37 | 0.37 | — | M:693 F:730 |
| Marti, 1988 | R | Q | 1 year | 428[i] | 172 | 0.40 | 0.40 | — | F |
| Marti et al., 1988 | R | Q | 1 year | 4,358[i] | 1,994 | 0.46 | 0.46 | — | M |
| Marti, 1989 | R | Q | 1 year | 4,786[i] | 2,166 | 0.45 | 0.45 | — | M:4,358 F:428 |
| Maughan, 1983 | R | Q | — | 497[e] | 287 | 0.58 | — | — | M:472 F:25 |
| McQuade, 1986 | — | Q | — | 214 | 96 | 0.45 | — | — | M:113 F:92 |
| Walter et al., 1988 | R | Q | 1 year | 476 | — | 0.57 | 0.57 | — | M:402 F:74 |
| Walter et al., 1989 | R | Q | 1 year retro & 1 year prosp | 1,288[c] | 637 | 0.50 | 0.50 | 0.56 | M:985 F:303 |
| *Range: Retrospective studies* | | | | | | 0.24-0.60 | 0.24-0.57 | 0.24-1.8 | |

[a]Limited or no running experience.

[b]Includes long distance, middle distance, and sprinters.

[c]Entrants in 4-km and 16-km runs.

[d]Recreational and competitive runners who wore orthotics.

[e]Entrants in a marathon.

[f]Respondents to a runner's survey.

[g]Danish national marathoners.

[h]Entrants in a 10,000-m run.

[i]Entrants in 16-km run.

**Table 22.2    A Comparison of Injury Rates in Running for Males**

| Study | Design Pros/Ret | Data collection Inter/Quest. | Duration inj. survey | # participants | # of injured athletes | # of inj. athletes/N | # of injuries/N |
|---|---|---|---|---|---|---|---|
| Prospective studies | | | | | | | |
| Macera et al., 1989 | P | | 1 year | 485[a] | 252 | 0.52 | 0.52 |
| Walter et al., 1989 | P & R | Q | 1 year retro & 1 year prosp | 985 | 483 P[c] | 0.49 P[c] | 0.49 |
| *Range: Prospective studies* | | | | | | 0.49-0.52 | 0.49-0.52 |
| Retrospective studies | | | | | | | |
| Koplan et al., 1982 | R | Q | 1 year | 693[b] | — | 0.37 | 0.37 |
| Marti et al., 1988 | R | Q | 1 year | 4,358[a] | 1,994 | 0.46 | 0.46 |
| Walter et al., 1988 | R | Q | 1 year | 402 | — | 0.56 | 0.56 |
| *Range: Retrospective studies* | | | | | | 0.37-0.56 | 0.37-0.56 |

[a]Entrants in a 16-km run.

[b]Entrants in a marathon.

[c]P = prospective.

**Table 22.3    A Comparison of Injury Rates in Running for Females**

| Study | Design Pros/Ret | Data collection Inter/Quest. | Duration inj. survey | # participants | # of injured athletes | # of inj. athletes/N | # of injuries/N |
|---|---|---|---|---|---|---|---|
| Prospective studies | | | | | | | |
| Macera et al., 1989 | P | | 1 year | 98 | 48 | 0.49 | 0.49 |
| Walter et al., 1989 | P & R[c] | Q | 1 year retro & 1 year prosp | 303 | 137 P 70 New | 0.46 P[a] 0.23 N[b] | 0.46 |
| *Range: Prospective studies* | | | | | | 0.46-0.49 | 0.46-0.49 |
| Retrospective studies | | | | | | | |
| Estok & Rudy, 1986 | R | Q | — | 57 | — | — | 1.8 |
| Koplan et al., 1982 | R | Q | 1 year | 730 | — | 0.38 | 0.38 |
| Marti, 1988 | R | Q | 1 year | 428 | 172 | 0.40 | 0.40 |
| Walter et al., 1988 | R | Q | 1 year | 74 | — | 0.53-62.5 | 0.53 -62.5 |
| Walter et al., 1989 | P & R[c] | Q | 1 year retro & 1 year prosp | 303 | 137 P 70 New | 0.46 P[a] 0.23 N[b] | 0.46 |
| *Range: Retrospective studies* | | | | | | 0.38-0.63 | 0.38-1.8 |

[a]P = prospective.

[b]N = new injuries at a race.

[c]R = retrospective.

the range of 8 to 23%. A study involving injured runners within a total city population yielded an incidence of only 5% (46). Most studies report the number of injured runners rather than the incidence rate for injuries. In a review of running injuries, Van Mechelen (246) reported various incidence rates ranging from 24 to 77% and annual incidence rates of 37 to 56%. For those studies that report the incidence rate of actual injuries, the injury rate is increased. This is demonstrated by the average incidence rate ranging from 40 to 151% in the prospective studies and 24 to 180% in the retrospective evaluations (Table 22.1).

• The annual incidence appears similar between male and female runners, although this interpretation should be cautiously accepted considering the limited number of studies that present separate data for the sexes (See Tables 22.2 & 22.3). The annual incidence rate for males ranged from 49 to 52% for prospective studies and 37 to 56% for retrospective ones. Female injury rates ranged from 46 to 49% of runners in prospective studies and 38 to 63% of runners in those that were retrospective (Table 22.3). The annual incidence rate for males and females may be influenced by sampling biases, since the studies typically contained a disproportionately higher number of males. A similar risk of injury between male and female runners has been substantiated in the literature (130, 131, 194, 255), but there is contradictory evidence to support higher rates of injury in male runners (180) or in female runners (136, 158).

There is little information on injured adolescent runners. One prospective study (178) evaluated 48 adolescent runners and reported that 40% of the runners incurred an injury. In two retrospective studies evaluating 16 (174) and 40 (208) adolescents, 25 and 18% of the adolescent runners reported injuries. Adolescent running injuries were reported to be lower than that seen for their adult counterparts.

# 3. Injury Characteristics

## 3.1 Injury Onset

While the onset of running injuries has not been extensively studied, there is some consensus that injuries develop gradually. Little or no distinction is made between acute and chronic injuries, and most injuries are considered to result from some cumulative effect of repetitive loading of the body during each running cycle. It has been suggested that injuries may develop slowly over time or result from one severe training session (239).

## 3.2 Injury Type

A comparison of injury types for adult runners, male runners, female runners, and adolescent runners is presented in Tables 22.4, 22.5, 22.6, and 22.7, respectively. These data were collected from prospective studies, retrospective studies, cross sectional, and case series data. These studies are summarized separately to distinguish between study designs, and data are reported as percentages of the total number of injured athletes or injuries regardless of study design. The section on injury type and location is an attempt to combine studies that report injury statistics using similar percentage calculations. There is still considerable variation in the classification of injury type or location, and these data should therefore be examined

with caution. Despite this major limitation, we have identified the following trends:

- Knee pain is the most reported injury for adult runners, regardless of gender, ranging from 12.7 to 29.5% of the injuries reported in the prospective studies, 17.0 to 32.0% in the retrospective studies, 23.2 to 40% in the cross-sectional data, and 5.0 to 41.7% in the case series studies (Table 22.4). The percentage of knee pain for males and females is similar: 14.0 to 41.0% for males and 14.0 to 50% for females according to the retrospective studies (see Tables 22.5 & 22.6). In adolescents, knee pain does not occur at the highest rate (11.3-19.5%) (Table 22.7).
- Tibial stress syndrome and knee pain was higher for females than males.
- The proportion of stress fractures also appear higher in females than males.
- In the adolescent runner, the most common injury types were strains, tibial stress syndrome, knee pain, apophyseal injuries, and tendinitis.

## 3.3 Injury Location

The percentage of injuries associated with anatomical locations is presented in Tables 22.8, 22.9, 22.10, and 22.11 for adult, male, female, and adolescent runners, respectively. The categories are derived from those commonly presented in retrospective, prospective, case series, and cross sectional studies on running injuries. The placement of an injury in these categories is not as variable across the studies as was the case for injury type, but considerable variability still exists. Given the limitations expressed earlier, the following observations are presented:

- Running-related injuries are primarily confined to the lower extremity and the low back.
- In adults, the knee is the area most often injured, followed by the leg (Table 22.8). Knee injury prevalence ranged from 12.7 to 29.5% in prospective studies, 23.0 to 31.7% in the retrospective studies, 26.0 to 38.2% in cross-sectional studies, and 14.2 to 41.7% in the case series.
- Adolescent runners tend to have more injuries in the knee and lower leg (Table 22.11).
- The location of injuries is similar between male and female runners (Tables 22.9 & 22.10). Females have slightly higher percentages of injury to the hip and groin, while males have slightly more injuries to the foot and ankle.

**Table 22.4  A Percent Comparison of Injury Types in Adult Runners**

| Study & study design (R, P, C, S)[a] | # partic. | Achilles tend. | Other tend. | Plantar fasciitis | IT band friction synd. | Nonspecific knee pain | Tibial stress synd. | Patello-femoral pain | Strain | Ankle sprain/strain | Low back/sciatica | Foot strain/sprain | Fracture | Bursitis |
|---|---|---|---|---|---|---|---|---|---|---|---|---|---|---|
| **Prospective studies** | | | | | | | | | | | | | | |
| Lysholm & Wiklander, 1987 P | 60 | 3.6 | 16.4 | 7.3 | 1.8 | 12.7 | 18.2 | 10.9 | 14.6 | 10.9 | 5.5 | 1.8 | — | 3.6 |
| Orava, 1978 P | 274 | 9.5 | 5.1 | 4.4 | 7.3 | 29.5 | 17.2 | — | — | | 2.6 | 4.7 | — | 3.6 |
| *Range: Prospective studies* | | 3.6-9.5 | 5.1-16.4 | 4.7-7.3 | 1.8-7.3 | 12.7-29.5 | 17.2-18.2 | | | | 2.6-5.5 | 1.8-4.7 | | |
| **Retrospective studies** | | | | | | | | | | | | | | |
| Hughes et al., 1985 R | 1,266 | 7.3 | — | — | — | 17.0 | 5.8 | — | 7.3 | 6.9 | 2.8 | 13.0 | — | — |
| Jacobs & Berson, 1986 R | 2,664 | 6.2 | — | 5.2 | — | 21.4 | 9.5 | — | — | 12.4 | — | — | — | — |
| Maughan, 1983 R | 497 | 11.0 | — | — | — | 32.0 | 6.0 | — | — | 12.0 | 3.0 | 13.0 | — | — |
| *Range: Retrospective studies* | | 6.2-11.0 | | | | 17.0-32.0 | 5.8-9.5 | | | 6.9-12.4 | 2.8-3.0 | | | |
| **Cross sectional studies** | | | | | | | | | | | | | | |
| Brubaker & James, 1974 S | 109 | — | 11.9 | — | — | — | 2.0 | 14.7 | 33.1 | — | 1.8 | — | 15.6 | 1.8 |
| Clough et al., 1987 S | 502 | 3.0 | — | — | — | 26.0 | 5.0 | — | — | 8.0 | 4.0 | 8.0 | — | — |
| Eggold, 1981 S | 146 | 8.0 | — | 15.0 | — | 39-40 | — | — | 18.0 | — | — | — | — | — |
| Garrick, 1985 S | 3,004 | — | — | — | — | — | — | — | — | — | — | — | 7.8 | — |
| Henderson, 1975 S | >1,000 | 12.4 | — | — | — | 23.2 | 14.6 | — | — | 6.7 | — | 8.3 | — | — |
| *Range: Cross sectional studies* | | 3.0-12.4 | | | | 23.2-40.0 | 2.0-14.6 | | 18.0-33.1 | 6.7-8.0 | 1.8-4.0 | 8.0-8.3 | 7.8-15.6 | |
| **Case series studies** | | | | | | | | | | | | | | |
| Apple, 1985 C | 648 | — | 19.0 | — | — | — | — | 12.0 | 22.0 | — | — | — | — | 6.0 |
| Brody, 1986 C | 8,000 | 15.0 | — | — | — | 40.0 | 15.0 | — | — | 10.0 | 5.0 | — | — | — |
| Clancy, 1974 C | 310 | 2.6 | 5.2 | 1.9 | — | — | 6.8 | 21.0 | 13.5 | — | — | — | 13.5 | — |
| Clement et al., 1981 C | 1,650 | 6.0 | 6.4 | 4.7 | 4.3 | 41.7 | 13.2 | 25.8 | — | — | 3.7 | 18.1 | 2.6 | — |
| Collins et al., 1989 C | 257 | 14.0 | — | 8.5 | 4.0 | 27.0 | 9.0 | — | 6.0 | 10.0 | 3.0 | — | 8.5 | — |
| D'Ambrosia, 1985 C | 100 | 2.0 | — | 19.0 | 7.0 | — | 27.5 | 3.0 | — | — | — | 15.0 | — | — |
| Gudas, 1980 C | 224 | 6.6 | — | 13.9 | — | 30.8 | 10.2 | 16.1 | — | 7.5 | — | 21.9 | 4.2 | — |
| James et al., 1978 C | 180 | 11.0 | — | 7.0 | 5.0 | 29.0 | 13.0 | — | — | — | — | — | 6.0 | — |
| Leadbetter, 1979 C | 456 | — | — | — | — | 35.0 | — | — | — | — | — | — | — | — |
| McBryde, 1982 C | 376 | 7.1 | — | 10.7 | — | 31.4 | 8.3 | — | — | — | 8.0 | — | 14.4 | — |
| McBryde et al., 1985 C | 1,000 | — | — | — | — | 32.1 | 7.3 | — | — | 13.2 | 7.4 | 17.2 | 9.6 | — |
| Pagliano & Jackson, 1980 C | 1,077 | 5.7 | 0.9 | 14.1 | 4.4 | — | 9.5 | 12.0 | 1.9 | 4.6 | 1.1 | 15.0 | 12.1 | — |
| Pagliano, 1986 C | 3,273 | 5.9 | — | 15.0 | 4.6 | 5.0 | 9.4 | 7.5 | — | 3.8 | — | 8.4 | 6.7 | — |
| Temple, 1983 C | 1,700 | 17.5 | — | — | — | 24.8 | 10.3 | — | 12.3 | 8.8 | — | 10.4 | — | — |
| *Range: Case series studies* | | 2.0-17.5 | 0.9-19.0 | 1.9-19.0 | 4.0-7.0 | 5.0-41.7 | 6.8-27.5 | 3.0-25.8 | 1.9-22.0 | 3.8-13.2 | 1.1-8.0 | 8.4-21.9 | 2.6-14.4 | |

[a]R, P, C, S = retrospective, prospective, case series, cross section, respectively.

**Table 22.5  A Percent Comparison of Injury Types in Male Runners**

| Study & study design (R, P, C, S)[a] | # partic. | Achilles tend. | Other tend. | Plantar fasciitis | IT band friction synd. | Nonspecific knee pain | Tibial stress synd. | Patello-femoral pain | Strain | Ankle sprain/strain | Low back/sciatica | Foot strain/sprain | Fracture | Bursitis |
|---|---|---|---|---|---|---|---|---|---|---|---|---|---|---|
| Retrospective studies | | | | | | | | | | | | | | |
| Estok & Rudy, 1987 R | 108 | 21.0 | — | — | — | 41.0 | 35.0 | — | — | 17.0 | 17.0 | — | 13.0 | — |
| Koplan et al., 1982 R | 693 | 3.0 | — | — | — | 14.0 | — | — | — | — | 4.0 | 8.0 | — | — |
| Marti et al., 1988 R | 4,358 | 11.6 | 17.0 | — | — | 27.9 | 29.9 | — | — | 15.0 | 2.2 | 5.0 | — | — |
| *Range: Retrospective studies* | | 3.0-21.0 | | | | 14.0-41.0 | 29.9-35.0 | | | 15.0-17.0 | 2.2-17.0 | 5.0-8.0 | | |
| Case series | | | | | | | | | | | | | | |
| Brunet et al., 1990 C | 1,130 | 18.0 | — | — | — | 49.0 | 31.0 | — | — | — | 35.0 | 14.0 | 8.0 | — |
| Clement et al., 1981 C | 987 | 7.9 | 7.6 | 5.3 | 4.6 | 42.2 | 10.7 | 24.3 | — | — | 3.3 | 19.5 | 2.4 | — |
| McBryde et al., 1985 C | 1,000 | — | — | — | — | 32.6 | 6.4 | — | — | 13.9 | 7.1 | 18.3 | 8.0 | — |
| *Range: Case series* | | 7.9-18.0 | | | | 32.6-49.0 | 6.4-31.0 | | | | 3.3-35.0 | 14.0-19.5 | 2.4-8.0 | |

[a]R, P, C, S = retrospective, prospective, case series, cross section, respectively.

**Table 22.6  A Percent Comparison of Injury Types in Female Runners**

| Study & study design (R, P, C, S)[a] | # partic. | Achilles tend. | Other tend. | Plantar fasciitis | IT band friction synd. | Nonspecific knee pain | Tibial stress synd. | Patello-femoral pain | Strain | Ankle sprain/strain | Low back/sciatica | Foot strain/sprain | Fracture | Bursitis |
|---|---|---|---|---|---|---|---|---|---|---|---|---|---|---|
| Retrospective studies | | | | | | | | | | | | | | |
| Estok & Rudy, 1986 R | 95 | 7.0 | — | — | — | 50.0 | 26.0 | — | — | — | 22.0 | — | 12.0 | — |
| Estok & Rudy, 1987 R | 112 | 21.0 | — | — | — | 48.0 | 47.0 | — | — | 13.0 | 13.0 | — | 17.0 | — |
| Koplan et al., 1982 R | 730 | 2.0 | — | — | — | 14.0 | — | — | — | — | 5.0 | 10.0 | — | — |
| Marti, 1988 R | 428 | — | — | — | — | 16.3 | 11.7 | — | — | 8.3 | — | — | — | — |
| *Range: Retrospective studies* | | 2.0-21.0 | | | | 14.0-50.0 | 11.7-47.0 | | | 8.3-13.0 | 5.0-22.0 | | 12.0-17.0 | |
| Case series studies | | | | | | | | | | | | | | |
| Brunet et al., 1990 C | 375 | 15.0 | — | — | — | 48.0 | 40.0 | — | — | — | 34.0 | 15.0 | 13.0 | — |
| Clement et al., 1981 C | 663 | 3.2 | 4.4 | 3.9 | 3.8 | 40.9 | 16.8 | 27.9 | — | — | 4.3 | 16.1 | 2.8 | — |
| McBryde et al., 1985 C | 1,000 | — | — | — | — | 30.8 | 9.4 | — | — | 11.5 | 8.0 | 14.3 | 13.6 | — |
| *Range: Case series studies* | | 3.2-15.0 | | | | 30.8-48.0 | 9.4-40.0 | | | | 4.3-34.0 | 14.3-16.1 | 2.8-13.6 | |

[a]R, P, C, S = retrospective, prospective, case series, cross section, respectively.

**Table 22.7  A Percent Comparison of Injury Types in Adolescent Runners**

| Study & study design (R, P, C, S)[a] | # partic. | Achilles tend. | Other tend. | Plantar fasciitis | Apophyseal | Nonspecific knee pain | Tibial stress synd. | Patello-femoral pain | Strain | Ankle sprain/strain | Low back/sciatica | Foot strain/sprain | Fracture | Bursitis |
|---|---|---|---|---|---|---|---|---|---|---|---|---|---|---|
| *Cross sectional and case series studies* | | | | | | | | | | | | | | |
| Orava & Saarela, 1978 P | 48 M: 26 F: 22 | 7.6 | — | 9.4 | 5.7 | 11.3 | 9.5 | — | — | 5.7 | 7.6 | — | 1.9 | — |
| Apple, 1985 C | 254 124 | — | 21.0 | — | 18.0 | — | — | 11.0 | 17.0[b] | — | — | — | 10.0 | 5.0 |
| | M: 95 | — | 5.0 | — | 20.0 | — | — | 2.0 | 15.0 | — | — | — | 9.0 | 5.0 |
| | F: 29 | — | 30.0 | — | 38.0 | — | — | 3.0 | 17.0 | — | — | — | 3.0 | 3.0 |
| Paty & Swafford, 1984 C | 19 | — | 3.7 | — | — | 14.8 | 29.6 | 3.4 | — | 3.4 | 7.4 | 7.4 | 14.8 | — |
| Watson & DiMartino, 1987 S | 257 | 2.4 M: 3.3 F: 0.0 | 9.8[c] M: 10.0 F: 9.8 | — | — | 19.5 M: 23.2 F: 9.1 | 19.5 M: 16.7 F: 27.2 | — | 23.4 M: 13.3 F: 18.2 | 17.1 M: 16.7 F: 27.2 | 7.3 M: 10.0 F: 0.0 | 2.4 M: 3.3 F: 0.0 | — | — |
| *Range: Cross sectional and case series studies* | | | 3.7-30.0 | | 18.0-38.0 | 14.8-19.5 | 19.5-29.6 | 2.0-11.0 | 15.0-23.4 | 3.4-17.1 | 7.3-7.4 | 2.4-7.4 | 3.0-14.8 | 3.0-5.0 |

[a]R, P, C, S = retrospective, prospective, case series, cross section, respectively.

[b]Includes sprains also.

[c]Patellar tendinitis only; included also in knee pain percentages.

**Table 22.8    A Percent Comparison of Injury Location in Adult Runners**

| Study & study design (R, P, C, S)[a] | # partic. | Back | Hip & groin | Thigh | Knee | Leg[b] | Ankle | Foot | Other |
|---|---|---|---|---|---|---|---|---|---|
| *Prospective studies* | | | | | | | | | |
| Lysolm & Wiklander, 1987 P | 39 | 5.5 | 7.3 | 18.2 | 12.7 | 27.3 | — | 12.7 | 10.9 |
| Orava, 1978 P | 274 | 2.6 | 7.7 | — | 29.5 | 17.1 | 24.1 | — | — |
| Walter et al., 1989 P & R | 1,288 | 11.0 | 9.0 | 7.0 | 27.0 | 12.0 | 15.0 | 16.0 | 4.0 |
| *Range: Prospective studies* | | 2.6-11.0 | 7.3-9.0 | 7.0-18.2 | 12.7-29.5 | 12.0-27.3 | 15.0-24.1 | 12.7-16.0 | 4.0-10.9 |
| *Retrospective studies* | | | | | | | | | |
| Blair et al., 1987 R | 438 | 5.0 | 2.0 | 10.0 | 31.0 | 22.0 | — | 15.0 | — |
| Henderson, 1975 R | > 1,000 | — | 10.1 | 7.5 | 23.2 | 34.0 | 6.7 | 19.5 | — |
| Jacobs & Berson, 1986 R | 210 | — | — | 9.8 | 31.7 | 32.4 | 18.3 | 7.7 | — |
| Krissof & Ferris, 1979 R | — | — | 7.0 | 6.0 | 25.0 | 40.0 | 11.0 | 24.0 | — |
| Marti et al., 1988 R | 4,358 | 2.2 | 5.5 | 5.0 | 27.9 | 29.9 | — | 28.5 | 0.9 |
| Walter et al., 1988 R | 476 | 6.0 | 11.0 | 9.0 | 23.0 | 12.0 | 10.0 | 12.0 | 5.0 |
| Walter et al., 1989 P & R | 1,288 | 11.0 | 9.0 | 7.0 | 27.0 | 12.0 | 15.0 | 16.0 | 4.0 |
| *Range: Retrospective studies* | | 2.2-11.0 | 2.0-11.0 | 5.0-10.0 | 23.0-31.7 | 12.0-40.0 | 6.7-18.3 | 7.7-28.5 | 0.9-5.0 |
| *Cross sectional studies* | | | | | | | | | |
| Clough et al., 1987 S | 2,462/502 | 4.0 | 5.0 | 1.0 | 26.0 | 7.0 | 8.0 | 8.0 | 9.0 |
| Garrick, 1985 S | 3,004 | 4.9 | 7.7 | 4.1 | 38.2 | 11.7 | 8.5 | 20.7 | 0.7 |
| *Range: Cross sectional studies* | | 4.0-4.9 | 5.0-7.7 | 1.0-4.1 | 26.0-38.2 | 7.0-11.7 | 8.0-8.5 | 8.0-20.7 | 0.7-9.0 |
| *Case series studies* | | | | | | | | | |
| Clement et al., 1981 C | 1,650 | 3.7 | 5.0 | 4.0 | 41.7 | 27.9 | — | 18.1 | — |
| Collins et al., 1989 C | 257 | 3.0 | 9.0 | 6.0 | 27.0 | 27.0 | 10.0 | 17.0 | 1.0 |
| Gudas, 1980 C | 224 | — | 4.9 | — | 30.8 | 16.8 | 7.5 | 35.0 | 4.2 |
| Kannus et al., 1987 C | 814 | 9.0 | 3.0 | — | 33.0 | 14.0 | 10.0 | 2.0 | — |
| McBryde et al., 1985 C | 1,000 | 7.4 | 8.8 | 2.8 | 32.1 | 7.3 | 13.2 | 17.2 | 11.2 |
| Pagliano & Jackson, 1980 C | 1,077 | 1.1 | 0.4 | 6.4 | 14.2 | 18.6 | 5.5 | 39.8 | 1.2 |
| Temple, 1983 C | 1,700 | — | 3.5 | 5.4 | 24.8 | 31.2 | 8.8 | 26.3 | — |
| *Range: Case series studies* | | 1.1-9.0 | 0.4-9.0 | 2.8-6.4 | 14.2-41.7 | 7.3-31.2 | 5.5-13.2 | 2.0-39.8 | 1.0-11.2 |

[a]R, P, C, S = retrospective, prospective, case series, cross section, respectively.

[b]Includes Achilles tendon.

**Table 22.9    A Percent Comparison of Injury Location in Male Runners**

| Study & study design (R, P, C, S)[a] | # partic. | Back | Hip & groin | Thigh | Knee | Leg[b] | Ankle | Foot | Other |
|---|---|---|---|---|---|---|---|---|---|
| *Retrospective studies* | | | | | | | | | |
| Estok & Rudy, 1987 R | 108 | 17.0 | 15.0 | — | 41.0 | 56.0 | 17.0 | — | — |
| Koplan et al., 1982 R | 693 | 4.0 | 2.0 | — | 14.0 | 7.0 | — | 8.0 | — |
| *Range: Retrospective studies* | | 4.0-17.0 | 2.0-15.0 | | 14.0-41.0 | 7.0-56.0 | | | |
| *Case series studies* | | | | | | | | | |
| Brunet et al., 1990 C | 1,130 | 35.0 | 24.0 | — | 49.0 | 48.0 | — | 14.0 | — |
| Clement et al., 1981 C | 987 | 3.3 | 4.2 | 3.5 | 42.2 | 27.2 | — | 19.5 | — |
| McBryde et al., 1985 C | — | 7.1 | 9.1 | — | 32.6 | — | 13.9 | 18.3 | — |
| *Range: Case series* | | 3.3-35.0 | 4.2-24.0 | | 32.6-49.0 | 27.2-48.0 | | 14.0-19.5 | |

[a]R, P, C, S = retrospective, prospective, case series, cross section, respectively.

[b]Includes Achilles tendon.

**Table 22.10   A Percent Comparison of Injury Location in Female Runners**

| Study & study design (R, P, C, S)[a] | # partic. | Back | Hip & groin | Thigh | Knee | Leg[b] | Ankle | Foot | Other |
|---|---|---|---|---|---|---|---|---|---|
| Retrospective studies | | | | | | | | | |
| Estok & Rudy, 1987 R | 112 | 13.0 | 21.0 | — | 48.0 | 68.0 | 13.0 | — | — |
| Koplan et al., 1982 R | 730 | 3.0 | 3.0 | — | 14.0 | 7.0 | — | 10.0 | — |
| *Range: Retrospective studies* | | 3.0-13.0 | 3.0-21.0 | | 14.0-48.0 | 7.0-68.0 | | | |
| Case series studies | | | | | | | | | |
| Brunet et al., 1990 C | 375 | 34.0 | 29.0 | — | 48.0 | 55.0 | — | 15.0 | — |
| Clement et al., 1981 C | 663 | 4.3 | 6.1 | 3.8 | 40.9 | 28.6 | — | 16.1 | — |
| McBryde et al., 1985 C | — | 8.0 | 8.0 | — | 30.8 | — | 11.5 | 14.3 | — |
| *Range: Case series* | | 4.3-34.0 | 6.1-29.0 | | 30.8-48.0 | 28.6-55.0 | | 14.3-16.1 | |

[a]R, P, C, S = retrospective, prospective, case series, cross section, respectively.

[b]Includes Achilles tendon.

**Table 22.11   A Percent Comparison of Injury Location in Adolescent Runners**

| Study & study design (R, P, C, S)[a] | # partic. | Back | Hip & groin | Thigh | Knee | Leg[b] | Ankle | Foot | Other |
|---|---|---|---|---|---|---|---|---|---|
| Nudel et al., 1989 R | 16 | 6.3 | — | — | 6.3 | 6.3 | — | 6.3 | — |
| Watson & DiMartino, 1987 S | 257 | 7.3 | 4.8 | 14.6 | 19.5 | 21.9 | 17.1 | 4.8 | — |
| Paty & Swafford, 1984 C | 19 | 3.7 | 7.4 | — | 37.0 | 29.6 | 3.7 | 11.1 | — |

[a]R, P, C, S = retrospective, prospective, case series, cross section, respectively.

[b]Includes Achilles tendon.

### 3.3.1 Head/Spine/Trunk

The reported proportion of injury to the spine and trunk in prospective studies ranges from 2.6 to 11% of injured runners (see Table 22.8). Injuries that are more common in the runner are centered in the low back region, which absorbs high levels of force during the support phase of running and is acted on by strong muscular contractions. Our literature review identified only a small number of articles that focused on the spine and trunk specifically. When examining case reports, case series, and cross-sectional studies that concentrated specifically on the running population, injuries such as fracture of the vertebral arch (1), sciatica and osteophyte formation (14), intraspinal cysts (15), and herniated discs (72) were identified.

### 3.3.2 Upper Extremity

Injuries to the upper extremity are rare unless a runner falls or is hit by an external object such as an automobile. Examples of rare injuries to the upper extremity are a radial palsy created by extreme flexion at the elbow (191), and a stress fracture of the scapula associated with poor running posture (248).

### 3.3.3 Lower Extremity

The lower extremity is subjected to repeated loading cycles that may or may not be accommodated by the musculoskeletal system. Alterations in running patterns also pose problems for the musculoskeletal system, sometimes making adaptation impossible and resulting in injury. Running patterns can be altered by changes in training, a change in the running surface, a change in running shoes, or any other factor that creates a functional change in the running action. Changes leading to injuries such as stress fractures can be caused by fatigue of specific muscle groups during a run, thereby increasing the load on the skeletal system (43).

The proportion of injury to the various locations in the lower extremity is highest for the knee joint, followed by the leg and foot (Table 22.8). The percentages vary considerably between designs.

Lower extremity injuries have been reported in several case reports, case series, and cross sectional studies. Examples of injuries to the hip, pelvis, and thigh, reported in these types of studies include the following: stress fracture of the pubis, sacrum, or femur, avulsion fracture of the anterior superior iliac spine, pubic symphysitis, or hamstring strain. The majority of the case reports, series, or cross-sectional studies report stress fractures more than any other injury. The most commonly reported was a stress fracture to the femoral neck, followed by stress fractures to the subtrochanteric femur, the pubis, and the sacrum (7, 26, 49, 59, 75, 96, 104, 112, 118, 121, 123, 124, 159, 172, 188, 197, 204, 212, 215, 224, 231, 264, 272).

Case reports and case series have provided a few examples of hip, pelvis, and thigh injuries to the adolescent runner, including avulsion fractures and apophysitis at the anterior or posterior iliac spine, and one case of a stress fracture of the distal femoral epiphysis (17, 35, 60, 66). These types of injury vary from the usual assortment of stress fractures seen in the adult runner.

There are only a few case studies that report on specific knee injuries. This may be related to the accepted importance placed on knee injuries and the documentation of such injuries reported in group statistics. Examples of individually reported knee injuries include iliotibial band friction syndrome, patellofemoral pain (chondromalacia), patellar tendinitis, medial or lateral knee pain, and stress fractures of the patella (5, 8, 47, 68, 119, 146, 151, 156, 167, 173, 196, 202, 217). Adolescent knee injuries, reported through case reports and case series studies, are similar to those seen in the adult and include examples such as nonspecific knee pain or patellar pain (61, 176, 230).

There are many cited case reports or case series studies on running injuries to the leg in adults, which can be categorized into posteromedial leg pain (shin splints), anterior compartment syndrome, stress fractures of the tibia or fibula, and tendinitis or rupture of the soleus, peroneus longus, or tibialis posterior (24, 44, 51, 64, 65, 82, 85, 87, 92, 97, 102, 103, 110, 114, 141, 152, 160, 164, 189, 207, 214, 222, 227, 250, 251, 252, 271). Injuries to the adolescent runner are similar, with reported case reports of stress fractures in the tibia and fibula (28, 43).

Case reports and case series on injuries to the foot of adult runners include the following: stress fractures of the medial malleolus, talus, navicular, or metatarsals, Achilles tendinopathy, avulsion fracture of the 5th metatarsal, tarsal tunnel syndrome or sural nerve entrapment, osteophyte formation on the tibia, talus, or navicular, and plantar fasciitis (29, 37, 50, 67, 74, 78, 87, 90, 93, 100, 111, 113, 122, 128, 157, 168, 183, 193, 211, 213, 226, 233, 238, 261). Likewise, the adolescent runner has been shown to experience epiphysitis or epiphyseal stress fractures at sites such as the calcaneal apophyseal insertion and the first metatarsal (31, 148, 190).

### 3.3.4 Systemic Alterations Associated With Running

Running, and especially long distance running or ultra-marathoning, can create problems outside the musculoskeletal system. There are many cases that illustrate the possible damaging effects of running (2, 10, 20, 27, 41, 53, 77, 89, 116, 125, 133, 139, 141, 143, 150, 165, 175, 199, 200, 201, 203, 205, 218, 220, 223, 235, 249, 259). For example, running in extreme temperatures or without proper hydration or nourishment can magnify the effects of the impact of running on other body functions. Although many adverse effects quickly revert to normal within a suitable rest period, the careful recognition and examination of the effects of running on general function is warranted.

The following generalizations are presented: (a) Gastrointestinal hemorrhage can occur in adult runners completing long distance runs. This bleeding can lead to iron deficiency anemia in runners (10, 41, 150, 201, 218). This has also been illustrated in the adolescent runner (216, 263). (b) Runners have experienced erosive gastritis leading to upper gastrointestinal symptoms (41, 200). (c) There are many reports of heat exhaustion and exertional heat stroke in runners (20, 199, 205). (d) Other system overload responses to running include the following: liver disturbances, hematuria and bladder lesions, the presence of urinary salts, increase in the basal serum CK activity, idiopathic edema, cerebral vasoconstriction, thrombosis, and hematopoietic bone marrow hyperplasia (27, 77, 175, 203, 220, 235, 249).

# 4. Injury Severity

## 4.1 Time Loss

Restricting running because of injury is common in the running population, but is poorly documented in the research literature. A runner should reduce mileage or rest following an injury, but there are very little data on the average time dedicated to recovery from a single injury. Fields and associates (58) in a study of psychological factors

**Table 22.12   A Percent Comparison of Absence From Running as a Result of Injury**

| Study | # participants | Sex | < 8 days | 8-21 days | 21 days |
|-------|---------------|-----|----------|-----------|---------|
| Blair et al., 1987 | 438 | M:76%<br>F:24% | 24% | | |
| Brody, 1986 | 8,000 | — | | 70% | |
| Marti, 1989 | 6,620 | M:91%<br>F:9% | | | 19.4% |
| Maughan, 1983 | 960 | M:472<br>F:25 | 12.7% | 18.1% | 12.6% |

associated with running injuries, reported an average time loss of 11.2 to 11.4 days per running injury. Lutter (127) has identified time periods ranging from 46 to 86 days of running cessation associated with injuries. A breakdown of time lost from running because of injury is presented in Table 22.12. Injured runners who discontinued running for 8 days or less ranged from 12.7 to 24%. Those who did not run for 8 to 21 days or more than 21 days ranged from 18.1 to 70% and 12.6 to 19.4%, respectively.

## 4.2 Catastrophic Injuries

There are no prospective studies that have monitored the incidence of catastrophic injuries. However, within the framework of case series and cross-sectional studies (11, 30, 76, 184, 210, 242, 253, 266, 267), we have identified the following associations with catastrophic injury:

- Categories of catastrophic injuries include the following: (a) those sustained by collisions with an automobile or other external object, and (b) those associated with heart failure.
- In one study, 65 joggers were injured over a one-year period; 30 of these were fatal (267).
- Chillag and associates (30) reported on 256 males and 15 females who died during exercise since 1940.
- The examination of individual case reports of running-related deaths has pointed out the common presence of predisposing coronary atherosclerosis or sinus bradycardia. There are a few case reports of deaths in runners who were asymptomatic.

## 5. Injury Risk Factors

An examination of risk factors associated with running injuries has been conducted by reviewing training techniques, measuring anthropometric and physical characteristics, and documenting the external environment of runners who are already injured. There are many studies that have identified factors presumed to be risk factors, but reported as anecdotal or speculative. However, there are factors identified within the framework of more robust study designs that should be given more emphasis. Given differences in the literature, the focus will be on the risk factors identified via prospective studies with less emphasis on other factors that are not supported by robust data.

We have reviewed and summarized specific analytic studies in Table 22.13. These offer comparisons between injured and noninjured runners, personality relationships to running injury, and an examination of various extrinsic or intrinsic factors related to specific running injuries. The studies are organized by study design, and should be interpreted with caution because of the following limitations:

- Most of the studies offer a descriptive comparison between groups, limiting the statistical interpretation of the differences. We identified no studies that specifically tested risk factors by using appropriate statistical analysis.
- The data were typically collected using a questionnaire format that influences response, response rate, and accuracy of the accrued information.
- Risk factors were commonly identified after injury was diagnosed, leading to a biased interpretation of the influence of the risk factor.

## 5.1 Intrinsic Factors

### 5.1.1 Physical Characteristics

There were no prospective studies that identified physical characteristics as a factor in injury. However, in the retrospective studies physical characteristics have been shown to play a very important

**Table 22.13   A Comparison of Analytical Epidemiological Injury Studies of Running**

| Study | Duration | Design | Method | n | Purpose | Results |
|---|---|---|---|---|---|---|
| Fields et al., 1990 | 1 year | Prospective | Questionnaire and training log | 40 | To assess type A behavior and running injuries. | A larger percentage of Type A runners experienced injury (57% vs. 34.6%) and had multiple injuries (57% vs. 15%) than runners who were not Type A. |
| Gardner et al., 1989 | 12 weeks | Prospective | Interview | 3,025 | To study the effect of insoles and age of running shoes on the incidence of stress fractures in marine recruits. | There was no significant difference in the incidence of stress fractures between recruits wearing polymer or standard insoles. There was a slight increasing trend of stress fractures with increasing age of running shoes. There was a strong trend for fewer stress fractures with a history of increasing physical activity. |
| Lindenberg et al., 1984 | 3 years | Prospective | Questionnaire | 36 | To identify factors associated with iliotibial band friction syndrome. | Seventy-eight percent of the runners with IT band syndrome ran 40-80 miles a week, 86% had 2-4 years of running experience, 69% ran on the road, 72% had no previous injury, 67% were running in hard running shoes, 50% had normal lower limb alignment, 42% had genu varum, and 56% had leg length discrepancies. |
| Macera et al., 1989 | 1 year | Prospective | Questionnaire | 583 | To identify risk factors associated with prediction of injury in runners. | Running 40 miles or more a week was the most important predictor of injury. Other risk factors were the presence of a previous injury and a running history of less than 3 years. |
| Ross & Schuster, 1983 | 5 years | Prospective | — | 63 | To determine the prediction of running injuries using preseason measures. | Running injuries could be predicted with a 75% rate using measures of the foot. |
| Viitasalo & Kvist, 1983 | 4 years | Prospective | — | 26 | To compare differences between runners with bad shin splints and those with mild shin splints. | Runners with bad shin splints had greater Achilles tendon angles and more pronation than the mild group. The mild shin splint group had lesser amounts of passive inversion and eversion. |
| Brunet et al., 1990 | — | Retrospective | Questionnaire | 1,505 | To determine relationships between running or physical characteristics and injury types. | There were more stress fractures, foot pain, Achilles tendinitis, and hip injuries in runners who ran more mileage per week. There was a high correlation between anatomical imbalance and the incidence of running injuries. Women have a special predisposition to stress fractures that is not related to conditioning. |
| Gross et al., 1991 | 23 months | Retrospective | Questionnaire | 347 | To evaluate the effectiveness of orthotics for the prevention and treatment of running injuries. | Seventy-five percent of the runners (n = 292) reported control or elimination of a malalignment or injury with the use of orthotics. Orthotics were effective in providing symptomatic relief. |
| Guyot, 1991 | — | Retrospective | Questionnaire | 370 | To evaluate significant medical symptoms as predictors of runners experiencing pain. | Runners with pain scored higher on 17 of 23 medical symptoms than nonpain runners. |

*(continued)*

**Table 22.13** (*continued*)

| Study | Duration | Design | Method | n | Purpose | Results |
|---|---|---|---|---|---|---|
| Jacobs & Berson, 1986 | — | Retrospective | Questionnaire | 2,664 | To compare training characteristics between injured (n = 210) and non-injured runners. | The injured runners ran more mileage per week, ran more days per week, and ran more races in the last year than the noninjured runners. There was no correlation with the length of the runs, the running surfaces, running intervals, running hills, or running sprints. |
| Lloyd et al., 1986 | — | Retrospective | Questionnaire | 367 | To compare differences in injuries between women with regular and irregular menses. | There were more injuries in women runners with absent menses. |
| McQuade, 1986 | — | Retrospective | Questionnaire | 214 | To compare runners with injury with those having no injury. | Runners who did not stretch had two times the risk of injury, and there was less risk if the stretch was after the run and not before. Twenty percent of the injured runners had more than one area of pain. There were more injuries in runners who ran 10-20 miles per week. |
| Diekhoff, 1984 | — | Case control | Questionnaire | 68 | To examine the relationship of personality and injury in runners. | The injured runners exhibited more Type A behaviors, were more addicted to running, ran more miles, and were more likely to participate in fun runs than the noninjured runners. |
| Garth & Miller, 1989 | — | Case control | — | 34 | To compare foot characteristics between runners with (n = 17) and without (n = 17) posteromedial shin pain. | Runners with symptomatic posteromedial shin pain had greater extension of the interphalangeal joints, less flexion of the toes, greater total range of motion, and less intrinsic strength than the control group. It was concluded that posteromedial shin pain was related to overuse of the flexor digitorum longus associated with mild claw foot deformity. |
| Gehlsen & Seger, 1980 | — | Case control | — | 20 | To examine differences between runners with (n = 10) and without (n = 10) shin splints. | Runners with shin splints had greater plantar flexion strength and greater angular displacement between the calcaneus and the midline of the lower leg during running. |
| Kirby & McDermott, 1983 | — | Case control | — | 14 | To measure anterior tibial compression pressures and to determine the influence of running style on the pressures. | There was significantly more anterior tibial compartment pressure in runners with accentuated rearfoot landing styles. |
| Kujala et al., 1993 | — | Case control | Questionnaire | 68 | To identify factors that differentiated between runners without knee pain (n = 17), with anterior knee pain (n = 16), and hospital patients with patellar subluxation (n = 16) or dislocation (n = 19). | Questions that differentiated between the four groups were related to: painful patella movements, presence of a limp, running, stair climbing, and prolonged sitting with knees flexed. |

| Study | Duration | Design | Method | N | Purpose | Results |
|---|---|---|---|---|---|---|
| Messier & Pittala, 1988 | 1 year | Case control | — | 74 | To compare anthropometric differences, gait, and injury histories between runners with no injuries (n = 19), runners with shin splints (n = 17), runners with plantar fasciitis (n = 15), and runners with iliotibial band friction syndrome (n = 13). | Using anthropometric, gait, and running histories, 69% were correctly assigned to groups using a discriminant analysis. The control group had been running more years than the other injury groups. Higher arches were found in the iliotibial group, and there was less range of motion in the ankles for the shin split and iliotibial groups. Fifty-three percent of the plantar fascia group had at least a 0.64 cm difference in leg lengths. Twenty percent of the injured groups ran hills. The control group had less pronation, less rearfoot motion, and smaller pronation velocity than all three injury groups. |
| Messier et al., 1991 | — | Case control | — | 36 | To compare differences between a patellofemoral pain group (n = 16) and an uninjured group of runners (n = 20). | The patellofemoral pain group had significantly greater Q angles, ran on crowned roads more, were weaker in the extensors, and were stronger in the flexors than the uninjured group. There were no differences in running pace. |
| Valliant, 1980 | — | Case control | Questionnaire | 64 | To compare personality traits between injured and noninjured male and female runners. | The injured female runners (n = 16) were more assertive, more practical, and less disciplined than the injured male runners (n = 32). The injured male runners were average on humbleness vs. assertiveness. |
| Valliant, 1981 | — | Case control | Questionnaire | 41 | To compare personality traits between injured (n = 26) and noninjured (n = 15) male runners. | Injured male runners were less toughminded, less forthright, heavier, and taller than the noninjured runners. |
| van Mechelen et al., 1992 | — | Case control | — | 32 | To compare injured and noninjured runners on flexibility parameters. | The injured runners had significantly less range of motion at the hip joint than the noninjured runners. There were no significant differences in flexibility of the ankle joint, and there were no significant bilateral differences in either group. |
| Wang et al., 1993 | — | | — | 40 | To compare the flexibility of runners (n = 20) and nonrunners (n = 20). | Runners had significantly tighter hamstrings, soleus than the nonrunners. There was no difference in the flexibility of the rectus femoris or the iliopsoas. |
| Warren & Jones, 1987 | — | Case control | Questionnaire | 91 | To compare running history and anthropometric differences between runners who presently are injured with plantar fasciitis (n = 31), those who have formerly had plantar fasciitis (n = 14), and noninjured runners (n = 46). | Runners who currently had plantar fasciitis had more dorsiflexion, more pronation, higher arches, weighed more, were taller and older, had been running the most years, ran the least per week, and ran for the longest time compared to the other two groups. |
| White & Malone, 1990 | — | Case control | — | 30 | To compare the effects of running on the intervertebral disc. | The vertebral column was measured in the morning and in the afternoon both before and after a 9-mile run. There was more loss in the height of the column after one hour of running than there was after 7.5 hours of static activity. |
| Herring & Richie, 1990 | — | Double blind | — | 35 | To compare the effect of running using different socks. | Runners who wore the 100% acrylic sock reported fewer and smaller blisters than runners who wore a 100% cotton sock. |

role in determining the potential for injury during running (Table 22.13). For example, Brunet et al. (23) identified a high correlation between anatomical imbalance and the incidence of running injuries.

Malalignment has been considered a contributing factor to running injuries in the retrospective studies. Alignment characteristics such as genu varum or leg length discrepancies have been associated with iliotibial band friction syndrome (119) and pelvic and hip injuries (121), and excessive Q angles have been related to patellofemoral problems (156). Higher arches and leg length inequalities have been implicated in iliotibial band friction syndrome and plantar fasciitis, respectively (155, 261) and shin splints have been tied to greater Achilles tendon angles (250).

Moreover, there are physical characteristics other than malalignment in the lower extremity that are contributors to running injuries. There may be an increased incidence of injury in older runners as suggested by Pagliano (180), who reported that runners over the age of 40 had more low-back and foot problems. However, other studies have found no increased predisposition to injury with increasing age (130, 138, 194).

Height and weight have been examined as contributing factors to running injury by Macera (130), Jackson and Matz (91), and Valliant (245). They report a higher rate of injury in taller individuals and in individuals who are heavier.

Gender differences have been observed for specific types of injuries. Men have been shown to incur more plantar fasciitis, Achilles tendinitis, and knee instability than women, and women experience more shin splints (180), are more susceptible to stress fractures (25, 144, 158) and are more prone to patellar and tibial pain (136). However, as reported in an earlier section, the epidemiological studies report that injury rates are similar across gender (130, 131, 194, 255).

One other physical characteristic identified with running injury is the presence of a previous injury. Most of the recent epidemiological studies report a greater risk of future injury if the runner has experienced a previous injury (94, 106, 131, 136, 255).

The running injury literature has also focused on the amenorrheic female runner as a special category of runners requiring special consideration (9, 52, 57, 166, 179). A cross-sectional study conducted by Estok and Associates (57) examined 112 female runners and found 32% with irregular or absent menses. Female runners who experience alterations in their menstrual cycle have been shown to experience stress fractures in the lower extremity, with incidences increasing from 29% in runners with normal menses to 49% in those with very irregular cycles (9). Within the limitations of the studies presented, irregular or absent menses in the female runner has been associated with stress fractures in the femoral shaft, the tibia, the navicular, the metatarsal, and the ribs.

Physical characteristics are also thought to play a significant role in running injuries presented in case series and case reports. A careful examination of this information is useful because it is offered mostly from the practical or clinical perspective of sport medicine practitioners. Moreover, these factors should not be considered true risk factors because they have not been substantiated by robust scientific study. Given the limited interpretation of this literature, we offer the following summaries:

- General anatomical malalignment (158), forefoot and rearfoot varus (47, 140, 239), genu varum and tibial varum (140), an increased Q angle (47), a cavus foot type (149, 209), a planus foot type (162), and leg length inequality (23, 36, 209, 268) have all been associated with stress fractures in the lower extremity.

- Malalignment of the lower extremity has also been associated with injury in the low back, hip, pelvis, and thigh. Leg length inequalities have been related to both hip and back pain (23, 36) and to bursitis at the hip joint (198). It is also speculated that trochanteric bursitis may be more common in individuals with a cavus foot type (149).

- There are many reports linking injuries to the knee joint with malalignment in the lower extremity. Iliotibial band friction syndrome has been related to valgus deformity (173), a cavus foot type (149, 173), genu varum (119, 187), leg length inequalities (36, 98, 192), and tibial varum (154, 269). Patellofemoral pain has been associated with the presence of a greater Q angle (42, 154) and may be related to planus foot types (149). Knee pain has been related to rearfoot varus (13, 196), rigid forefoot valgus (13), the combination of coxa vara and genu valgum (13), the combination of coxa valga and genu varum (13), and an excessive Q angle (13).

- Leg injuries associated with malalignment are anterior tibial strain, which may be associated with a short, tight Achilles tendon (147), medial tibial stress syndrome associated with a planus foot type (149), and posterior tibial tendinitis associated with a planus foot type (149).

Injuries specifically identified as shin splints have been related to leg length inequalities (192) and varus deformities (209).

- In the foot and ankle, Achilles tendinitis is a common injury associated with the presence of varus alignment (36), both cavus and planus foot types (149), and rearfoot valgus or heel or forefoot varus (170, 269). Plantar fasciitis has been associated with cavus foot types (128, 134, 135, 149), planus foot types (149), and forefoot varus or rearfoot valgus (269). Retrocalcaneal bursitis is an injury that may be related to tibia varum or cavus foot types (198).
- Finally, anatomical factors associated with calcaneal epiphysitis in the adolescent runner include genu varum, subtalar varus, and forefoot varus (148).

### 5.1.2 Motor/Functional Characteristics

A review of Table 22.13 has identified some selected functional characteristics related to running injuries. For example, posteromedial shin pain has been attributed to flexibility and strength abnormalities in the toes (64) and shin splints have been associated with greater plantar flexion strength and a greater angular displacement between the calcaneus and the lower leg (65). Runners with patellofemoral pain have been shown to be stronger in the knee flexors and weaker in the extensors than a noninjured group (156) and injured runners had significantly less range of motion at the hip joint than noninjured runners (247). Likewise, runners as a group had tighter hamstrings and soleus muscles than a nonrunning population (258).

There have been no prospective or retrospective studies that have identified motor or functional characteristics as risk factors for injury. For example, no retrospective or prospective running injury study has identified stretching as a factor in preventing running injury. In the few studies published, there were no differences in injury occurrence between runners who regularly stretched, and those who did not (106, 131, 255).

A review of the case series studies and other general running literature yields several references on the role of functional parameters in the development of running injury. Recognizing that the information presented in this literature does not confirm a risk factor, we offer the following summary of the general literature.

Functional variables that may be associated with stress fractures include excessive pronation (140, 209), tight hamstrings, gastrocnemius, or quadriceps (47), a bilateral strength imbalance (47), an

increase in soleus tension with dorsiflexion (102), and an excessive arm swing during running (59). Motor and functional variables that may be associated with hamstring strain include a lack of overall strength and flexibility, an inequality of bilateral hamstring strength, and a strength imbalance between the quadriceps and the hamstrings (3).

At the knee joint, the iliotibial band friction syndrome may be related to excessive pronation (98, 154), and patellofemoral pain may be related to a tight vastus lateralis and a weak vastus medialis (42, 154). Knee pain, in general, has been related to an imbalance in the strength of the quadriceps and the hamstrings (196) while medial knee pain, in particular, has been attributed to a weakness in the vastus medialis obliquus, tight hamstrings, and excessive pronation (13).

In the leg, anterior tibial strain has been related to an imbalance between the anterior and posterior musculature (147), and posterior tibial tendinitis and shin splints have been associated with hyperpronation (65, 98, 209, 250, 269), inversion and eversion range of motion (98), and excessive external rotation at the hip joint (209).

Achilles tendinitis may occur in runners who have limited subtalar mobility or ankle range of motion (109), a gastrocnemius and soleus insufficiency (37, 170), or foot hyperpronation (147, 170). Plantar fasciitis may be related to hyperpronation (128, 134, 135, 269) and retrocalcaneal bursitis has been associated with hamstring tightness (198).

### 5.1.3 Psychological and Psychosocial Characteristics

There is some suggestion that psychological characteristics may influence the occurrence of running injuries. Both Diekhoff (48) and Fields and associates (58) have reported a higher rate of injury in runners categorized as exhibiting Type A behavior (Table 22.13). However, further explorations of this association are required.

## 5.2 Extrinsic Factors

### 5.2.1 Exposure

The incidence of running injuries has been calculated relative to exposure and has been reported in the range of 2.2 to 12.1 injuries per 1,000 hours of running (18, 129). Because there is limited information on exposure calculated in hours of running, exposure considerations relating to risk of running injuries are presented in this section as a function of total mileage run per week rather than time spent while running. Injuries such as stress fractures, foot pain, Achilles tendinitis, and hip injuries have been identified by Brunet et al. (23) to be more common in runners with higher weekly mileages (Table 22.13). Other researchers have also mentioned high running mileage as a risk factor for running injuries (48, 94, 119, 131).

In the epidemiological literature, the relationship between high mileage and running injuries has been supported by some but not by others. Walter and associates (255) have reported a greater risk of injury in runners who run more than 40 miles per week. Macera and associates (131) and Powell and associates (194) also documented more injuries in runners running more miles per week. However, Jackson and Matz (91) indicated that 48% of injured runners in their study were running less than 20 miles per week, and only 2% of the injured runners were running more than 80 miles per week. Macera (130) explains that there is typically a higher injury rate with an increase in weekly mileage but the injury rate per exposure decreases with increased distance.

The seemingly inconclusive information about the influence of exposure on injury rates in running may be confounded by the variable fitness levels or experience of the runners studied. Runners who have been running for less than 3 years or who are generally inexperienced may be at a greater risk of injury (130, 131, 136). However, Powell and associates (194) have stated that years of experience have no relationship with injury, and Walter and associates (255) have reported that the more competitive runners have the highest incidence of injuries.

Linkages between exposure and running injuries have also been proposed in case series and case reports. Recognizing that this information does not imply an actual risk factor, the following components of exposure have been identified. Increases in weekly mileage have been associated with stress fractures in the lower extremity (26, 87, 88, 195). Other lower extremity injuries attributed to an increase in running mileage are Achilles tendinitis (170, 187), iliotibial band friction syndrome (68, 151, 187), nonspecific knee pain (167, 196), patellofemoral pain (187), plantar fasciitis (260), and pes anserinus bursitis (198).

### 5.2.2 Training Methods or Conditions

A sudden change in training is one of the most often mentioned risk factors identified with running injuries (194). A review of Table 22.13 identified running more days per week (94), hill running

(155), and running for longer periods (261) as training techniques that lead to more injuries. Specifically, hill running has been identified as a training method that increases risk of injury because of the strain on the anterior and lateral compartments when going downhill and the strain on the gastrocnemius and plantar fascia in uphill running (225).

The runner usually focuses on training considerations, including frequency of running, the distance of the run, and the running pace. In terms of frequency, the injury rate is greater if the same weekly mileage is run over fewer days (130). Injury risk is higher if individuals run more miles per day and more days per week and the risk significantly increases at distances greater than 40 km per week (255).

Running pace is also an important training consideration. Macera (130) indicates that running pace has no influence on the rate of injury, and Powell and associates (194) agree that running pace is not a factor if the number of miles per week is considered. Finally, the frequent use of interval training may also be associated with a higher rate of injury (33, 34).

Training methods or conditions that might be related to running injuries in case studies or the general literature are presented as follows:

- Specific injuries that may be associated with training errors include stress fractures following interval training (87), iliotibial band friction syndrome related to a single severe training session (151) or hill running (94, 98, 187), and popliteal tendinitis also associated with hill running (154). Nonspecific knee pain has been associated with hill running (13, 196) and interval training (196), and patellofemoral pain has been associated with hill running (181). Hill running was also related to plantar fasciitis (181, 260). Pagliano reported more injuries in long slow runs (182). Breyne (19) suggests that the injury-causing component in the slow run is related to a significant increase in the number of footstrikes.

### 5.2.3 Environment

Running takes place in an outdoor environment and is subjected to a great deal of influence by weather, running surfaces, and running terrain. These factors might all play a role in determining the incidence of running injury.

Running injury has been attributed to a change in running surface (91). Macera (130) reported that women have a five times greater risk of injury running on concrete versus no concrete, even when mileage is controlled. She also notes that, for males, the running surface does not influence the injury rate if controlled for by weekly mileage. Epidemiological studies have identified no other training variables (such as running surface or time of day) as risk factors for running injury.

Environmental factors implicated as risk factors in case series or case reports are numerous. These studies have shown that running on hard surfaces may be related to stress fractures (51, 87, 88, 91, 195, 234), posterior tibial tendinitis (187), shin splints (209), Achilles tendinitis (170, 269), medial knee pain (13), and plantar fasciitis (260). Also, it is speculated that running on sand may be related to injuries such as Achilles tendinitis (209), medial knee pain (13), and plantar fasciitis (260).

Another consideration in the environment is the slant of the running surface. Running on a cambered road may increase the risk of injury because of the functional asymmetry created. On a slanted road, the uphill foot must pronate more, which imposes a change in the running pattern (225). Running on slanted or cambered roads is related to shin splints (209), iliotibial band friction syndrome (187, 225), knee pain (13), plantar fasciitis (225), hip bursitis (225), and adductor strain (225).

Running in a hot environment increases the risk of heat exhaustion, heatstroke, and dehydration (20, 116, 199, 205). Likewise, a runner can experience frostbite or hypothermia if running in extreme cold temperatures without taking precautionary steps (225).

### 5.2.4 Equipment
Shoes have been identified as influencing the type and incidence of injury in runners. Shoes have been used to reduce pronation, increase shock absorption, and control torsion in the forefoot (228). However, the effect of shoes on running injuries has been questioned by Marti (137, 138), who reported no relationship between injury occurrence and shoe selection.

## 6. Suggestions for Injury Prevention

The purpose of the present review is to evaluate the risk of running injury and identify some specific considerations for prevention. Given the variability of studies on running injuries, suggestions for injury prevention can only be offered in a generalized way. Based on a small number of epidemiological studies, it has been shown that injury risk increases with increases in training mileage, previous running injury, and possibly the experience level of the runner. Given this limited perspective on risk factors, preventive measures should be incorporated that monitor the changes in training mileage and give special attention to the avoidance of future injuries.

To go beyond the epidemiological literature, there are many preventive suggestions for reduction of injury that are based on speculation about the cause of injury. Some of these recommendations may prove useful and we summarize them in Table 22.14. They should be cautiously interpreted and implemented given their lack of robust evaluation.

**Table 22.14  Suggestions for Injury Prevention**

| Preventive measures | Examples/suggestions |
| --- | --- |
| **Runners** | |
| Correct training errors | Van Mechelen (246) recommends that training be built up gradually, alternate day running is suggested for beginning runners, and running speeds should be such that the runner can speak without being short of breath. |
| | Monitor the number of days of high intensity workouts and the increase in the training program (33, 34, 171). Alternate days of high effort with days of less effort (33, 34). To prevent iliotibial friction syndrome, runners should avoid training errors such as excessive distances, hill running, and speed work (173). |
| | It is impossible to set safe distance guidelines. Stamford (229) suggests that a runner train at one half the distance he/she plans to race. If a runner wants to increase mileage, a beginning runner can do so safely by gradually increasing mileage from 1 to 2 miles/session over several weeks (229) and still be injury free. If an experienced runner attempts to double mileage from 5 to 10 miles per session in a short time, injury may result. A general guideline is to increase the individual session mileage by 10% per week (229). |

*(continued)*

**Table 22.14**  *(continued)*

| Preventive measures | Examples/suggestions |
|---|---|
| **Runners** *(continued)* | |
| | To prevent running injuries Wischnia (270) suggests that runners discontinue training hard if tired. Also, don't experiment with shoes in a race, don't run through pain, don't make up for lost miles, don't increase mileage more than 10% a year, don't do more than one hard workout on successive days, don't plunge into a greater level of training, and rest. |
| | Mirkin (161) suggests that runners allow a period of recovery after a hard workout and substitute an easy run the next day. It is also suggested that if it takes more than 48 hours to recover, the workout is too hard. |
| | To prevent excessive compressive loading of the intervertebral disks, White & Malone (265) suggest doing high impact activities in the morning when the disc height is greater. Also, uphill running should be used at a minimum because it creates more lumbar flexion, which is problematic for the low back. When the discs lose height over the course of a run, spinal motion is reduced, which shortens the length of the stride. |
| Correct muscle imbalance | Prevention of injuries may be facilitated by incorporating exercises that balance out the strength of the musculature (171). It is especially important to strengthen the anterior compartment (161). Medial knee pain has been associated with weakness of the vastus medialis oblique, which is related to irritation of the patella, and also an anterior posterior muscular imbalance, which can be brought on by tight hamstrings, uphill running, and stair climbing (13). |
| Identify structural abnormalities and correct | To prevent injuries, structural abnormalities should be identified and corrected if possible (161, 171). Malalignments that should be identified and reduced if possible are coxa vara and genu valgum, coxa valga and genu varum, an excessive Q-angle, and excessive motion at the subtalar and midtarsal joints (13). |
| | To prevent injury in a runner with cavus feet, good shock absorbing shoes should be worn, the runner should not run on cement, and should keep the mileage down on asphalt roads (135). |
| | Orthotics have been successfully prescribed for the prevention or treatment of injuries in runners with excessive or prolonged pronation. Limited success with the use of orthotics has also been seen in the runner with cavus feet (69). |
| Correct running style | Imperfections in running style should be corrected if possible. Imperfections in running style are magnified as the distance increases, so a runner with more imperfections should run shorter distances (229). |
| | To prevent iliotibial band friction syndrome, it may help to shorten the stride (173). |
| Improve the runner's fitness | For runners with back pain, 1-2 sets of stretching and strengthening exercises are prescribed. Examples of stretches include alternating knees or both knees to chest, toe touches, abdominal flexes, and low-back flattening exercises. Examples of strengthening exercises include dumbbell swing, stiff legged dead lift with light dumbbells, windmill exercise, elbow to knee, hamstring curls, quad stretch, and bent knee sit ups. The exercises can be increased in resistance to include the good morning exercise, back hyperextensions, hamstring curls, quad stretch, hanging stretch, and the seated knee to chest (163). |
| | To prevent the occurrence of stress fractures, Micheli (158) recommends a slow and progressive training program and attention to increasing the strength and endurance of the back and lower extremities. |
| **Sport** | |
| Running shoes | To prevent running injury, excessive wear of the sole of the running shoe should be avoided (40). Because the shock absorbing capacity of the shoe decreases with increasing mileage, runners should purchase new shoes regularly. A shoe should offer good stability to the foot, have a good heel counter and heel counter support to prevent overpronation (40). |
| | Shoes should offer the proper amount of support and shock absorption (13). The heel counter, insert, and the heel leverage are important components to evaluate. Runners should also consider the stiffness in the longitudinal area (torsional stiffness), which is important in the touchdown phase of running (228). |
| | McKenzie et al. (149) recommend a slip last, curved last, softer EVA or air, and a narrow flare shoe for runners with pes cavus feet. They recommend a board last, straight last, a motion control heel counter, medial support, high density material on the medial insole, and a wider flare for runners with pes planus feet. |
| **External environment** | |
| Altitude | To run at higher altitudes, a 3-4 week acclimatization is needed to avoid hypoxia during acute exposure (225). |

| Preventive measures | Examples/suggestions |
|---|---|
| **External environment** *(continued)* | |
| Running surface | The ideal running surface is a flat, smooth, soft, and resilient running surface (225). Running surfaces such as cement or soft sand should be avoided (13). Hard, rigid surfaces should be avoided (91). |
| Running terrain | Uneven ground and slanted roads should be run on with caution because of the valgus force created in the lower extremity (13). Runners should alternate running on each side of the road or run different directions on the same road if it is slanted. Slanted surfaces are responsible for increases in pronation, plantar fascia stress, adductor strain, iliotibial strain, and bursitis of the hip (225). Downhill and uphill running should be used with moderation because of the stress placed on the anterior and lateral compartments (DH) and on the gastrocnemius and the plantar fascia (UH) (225). |
| Weather: Cold | When running in cold weather, wear wind breakers, cover both head and hands, and wear a face mask (225). A runner can tolerate −30 °F for 0.5 hours every 4 hours (225). |
| Weather: Hot | Heat acclimatization is possible, and it increases the sweating mechanism by decreasing the threshold, increasing the cooling, and decreasing the cardiac output (225). Acclimatization can be obtained by running in hot weather and it lasts for several weeks. It can be maintained by running in a sweatsuit or in a hot temperature (225). |
| | To prevent heat injuries, the American College of Sports Medicine recommends that races > 16 km or 10 miles should not be run in temperatures > 28 °C or 82.4 °F. If the temperature exceeds 27 °C, the race should be run before 9:00 a.m. or after 4:00 p.m. Also, fluids should be provided and runners should be encouraged to ingest fluids in the race and 400-500 ml, 10-15 minutes before competing. Water stations should be placed at 3-4 km intervals. Finally, runners should be trained to recognize early signs of heat injury (4). |
| | Sherwood and Strong (221) recommend the following for the preparing for a race and preventing of heat injuries: train adequately by completing 2 runs in previous month that are at least 2/3rds the length of the race, do not run to exhaustion the week before the race, emphasize carbohydrates in the previous day's meal, maintain adequate hydration during the race, and don't forget the pre-run warmup. |
| **Health support system** | |
| Early identification of symptoms | To prevent running injuries, health education is important. Runners and health professionals should focus on the early recognition of symptoms of overuse (246). |
| Treat injuries properly and completely | A recommended treatment for patellofemoral problems can include anti-inflammatory drugs, patellar stabilization, orthotics, ice and heat, a change in the running terrain, quadriceps femoris exercises, iliotibial band stretching, and muscle stimulation (42). |
| | Treatment of knee pain should include the avoidance of downhill running and a progressive resistance program for the hamstrings and the quadriceps (117). |
| | Treatment for iliotibial band friction should consider the reduction of the running mileage, level surface running, and no roadside running (117). |
| | It is recommended that shin splints be treated with rest and graduated exercise (117). |
| | Stress fractures should be treated with rest, protected weight bearing, and bicycling or swimming (117). |
| | When injured, the runner should be treated immediately, using conventional treatments. The runner should go to a softer surface and a firmer sole in the shoe, run more erect, take more recovery days, use supplemental exercises, and take one easy week for every hard week. The cause of the injury needs to be corrected and exercises prescribed (270). |
| Prescription of orthotics | D'Ambrosia (45) identifies that the injuries most helped by orthotics are posterior tibial tendinitis, pes planovalgum, metatarsalgia, and calcaneal spurs. |
| Physical examination | A physical examination of a runner should include an assessment and identification of any kinetic chain dysfunction and identification of prior overuse injuries (132). |
| | Paty (185) recommends a physical examination of runners that would measure anthropometric and functional characteristics associated with risk of running injury. Acceptable values are leg length differences of 1 cm or less, 90 degrees or more of hip external and internal rotation, minimum of 10 degrees of dorsiflexion with the knee extended, 0-4 degrees of subtalar varus, 10 degrees of eversion and 20 degrees of inversion of the subtalar joint, forefoot perpendicular to the calcaneus, and a Q angle less than 20 degrees. |
| Orthotic prescription | It is recommended that orthotics for the runner with pes cavus feet include a heel lift, a neoprene or sorbothane insole, and soft orthotics. For the pes planus foot type, a medial wedge and a soft or semirigid orthotic is recommended (149). |

# 7. Suggestions for Further Research

The review of the literature on running injuries has identified numerous areas for future study. Some of these research questions and future directions are presented in Table 22.15. One of the most important recommendations is that running injury studies incorporate epidemiological designs that are denominator based and thereby allow calculations of absolute or relative risk of injury in the target population. Prospective studies are preferred because they allow the examination of present risk factors as they relate to subsequent injury. The research team for evaluation of running injuries could benefit by the inclusion of an epidemiologist who could establish techniques and suggest designs from which more reliable and valid running injury statistics could be derived. This is lacking within the framework of most studies. Also, the sample populations should be expanded to reduce sample bias and to allow for computation

**Table 22.15  Suggestions for Further Research**

| Research component | Research directions/questions |
| --- | --- |
| **Incidence of injury** | |
| Injury rates | What is the injury rate in the general running population? Denominator-based injury rates for the general running population need to be expanded. |
| | What is the incidence of injuries or the number of new injuries over a time period (81)? Most studies report incidence of injured runners, and research on the incidence of injuries should be expanded. |
| | What is the prevalence of running injuries (# of total injuries in a time period) (81)? This information is lacking in the literature. |
| | It is recommended that more prospective studies be conducted to determine the incidence of new injuries, to identify the number of individuals in the population who are at risk, and to identify absolute risk factors in the population. |
| Reinjury rates | There is very little information of reinjury rates in the literature. Future studies should include the calculation of reinjury rates. |
| **Injury characteristics** | |
| Nature of injury onset | What are the actual injury mechanisms for specific injuries incurred during running? Mechanisms of injuries should be evaluated both in isolation and in combination to develop a multifactorial explanation of the development of running injuries. |
| Injury type | The definition of injury and of injury types needs to be standardized across studies on running injuries. Additionally, the method of reporting the injuries has relied almost exclusively on the use of a questionnaire, which limits the accuracy of the injury data. It is recommended that a uniform system of reporting be developed that would eliminate the bias of the self-report mechanism. |
| | What are some of the intrinsic or extrinsic factors that are discriminants of specific types of injuries? |
| Injury location | The information on injury location needs to be standardized with respect to group classification. For example, should Achilles tendinitis be considered in the foot/ankle region or in the lower leg? Likewise, is iliotibial band friction to be considered with the knee or the thigh? |
| | What are the reasons certain locations are injured more frequently than others? |
| | What are the special risk factors or running injury considerations that should be examined in the adolescent or female runner? |
| Lower extremity | What are the causes of specific injuries in the lower extremity? |
| Systemic alterations associated with running | Are there any long-term systemic effects from running? What are the actual physiological changes in the muscles that occur with long distance running? |
| **Injury severity** | |
| Time loss | More studies should include data on time loss as a result of injury. Specifically, what is the time loss associated with specific injuries sustained in running? What factors influence the amount of time loss? Finally, how is time loss related to the type of rehabilitation that the athlete receives? |
| Catastrophic injuries | What is the incidence of fatality in running? What are the causes of fatalities in running, and are certain individuals more susceptible? |

| Research component | Research directions/questions |
|---|---|
| Injury risk factors | Risk of injury in running can only be calculated from epidemiological studies. More studies should be conducted and less emphasis should be placed on information presented in case series designs where risk cannot be assessed. |
| Intrinsic factors | |
|    Physical characteristics | What are the specific malalignments in the lower extremity that contribute to specific running injuries? Why are there specific risks associated with height and weight? How does the presence of a previous injury increase the risk of a new injury? Further studies should attempt to clarify the risk factors associated with gender and age, which are not clearly established. |
|    Motor/functional characteristics | What specific strength and flexibility characteristics are related to running injury? |
|    Psychosocial characteristics | A limited number of studies have established a link between personality characteristics and running injuries. Further study to clarify these relationships should be conducted. |
| Extrinsic factors | |
|    Exposure | Exposure rates as a function of running hours needs to be calculated in future studies. This should include consideration of the total number of running hours and how the hours are dispersed over the course of a week. |
|    Training methods or conditions | Studies on running injury should include attention to durations of runs, pace of runs, and days running per week. These factors should be related to specific types of injuries. Optimal training techniques should be tested to determine effects on performance and injury. |
|    Environment | What are the differences in injury rates of individuals who run on the road, cross country, or on the track? How do different running surfaces relate to specific types of running injuries? What are the special precautions that should be taken before running in an extreme hot or cold temperature? |
|    Equipment | What specific shoe types are best for specific foot types? What shoes are best for a specific running style? Can running shoes or orthotics correct dysfunction or lower extremity malalignment enough to reduce the risk of injury? What are the characteristics of the shoe that would be best for different running surfaces? |
| Injury prevention | What factors can be identified for the prevention of running injury that can be substantiated through prospective studies using a control group? |

of risks across an expanded population of interest. Finally, there is much to do in the area of injury etiology as it relates to specific intrinsic and extrinsic risk factors.

# References

1. Abel, M.S. Jogger's fracture and other stress fractures of the lumbosacral spine. Skeletal Rad. 13:221-227; 1985.
2. Adno, J. Jogger's testicles in marathon runners, (letter). S. African Med. J. 65:1036; 1984.
3. Agre, J.C. Hamstring injuries: proposed aetiological factors, prevention and treatment. Sports Med. 2(1):21-33; 1985.
4. American College of Sports Medicine. The prevention of thermal injuries during distance running. In: The Official Position Papers of the American College of Sports Medicine (5th ed.). Indianapolis: American College of Sports Medicine; 1990:15-20.
5. Antich, T.J.; Randal, C.C.; Westbrook, F.A.; Morrissey, M.C.; Brewster, C.E. Evaluation of knee extensor mechanism disorders: clinical presentation of 112 patients. J. Orth. Sports Phys. Ther. 8(5):248-254; 1986.
6. Apple, D.F. Adolescent runners. Clin. Sports Med. 4(4):641-655; 1985.
7. Atwell, A.E.; Jackson, D.W. Stress fracture of the sacrum in runners. Amer. J. Sports Med. 19(5):531-533; 1991.
8. Barber, F.A.; Sutker, A.N. Iliotibial band syndrome. Sports Med. 14(2):144-148; 1992.
9. Barrow, G.W.; Saha, S. Menstrual irregularity and stress fractures in collegiate female distance runners. Amer. J. Sports Med. 16(3):209-216; 1988.
10. Baska, R.S.; Moses, F.M.; Graeber, G.; Kearney, G. Gastrointestinal bleeding during a marathon. Dig. Dis. Sci. 35(2):276-279; 1990.
11. Bharati, S.; Dreifus, L.S.; Chopskie, E.; Lev, M. Conduction system in a trained jogger with sudden death. Chest. 93(2):348-351; 1988.
12. Blair, S.N.; Kohl, H.W.; Goodyear, N.N. Rates and risks for running and exercise injuries: studies in three populations. Res. Quart. Exerc. Sport. 58(3):221-228; 1987.
13. Blake, R.L.; Burns, D.P.; Colson, J.P. Etiology of a traumatic medial knee pain. J. Amer. Pod. Assoc. 7(10):580-583; 1981.

14. Blake, R.L.; Fettig, M.H. Chronic low back pain in a long distance runner. A case report. J. Amer. Pod. Assoc. 73(11):598-601; 1983.

15. Bland, J.H.; Schmidek, H.H. Symptomatic intra-spinal synovial cyst in a 66-year-old marathon runner. J. Rheum. 12(5):1006-1010; 1985.

16. Blatz, D.J. Bilateral femoral and tibial shaft stress fractures in a runner. Amer. J. Sports Med. 9(5):322-325; 1981.

17. Blatz, D.J. Multiple epiphyseal fractures in an athlete. Orthop. Rev. 8(9):980-982; 1989.

18. Bovens, A.M.; Janssen, G.M.; Vermeer, H.G.; Hoeberigs, J.H.; Janssen, M.P.; Verstappen, F.T. Occurrence of running injuries in adults following a supervised training program. Int. J. Sports Med. 10(Suppl. 3):186-190; 1989.

19. Breyne, R. Relative risks of running. Runner's World. 10(2):22-23; 1975.

20. Brodeur, V.B.; Dennett, S.R.; Griffin, L.S. Exertional hypothermia, ice baths, and emergency care at the Falmouth Road Race. J. Emerg. Nurs. 15(4):304-312; 1989.

21. Brody, D.M. Running injuries. In: Nicholas, J.A.; Hershman, E.B., eds. The Lower Extremity and Spine in Sports Med. St. Louis: Mosby Company; 1986:1534-1579.

22. Brubaker, C.E.; James, S.L. Injuries to runners. J. Sports Med. 2(4):189-198; 1974.

23. Brunet, M.E.; Cook, S.D.; Brinker, M.R.; Dickinson, J.A. A survey of running injuries in 1505 competitive and recreational runners. J. Sports Med. Phys. Fit. 30(3):307-315; 1990.

24. Burgess, I.; Ryan, M.D. Bilateral fatigue fractures of the distal fibulae caused by a change of running shoes. Med. J. Australia. 143(7):304-305; 1985.

25. Burfoot, A. Differences between sexes: often they mean more injuries. Runner's World. 18(7):46-48,71; 1983.

26. Butler, J.E.; Brown, S.L.; McConnell, B.G. Subtrochanteric stress fractures in runners. Amer. J. Sports Med. 10(4):228-232; 1982.

27. Byrnes, W.C.; Clarkson, P.M.; White, J.S.; Hsieh, S.S.; Frykman, P.N.; Mayghan, R.J. Delayed onset muscle soreness following repeated bouts of downhill running. J. Applied Phys. 59(3):710-715; 1985.

28. Cahill, B.R. Stress fractures of the proximal tibial epiphysis: a case report. Amer. J. Sports Med. 5(5):186-187; 1977.

29. Campbell, G.; Warnekros, W. A tarsal stress fracture in a long distance runner, a case report. J. Amer. Pod. Assoc. 73(10):532-535; 1983.

30. Chillag, S.; Bates, M.; Voltin, R.; Jones, D. Sudden death: myocardial infarction in a runner with normal coronary arteries. Phys. & Sports Med. 18(3):92-94; 1990.

31. Cibulka, M.T. Management of a patient with forefoot pain: a case report. Phys. Ther. 70(1):41-44; 1990.

32. Clancy, W.G. Lower extremity injuries in the jogger and distance runner. Phys. Sports Med. 2(6):46-50; 1974.

33. Clancy, W.G. Runners' injuries, part 1. Amer. J. Sports Med. 8(2):137-138; 1980a.

34. Clancy, W.G. Runners' injuries, part 2. Evaluation and treatment of specific injuries. Amer. J. Sports Med. 8(4):287-289; 1980b.

35. Clancy, W.G.; Foltz, A.S. Iliac apophysitis and stress fractures in adolescent runners. Amer. J. Sports Med. 4(5):214-218; 1976.

36. Clement, D.B.; Taunton, J.E.; Smart, G.W.; McNicol, K.L. A survey of overuse running injuries. Phys. Sports Med. 9(5):47-50, 52-53, 56-58; 1981.

37. Clement, D.B.; Taunton, J.E.; Smart, G.W. Achilles tendonitis and peritendinitis: etiology and treatment. Amer. J. Sports Med. 12(3):179-184; 1984.

38. Clough, P.J.; Dutch, S.; Maughan, R.J.; Shepherd, J. Pre-race drop-out in marathon runners: reasons for withdrawal and future plans. British J. Sports Med. 21(4):148-149; 1987.

39. Collins, K.; Wagner, M.; Peterson, K.; Storey, M. Overuse injuries in triathletes: a study of the 1986 Seafair triathalon. Amer. J. Sports Med. 17(5):675-680; 1989.

40. Cook, S.D.; Brinker, M.R.; Roche, M. Running shoes: their relationship to running injuries. Sports Med. 10(1):1-8; 1990.

41. Cooper, B.T.; Douglas, S.A.; Firth, L.A.; Hannagan, J.A.; Chadwick, V.S. Erosive gastritis and gastrointestinal bleeding in a female runner. Gastroenterology. 92:2019-2023; 1987.

42. Cox, J.S. Patello-femoral problems in runners. Clinics in Sports Med. 4(4):699-715; 1985.

43. Daffner, R.H.; Martinez, S.; Gehweiler, J.A.; Harrelson, J.M. Stress fractures of the proximal tibia in runners. Radiology. 142(1):63-65; 1982.

44. D'Ambrosia, R.D.; Zelis, R.F.; Chuinard, R.O.; Wilmore, J. Interstitial pressure measurements in the anterior and posterior compartment in athletes with shin splints. Amer. J. Sports Med. 5:127-131; 1977.

45. D'Ambrosia, R.D. Orthotic devices in running injuries. Clinics in Sports Med. 4(4):611-618; 1985.

46. DeLoes, M.; Goldie, I. Incidence and rate of injuries during sport activity and physical exercise in a rural Swedish municipality: incidence rates in 17 sports. International J. Sports Med. 9(6):461-467; 1988.

47. Dickoff, S.A. A case report: longitudinal stress fracture of the patella—a cause of peripatellar pain in a runner. J. Orthopaedic and Sports Physical Therapy. 9(5):194-197; 1987.

48. Diekhoff, G.M. Running amok: injuries in compulsive runners. J. Sport Behavior. 7(3):120-129; 1984.

49. Draper, D.O.; Dustman, A.J. Avulsion fracture of the anterior superior iliac spine in a collegiate distance runner. Archives of Physical Med. and Rehabilitation. 73(9):881-882; 1992.

50. Drez, D.; Young, J.C.; Johnson, R.D.; Parker, W.D. Metatarsal stress fractures. Amer. J. Sports Med. 8(2):123-125; 1980.

51. Dugan, R.C.; D'Ambrosia, R. Fibular stress fractures in runners. J. Family Practice. 17(3):415-418; 1983.

52. Dugowson, C.E.; Drinkwater, B.L.; Clark, J.M. Nontraumatic femur fracture in an oligomenorrheic athlete. Med. and Science in Sports and Exercise. 23(12):1323-1325; 1991.

53. Dyck, P.J.; Classen, S.M.; Stevens, J.C.; O'Brien, P.C. Assessment of nerve damage in the feet of long distance runners. Mayo Clinic Proceedings. 62(7): 568-572; 1987.

54. Eggold, J.F. Orthotics in the prevention of runners' overuse injuries. Physician Sports Med. 9(3):124-127, 131; 1981.

55. Estok, P.J.; Rudy, E.B. Physical, psychosocial, menstrual changes/risks and addiction in the female marathon runner and non marathon runner. Health Care for Women. 7(3):187-202; 1986.

56. Estok, P.J.; Rudy, E.B. Marathon running: comparison of psychological risks for men and women. Research in Nursing and Health. 10(2):79-85; 1987.

57. Estok, P.J.; Rudy, E.B.; Just, J.A. Body-fat measurements and athletic menstrual irregularity. Health Care Women International. 12(2):237-248; 1991.

58. Fields, K.B.; Delaney, M.; Hinkle, R. A prospective study of type A behavior and running injuries. J. Family Practice. 30(4):425-429; 1990.

59. Fink-Bennett, D.M.; Benson, M.T. Unusual exercise related stress fractures. Two case reports. Clinical Nuclear Med. 9(8):430-434; 1984.

60. Fox, I.M. Iliac apophysitis in teenage distance runners. J. Amer. Podiatry Association. 76(5):294-296; 1986.

61. Gamble, J.R. Symptomatic dorsal defect of the patella in a runner. Amer. J. Sports Med. 14(5):425-427; 1986.

62. Gardner, L.I.; Dziados, J.E.; Jones, B.H.; Brundage, J.F.; Harris, J.M.; Sullivan, R.; Gill, P. Prevention of lower extremity stress fractures: a controlled trial of shock absorbent insole. Am. J. Public Health. 78(12):1563-1567; 1989.

63. Garrick, J.G. Characterization of the patient population in a sports med. facility. Physician and Sports Med. 13(10):73-76; 1985.

64. Garth, W.P.; Miller, S.T. Evaluation of claw toe deformity, weakness of the foot intrinsics and posteromedial shin pain. Amer. J. Sports Med. 17(6):821-827; 1989.

65. Gehlsen, G.M.; Seger, A. Selected measures of angular displacement, strength and flexibility in subjects with and without shin splints. Research Quarterly for Exercise and Sport. 51(3):478-485; 1980.

66. Godshall, R.W.; Hansen, C.A.; Rising, D.C. Stress fractures through the distal femoral epiphysis in athletes. Amer. J. Sports Medicine. 9(2):114-116; 1981.

67. Gould, W.; Trevino, S. Sural nerve entrapment by avulsion fracture of the fifth metatarsal bone. Foot and Ankle. 2(3):153-155; 1981.

68. Grana, W.A.; Coniglione, T.C. Knee disorders in runners. Physician and Sports Med. 13(5):127-133; 1985.

69. Gross, M.L.; Napoli, R.C. Treatment of lower extremity injuries with orthotic shoe inserts. An overview. Sports Med. 15(1):66-70; 1993.

70. Gross, M.L.; Davlin, L.B.; Evanski, P.M. Effectiveness of orthotic shoe inserts in the long-distance runner. Amer. J. Sports Med. 19(4):409-412; 1991.

71. Gudas, C.J. Patterns of lower extremity injury in 224 runners. Comprehensive Therapy. 6(9):50-59; 1980.

72. Guten, G. Herniated lumbar disk associated with running: a review of 10 cases. Amer. J. Sports Med. 9(3):155-159; 1981.

73. Guyot, W.G. Psychological and medical factors associated with pain in running. J. Sports Med. & Physical Fitness. 31(3):452-460; 1991.

74. Ha, K.I.; Hahn, S.H.; Chung, M.Y.; Yang, B.K.; Yi, S.R. A clinical study of stress fractures in sports activities. Orthopedica. 14(10):1089-1095; 1991.

75. Hajek, M.R.; Noble, H.B. Stress fractures of the femoral neck in joggers: a case report and review of the literature. Amer. J. Sports Med. 10(2):112-116; 1982.

76. Hanzlick, R.L.; Stivers, P.R. Sudden death due to anomalous right coronary artery in a 26-year-old marathon runner. Amer. J. Forensic Med. and Pathology. 4(3):265-268; 1983.

77. Hart, L.E.; Egier, B.P. Exertional heat stroke: the runner's nemesis. Canadian Med. Association J. 122(10):1144, 1147-1150; 1980.

78. Hawkins, R.B. Arthroscopic treatment of sports-related anterior osteophytes in the ankle. Foot and Ankle. 9(2):87-90; 1988.

79. Henderson, J. The 6 in 10 who breakdown. Runner's World. 10(12):34-35; 1975.

80. Herring, K.M.; Richie, D.H. Friction blisters and sock fiber composition. A double blind study. J. Amer. Podiatric Med. Association 80(2):63-71; 1990.

81. Hoeberigs, J.H. Factors related to the incidence of running injuries. A review. Sports Med. 13(6):408-422; 1992.

82. Holder, L.E.; Michael, R.H. The specific scintigraphic pattern of "shin splints" of the lower leg. J. Nuclear Med. 25:865-869; 1984.

83. Holmich, P.; Christensen, S.W.; Darre, E.; Jahnsen, F.; Hartvig, T. Non-elite marathon runners: Health, training and injuries. British J. Sports Med. 23(3):177-178; 1989.

84. Holmich, P.; Darre, E.; Jahnsen, F.; Hartvig-Jensen, T. The elite marathon runner: Problems during and after competition. British J. Sports Med. 22(1):19-21; 1988.

85. Hoover, J.A. Exertional anterior compartment syndrome with fascial hernias. J. Foot Surgery. 22(3): 271-272; 1983.

86. Hughes, W.A.; Noble, H.B.; Porter, M. Distance race injuries: analysis of runner's perceptions. Physician Sports Med. 13(11):43-46, 50-53, 57-58; 1985.

87. Hulkko, A.; Orava, S. Stress fractures in athletes. International J. Sports Med. 8(3):221-226; 1987.

88. Hulkko, A.; Alen, M.; Orava, S. Stress fractures of the lower leg. Scandinavian J. Sports Sciences. 9(1):1-8; 1987.

89. Hunding, A.; Jordal, R.; Pauley, P.E. Runner's anemia and iron deficiency. Acta Medica Scandinavica. 209(4):315-318; 1981.

90. Hunter, L.Y. Stress fracture of the tarsal navicular. More frequent than we realize? Amer. J. Sports Med. 9(4):217-219; 1981.

91. Jackson, D.W.; Matz, S.O. Prevention of running injuries. J. Musculoskeletal Med. 3(4):10-19; 1986.

92. Jackson, M.A.; Gudas, C.J. Peroneus longus tendonitis: a possible biomechanical etiology. J. Foot Surgery. 21(4):344-348; 1982.

93. Jackson, D.L.; Haglund, B. Tarsal tunnel syndrome in athletes. Amer. J. Sports Med. 19(1):61-65; 1991.

94. Jacobs, S.J.; Berson, B.L. Injuries to runners: a study of entrants to a 10,000 meter race. Amer. J. Sports Med. 14(2):151-155; 1986.

95. James, S.L.; Bates, B.T.; Osternig, L.R. Injuries to runners. Amer. J. Sports Medicine. 6(2):40-50; 1978.

96. Johansson, C.; Ekenman, I.; Tornkvist, H.; Eriksson, E. Stress fractures of the femoral neck in athletes. The consequence of a delay in diagnosis. Amer. J. Sports Med. 18(5):524-528; 1990.

97. Johnell, O.; Rausing, A.; Wendelberg, B.; Westin, N. Morphological bone changes in shin splints. Clinical Orthopaedics. 167:180-184; 1982.

98. Jones, D.C.; James, S.L. Overuse injuries of the lower extremity: shin splints, iliotibial band friction syndrome, and exertional compartment syndromes. Clinics in Sports Med. 6(2):273-289; 1987.

99. Kannus, V.P.; Aho, H.; Jarvinen, M.; Niittymakis, S. Computerized recording of visits to an outpatient sports clinic. Amer. J. Sports Med. 15(1):79-85; 1987.

100. Kibler, W.B.; Goldberg, C.; Chandler, T.J. Functional biomechanical deficits in running athletes with plantar fasciitis. Amer. J. Sports Med. 19(1):66-71; 1991.

101. Kibler, W.B. Clinical aspects of muscle injury. Med. and Science in Sports and Exercise. 22(4):450-452; 1990.

102. King, W.D.; Wiss, D.A. Isolated fibular shaft fracture in a sprinter. Am. J. Sports Med. 18(2):209-210; 1990.

103. Kirby, R.L.; McDermott, A.G.P. Anterior tibial compartment pressures during running with rearfoot and forefoot landing styles. Archives of Physical Med. and Rehabilitation. 64(7):296-299; 1983.

104. Koch, R.A.; Jackson, D.W. Pubic symphysitis in runners. A report of two cases. Amer. J. Sports Med. 9(1):62-63; 1981.

105. Konradsen, L.; Hansen, E.B.; Sondergaard, L. Long distance running and osteoarthrosis. Amer. J. Sports Med. 18(4):379-381; 1990.

106. Koplan, J.P.; Powell, K.E.; Sikes, R.K.; Shirley, R.W.; Campbell, C.C. An epidemiologic study of the benefits and risks of running. J. Amer. Med. Association. 248(23):3118-3121; 1982.

107. Krissoff, W.B.; Ferris, W.D. Runner's injuries. Physician Sports Med. 7(12):53-64; 1979.

108. Kujala, U.M.; Jaakkola, L.H.; Koskinen, S.K.; Taimela, S.; Hurme, M.; Nelimarkka, O. Scoring of patellofemoral disorders. Arthroscopy. 9(2):159-163; 1993.

109. Kvist, M. Achilles tendon injuries in athletes. Anna Chir. Gynaecol. 80(2):188-201; 1991.

110. Lacroix, H.; Keeman, J.N. An unusual stress fracture of the fibula in a long-distance runner. Archives of Orthopaedic and Traumatic Surgery. 111(5):289-290; 1992.

111. Larsen, L.; Lauridsen, F. Dislocation of the tibialis posterior tendon in two athletes. Amer. J. Sport Med. 12(6):429-430; 1984.

112. Latshaw, R.F.; Kantner, T.R. Pelvic stress fracture in a female jogger. A case report. Amer. J. Sports Med. 9(1):54-56; 1981.

113. Leach, R.E.; James, S.; Wasilewski, S. Achilles tendonitis. Amer. J. Sports Med. 9(2):93-98; 1981.

114. Leach, R.E.; Purnell, M.B.; Satio, A. Peroneal nerve entrapment in runners. Amer. J. Sports Med. 17(2):287-291; 1989.

115. Leadbetter, W.B. Getting ahead of the injury. Emergency Med. 11(6):27-29, 34-37, 39; 1979.

116. Lee, R.P.; Bishop, G.F. Severe heat stroke in an experienced athlete. Med. J. Aust. 153(2):100-104; 1990.

117. Lehman, W.L. Overuse syndromes in runners. Amer. Family Physician. 29(1):157-161; 1984.

118. Leinberry, C.F.; McShane, R.B.; Stewart, W.G.; Hume, E.L. A displaced subtrochanteric stress fracture in a young amenorrheic athlete. Amer. J. Sports Med. 20(4):485-487; 1992.

119. Lindenberg, G.; Pinshaw, R.; Noakes, T.D. Iliotibial band friction syndrome in runners. Physician Sports Med. 12(5):118-124, 127-128, 130; 1984.

120. Lloyd, T.; Triantafyllou, S.J.; Baker Houts, P.S.; Whiteside, J.A.; Kalenak, A.; Stumpf, P.G. Women athletes with menstrual irregularity have increased musculoskeletal injuries. Med. and Science in Sports and Exercise. 18(4):374-379; 1986.

121. Lloyd-Smith, R.; Clement, D.B.; McKenzie, D.C.; Taunton, J.E. A survey of overuse and traumatic hip and pelvic injuries in athletes. Physician Sports Med. 13(10):131-137,141; 1985.

122. Lombardo, J.A.; Bergfeld, J.A.; Micheli, L.J. Cross country runner with pain in the dorsum of the foot. Physician Sports Med. 16(3):85-88; 1988.

123. Lombardo, S.J.; Benson, D.W. Stress fractures of the femur in runners. Amer. J. Sports Med. 10(4):219-227; 1982.

124. Luchini, M.A.; Sarakhhan, A.J.; Micheli, L. Acute displaced femoral shaft fractures in long distance runners. Two case reports. J. Bone and Joint Surgery. 65(5):689-691; 1983.

125. Lundell, C.; Kadir, S. Jogger's aneurysm: unusual presentation of popliteal artery trauma. Cardiovascular and Interventional Radiology. 4(4):239-241; 1981.

126. Lutter, L. Injuries in the runner and jogger. Minnesota Med. 63(1):45-51; 1981.

127. Lutter, L.D. Cavus foot in runners. Foot and Ankle. 1(4):225-228; 1981.

128. Lutter, L.D. Surgical decisions in athletes' subcalcaneal pain. Amer. J. Sports Med. 14(6):481-485; 1986.

129. Lysholm, J.; Wiklander, J. Injuries in runners. Amer. J. Sports Med. 15(2):168-171; 1987.

130. Macera, C.A. Lower extremity injuries in runners. Advances in prediction. Sports Med. 13(1):50-57; 1992.

131. Macera, C.A.; Pate, R.R.; Powell, K.E.; Jackson, K.L.; Kendrick, J.S.; Cravery, T.E. Predicting lower extremity injuries among habitual runners. Archives Internal Med. 149:2565-2568; 1989.

132. MacIntyre, J.; Lloyd-Smith, R. Overuse running injuries. In: Renstrom, P.A.F., ed. Sports Injuries: Basic Principles of Prevention and Care. London: Blackwell Scientific; 1993:139-160.

133. Mackie, J.W.; Webster, J.A. Deep vein thrombosis in marathon runners. Physician Sports Med. 9(5):91-96; 1981.

134. Mann, R.A.; Baxter, D.E.; Lutter, L.D. Running symposium. Foot and Ankle. 1(4):190-224; 1981.

135. Marshall, P. The rehabilitation of overuse foot injuries in athletes and dancers. Clin. Podiatr. Med. Surg. 6(3):639-655; 1989.

136. Marti, B. Benefits and risks of running among women: an epidemiologic study. International J. Sports Med. 9(2):92-98; 1988.

137. Marti, B. Relationships between running injuries and running shoes: results of a study of 5000 participants of a 16 Km run—May 1984 Bern Grand Prix. In: Segasser, B.; Pfoerringer, W., eds. The Shoe in Sport. Chicago: Yearbook Med. Publishers; 1989:256-265.

138. Marti, B.; Vader, J.P.; Minder, C.E.; Abelin, T. On the epidemiology of running injuries: the 1984 Bern Grand-Prix study. Amer. J. Sports Med. 16(3):285-294; 1988.

139. Massey, E.W. Effort headache in runners. Headache. 22(3):99-100; 1982.

140. Matheson, G.O.; Clement, D.B.; McKenzie, D.C.; Taunton, J.E.; Lloyd-Smith, D.R.; MacIntyre, J.G. Stress fractures in athletes: a study of 320 cases. Amer. J. Sports Med. 15(1):46-58; 1987.

141. Matin, P.; Lang, G.; Carretta, R.; Simon, G. Scintigraphic evaluation of muscle damage following extreme exercise: concise communication. J. Nuclear Med. and Allied Sciences. 24(4):308-311; 1983.

142. Maughan, R.J. Incidence of training related injuries among marathon runners. British J. Sports Med. 17(3):162-165; 1983.

143. Maughan, R.J. Exercise induced muscle cramp: a prospective biochemical study in marathon runners. J. Sport Sciences. 4(1):31-34; 1986.

144. McBryde, A.M. Stress fracture in runners. In: D'Ambrosia. R.D.; Drez, D., eds. Prevention and Treatment of Running Injuries. Thorofare, NJ: C.B. Slack; 1982:21-42.

145. McBryde, A.M.; Jackson, D.W.; James, C.M. Injuries in runners and joggers. In: Schneider, R.C., ed. Sports Injuries: Mechanisms, Prevention, and Treatment. Baltimore: Williams & Wilkins; 1985; 395-416.

146. McDermott, M.; Freyne, P. Osteoarthritis in runners with knee pain. British J. Sports Med. 17(2):84-87; 1983.

147. McKeag, D.B.; Dolan, C. Overuse syndromes of the lower extremity. Physician Sports Med. 17(7):108-112, 114-116, 121-123; 1989.

148. McKenzie, D.C.; Taunton, J.E.; Clement, D.B.; Smart, G.W.; McNicol, K.L. Calcaneal epiphysitis in adolescent athletes. Canadian J. Applied Sport Sciences. 6(3):123-125; 1981.

149. McKenzie, D.C.; Clement, D.B.; Taunton, J.E. Running shoes: orthotics and injuries. Sports Med. 2(5):334-347; 1985.

150. McMahon, L.F.; Ryan, M.J.; Larson, D.; Fisher, R.L. Acute gastrointestinal blood loss in marathon runners. Annals of Internal Med. 100(6):846-847; 1984.

151. McNichol, K.; Taunton, J.E.; Clement, D.B. Iliotibial tract friction syndrome in athletes. Canadian J. Applied Sport Sciences. 6(2):76-80; 1981.

152. McPoil, T.G.; Cornwall, M.W. Rigid versus soft foot orthoses. A single subject design. J. Amer. Podiatric Med. Association. 81(12):638-642; 1992.

153. McQuade, K.J. A case-control study of running injuries: comparison of patterns of runners with and without running injuries. J. Orthopaedic and Sports Physical Therapy. 8:81-84; 1986.

154. Medhat, M.A.; Redford, J.B. Knee injuries. Damage from running and related sports. J. Kansas Med. Society. 84(7):379-383, 413; 1983.

155. Messier, S.P.; Pittala, K.A. Etiologic factors associated with selected running injuries. Med. and Science in Sports and Exercise. 20(5):501-505; 1988.

156. Messier, S.P.; Davis, S.E.; Curl, W.W.; Lowery, R.B.; Pack, R.J. Etiologic factors associated with patellofemoral pain in runners. Med. and Science in Sports and Exercise. 23(11):1233; 1991.

157. Meyer, J.M.; Hoffmeyer, P.; Borst, F. The treatment of hallux valgus in runners using a modified McBride procedure. International Orthopaedics. 11(3):197-200; 1987.

158. Micheli, L. Female runners. In: D'Ambrosia, R.D.; Drez, D., eds. Prevention and Treatment of Running Injuries. Thorofare, NJ: C.B. Slack; 1982:125-134.

159. Miller, M.L. Avulsion fractures of the anterior superior iliac spine in high school track. Athletic Training. 17(1):57-59; 1982.

160. Mills, G.Q.; Marymount, J.H.; Murphy, D.A. Bone scan utilization in the differential diagnosis of exercise-induced lower extremity pain. Clinical Orthopaedics. 149:207-210; 1980.

161. Mirkin, G. Prevention and treatment of running injuries. J. Amer. Podiatry Association. 66(11):880-884; 1976.

162. Montgomery, L.C.; Nelson, F.R.T.; Norton, J.P.; Deuster, P.A. Orthopedic history and examination in the etiology of overuse injuries. Med. and Science in Sports and Exercise. 21(3):237-243; 1989.

163. Mozee, G.; Prokop, D. You can fight lower back pain: the constant jarring of running can be hard on the back, but there are tried and true methods to strengthen the back against injury. Runner's World. 19(5):66-69, 130; 1984.

164. Mubarak, S.J. Exertional compartment syndromes. In: D'Ambrosia, R.D.; Drez, D., eds. Prevention and Treatment of Running Injuries, 2nd ed. Thorofare, NJ: Slack; 1982:133-153.

165. Nagel, D.; Seiler, D.; Franz, H.; Jung, K. Ultra long distance running and the liver. Int. J. Sports Med. 11(6):441-445; 1990.

166. Nelson, M.E.; Fisher, E.C.; Catsos, P.D.; Meredith, C.N.; Turksoy, R.N.; Evans, W.J. Diet and bone status in amenorrheic runners. Amer. J. Clinical Nutrition. 43:910-916; 1986.

167. Newell, S.G.; Bramwell, S.T. Overuse injuries to the knee in runners. Physician Sports Med. 12(3):80-85, 88, 90-92; 1984.

168. Newman, N.M.; Fowles, J.V. A case of "trigger toe." Canadian J. Surgery. 27(4):378-379; 1984.

169. Nicholl, J.P.; Williams, B.T. Injuries sustained by runners during a popular marathon. British J. Sports Med. 17(1):10-15; 1983.

170. Nichols, A.W. Achilles tendinitis in running athletes. J. Am. Board Fam. Prac. 2(3):196-203; 1989.

171. Nilsson, S. Overuse knee injuries in runners. International J. Sports Med. Nov(supp.5):145-148; 1984.

172. Noakes, T.D.; Smith, J.A.; Lindenberg, G.; Wills, C.E. Pelvic stress fractures in long distance runners. Amer. J. Sports Med. 13(2):120-123; 1985.

173. Noble, C. Iliotibial band friction syndrome in runners. Amer. J. Sports Med. 8(4):232-234; 1980.

174. Nudel, D.B.; Hassett, I.; Gurian, A.; Diamant, S.; Weinhouse, E.; Goodman, N. Young long distance runners. Physiological and psychological characteristics. Clin. Pediatr. 28(11):500-505; 1989.

175. O'Brien, C.J.; Hopkinson, J.M.; Bastable, J.R. Haematuria after strenuous exercise. British J. Urology. 59(5):478; 1987.

176. Ogden, J.A.; McCarthy, S.M.; Jokl, P. Painful bipartite patella. J. Pediatric Orthopaedics. 2(3):263-269; 1982.

177. Orava, S. Overexertion injuries in keep-fit athletes. A study on overexertion injuries among non-competitive keep-fit athletes. Scandinavian J. Rehabilitative Med. 10(4):187-191; 1978.

178. Orava, S.; Saarela, J. Exertion injuries to young athletes. Amer. J. Sports Med. 6(2):68-74; 1978.

179. Otis, C.L.; Puffer, J.C.; Mandelbaum, B.R. Tibial pain in an amenorrheic runner. Physician Sports Med. 16(5):115-118, 122; 1988.

180. Pagliano, J.W. You don't have to hurt: a guide to understanding, treating and avoiding the 10 most common running injuries. Runner's World. 21(6):30-32, 34, 36, 38-39; 1986.

181. Pagliano, J.W.; Jackson, D.W. The ultimate study of running injuries. Runner's World. 15(11):42-50; 1980.

182. Pagliano, J.W.; Jackson, D.W. A clinical study of 3,000 long distance runners. Annals Sports Med. 3(2):88-91; 1987.

183. Panni, A.S.; Maiotti, M.; Burke, J. Osteoid osteoma of the neck of the talus. Amer. J. Sports Med. 17(4):584-588; 1989.

184. Parsons, M.A.; Anderson, P.B.; Williams, B.T. An "unavoidable" death in a people's marathon. British J. Sports Med. 18(1):38-39; 1984.

185. Paty, J.G. Diagnosis and treatment of musculoskeletal running injuries. Semin. Arthritis Rheum. 18(1):48-60; 1988.

186. Paty, J.G.; Swafford, D. Adolescent running injuries. J. Adolescent Health Care. 5(2):87-90; 1984.

187. Paul, G.R. Injury prevention and rehabilitation in track. In: Cantu, R.C., ed. Clinical Sports Med. Lexington, MA: Collamore Press, D.C. Heath; 1984:193-201.

188. Pavlov, H.; Nelson, T.; Warren, R.F.; Torg, J.S.; Burstein, A.H. Stress fractures of the pubic ramus. A report of twelve cases. J. Bone and Joint Surgery. 64(7):1020-1025; 1982.

189. Pearl, A.J. Anterior compartment syndrome: a case report. Amer. J. Sports Med. 9(2):119-120; 1981.

190. Percy, E.C.; Gamble, F.O. Epiphyseal stress fracture of the foot and shin splints in an anomalous calf muscle in a runner. Case report. British J. Sports Med. 14(2/3):110-113; 1980.

191. Pickering, T.G. Runner's radial palsy (letter). New England J. Med. 305(13):768; 1981.

192. Pinshaw, R.; Atlas, V.; Noakes, T.D. The nature and response to therapy of 196 consecutive injuries seen at a runners' clinic. South African Med. J. 65(8):291-298; 1984.

193. Pittman, M.I.; Norman, A. Value of CT scanning in differential pain diagnosis in runners. Amer. J. Sports Med. 14(4):324-326; 1986.

194. Powell, K.E.; Kohl, H.W.; Caspersen, C.J.; Blair, S.N. An epidemiological perspective on the causes of running injuries. Physician Sports Med. 14(6):100-103, 106-108, 111-114; 1986.

195. Prescott, L. Pelvis stress fractures more common in women. Physician Sports Med. 11(5):25-26; 1983.

196. Pretorius, D.M.; Noakes, T.D.; Irving, G.; Allerton, K. Runner's knee: What is it and how effective is conservative management? Physician Sports Med. 14(12):71-81; 1986.

197. Puranen, J.; Orava, S. The hamstring syndrome: a new diagnosis of gluteal sciatic pain. Amer. J. Sports Med. 16(5):517-521; 1988.

198. Reilly, J.P.; Nicholas, J.A. The chronically inflamed bursa. Clinics in Sports Med. 6(2):345-369; 1987.

199. Richards, D.; Richards, R.; Schofield, J.; Ros, V.; Sutton, J.R. Management of heat exhaustion in Sydney's the Sun-City-to-Surf fun runners. Med. J. Australia. 2:457-461; 1979.

200. Riddoch, C.; Trinick, T. Gastrointestinal disturbances in marathon runners. British J. Sports Med. 22(2):9-11; 1988.

201. Robertson, J.D.; Maughan, R.J.; Davidson, R.J. Fecal blood loss in response to exercise. British Med. J. 295(6593):303, 305; 1991.

202. Rockett, J.F.; Magill, H.L.; Moinuddin, M.; Buchignani, J.S. Scintigraphic manifestation of iliotibial band injury in an endurance athlete. Clinical Nuclear Med. 16(11):836-838; 1991.

203. Rodgers, A.L.; Greyling, K.G.; Irving, R.A.; Noakes, T.D. Crystalluria in marathon runners. II Ultra-marathon-males and females. Urological Research. 16(2):89-93; 1988.

204. Rold, J.F.; Rold, B.A. Pubic stress symphysitis in a female distance runner. Physician Sports Med. 14(6):61-63, 65; 1986.

205. Rose, R.C.; Hughes, R.D. Heat injuries among recreational runners. Southern Med. J. 73(8):1038-1040; 1980.

206. Ross, C.F.; Schuster, R.O. A preliminary report on predicting injuries in distance runners. J. Amer. Podiatry Association. 73(5):275-277; 1983.

207. Roub, L.W.; Gummerman, L.W.; Hanley, E.N.; Clark, M.W.; Goodman, M.; Herbert, D.L. Bone stress: a radionuclide imaging perspective. Radiology. 132:431-438; 1979.

208. Rowland, T.W.; Walsh, C.A. Characteristics of child distance runners. Physician Sports Med. 13(9):45-48, 52-53; 1985.

209. Rzonca, E.C.; Baylis, W.J. Common sports injuries to the foot and leg. Clin. Podiatr. Med. Surg. 5(3):591-612; 1988.

210. Sadaniantz, A.; Clayton, M.A.; Sturner, W.Q.; Thompson, P.D. Sudden death immediately after a record-setting athletic performance. Amer. J. Cardiology. 63(5):375; 1989.

211. Schepsis, A.A.; Leach, R.E. Surgical management of achilles tendonitis. Amer. J. Sports Med. 15(4):308-315; 1987.

212. Schils, J.; Hauzeur, J.P. Stress fracture of the sacrum. Amer. J. Sports Med. 20(6):769-770; 1992.

213. Schils, J.P.; Andrish, J.T.; Piraino, D.W.; Belhobek, G.H.; Richmond, B.J.; Bergfeld, J.A. Medial malleolar stress fractures in seven patients: review of the clinical and imaging features. Radiology. 185(1):219-221; 1992.

214. Schlefman, B.S.; Arenson, D.J. Recurrent tibial stress fractures in a jogger. J. Amer. Podiatry Association. 71(100):577-579; 1981.

215. Schneider, R.; Kaye, J.; Ghelman, B. Adductor avulsive injuries near the symphysis pubis. Radiology. 120(3):567-569; 1976.

216. Schoch, D.R.; Sullivan, A.L.; Grand, R.J.; Eagan, W.F. Gastrointestinal bleeding in an adolescent runner. J. Pediatrics. 111(2):302-304; 1987.

217. Schranz, P.J. Stress fracture of the patella (letter). Br. J. Sports Med. 22(4):169; 1988.

218. Schwartz, A.E.; Vanagunas, A.; Kamel, P.L. Endoscopy to evaluate gastrointestinal bleeding in marathon runners. Annals Internal Med. 113(8):632-633; 1990.

219. Shellock, F.G.; Deutsch, A.L.; Mink, J.H.; Kerr, R. Do asymptomatic marathon runners have an increased prevalence of meniscal abnormalities? An MR study of the knee in 23 volunteers. Amer. J. Roentgenology. 157(6):1239-1241; 1991.

220. Shellock, F.G.; Morris, E.; Deutsch, A.L.; Mink, J.H.; Kerr, R.; Boden, S.D. Hematopoietic bone marrow hyperplasia: high prevalence on MR images of the knee in asymptomatic marathon runners. Amer. J. Roentgenology. 158(2):335-338; 1992.

221. Sherwood, B.K.; Strong, W.B. Heat stress in athletes. J. Med. Association of Georgia. 74(7):478-480; 1985.

222. Simpson, R.R.; Gudas, C.J. Posterior tibial tendon rupture in a world class runner. J. Foot Surgery. 22(1):74-77; 1983.

223. Sjostrom, M.; Johansson, C.; Lorentzon, R. Muscle pathomorphology in m. quadriceps of marathon runners. Early signs of strain disease or functional adaptation? Acta. Physiol. Scand. 132(4):537-541; 1988.

224. Skinner, H.B.; Cook, S.D. Fatigue failure stress of the femoral neck: a case report. Amer. J. Sports Med. 10(4):245-247; 1982.

225. Smith, W.B. Environmental factors in running. Amer. J. Sports Med. 8(2):138-140; 1980.

226. Smith, L.S.; Tillo, T.H. Haglund's deformity in long distance runners. Nine surgical cases. J. Amer. Podiatric Association. 78(8):419-422; 1988.

227. Spector, F.C.; Karlin, J.M.; DeValentine, S.; Scurran, B.L.; Silvani, S.L. Spiral fracture of the distal tibia: An unusual stress fracture. J. Foot Surgery. 22(4):358-361; 1983.

228. Stacoff, A.; Kalin, X.; Stussi, E. The effects of shoes on the torsion and rearfoot motion in running. Med. and Science in Sports and Exercise. 23(4):482-490; 1991.

229. Stamford, B. Sportsmedicine advisor: training distance and injury in runners. Physician Sports Med. 12(8):160; 1984.

230. Stanitski, C.L. Knee pain in a young female runner. In: Smith, N.J., ed. Common Problems in Pediatric Sports Med. Chicago: Year Book Med. Publishers; 1989:242-248.

231. Sterling, J.C.; Webb, R.F., Jr.; Meyers, M.C.; Calvo, R.D. False negative bone scan in a female runner. Med. Sci. Sports Excer. 25(2):179-185; 1993.

232. Subotnick, S.I. The biomechanics of running implications for the prevention of foot injuries. Sports Med. 2(2):144-153; 1985.

233. Subotnick, S.I.; Sisney, P. Treatment of achilles tendinopathy in the athlete. J. Amer. Podiatric Med. Association. 76(10):552-557; 1986.

234. Sullivan, D.; Warren, R.F.; Pavlov, H.; Kelman, G. Stress fractures in 51 runners. Clinical Orthopaedics and Related Research. 187:188-192; 1984.

235. Sutherland, I.H. Idiopathic edema in the athletic woman. Singapore Med. J. 27(3):253-255; 1986.

236. Sutker, A.N.; Barber, F.A.; Jackson, D.W.; Pagliano, J.W. Iliotibial band syndrome in distance runners. Sports Med. 2(6):447-451; 1985.

237. Sutton, J.R.; Nilson, K.L. Repeated stress fractures in an amenorrheic marathoner. Physician Sports Med. 17(4):65-71; 1989.

238. Taunton, J.E.; Clement, D.B.; McNicol, K. Plantar fasciitis in runners. Canadian J. Applied Sport Sciences. 7(1):41-44; 1982.

239. Taunton, J.E.; Clement, D.B.; Webber, D. Lower extremity stress fractures in athletes. Physician Sports Med. 9(1):77-81, 85-86; 1981.

240. Taunton, J.E.; Clement, D.B.; Smart, G.W.; McNicol, K.L. Non-surgical management of overuse knee injuries in runners. Canadian J. Sports Science. 12(1):11-18; 1987.

241. Temple, C. Sports injuries. Hazards of jogging and marathon running. British J. Hospital Med. 29(3):237-239; 1983.

242. Thompson, P. Death during jogging or running: A study of 18 cases. J. Amer. Med. Association. 242:1265-1267; 1979.

243. Tunstall-Pedoe, D. Medical support for marathons in the United Kingdom The London Marathon. In: Sutton, J.R.; Brock, R.M., eds. Sports Medicine for the Mature Athlete. Indianapolis: Benchmark Press; 1986:181-192.

244. Valliant, P.M. Injury and personality traits in non-competitive runners. J. Sports Med. and Physical Fitness. 20(3):341-346; 1980.

245. Valliant, P.M. Personality and injury in competitive runners. Perceptual and Motor Skills. 53(1):251-253; 1981.

246. van Mechelen, W. Running injuries: A review of the epidemiological literature. Sports Med. 14(5):320-325; 1992.

247. van Mechelen, W.; Hlobil, H.; Zijilstra, W.P.; de Ridder, M.; Kemper, H.C. Is range of motion of the hip and ankle joint related to running injuries? A case control study. Int. J. Sports Med. 13(8):605-610; 1992.

248. Veluvolu, P.; Kohn, H.S.; Guten, G.N.; Donahue, P.M.; Isitman, A.T.; Whalen, J.P.; Collier, B.D. Unusual stress fracture of the scapula in a jogger. Clin. Nucl. Med. 13(7):531-532; 1988.

249. Verde, T.; Thomas, S.; Shephard, R.J. Potential markers of heavy training in highly trained distance runners. British J. Sports Med. 26(3):167-175; 1992.

250. Viitasalo, J.T.; Kvist, M. Some biomechanical aspects of the foot and ankle in athletes with and without shin splints. Amer. J. Sports Med. 11:125-130; 1983.

251. Wallenstein, R.; Eriksson, E. Is medial lower leg pain (shin splint) a chronic compartment syndrome? In: Mack, R.P., ed. Symposium on the Foot and Leg in Running Sports. Coronado, CA: 1982; 135-140.

252. Wallenstein, R.; Karlsson, J. Histochemical and metabolic changes in lower leg muscles in exercise-induced pain. International J. Sports Med. 5(4): 202; 1984.

253. Waller, B.F.; Csere, R.S. Running to death. Chest. 79(3):346-349; 1981.

254. Walter, S.D.; Hart, L.E. Application of epidemiological methodology to sports science research. Exercise and Sports Science Reviews. 18(14):417-448; 1990.

255. Walter, S.D.; Hart, L.E.; McIntosh, J.M.; Sutton, J.R. The Ontario cohort study of running related injuries. Archives Internal Med. 149:2561-2564; 1989.

256. Walter, S.D.; Hart, L.E.; Sutton, J.R.; McIntosh, J.M.; Gauld, M. Training habits and injury experience in distance runners: Age- and sex-related factors. Physician Sport Med. 16(6):101-113; 1988.

257. Walter, S.D.; Sutton, J.R.; McIntosh, J.M.; Connolly, C. The aetiology of sport injuries. A review of methodologies. Sports Med. 2:47-58; 1985.

258. Wang, S.S.; Whitney, S.L.; Burdett, R.G.; Janosky, J.E. Lower extremity muscular flexibility in long distance. J. Orthop. Sports. Phys. Therapy 17(2): 102-107; 1993.

259. Warhol, M.J.; Siegel, A.J.; Evans, W.J.; Silverman, L.M. Skeletal muscle injury and repair in marathon runners after competition. Amer. J. Pathology. 118(2):331-339; 1985.

260. Warren, B.L. Plantar fasciitis in runners: treatment and prevention. Sports Med. 10(5):338-345; 1990.

261. Warren, B.L.; Jones, C.J. Predicting plantar fasciitis in runners. Med. and Science in Sports and Exercise. 19(1):71-73; 1987.

262. Watson, M.D.; DiMartino, P.P. Incidence of injuries in high school track and field athletes and its relation to performance ability. Amer. J. Sports Med. 15(3):251-254; 1987.

263. Weiss, R.F. The anemic runner. J. Amer. Podiatric Medical Association. 76(10):584-585; 1986.

264. Whieldon, T.J.; Wihiewicz, T.W. Sacroiliac dysfunction in runners. Athletic Training. 21(1):15-19; 1986.

265. White, T.L.; Malone, T.R. Effects of running on intervertebral disc height. J. Orthopaedic Sports Physical Therapy. 12(4):139-146; 1990.

266. Whitworth, J.A.; Wolfman, M.J. Fatal heat stroke in a long distance runner. British Med. J. 287(6397): 948; 1983.

267. Williams, A.F. When motor vehicles hit joggers: an analysis of 60 cases. Public Health Reports, 96(5):448-451; 1981.

268. Williams, K.R. Biomechanics of running. Exercise and Sport Sciences Reviews. 13:389-441; 1985.

269. Winter, D.A.; Bishop, P.J. Biomechanical factors associated with chronic injury to the lower extremity. Sports Med. 14:149-156; 1992.

270. Wischnia, B. Runners who never get injured. Runner's World. 19:59-62; 1984.

271. Woods, L.; Leach, R.E. Posterior tibial tendon rupture in athletic people. Amer. J. Sports Med. 19:495-498; 1991.

272. Zacharias, C.K.; Marsh, H.O. Jogging: a non-traumatic exercise? J. Kansas Med. Society. 81:563-565; 1980.

# 23

# Soccer

*Melinda Larson, Arthur J. Pearl,*
*Rey Jaffet, and Andrew Rudawsky*

## 1. Introduction

Soccer is the most popular sport in the world with about 200 million players in 186 countries registered with the International Federation of Football Association, FIFA (19). Since 1970, the popularity of this sport has increased considerably in the United States. This trend is most apparent in women's and youth soccer. With the increased popularity, the number of soccer injuries has also likely increased.

The purpose of this review is to explore the nature and incidence of soccer injuries and possible risk factors, suggesting preventive measures and avenues for further study. An overview of the epidemiologic literature, for soccer injuries at all levels of participation, was accomplished. This literature review encompassed the years 1976-1994 and was limited to English language publications. We used Medline, Soccer Industry Council of America, NCAA soccer injury surveillance reports from 1976-1993[1], and the database for the National Library of Congress in compiling this study. The key words in this search were soccer, football, injury, prevention, and epidemiology.

A comparison of the nature and incidence of injuries across studies was limited by the following:

- Inconsistency in the definition of an injury.
- A wide diversity in the backgrounds of the evaluators of these injuries.
- A lack of common terms for the description of injuries.
- Varied use of time loss as a criterion for injury severity.

- A small number of athletes in some studies.
- Failure to address the difference between chronic and acute injuries.
- Playing time per athlete was not recorded.

## 2. Incidence of Injury

### 2.1 Injury Rates

The data on injury rates for senior amateur and professional males and females are shown in Table 23.1. A review of these data suggests the following observations:

- Among studies reporting the number of injuries per 1,000 exposures, university age males had a higher rate of injury than senior amateur males.
- In studies reporting the number of injuries per hours of practice, elite and college age females had slightly higher injury rates than males, with the exception of senior amateur males studied by Ekstrand et al. (11).
- Injury rates per hour in games were highest in elite senior females, followed by college males. Senior amateur males and college females had similar rates, with semipro males reporting the lowest injury rates in games.

Injury rates for youth soccer are shown in Table 23.2. Reported injury rates in youth soccer yield conflicting results primarily because of differences in data collection and definition of injury. A review of Table 23.2 suggests the following observations:

---

[1]Conclusions drawn from or recommendations based on the data provided by the National Collegiate Athletic Association are those of the authors based on analyses/evaluations of the authors and do not represent the views of the officers, staff, or membership of the NCAA.

**Table 23.1  Injury Rates**

| Reference | Study period | Population | Sample size | No. of injuries | Study design | Data collection method | Injuries per 1,000 hours of practice or game | Injuries per 1,000 exposures |
|---|---|---|---|---|---|---|---|---|
| Albert, 1983 | 3 outdoor seasons 1 indoor season | Professional males age 19-38 | 56 players | 142 | Prospective | Exam by athletic trainer | 9.3 | |
| Ekstrand et al., 1983b | 1 season | Senior amateur males | 180 players | 156 | Prospective | Coach | Practice, 7.6 Game, 16.9 | |
| Ekstrand & Tropp, 1990 | 1 year | Senior amateur males age 17-35 | 639 players | 913 | Prospective | Weekly interview with coach | | 9.1 |
| Engström et al., 1990 | 1 season | Semi-professional males | 64 players | 85 | Prospective | Exam by athletic trainer | Practice, 3 Game, 13 | |
| Engström et al., 1991 | 1 year | Elite senior females | 41 players | 78 | Prospective | Medical students | Practice, 7 Game, 24 | |
| NCAA Men, 1992 | 6 seasons | College males | 451 teams | 5,173 | Prospective | Exam by athletic trainer | Practice, 4.72 Game, 19.67 | |
| NCAA Women, 1992 | 6 seasons | College females | 270 teams | 2,505 | Prospective | Exam by athletic trainer | Practice, 5.32 Game, 16.42 | |
| Nielsen & Yde, 1989 | 1 season | Males | 123 | 109 | Prospective | Coach | Practice, 3.6 Game, 14.3 | |
| Poulsen et al., 1991 | 1 season | Amateur males age 21-30 | 55 players | 57 | Prospective | Author interviews with players | | 8.4 |
| Resnick, 1980 | 3 seasons | University males | 1,090 | | Prospective | Exam by athletic trainer | | 1975, 18.1 1976, 17.6 1977, 17.4 |

- Injury rates for females are consistently greater than for males.
- Injury rates appear to be highest at higher competitive levels, for example, international tournaments.
- Injury rates from studies conducted over an entire season are lower than studies done during summer camps or tournaments, and this is consistent with research shown in Table 23.1, which suggests higher rates for games than practice.

## 2.2 Injury Rates in Practice vs. Competition

Keller, Noyes, and Buncher (21) noted an equal distribution of injuries during games and practices in the senior players. However, when exposure information was taken into account and injury rates for games versus practice calculated, the picture was different. In studies reporting separate injury rates for practices and games, injury rates in games were higher than during practices. This finding was consistent for senior amateur males (11), semiprofessional males (14), elite senior females (15), college males and females (29), and for youth (3, 18, 21).

Ekstrand and Gillquist's (7) study of 12 male teams in Sweden and Engström, Johansson, and Törnkvist's (15) study of two female Swedish teams indicated that traumatic injuries occurred more frequently in games, and overuse injuries occurred during practices.

## 3. Injury Characteristics

### 3.1 Injury Onset

A review of Table 23.3 reveals that most soccer injuries have acute onset, probably because the

**Table 23.2   Youth Injury Rates**

| Reference | Study period | Population | No. of injuries | Ages (years) | Data collection method | Study design | Injury definition | Injuries per 1,000 hours of practice or game |
|---|---|---|---|---|---|---|---|---|
| Backous et al., 1988 | 5 one-week summer camps | 458 girls<br>681 boys | 107<br>105 | 6-17<br>6-17 | Exam by athletic trainer | Prospective | Time loss of one or more 2-hour sessions | 10.6<br>7.3 |
| Backx et al., 1991 | 7 months | 361 boys and girls | | 8-17 | School children self reporting | Prospective | Time loss | Practice 1.6<br>Games, 8 |
| Kristiansen, 1983 | Tournament, 35 games | boys | 114 | 6-11 | Observation and personal interview | Prospective | Time loss | 6.7 |
| Maehlum et al., 1986 | 6-day international tournament | 332 girls teams<br>1,016 boys teams | 145<br>266 | Under 18<br>Under 18 | Exam by on-site paramedic or physician | Prospective | Any injury reported | 17.6<br>9.9 |
| Nilsson and Roaas, 1978 | 2 6-day international tournaments | 25,000 boys and girls | 1,534 | Under 18 | Exam by on-site health professional | Prospective | Any injury reported | Girls, 32[a]<br>Boys, 14[a] |
| Schmidt-Olsen et al., 1985 | 2 5-day international tournaments | 1,325 girls<br>5,275 boys | 117<br>229 | 9-19<br>9-19 | Exam by on-site health professional | Prospective | Advice of reduced activity given | 17.6<br>7.4 |
| Schmidt-Olsen et al., 1991 | 1 year | 496 boys | 312 | 12-18 | Self registration by players and coach | Prospective | Time loss | 3.7 |
| Sullivan et al., 1980 | One season | 341 girls<br>931 boys | 15<br>19 | 7-18<br>7-18 | Author interview with coach | Prospective | Time loss | 1.1<br>0.51 |
| Yde and Nielsen, 1990 | One season | 152 boys | 119 | 6-18 | Author interview with athletes | Prospective | Time loss | 5.6 |
| Hoff and Martin, 1986 | 1 outdoor season 1 indoor season | 455 males<br>366 males | 46<br>74 | 8-16<br>8-16 | Mailed questionnaire | Retrospective | Time loss | 7.4<br>45.2 |

[a]All injuries and illnesses except blisters and minor skin abrasions.

**Table 23.3   Injury Onset**

| Reference | Population | Sample size | No. of injuries | Type of study | Acute injuries (%) | Overuse injuries (%) |
|---|---|---|---|---|---|---|
| Albert, 1983 | Professional males age 19-34 | 56 | 142 | Prospective | 136 (96) | 6 (4)[a] |
| Ekstrand et al., 1983b | Senior males age 17-38 | 180 | 256 | Prospective | 177 (69) | 79 (31) |
| Engström et al., 1991 | Elite females age 16-28 | 41 | 78 | Prospective | 56 (72) | 22 (28) |
| Brynhildsen et al., 1990 | Senior females age 15-34 | 150 | 248 | Retrospective | 209 (85) | 39 (15) |

[a]Inflammatory/overuse.

game of soccer demands bursts of speed and power and includes frequent collisions with other players, the ball, and the playing surface. However, the results in the table may not be entirely accurate because of varying definitions of acute and overuse injuries. Most authors were vague on what classified as a chronic injury, for example, inflammatory, overuse, and tendinitis. Ekstrand

and Gillquist (7) stated that overuse injuries were most often seen during preseason training and that adductor tenosynovitis and Achilles tendinitis were the most common types of overuse injury. Shin splints and iliotibial tract tendinitis were common overuse injuries in female players (4).

## 3.2 Injury Type

A review of the prospective studies in Table 23.4 suggests that the most common injuries in soccer are sprains (27.6-35.0%), strains (10.0-47%), and contusions (8.3-21.3%).

In youth soccer players, on the other hand, the most common injury type appears to be contusion (32.9-47.0%), followed by sprains (19.4-35.3%), strains (8.8-27.8%), and wounds (6.5-39.0%), as reported by prospective studies. In Hoff and Martin's retrospective study (18), the most common injury found was sprain (38.3%), followed by strain (23.3%) and contusion (18.3%). The variation in the different studies as to the frequency of sprains and

**Table 23.4   Injury Type (Percent of Total Injuries)**

| Study type | Albert, 1983 N=56 Prospective | Ekstrand & Gillquist, 1983b N=180 Prospective | Engström et al., 1991 N=41 Prospective | McMaster & Walter, 1978 N=15 Prospective | NCAA men, 1992 N=105 teams Prospective | NCAA women, 1992 N=61 teams Prospective | Poulsen et al., 1991 N=55 Prospective |
|---|---|---|---|---|---|---|---|
| Total number of injuries | 142 | 256 | 78 | 60 | 1,221 | 594 | 57 |
| Sprain | 27.6 | 29 | 33 | 35.0 | 58.2 | 54.0 | 71.8 |
| Strain | 31.0 | 18 | 10 | 47.0 | | | |
| Contusion | 17.6 | 20 | 15 | 8.3 | 11.6 | 21.3 | 12.3 |
| Dislocation/ subluxation | 3.5 | 2 | 3 | 5.0 | 2.2 | 1.7 | — |
| Fracture | 3.5 | 4 | 1 | 1.7 | 5.5 | 5.7 | 7.0 |
| Wound | — | — | — | 3.3[b] | 1.3 | 2.4 | 3.5 |
| Bursitis/ tendinitis | 4.2[a] | 23 | 24 | — | 4.5 | 3.2 | — |
| Concussion | 2.1 | — | — | — | 2.9 | 3.7 | — |
| Other | 10.5 | 4 | 13 | — | 1.3 | 1.0 | 5.3 |

[a]Overuse.

[b]Laceration.

**Table 23.5   Youth Injury Type (Percent of Total Injuries)**

| Study type | Backous et al., 1988 N=1,129 Prospective | Maehlum et al., 1986 N=1,348 Prospective | Nilsson & Roaas, 1978 N=25,000 Prospective | Schmidt-Olsen et al., 1985 N=6,600 Prospective | Sullivan et al., 1980 N=1,272 Prospective | Hoff & Martin, 1986 N=821 Retrospective |
|---|---|---|---|---|---|---|
| Total number of injuries | 216 | 411 | 1,534 | 340 | 34 | 120 |
| Sprain | 19.4 | 21.7 | 20.0 | 20.2 | 35.3 | 38.3 |
| Strain | 27.8 | — | | 9.8 | 8.8 | 23.3 |
| Contusion | 35.2 | 47.0 | 36.0 | 32.9 | 38.2 | 18.3 |
| Dislocation | — | 1.0 | — | 1.1 | 2.9 | 0.8 |
| Fracture | — | 5.6 | 3.5 | 4.0 | 5.9 | 5.9 |
| Wound | 6.5 | 18.0[a] | 39.0[b] | 24.2 | — | — |
| Overuse | — | — | — | 5.2 | — | — |
| Concussion | — | — | — | 1.2 | — | — |
| Other | 17.1 | 6.8 | 1.5 | 1.4 | 8.8 | 13.5 |

[a]Laceration.

[b]Skin abrasion/blister.

strains may be attributable to a difference in classification and terminology between the examiners and authors.

## 3.3 Injury Location

Data on injury location are shown in Table 23.6. A review of the table suggests the following observations:

- The data from all types of studies are similar.
- The majority of injuries in prospective studies involve the lower extremity (75.4-93.0%); this was also the case in the retrospective studies (64.0-86.8%).
- Both prospective and retrospective studies indicate that head/spine/trunk injuries appear to occur more often than upper extremity injuries.
- Data from prospective studies indicate the most frequently injured areas in the lower extremity were the ankle (17.0-26.0%) and knee (17.0-23.0%); this was also true in the retrospective studies (20.0-39.5% and 20.1-22.0%, respectively).

Data on youth injury location is shown in Table 23.7. A review of the table reflects similar injury patterns to those of adult players:

- Prospective data indicate that the body region most affected by injury was the lower extremity (61-89%), followed by the upper extremity (4.0-17.6%) and head/spine/trunk (9.7-24.8%); this trend was also evident in the retrospective studies.
- Prospective studies indicate that the ankle (16.0-41.2%) was the most frequently injured body part.

### 3.3.1 Head/Spine/Trunk

The ranges of the total injuries attributable to the head, spine, and trunk areas are 4 to 16.8% in adults and 9.7 to 24.8% in youth, as reported in prospective studies (see Tables 23.6 and 23.7). Fields (16) outlines the most common ways soccer players may sustain head trauma: (a) when a player heads the ball, particularly if they use incorrect form, (b) when a forcefully kicked ball strikes the head, and (c) head-to-head contact, which happens most often when two players attempt to head the ball simultaneously. Common head injuries in soccer resulting from these mechanisms include lacerations and concussions.

Eye injuries have been reported in soccer; however, the incidence of these injuries is unclear. Burke, Sanitato, Vinger, Raymond, and Kulwin (5) reported a series of 24 eye injuries resulting from soccerball impact. Fifty percent resulted in hyphema, 29% vitreous hemorrhage, 21% corneal abrasion, 8% angle recession, and 4% retinal tear. All but two of the patients recovered with normal visual acuities.

### 3.3.2 Upper Extremities

Upper extremity injuries are infrequent in soccer. Prospective studies in Table 23.6 indicate that from 5.9 to 7.8% of all injuries in adult soccer players occur in the upper extremity. In youth soccer players, 4 to 17.6% of all injuries occur in the upper extremity (see Table 23.7). Retrospective studies in both adult and youth players show slightly higher incidence of upper extremity injuries.

### 3.3.3 Lower Extremity

The nature of the game of soccer, in which players make hard cuts, sharp turns off a planted foot, and intense contact with the ball and other players, makes them more vulnerable to lower extremity injury. As indicated in the prospective data in Table 23.6, injuries in the lower extremity occur most frequently in the ankle (17-26.0%) and knee (17.0-23%), followed closely by injuries to the upper leg (14.0-18.3%). In youth, ankle injuries were also the most common lower extremity injury (16-41.2%) with injuries to other areas closely distributed (see Table 23.7).

## 4. Injury Severity

### 4.1 Time Loss

Many epidemiological studies of soccer injuries reported the amount of time loss due to injury. Time loss is an effective indicator of injury severity, but it is dependent on who makes the decision governing when the athlete is able to return to play and by what criteria they make that judgment. Another variable affecting reported time loss is whether the athlete has any days off, and whether those days were included in the reported time lost. There is little uniformity in the establishment of time loss/injury criteria, and this variation makes the data in Table 23.8 difficult to interpret. With these limitations in mind, it is suggested by Table 23.8 that the majority of soccer injuries require less than one week of time loss.

**Table 23.6  Injury Location (Percent of Total Injuries)**

| | Albert, 1983 N=56 | Ekstrand & Gillquist, 1983b N=180 | Engström et al., 1991 N=41 | NCAA men 1991-1992 N=105 teams | NCAA women 1991-1992 N=61 teams | Poulsen et al., 1991 N=55 | Brynhildsen et al., 1990 N=150 | Sandelin et al., 1985 N=35,500 |
|---|---|---|---|---|---|---|---|---|
| Study type | Prospective | Prospective | Prospective | Prospective | Prospective | Prospective | Retrospective | Retrospective |
| Total number of injuries | 142 | 256 | 78 | 1,221 | 595 | 57 | 248 | 2,072 |
| Head/spine/trunk | 16.8 | 5 | 4 | 14.2 | 11.3 | — | 4.8 | 22 |
| Upper extremity | 7.8 | — | — | 6.6 | 5.9 | — | 5.6 | 14 |
| Lower extremity | 75.4 | 88 | 88 | 76.3 | 81.3 | 93 | 86.8 | 64 |
| Hip/groin | 11.3 | 13 | 6 | 5.6 | 5.4 | 10 | 3.6 | 9 |
| Upper leg | 17.7 | 14 | 15 | 17.0 | 18.3 | 18 | 6.0 | 0 |
| Knee | 17.6 | 20 | 23 | 18.0 | 17.0 | 23 | 20.1 | 22 |
| Lower leg | 4.2 | 12 | 9 | 6.6 | 8.9 | 2 | 14.0 | 6 |
| Ankle | 24.6 | 17 | 26 | 21.4 | 22.2 | 19 | 39.5 | 20 |
| Foot/toe | | 12 | 9 | 7.9 | 9.6 | 21 | 3.6 | 7 |
| Other | — | 7 | 8 | 2.9 | 1.5 | 7 | 2.8 | 0 |

**Table 23.7  Youth Injury Location (Percent of Total Injuries)**

| | Backous et al., 1988 N=1,139 | Maehlum et al., 1986 N=1,348 teams | Nilsson & Roaas, 1978 N=25,000 | Schmidt-Olsen et al., 1985 N=6,600 | Sullivan et al., 1980 N=1,272 | Yde & Nielsen, 1990 N=152 | Hoff & Martin, 1986 N=821 | Pritchett, 1987 N=10,634 |
|---|---|---|---|---|---|---|---|---|
| Study type | Prospective | Prospective | Prospective | Prospective | Prospective | Prospective | Retrospective | Retrospective |
| Total number of injuries | 216 | 411 | 351 | 169 | 34 | 119 | 120 | 436 |
| Head/spine/trunk | 9.7 | 24.8 | 17 | 10.7 | 17.6 | — | 25.8 | 9.2 |
| Upper extremity | 4.7 | 14.1 | 15 | 14.8 | 17.6 | 4 | 14.2 | 26.1 |
| Lower extremity | 68.7 | 61.0 | 68 | 74.6 | 64.7 | 89 | 60.0 | 57.6 |
| Hip/groin | 2.8 | — | — | 2.4 | — | — | — | — |
| Upper leg | 8.3 | — | 12 | 14.8 | — | 24[a] | — | — |
| Knee | 12.6 | — | 14 | 13.6 | 11.8 | 19 | — | 11.7 |
| Lower leg | 15.7 | — | 13 | 9.5 | — | — | — | — |
| Ankle | 19.1 | — | 16 | 29.0 | 41.2 | 27 | — | — |
| Foot/toe | 10.2 | — | 13 | 5.3 | — | 19 | — | — |
| Other | 17.1 | — | — | — | 11.8 | 7 | — | — |

[a]Upper and lower leg.

**Table 23.8    Time Loss (Percent of Total Injuries)**

| | Albert, 1983 N=56 | McMaster & Walter, 1978 N=15 | Ekstrand & Gillquist 1983b N=180 | Nielsen and Yde, 1989 N=123 | Engström et al., 1990 N=64 | Engström et al., 1991 N=41 | NCAA men, 1992 N=105 teams | NCAA women, 1992 N=61 teams |
|---|---|---|---|---|---|---|---|---|
| Total number of injuries | 142 | 60 | | | | | | |
| 1-7 days | 72 | 88.3 | | | | | | |
| 8-21 days | 24 | 11.7 | | | | | | |
| >21 days | 4 | 11.7 | | | | | | |
| Total number of injuries | | | 256 | 109 | 85 | 78 | | |
| <1 week | | | 62 | 46 | 27 | 49 | | |
| 1 week-1 month | | | 27 | 19 | 39 | 36 | | |
| >1 month | | | 11 | 35 | 34 | 15 | | |
| Total number of injuries | | | | | | | 5,179 | 2,530 |
| 1-2 days | | | | | | | 42.2 | 39.5 |
| 3-6 days | | | | | | | 32.0 | 32.2 |
| 7-9 days | | | | | | | 8.8 | 9.2 |
| >10 days | | | | | | | 17.0 | 19.1 |

*Note.* All studies indicated in this table are prospective.

Albert (1), in a study of 142 reportable injuries in one season of professional soccer, found that the predominant injuries causing a time loss of one week or more were sprains and strains. He recorded six major injuries (out more than 21 days) with an average time loss of 36 weeks. The overall average time loss per injury was 2.38 games and 8.59 practices.

Yde and Nielsen's (44) study of 152 males under 18 years of age in a Danish sports club revealed similar rates to college-age players and professional males. Of the 24% of all injuries resulting in time loss of 4 weeks or more, four were fractures, seven were knee injuries, and five were ankle sprains.

### 4.2 Catastrophic Injuries

In the six seasons of men's and women's soccer, from 1986 to 1992, the NCAA Soccer Injury Surveillance System recorded only four catastrophic injuries (.05% of all injuries), none of which were fatal.

### 4.3 Clinical Outcome/Residual Symptoms

Serious injuries in soccer may result in persistent symptoms and cause permanent physical damage or disability. If the residual symptoms are severe enough they may force the player to drop to a lower level of play, choose a different activity, or quit playing sports altogether.

Of 180 players examined by Ekstrand and Gillquist (9) 52 players (28.9%) had clinical instability, and 31 (17.2%) had persistent symptoms from previous ankle injury. Twenty-six players (14.4%) also had persistent knee instability from past injury. Tropp et al. (42) found a combined functional and mechanical instability in 7% of senior amateur soccer players.

In a retrospective study of female players, Brynhildsen et al. (4) report that 22% of the players had sustained an overuse injury during their career. Half of those who had suffered shin splints and 100% of those that had patellofemoral pain or iliotibial tendinitis continued to have chronic pain. Of the players who had sustained an ankle injury, 13.3% had mechanical instability and 9.3% had persistent symptoms. Eleven players (7.3%) with previous knee sprains had residual symptoms and four players had mechanical instability (positive Lachman test).

Studies comparing former soccer players with those who are still active or never played found that the former players seemed to be at a higher risk for developing osteoarthrosis of the hip (24, 43) and knee (24). It was also found that elite soccer players had an increased risk of osteoarthritis over amateur players and nonplayers (24, 43).

## 5. Injury Risk Factors

### 5.1 Intrinsic Factors

#### 5.1.1 Physical Characteristics

The incidence of soccer injuries appears to increase with the age of the players (2, 18, 26, 36, 37). The increased rate of injury in the older groups was mainly due to injuries from player contact because increased strength, speed, and aggressiveness in older players led to higher joint reaction forces and higher impact forces on collision (21). In younger age groups, a higher incidence of head, face, and upper extremity injuries in youth players was documented by Keller et al. (21), possibly because of more frequent falls on outstretched hands, illegal ball contact, increased fragility of the upper extremity epiphyses, insufficient technical expertise in heading the ball, mechanical weakness of growing dental tissue, and increased ball-weight to head-weight ratio. Within age groups, adolescents who lagged behind in skeletal maturity were found to be at greater risk than their competitors (2).

Players with a history of previous injury may be at increased risk of reinjury. In a study of soccer injury mechanisms, Ekstrand and Gillquist (8) found that ankle sprains were significantly more common in those with a history of sprains than in those without, suggesting that incomplete rehabilitation is an injury risk factor. They also found that players who sustained a noncontact knee sprain more commonly had a previous knee sprain with residual mechanical instability than players injured during collisions. Ekstrand and Tropp (13) report that soccer players with previous ankle problems are at 2.3 times greater risk for ankle injuries (almost 48% of all players). Only 10% of previously uninjured players will suffer ankle sprains. Nielsen and Yde (30) found that 56% of ankle injuries occurred in players with a history of ankle sprains.

Gender may also be related to injury risk. Engström et al. (15) found that elite female soccer players sustained a higher injury rate than professional, amateur, and college-age males. However, the NCAA Injury Surveillance System (28, 19) reported that the injury rate between male and female soccer players was similar (see Table 23.1). Yet, in youth soccer, as seen in Table 23.2, females sustained a higher rate of injury than males (2, 25, 31, 36, 39). This has been attributed to the females' unfamiliarity and inferior technical skills when compared with males of the same age (25, 31, 36).

### 5.1.2 Motor/Functional Characteristics

Taimela, Osterman, Kujala, Lehto, Korhonen, and Alaranta (40) concluded from a study of 37 male soccer players that there was an association between injury and weakness of motor ability skills as well as personality types. Lack of strength and

flexibility are proposed risk factors for injury in soccer as proposed by Ekstrand and Gillquist (8), who found that players who suffered noncontact knee injuries had less quadriceps strength in the injured leg compared with uninjured players. In another study, Ekstrand and Gillquist (9) found a correlation between muscle tightness in the lower extremity and strains and tendinitis injuries.

## 5.2 Extrinsic Factors

### 5.2.1 Exposure

In Ekstrand, Gillquist, and Liljedahl (10) and Ekstrand, Gillquist, Möller, Öberg, and Liljedahl (11) teams with a higher practice-to-game ratio had fewer injuries, possibly because of superior physical conditioning.

Two studies (32, 35) reported conflicting results with respect to the level of play and injury occurrence. Research conducted prospectively in Scandinavia on one high and two lower ranked teams over the course of a season found no statistically significant difference in the number of injuries that occurred (32), although a retrospective investigation of insurance company records of acute soccer injuries in Finland (35) revealed significantly more injuries occurring in the top two divisions compared with the lower ones. In the latter study, however, the rate of injury with respect to exposure was not calculated, and it was stated that players in the top divisions spend more time practicing and playing games so they would have an increased exposure to injury.

The incidence of injury according to playing position must take into account the unequal and often variable number of players at each position. Although there is only one goalkeeper, the number of players at defense, midfield, and forward will depend upon the formation and strategy employed by the coach. Players are exposed to different situations based upon their relative field positions. Two prospective studies (1, 21) and one retrospective study (35) reported no significant differences between injury rates of players at different positions. However, other studies have found differences. Keller et al. (21) cited a study in which youth soccer goalkeepers sustained significantly more injuries than the remainder of positions, and the midfielders had a low injury number. Jorgensen's (20) retrospective study of 383 adult male players over one season was the only one to find a significant difference in injury incidence with goalkeepers and defenders sustaining more injuries than attackers. In female elite soccer,

Engström et al. (15) found the highest percentage of injuries occurred to backs and midfielders (36% each) whereas forwards and goalkeepers sustained 18% and 9%, respectively.

### 5.2.2 Environment

In both women's and men's NCAA soccer, the rate of injury occurrence on artificial surface is higher than on natural surfaces (28, 29). The college-age men sustained 11.45 injuries to 7.65 injuries per 1,000 exposures and college-age females incurred 9.99 and 7.71 injuries per 1,000 exposures on artificial and natural surfaces, respectively.

In their review of the role that surface type plays in soccer injuries, Ekstrand and Nigg (12) cited a 2-year study of the first artificial soccer surface in Sweden. No difference in injury frequency was found between the natural grass or gravel and the artificial turf. However, they reported that playing with cleated shoes on artificial turf was associated with an increase in the rate of injury. A difference in injury patterns between playing on natural surfaces and artificial surfaces was noted. On artificial surfaces there were more injuries affecting midfielders, more injuries in tackling and sliding, and more abrasions. Ekstrand and Nigg (12) postulate that the two main factors involved in surface-related soccer injuries are surface stiffness and frictional forces between the surface and the shoe, although there is no hard evidence to support this.

# 6. Suggestions for Injury Prevention

The soccer injury literature is primarily descriptive in nature and design, thus lacking the depth that analytical studies can provide. Because of this lack, risk factors have been identified with little confidence, and evaluation of the effectiveness of injury prevention measures has been all but ignored. Thus, the following discussion of injury prevention strategies should be viewed with caution.

## 6.1 Players

Individual player factors are often related to soccer injuries and can be prevented through corrections in training and conditioning. Several authors reviewed (2, 8, 9, 40) agreed that musculoskeletal deficiencies contributed to soccer injuries. Ekstrand and Gillquist (8) in their assessment of etiologic factors in soccer injuries found that 42% of all injuries were due to player factors such as joint instability, muscle tightness, inadequate rehabilitation, or lack of training.

## 6.2 Sport

Ekstrand (6) suggests correction of training, warm-up, cool-down, and stretching techniques. He states that flexibility exercises for the lower extremity should be included in the warm-up and cool-down and that players with muscle tightness detected in the preseason examination be given additional exercises. Ekstrand et al. (11) observed that the duration of warm-up seems adequate but the content is less than ideal. Shooting at the goal before warm-up should be avoided because it is related to quadriceps strain (8).

## 6.3 External Environment

The use of proper equipment is a valuable injury prevention measure. It is the consensus of the authors reviewed (8, 17, 38) that shock-absorbent, anatomically shaped shin guards that cover a large area of the lower leg can prevent injuries to the shin in soccer players. Shoes should have enough traction to prevent slipping, but not create excessive friction forces that put stress on the knees and ankles.

Fields (16) suggests that rule changes and padding of the goalposts may be appropriate steps in decreasing the incidence of head injury.

## 6.4 Health Support System

Ekstrand (6) suggests that a preseason examination, besides a routine history and physical examination, include measurements of flexibility and muscle strength so that any deficiencies can be corrected. The exam should focus on the lower extremity with tests for mechanical and functional instability of the ankle, knee, and hip. Players with mechanical instabilities should be recommended for taping or bracing. Functional instabilities can be reduced or eliminated through exercises for muscular strength, coordination, and proprioception.

In an investigation of soccer injury mechanisms, Ekstrand and Gillquist (7) found that a minor injury was often followed within two months by a major one to the same area and of the same type. Reinjuries are frequently an indication of neglect in the rehabilitation of the initial injury and premature return to play. In the same study, it was observed that some major injuries were preceded by minor ones of different type and location. They hypothesized that impairment of timing or neuromuscular coordination may be involved. For these reasons the authors suggest that the medical and coaching staff insist upon controlled rehabilitation and strict adherence to programs for rehabilitation.

A prophylactic program intended to reduce soccer injuries was instituted by Ekstrand, Gillquist, and Liljedahl (10) in Sweden. Twelve teams in a male senior soccer division were randomly divided into two groups of six teams each. The program was administered to one group. It comprised (a) correction of training; (b) provision of optimum equipment; (c) prophylactic ankle taping; (d) controlled rehabilitation; (e) exclusion of players with grave knee instability; (f) information about the importance of disciplined play and the increased risk of injury at training camps; and (g) correction and supervision by doctor(s) and physiotherapist(s). Six months later the test teams had sustained 75% fewer injuries than the controls.

Tropp, Askling, and Gillquist (42) found that ankle disk training seems to reduce the incidence of recurrent ankle injuries in players with a history of ankle problems. They also found that the use of a semirigid ankle orthosis during the rehabilitation period of an ankle injury provided a prophylactic effect.

# 7. Suggestions for Further Research

Further research in the epidemiology of soccer injuries will provide important information for the prevention of injuries. The fundamental problem with epidemiological assessment of data on soccer injuries is the inconsistent manner in which injury is defined and information collected and recorded (7, 21). Prospective studies yield more accurate data regarding exposure time, mechanism, severity, and type of injury. One exposure should be recorded for every hour of activity because of the varying length of games and practices. The ideal study would have the capability of recording the specific amount of actual playing time for each soccer player for both the practice sessions and games. Keller et al. (21) suggest that only injuries resulting in lost time from practice or play be included in statistics and that the duration of restricted activity should be reported as a measure of the severity of injury. Other meaningful measures of injury severity are lost time from school or work, disability during activities of daily living and financial cost of medical care. Poulsen et al. (32) recommended that accurate data collection could be obtained best by direct supervision and examination of the players on the field. Future

studies should include these measures if the impact of the injury on the life of the athlete is to be fully appreciated (21). There is scant literature available that addresses the long-term effects of injuries sustained in soccer, in particular, looking at the soccer players who have discontinued playing for various reasons. This study would need to establish a database with broad participation by all the different leagues, trained data gatherers, the ability for follow-up of all players, and a standardization of the definitions of injury and disability.

According to a study by Kibler (22), injury rates in female soccer players appear to be higher than in their male counterparts. In a prospective study of 4 years of a youth soccer tournament, Kibler states that since females seem to be at a higher risk of injury, equipment such as ball size, refereeing, and physical conditioning need to be looked at. These recommendations, although addressed to the female soccer player, seem applicable to all players and all ages.

The studies referred to in the section on prevention of ankle injuries and reinjuries were in sports other than soccer; a similar study of the use of semirigid orthosis, taping, and lace-up ankle support should be carried out in the soccer player. Another factor that has been mentioned is the relationship between the soccer shoes and playing surface. Does this play a role in lower extremity injury?

There is a need for better knowledge about the psychosocial maturity and its relationship to soccer injuries. Conditioning has been said to be important in reducing the incidence of soccer injuries, but there is a paucity of related studies that address the types, methods, and frequency of conditioning.

A vital factor in accurate injury reporting is the personal surveillance and evaluation of each injury by a knowledgeable health professional, preferably the same individual for each injury. Consistent injury evaluation and diagnosis are necessary for internal reliability as well as comparison of epidemiological studies.

There is also a need for better knowledge of the relationship between soccer injuries and physiological factors such as gender, muscle strength, range of motion, and joint laxity. With the high proportion of youth soccer players, more research regarding the physical maturity level of adolescents and injury etiology in younger players is warranted. Other factors that have been considered but require more in-depth investigation include level of play and player position. Often preventive measures are proposed but require more research to assess their effectiveness.

# References

1. Albert, M. Descriptive three year data study of outdoor and indoor professional soccer injuries. Ath. Train. 18(3):218-220; 1983.

2. Backous, D.D.; Friedl, K.E.; Smith, N.J.; Parr, T.J.; Carpine, W.D., Jr. Soccer injuries and their relation to physical maturity. Sports Med. 142:839-842; 1988.

3. Backx, F.J.G.; Beijer, J.J.M.; Bol, E. Injuries in high risk persons and high risk sports. Am. J. Sports Med. 19:124-30; 1991.

4. Brynhildsen, J.; Ekstrand, J.; Jeppsson, A.; Tropp, H. Previous injuries and persisting symptoms in female soccer players. International Journal Sports Med. 11:489-492; 1990.

5. Burke, M.J.; Sanitato, J.J.; Vinger, P.F.; Raymond, L.A.; Kulwin, D.R. Soccerball-induced eye injuries. J. Am. Med. Assoc. 249(19):2682-2685; 1983.

6. Ekstrand, J. Injuries in Soccer: Prevention. In: Renström, P.A.F.H., ed. Clinical practice of sports injury prevention and care. Boston: Blackwell Scientific Publications; 1994:285-293.

7. Ekstrand, J.; Gillquist, J. Soccer injuries and their mechanisms: A prospective study. Med. Sci. Sports. 15(3):267-270; 1983b.

8. Ekstrand, J.; Gillquist, J. The avoidability of soccer injuries. International Journal Sports Med. 4:124-128; 1983a.

9. Ekstrand, J.; Gillquist, J. The frequency of muscle tightness and injuries in soccer players. Am. J. Sports Med. 10:75-78; 1982.

10. Ekstrand, J.; Gillquist, J.; Liljedahl, S. Prevention of soccer injuries. Am. J. Sports Med. 11(3):116-120; 1983a.

11. Ekstrand, J.; Gillquist, J.; Möller, M.; Öberg, B.; Liljedahl, S. Incidence of soccer injuries and their relation to training and team success. Am. J. Sports Med. 11(2):63-67; 1983b.

12. Ekstrand, J.; Nigg, B. Surface-related injuries in soccer. Sports Med. 8(1):56-62; 1989.

13. Ekstrand, J.; Tropp, H. The incidence of ankle sprains in soccer. Foot Ankle. 11(1):41-44; 1990.

14. Engström, B.; Forssblad, M.; Johansson, C. Does a major knee injury definitely sideline an elite soccer player? Am. J. Sports Med. 18:101-105; 1990.

15. Engström, B.; Johansson, C.; Törnkvist, H. Soccer injuries among elite female players. Am. J. Sports Med. 19(4):372-375; 1991.

16. Fields, K.M. Head injuries in soccer. Physician Sportsmed. 17(1):69-73; 1989.

17. Greene, T.A.; Hillman, S.K. Comparison of support provided by a semirigid orthosis and adhesive ankle taping before, during and after exercise. Am. J. Sports Med. 18(5):498-506; 1990.

18. Hoff, G.L.; Martin, T.A. Outdoor and indoor soccer: Injuries among youth players. Am. J. Sports Med. 14(3):231-233; 1986.

19. Inklaar, H. Soccer injuries: Incidence and severity. Sports Med. 18:55-73; 1994.

20. Jorgensen, U. Epidemiology of injuries in typical Scandinavian team sports. Brit. J. Sports Med. 18(2):59-63; 1984.

21. Keller, C.S.; Noyes, F.R.; Buncher, C.R. The medical aspects of soccer injury epidemiology. Am. J. Sports Med. 15(3):230-237; 1987.

22. Kibler, W.B. Injuries in adolescent and preadolescent soccer players. Med. Sci. Sports. 25(12):1330-1332; 1993.

23. Kristiansen, B. Association football injuries in schoolboys. Scand. J. Sports Sci. 5(1):1-2; 1983.

24. Lindbert, H.; Roos, H.; Gärdsell, P. Prevalence of coxarthrosis in former soccer players. Acta. Orthop. Scand. 64(2):165-167; 1993.

25. Maehlum, S.; Dahl, E.; Daljord, O.A. Frequency of injuries in a youth soccer tournament. Physician Sportsmed. 14(7):73-79; 1986.

26. McCarroll, J; Meaney, C.; Sieber, J.M. Profile of youth soccer injuries. Physician Sportsmed. 12(2):113-117; 1984.

27. McMaster, W.C.; Walter, M. Injuries in soccer. Am. J. Sports Med. 6(6):354-357; 1978.

28. National Collegiate Athletic Association Men's Soccer Injury Surveillance System. 1991-1992.

29. National Collegiate Athletic Association Women's Soccer Injury Surveillance. 1991-1992.

30. Nielsen, A.B.; Yde, J. Epidemiology and traumatology of injuries in soccer. Am. J. Sports Med. 17:803-807; 1989.

31. Nilsson, S.; Roaas, A. Soccer injuries in adolescents. Am. J. Sports Med. 6(6):358-361; 1978.

32. Poulsen, T.D.; Freund, K.G.; Madsen, F.; Sandvej, K. Injuries in high-skilled and low-skilled soccer: a prospective study. Brit. J. Sports Med. 25(3):151-153; 1991.

33. Pritchett, J.W. Cost of high school soccer injuries. Am. J. Sports Med. 9(1):64-66; 1981. 15(5):500-502; 1987.

34. Resnick, E.J. Etiology and pathogenesis of football knee injuries. In: Vecchiet, L., ed. Proceedings 1st International Congress on Sports Medicine Applied to Football. Vol II. Rome: D Guanella, 1980: 481-489.

35. Sandelin, J.; Santavirta, S.; Kiviluoto, O. Acute soccer injuries in Finland in 1980. Brit. J. Sports Med. 19(1):30-33; 1985.

36. Schmidt-Olsen, S.; Bünemann, L.K.H.; Lade, V.; Brassoe, J.O.K. Soccer injuries of youth. Brit. J. Sports Med. 19(3):161-164; 1985.

37. Schmidt-Olsen, S.; Jörgensen, U.; Kaalund, S. Injuries among young soccer players. Am. J. Sports Med. 19:273-275; 1991.

38. Shapiro, M.S.; Kabo, J.M.; Mitchell, P.W.; Loren, G.; Tsepter, M. Ankle sprain prophylaxis: An analysis of the stabilizing effects of braces and tapes. Am. J. Sports Med. 22(1):78-82; 1994.

39. Sullivan, J.A.; Gross, R.H.; Grana, W.A.; Garcia-Moral, C.A. Evaluation of injuries in youth soccer. Am. J. Sports Med. 8(5):325-327; 1980.

40. Taimela, S.; Osterman, L.; Kujala, U.; Lehto, M.; Korhonen, T.; Alaranta, H. Motor ability and personality with reference to soccer injuries. J. Sports Med. and Physical Fitness. 30(2):194-201; 1990.

41. Tenvergert, E.M.; Ten Duis, H.J.; Klasen, H.J. Trends in sports injuries, 1982-1988: an in-depth study of four types of sport. J. Sports Med. and Physical Fitness. 32(2):214-220; 1992.

42. Tropp, M.; Askling, C.; Gillquist, J. Prevention of ankle sprains. Am. J. Sports Med. 13:259-262; 1985.

43. Vingard, E.; Alfredsson, L.; Goldie, I. Sports and osteoarthrosis of the hip. An epidemiologic study. Am. J. Sports Med. 21:195-200; 1993.

44. Yde, J.; Nielsen, A.B. Sports injuries in adolescents' ball games: soccer, handball and basketball. Brit. J. Sports Med. 24(1):51-54; 1990.

# 24

# Volleyball

*Koenraad J. Lindner and Andrea Ferretti*

## 1. Introduction

Volleyball-like games have been played for many centuries in China, in other Southeast Asian areas and in Central and South American regions (3). Modern volleyball was developed in Holyoke, Massachusetts before the turn of the century and has experienced an explosive growth and development in less than half a century. From the 14 founding national federations in 1947, the number of affiliated members of the Fédération Internationale de Volley-ball (F.I.V.B.) has risen to 175 in 1988 with an estimated 150 million active players worldwide (3). Volleyball was the most popular sport for school girls and the fifth most popular sport for boys in Canada (63), and in many countries around the globe its popularity is this great or even greater.

The recreational version of the original volleyball game is still popular because of its relatively simple rules, inexpensive equipment, and adaptability, which make playing the game enjoyable for anyone at widely varying levels of proficiency and intensity. There is the immensely popular beach volleyball, family volleyball with its own rules, volleyball for senior citizens and for recuperating heart patients, co-ed volleyball with adjusted regulations, minivolleyball for children, and wheelchair volleyball for the disabled (3). Great strides were made in the competitive type of volleyball, often called "power volleyball." This grew into a highly technical and physically demanding sport, whose standing as an Olympic Sport dates from the 1964 Tokyo Games, and is now played at professional levels in many countries.

The many variations of volleyball have allowed an enormous increase in the number of active participants. Although the benefits of the activity are available to the masses, the risk of injury is by necessity also run by the millions of participants. Because the rate and severity of injuries in recreational and lower level competitive volleyball are rather low, these variations of the sport cannot be regarded as high risk. In contrast, certain types of sports injuries in power volleyball are of great concern, because of their frequent severity and their high incidence rates. The incidence of injury, particularly the overuse type, has risen with the sport's higher intensity and increased technical demands, which require longer, more frequent, and more intense training. In addition, changes in commonly used skills and alterations of the rules of the sport have affected the nature and numbers of injuries. For example, the incidence of "volleyball finger" declined dramatically after the introduction of the forearm passing technique. On the other hand, the change in rule that allowed players to land on or mostly over the center line under the net was accompanied by a rise in ankle sprain injuries.

In volleyball, as in other sports, injuries have been modified by the evolution of the rules, techniques, and training methods of the game. Attempts to reach ever more spectacular solutions are often associated with greater risk for the athlete. A deeper knowledge of the etiopathogenic mechanisms of volleyball injuries will improve methods of prevention and treatment by changing training techniques, adopting and adapting protective devices, and by arriving at new technical solutions.

The purpose of this chapter is to provide an overview of the information currently available on injuries in the sport of volleyball. In view of the sport's worldwide popularity, the epidemiological literature on volleyball injuries is surprisingly limited in terms of volume and the research methodology generating it. The case literature, although more voluminous, has concentrated primarily on a few injury types typical for the sport. There is still a great deal of uncertainty about the specific causes of the injuries, and there are conflicting conclusions with regard to risk factors, treatment methods, and preventive measures. Literature searches for this chapter involved the Sport Discus (descriptors were volleyball injuries and accidents; search period was from 1972 to 1992) and Medline (descriptors were volleyball and volleyball injuries; search period was from 1983 to 1992) databases, and references found in published articles and reviews. Only articles dealing with incidence and cause of injury are included, whereas articles pertaining to treatment are not reviewed here. We conducted a thorough review of the available English and Italian literature, the latter because of its large contribution to the body of knowledge pertaining to volleyball injuries. We also incorporated materials from abstracts written in French and German in this chapter.

## 2. Incidence of Injury

### 2.1 Injury Rates

Reported injury rates in the sport of volleyball vary widely. The main reasons for this variability are the different injury definitions that were used, different levels of competition, different age levels, and different times of the season the investigation

covered. Injury rates should therefore be considered with caution, and they are not easily comparable across sports. For instance, Schafle et al. (84) monitored a 6-day USVBA national championships tournament and arrived at an extreme rate of nearly 20 injuries per 1,000 hours of exposure (20/1,000HrE). Similarly, Backx et al. (5) found a high injury rate because it was based on a 6-week retrospective surveillance period, which fell at the start of the volleyball season, a time when the incidence of injuries tends to be highest (26), and because they used a broad injury definition.

Information about volleyball injury incidence in schools has come from studies that surveyed populations across all sports, and the reports provide few data specific to volleyball. Volleyball tends to rank low in terms of injury risk and incidence in these studies (4, 43, 88, 94, 97). Particulars for these studies and reported injury rates are presented in Table 24.1.

There also have been no specific volleyball injury studies at the college level. In multisport studies, volleyball ranked average (17) to above average (60).

At the club level, where the elite volleyball players are studied, there have been a few epidemiological investigations specific to volleyball. Retrospective studies of career injuries by Candela et al. (15) and Giacomelli et al. (45) indicate that a very high percentage of participants sustain injuries in

**Table 24.1   A Comparison of Injury Rates in Volleyball**

| Study | Design[a] | Data collection[b] | Duration | # injuries | Sample # participants | # teams | Rate inj/100 part-seasons | Rate inj/1,000 HrE | Rate inj/1,000 A-E |
|---|---|---|---|---|---|---|---|---|---|
| School |
| Zaricznyj et al. (1980) | P | Q | 1 year | 4[c] | 105 M, F | — | 3.8 | 0.13 | — |
| Garrick & Requa (1978) | P | Q | 2 years | 17 | 174 M, F | 3/yr | 4.9 | — | — |
| Backx et al. (1991) | P | Q | 7 months | 18 | 55 M, F | — | 54.8 | 6.70[d] | — |
| College |
| Clarke & Buckley (1980) | P | NAIRS | 3 years | — | Intercoll, W | 16/yr | 10.9 | — | 2.1 |
| Lanese et al. (1990) | P | Med. records | 1 year | 7 | 13 intercoll, W | 1 | 54.8 | 1.50 | — |
| Lanese et al. (1990) | P | Med. records | 1 year | 13 | 17 intercoll, W | 1 | 76.0 | 1.90 | — |
| Club |
| Backx et al. (1991) | R | Q | 6 weeks | 11 | 188 M, F | — | 50.7 | — | — |
| Schafle et al. (1990) | P | Q | 6-day tourney | 154 | 1,520 M, F | — | — | 19.7 | — |
| Jacchia et al. (1990) | P | I | 4 years | 58 | 100 M, F | — | 14.5 | — | — |

[a]P = prospective, R = retrospective.

[b]I = interview, Q = questionnaire.

[c]Calculations based on number of organized sport participants only.

[d]Hours of practice only.

this sport in the course of their career. Jacchia et al. (53) have published the only prospective epidemiological study of injuries in volleyball club teams. Their rather low injury rate for this level must be ascribed to a stringent injury definition (which was not specified).

The currently available data on injury rates in volleyball show a trend of increasing incidence along two parameters:

- There is an increase in injury rates with level of play from school to college to club and professional volleyball.
- There is an increase over time, whereby older studies tend to report lower rates than more recent ones.

This likely corresponds with the change in the nature of volleyball from a low-level, largely recreational pastime to the highly technical, intense, and physically demanding sport now played by professionals and semiprofessionals in many countries.

## 2.2 Reinjury Rates

There is no information available on the extent of injury recurrence in volleyball. Some authors have grouped recurrent and chronic injuries together under the classification "overuse injuries" (53), but most studies have not examined whether injuries were of the same type and to the same body part as antecedent injuries. Since shoulder and knee problems in volleyball frequently plague the

player repeatedly, it is difficult to distinguish between a chronic condition and a recurrence of a previously healed injury. Nevertheless, attempts should be made in prospective injury studies to assess the rate of reinjury in volleyball.

## 2.3 Practice Versus Competition

Whether injuries are more frequently sustained during practice or during games cannot be determined with any degree of confidence from the available literature. Data reported from school studies (Table 24.2) vary widely. Zaricznyj et al. (97) found that all of the injuries in volleyball had occurred during competition, but Garrick and Requa (43) reported that nearly all injuries were sustained during practice. Ferrari et al. (26) found that 32 of 50 hand and wrist injuries that did not occur in recreational play were sustained in practice in a group of players under 15 years of age.

At the club level, Ferretti et al. (35) reported that the majority of knee ligament injuries (32 injuries) had occurred under game conditions, even though the players spent about 3.5 hours of practicing for each hour of competition. In a previous article (34) the estimate was a 55% to 45% division for injuries to occur in game or practice conditions, respectively. Byra and McCabe (12) found that females were injured more often during practice, but men suffered a larger percentage of injuries during match play. There is no information on injury in practice versus competition at the college level.

It should be realized that the origin of a so-called acute injury that occurs in competition may well

**Table 24.2 A Percentage Comparison of Injuries in Practice vs. Competition**

| Study | # of partic.[a] | # inj. | Practice % of total # of inj. | Practice Inj. per 1,000 A-E | Competition % of total # of inj. | Competition Inj. per 1,000 A-E |
|---|---|---|---|---|---|---|
| School | | | | | | |
| Garrick & Requa (1978) | 174 | 17 | 93 | — | 7 | — |
| Zaricznyj et al. (1980) | 105 | 4 | 0 | — | 100 | — |
| Backx et al. (1991) | 55 | 18 | — | 6.7 | — | — |
| Ferrari et al. (1990)[b] | 100 | 100 | 64 | — | 36 | — |
| Club | | | | | | |
| Byra & McCabe (1982) | — | — | 43 | — | 57 | — |
| Ferretti et al. (1990a)[c] | 42 | 42 | 45 | — | 55 | — |
| Ferretti et al. (1992)[c] | 55 | 55 | 38.5 | — | 61.5 | — |

[a]Absolute # of participants surveyed.

[b]Hand injuries only.

[c]Case series of knee ligament injuries.

be in practice, and that maximum effort typical for intense game conditions may merely aggravate an already existing condition. Conversely, an acute injury may lead to a chronic condition. The paucity of information on the practice versus competition issue may stem from this realization.

## 3. Injury Characteristics

### 3.1 Injury Onset

The type of injury that appears to have increased most during the technical advancement of the sport of volleyball is the overuse injury. The desirability of greater jumping height gave impetus to the development of jump training techniques, such as plyometric exercises, which involve extraordinarily strong and repetitive forces in the knee and ankle joints. The growing use of the jump serve added to the heavy use of the knee extensors and put more strain on the shoulder joint, already taxed by the frequent spiking actions. Common injuries seen in high-level players include "jumper's knee," an insertional tendinopathy, tears of the cruciate ligaments, rotator cuff problems in the shoulder, and paresis of the infraspinatus muscle resulting from repetitive stretching of the suprascapular nerve at the base of the scapular spine. However, very few epidemiological data have been published regarding the onset of injuries in volleyball. It appears that the acute injuries are more numerous than the overuse types when considering all volleyball-related injuries, but it is not always clear whether traumatic injuries were checked for long-term antecedents. The incidence of overuse injuries seems to rise with level of play and age, and is dependent upon specialization and gender. We will discuss this in the section dealing with risk factors. Candela et al. (15) reported that 58% of the injuries in high-level players were overuse syndromes and that female players had a much higher

incidence of overuse injuries than men. Ferretti and Di Rosa (30) observed an about equal division of traumatic and overuse injuries in the 214 injuries they treated in volleyball players.

Ferretti et al. (35) reported that 58% of the knee ligament injuries they treated and followed up in volleyball players were acute injuries with ACL tears, whereas the chronic instability cases had meniscal tears and ruptures combined with ACL tears. Most of the knee injuries involving the extensor mechanisms appear to be of a chronic nature. Kujala et al. (59) registered 76% of knee complaints as exertion injuries, and 24% were labeled as single trauma injuries. Schafle et al. (84) found that almost two thirds of the knee injuries they encountered were overuse and degenerative problems. Ferretti et al. (37) estimated that nearly 30% of all knee injuries were jumper's knee syndromes and that the incidence of this syndrome in high-level players may be as high as 40%. They cited overload on tendons and ligaments during jumping and landing and the emphasis on jump training as the leading cause for knee injuries.

### 3.2 Injury Type

The incidence of injury types in volleyball at the school and college levels is not known because no studies have reported injury types specifically for this sport. Whiteside et al. (95) reported on fractures exclusively in intercollegiate sports over an 11-year period. Women's volleyball was second in female teams and fourth overall in percentage of players sustaining fractures. There were no fractures in men's volleyball. For club volleyball, primarily Italian studies have provided insight into the distribution of injuries over the various kinds of trauma (Table 24.3). The sprain is the most common kind, and the majority are ankle sprains, followed by knee sprains. Overuse injuries and muscle strains make up the bulk of the remaining

**Table 24.3  A Percentage Comparison of Injury Types in Volleyball**

| Study | # partic.[a] | # inj. | Contus. | Disloc. | Fract. | Inflam. | Lacer. | Nonspec. | Strain | Sprain | Other |
|---|---|---|---|---|---|---|---|---|---|---|---|
| Club |  |  |  |  |  |  |  |  |  |  |  |
| Mollica et al. (1979) | 251 | 251 | 1 | 2 | 9 | 4 | — | — | 8 | 73 | 3 |
| Gangitano et al. (1981) | 698 | ? | 2 | 2 | 9 | — | 0 | 28 | 4 | 55 | 0 |
| Schafle et al. (1990) | 1,520 | 154 | 5 | 3 | 3 | — | 2 | 20 | 36 | 28 | 3 |
| Candela et al. (1990) | 89 | 128 | — | — | 6 | — | — | 8 | 58 | 26 | — |

[a]Absolute # of participants surveyed.

injury types, whereas fractures, dislocations, inflammations, and contusions comprise only a small percentage of all injuries. There is a need to analyze volleyball injuries in controlled prospective studies particularly at the school and college levels.

## 3.3 Injury Location

There is also a paucity of information on the distribution of injuries over anatomical locations, particularly at the school and college level. Only one school study has analyzed injury location percentages. Zaricznyj et al. (97) found that of school-aged players nearly 50% of volleyball injuries were to the hand and fingers and 20% to the ankles. Knee injuries accounted for less than 6% of the cases, and there were no back injuries. No college-level data are available for injury locations, except Whiteside et al.'s study (95) on sports fractures at Pennsylvania State University in which 3 of 58 women volleyball players suffered fractures: to the nose, foot, and fibula.

There are a substantial number of reports at the club level that list the distribution of injuries over the various locations (Table 24.4).

From the averages calculated on the nine club level studies it is clear that

- traumas to the lower extremities make up the majority of the volleyball injuries;
- the percentage of injuries is generally higher for the ankle than for the knee, but in some studies the knee is reported to have more than twice the incidence rate of the ankle; and
- hand and finger injuries rank next at a substantially lower incidence, followed by spinal injuries and shoulder problems.

Additional information on injury location can be gleaned from an overview of the case report, case series, and cross-sectional study literature. Although these reports do not provide statistics on incidence rates in predetermined populations, they are useful for an appreciation of the type and frequency of injuries in the various anatomical locations. Case reports and case series allow detailed description of observed medical conditions and are often accompanied by an appraisal of the effectiveness of the treatment applied. Cross-sectional studies usually survey an available group at a given point in time to examine any prevalence of one or more selected traumata along with information of risk factors. These types of injury studies are prevalent in volleyball to date, and a substan-

tial body of literature is available describing injuries to specific sites on the body, particularly for the knee. We summarize this literature below in table form (Tables 24.5-24.8) and briefly discuss it by body region: head/spine/trunk, upper extremity, and lower extremity.

### 3.3.1 Head/Spine/Trunk

Nearly all of the trunk injuries in volleyball are traumas to the spine. Although these injuries represent almost 8% of volleyball injuries, they have not received much attention in the case literature. Case reports describe lumbo-sacral complaints, fractures to the lumbar and cervical spine, vertebral disk alterations, and restricted mobility (Table 24.5).

### 3.3.2 Upper Extremity

As was evident from the epidemiological literature, injuries to the upper extremities account for nearly 30% of the injuries in volleyball. Overviews of common *shoulder* injuries in volleyball have been published by Costa et al. (20), who described acute and overuse injuries involving the supraspinatus tendon, the rotator cuff, the glenoid labrum, and the acromion; and by Cooney (19), who discussed recurrent microstresses, overstretching, and "rubbing" of tendons leading to overuse injuries. Two conditions are particularly well documented in the volleyball case literature. These are the impingement and the entrapment syndromes, the former referring to tendinous pathology (7, 54, 71, 79), and the latter to pressure exerted on nerves resulting in atrophy and/or paresis of the muscles they innervate (47).

Whether shoulder joint instability can be regarded as a common condition in volleyball players is controversial. Jerosch et al. (54) described this condition as a common result of repetitive stress on anterior shoulder joint structures, but Lanzetta (61) only found one case of instability in 66 volleyball players with shoulder pain complaints. He concluded that true shoulder instability is rarely a result of progressive stretching of the anterior joint capsule (Table 24.6).

Repetitive contact between the ball and the *forearms* of volleyball players is frequent in games and particularly in practice conditions. Several cases have been cited in which this has led to trauma (56, 62, 74). No case studies are known to exist describing elbow injuries in volleyball players. *Wrist and hand* injuries include interphalangeal or metacarpo-phalangeal sprains, and metacarpal and wrist fractures (26), radial, metacarpal and

**Table 24.4   A Percentage Comparison of Injury Locations in Club Volleyball**

| | Mollica et al. (1979) N$^a$ = 251 # inj = 251 | Ferretti & DiRosa (1980) N$^a$ = 214 # inj = 214 | Gangitano et al. (1981) N$^a$ = 698 # inj = ? | Hell & Schoenle (1985) N$^a$ = 224 # inj = ? | Giacomelli et al. (1986) N$^a$ = 202 # inj = 98 | Gerberich et al. (1987) N$^a$ = 106 # inj = 106 | Schafle et al. (1990) N$^a$ = 1,520 # inj = 154 | Candela et al. (1990) N$^a$ = 89 # inj = 128 | Jacchia et al. (1990) N$^a$ = 100 # inj = 54 |
|---|---|---|---|---|---|---|---|---|---|
| Trunk & head | (3) | (15.9) | (3) | (3.5) | (10.4) | (2.5) | (26) | (13) | (8.6) |
| Skull/face | — | — | 0 | 2 | — | 0 | 4 | — | — |
| Neck | — | — | 0 | 0 | — | 0 | 0 | — | — |
| Back | 3 | 15.9 | 3 | 1.5 | 10.4 | 2.5 | 22 | 13 | 8.6 |
| Chest/stomach | — | — | 0 | 0 | — | 0 | 0 | — | — |
| Upper extremity | (31.8) | (16.9) | (33.5) | (30) | (27.0) | (12.5) | (26) | (24) | (27.5) |
| Shoulder | 6 | 9.7 | 6 | 2 | 8 | 7 | 8 | 16 | 3.4 |
| Upper arm | 0.8 | — | 0 | 0 | — | 1.5 | 0 | — | — |
| Elbow | 0.8 | — | 3 | 3 | — | 1.5 | 4 | — | — |
| Forearm | 0.8 | — | 0 | 0 | — | 0 | 3 | — | — |
| Wrist | 1.2 | 2.6 | 0 | 1 | 2.3 | 2.5 | 0 | — | — |
| Hands/finger | 23 | 4.6 | 24.5 | 24 | 16.7 | 0 | 11 | 8 | 24.1 |
| Lower extremity | (65.2) | (61.0) | (54.5) | (73.5) | (62.8) | (85) | (48) | (53) | (63.7) |
| Pelvis | — | — | 0 | 3 | — | 0 | 3 | — | — |
| Thigh | 0.8 | — | 0 | 2.5 | — | 1.5 | 3 | — | — |
| Knee | 20 | 40.0 | 10.5 | 10 | 20 | 58 | 11 | 33 | 17.2 |
| Lower leg | — | — | 0 | 0.5 | — | 1.5 | 7 | — | — |
| Ankle | 42 | 21.0 | 42 | 55 | 30.5 | 21 | 18 | 20 | 43.1 |
| Foot/toe | 2.4 | — | 2 | 2.5 | 12.3 | 3 | 6 | — | 3.4 |

$^a$Absolute # of participants surveyed.

**Table 24.5  Case Reports, Case Series, and Cross-Sectional Studies of Injuries of the Spine/Trunk in Volleyball Players**

| Study | Design | Subjects | Age | Level | Condition/diagnosis |
|---|---|---|---|---|---|
| **Spine** | | | | | |
| Oudot et al. (1982) | Case series | 157 M, F | Adults | Top level | Various overuse injuries in the lumbo-sacral region |
| Sommer (1988) | Cross-sectional | 15 M[a] | Adults | High level | Many showed movement restrictions in spine as well as lordotic/kyphotic and scoliotic deviations |
| Jacchia et al. (1990) | Case | 2 M | Adults | ? | Minor fractures of the cervical and lumbar spine |
| Bartolozzi et al. (1991) | Case series | 45 | Adults | Professional | 44% had intervertebral disk alterations: bulging (11 cases), disk herniation (9), and disk degeneration (11) |

[a]Volleyball and basketball players.

**Table 24.6  Case Reports, Case Series, and Cross-Sectional Studies of Injuries of the Upper Extremities in Volleyball Players**

| Study | Design | Subjects | Age | Level | Condition/diagnosis |
|---|---|---|---|---|---|
| **Shoulder** | | | | | |
| Ferretti et al. (1987) | Cross-sectional | 69 M, F | Adults | Top level | 12 had atrophy of infraspinatus muscle; subscapular nerve damage |
| Holzgräfe et al. (1988) | Case series | 36 | Adults | ? | 28% showed suprascapular neuropathy |
| Distefano (1989) | Case | 1 | Adolescent | ? | Paresis of serratus anterior due to entrapment of long thoracic nerve |
| Melzer & Wirth (1989) | Case series | 27[a] | Adults | Recr. + comp. | Complete rotator cuff lesions |
| Bracker et al. (1990) | Case | 1 F | 14 yrs | School | Synovial chondromatosis |
| Bonsignore & Giombini (1990) | Case series | 17 M | Adults | ? | Shoulder pain identified as impingement syndrome |
| Lanzetta (1990) | Case series | 66 | Adults | ? | One in 66 cases of shoulder pain diagnosed as instability |
| **Forearm and elbow** | | | | | |
| Mutoh et al. (1982) | Case[b] | 1 F | 14 yrs | Beginner | Stress fracture of the ulna |
| Kostianen & Orava (1983) | Case | 3 | Adults | ? | Antebrachial-palmar hammer syndrome |
| Lanzetta & Fox (1990) | Case | 1 F | 28 yrs | Club | Aneurism of ulnar artery |
| **Wrist, hand, and finger** | | | | | |
| Watson (1983) | Case | 1 M | 28 yrs | ? | Double interphalangeal dislocation in single finger |
| Shen (1983) | Case series | 11 M, F | Adolescents | School | 10 fractures and 2 avascular bone changes |
| Ferrari et al. (1990) | Case series | 100 M, F | Under 15 yrs | Recr. + club | Most were sprains |
| Curti & D'Amato (1990) | Case | 3 | Adults | Top level | Obstructive digital arteriopathy |

[a]From various sports including volleyball.

[b]Obtained from case series data.

scaphoid bone fractures (85), vascular problems (21), and finger dislocations (93). Kruger-Franke (57) discussed mechanisms and types of injuries to the metacarpal III, which are considered rare in volleyball. Montorsi et al. (72) grouped the fingers into three locations with distinct types of injuries. The thumb injuries usually affect the metacarpal proximal joint; the three middle fingers frequently have the proximal and distal interphalangeal joints

involved with "mallet-" or "volleyball finger" a rather common occurrence; and on the little finger typically the proximal phalanx and proximal IP joint are affected. The volleyball finger was first described in the oldest known article on volleyball injuries by Amorth and Tosatti (2). They estimated that one third of all volleyball players were affected by this condition, but they wrote this at a time when the forearm pass was not normally used for receiving serves and spikes and fingers were at great risk of injury. The decreased incidence of the volleyball finger was observed in a paper by Ferretti and Puddu (38). Nevertheless, finger injuries, even though not usually severe, are quite common. Moraldo et al. (73) reported that 44% of all the volleyball injuries involved the fingers and more than half of these were thumb injuries.

### 3.3.3 Lower Extremity

The majority of the injury case literature pertaining to volleyball is devoted to the description and discussion of knee pathology. There are relatively few reports of volleyball injuries affecting the hip, upper leg, lower leg, and foot (Table 24.7). High-level basketball and volleyball players were found to have a high incidence of pelvis and hip abnormalities (86). No studies have been found on femur or upper leg muscular or tendinous injuries, and the lower leg injury studies were limited to one each of stress fractures, fibula fractures, and chronic leg pain syndrome.

Three studies on foot injuries have been published, two case studies and one cross-sectional study. Achilles tendon problems are relatively rare in volleyball players. Low-level and older players appear more frequently affected, and beach volleyball had a higher percentage than indoor volleyball (78).

The case, case series, and cross-sectional literature on knee problems in volleyball is fairly exten-sive and we summarize it below and in Table 24.8. Injuries to the knee in volleyball can be grouped into three main types, that is, knee ligament injuries, meniscus problems, and the pathology involving the quadriceps and patellar tendons often referred to as "jumper's knee." *Knee Ligament Injuries* usually involve the anterior cruciate ligament (ACL), often with additional damage to the medial collateral ligament and the joint capsule. The PCL is rarely involved (34, 36). Chronic instability associated with meniscal tears and ruptures, and ACL problems are frequently seen (28, 35-37).

Although the reports on *meniscal injuries* in volleyball are not encouraging (52, 59), Volpi and Vanni (92) concluded that although volleyball is a high-risk sport for the knee joint, meniscus tears in isolation occur rarely and much less frequently than extensor mechanism problems and ligamental damage.

In one of the earliest reports of *jumper's knee* syndrome in volleyball, Maurizio (69) described six cases of patellar tendinitis. The syndrome involving the knee's tendons was so frequent in sports such as basketball, volleyball, high- and long jumping, cross-country running, and diving, all of which involve functional stress overload on the knees, that the name "jumper's knee" became commonly accepted (8). Initially it referred to quadriceps tendinitis only, but later symptoms of the patellar tendon and the tibial tuberosity were also included (67, 80). Heckman and Alkire (49) recommended that patellar distal pole fractures also be recognized as a form of jumper's knee.

**Table 24.7   Case Reports, Case Series, and Cross-Sectional Studies of Injuries of the Lower Extremities in Volleyball Players**

| Study | Design | Subjects | Age | Level | Condition/diagnosis |
|---|---|---|---|---|---|
| Pelvis/hip | | | | | |
| Sommer (1988) | Cross-sectional | 15 M[a] | Adults | High level | Unfavorable pelvic stabilization; hip extension deficits; relative weakness in gluteal and abdominal muscles; vastus medialis hypertrophy |
| Lower leg | | | | | |
| Whiteside et al. (1981) | Case | 1 F | Adult | College | Fractured fibula |
| Martens et al. (1984) | Case[b] | 2 | Adults | ? | Chronic leg pain due to compartment syndrome |
| Ha et al. (1991) | Case series | 33 M, F | Adults | Recr.-prof. | 26 stress fractures of the tibia; 7 other locations |
| Foot/ankle | | | | | |
| Whiteside et al. (1981) | Case | 1 F | Adult | College | Recurrence of fracture of fifth metatarsal bone |
| Julsrud (1983) | Case | 1 F | Adult | College | Osteochondritis in first metatarsal sesamoid bone |
| Pace et al. (1990) | Case series | 700 | Adults | Recr.-prof. | 15 cases of Achilles tendon pathology |

[a]Volleyball and basketball players.

[b]Obtained from case series data.

**Table 24.8   Case Reports, Case Series, and Cross-Sectional Studies of Injuries Occurring in the Knees of Volleyball Players**

| Study | Design | Subjects | Age | Level | Condition/diagnosis |
|---|---|---|---|---|---|
| **Chondromalacia** | | | | | |
| Kujala et al. (1986) | Case series | 103 M, F | Adol. + adults | Various | 14 had patellar chondropathy |
| Kujala et al. (1989) | Cross-sectional | 32 M | Adults | High level | 5 had patellar chondromalacia |
| **Jumper's knee** | | | | | |
| Maurizio (1963) | Case series | 5 | Adults | ? | 6 knees diagnosed with patellar tendinitis |
| Roels et al. (1978) | Case series | 12 M, F | Adults | ? | All jumper's knee symptoms; 4 surgically treated |
| Ferretti et al. (1983) | Case series | 9 M, F | Adults | ? | 4 had poor results after surgery, 2 good, 3 very good |
| Ferretti et al. (1984, 1986) | Cross-sectional | 407 M, F | Adol. + adults | Various | 93 (22.8) had jumper's knee symptoms |
| Kujala et al. (1986) | Case series | 103 M, F | Adol. + adults | Various | 39 had patellar apicitis |
| Kujala et al. (1989) | Cross-sectional | 32 M | Adults | High level | 10 had jumper's knee syndrome: 9 lower pole, 4 upper pole, 2 cartilage |
| **Other** | | | | | |
| Hoshikawa et al. (1983) | Case[a] | 4 F | Adol. + adults | Elite | Poorest clinical scores after meniscectomy among 8 sports |
| Kujala et al. (1986) | Case series | 103 M, F | Adol. + adults | Various | 6 meniscus tears, 5 contusions, 2 sprains, 24 other knee disorders |
| Ferretti et al. (1988) | Case series | 42 M, F | Adults | Various | Mostly ACL, some with medial collateral ligs. and knee capsules |
| Kujala et al. (1989) | Cross-sectional | 32 M | Adults | High level | 7 had Osgood-Schlatter Disease during growth spurt |
| Volpi & Vanni (1990) | Case series | 36 M, F | Adol. + adults | ? | Of 36 arthroscopies, only 7 cases of meniscal tears |
| Ferretti et al. (1992) | Case series | 52 M, F | Adol. + adults | Amat.-prof. | Knee lig. instability: 42% chronic, 58% acute |

[a]Obtained from case series data.

Among the case series involving jumper's knee, volleyball players are usually highly represented (27, 31, 39, 80). Kujala concluded that knee injuries including jumper's knee have a high incidence in volleyball particularly at high levels, as a result of frequent jumping and striking of the knee on the floor (58, 59).

## 3.4 Injury Mechanism

There is general agreement that the high incidence of injuries to the lower extremities in volleyball is the result of frequent jumping and landing, as well as striking the leg on the floor during defensive maneuvers (4, 39, 44, 52, 58, 75). The occasional direct blows to the patella in falls or contact with other players are not believed to be a direct cause of jumper's knee, according to Ferretti (29), but likely an aggravating factor. Nearly all acute injuries occur during jumping and more often during offensive than defensive jumping. The landing after loss of balance during the jump was frequently implicated. Meniscus injuries were most

often the consequence of defensive moves in which rapid twisting motions occur in deep ready positions.

Blocking and spiking appear to be the most injury-producing actions in volleyball, being responsible for 64% of all injuries according to Byra and McCabe (12). However, there is uncertainty about which volleyball maneuvers are likely to underlie what specific traumas. The limited information on injury percentages associated with the various skills is summarized in Table 24.9. From this table it appears that blocking is by far the most risk-producing action overall, whereas spiking and defense maneuvers contribute about equally to the injury totals. Hand injuries result mainly from passing and defensive actions including blocking; the knee injuries predominantly occur during spiking.

Other information gleaned from the injury mechanism literature can be summarized as follows:

- Jumping and landing with the knees in valgus position and the forefoot on abduction and/

**Table 24.9    A Percentage Comparison of Injury Mechanisms in Club Volleyball**

| Study | # of partic. | # of inj. | Spiking | Blocking | Defense | Pass/set |
|---|---|---|---|---|---|---|
| Gangitano et al. (1981) | 698 | ? | 10 | 70 | 15 | 5 |
| Hell & Schoenle (1985) | 224 | ? | 19 | 53 | 14 | 3 |
| Schafle et al. (1990) | 1,520 | 154 | 31 | 33 | 30 | 6 |
| Ferrari et al. (1990)[a] | 100 | 100 | 13 | —[b] | 43 | 44 |
| Ferretti et al. (1992)[c] | 52 | 52 | 73 | 19 | 8 | — |

[a]Hand injuries only.

[b]Blocking not separately listed.

[c]Knee ligament injuries only.

or supination appear to increase the chances of injury (86).

- Jumping-related injuries to the knee occur predominantly during the landing phase and particularly where there are twisting motions (35, 87).
- One-legged take-offs and landings in volleyball jumps will exert very high strain on hip, knee, and ankle and increase the risk of injury (90).
- Collision with other players, particularly under the net, is a major cause of injuries, notably ankle traumas in blocking and spiking (25, 50, 84).
- The spiking and jump-serve actions produce a variety of shoulder injuries, such as shoulder instability (89), supraspinatus tendinopathy (61), rotator cuff disease and impingement syndrome (7), and entrapment syndrome (29, 47).
- The "volleyball finger" is now rarely seen (38), but the fingers are at risk during blocking (72).

# 4. Injury Severity

## 4.1 Time Loss

There is very little published information on the severity of volleyball injuries, the time lost because of injury, and incidence of catastrophic injuries. The majority of the injuries in the sport as a whole, such as the hand/finger injuries and the ankle sprains, are not severe and require relatively little recovery time. However, the knee injuries, in particular the chronic tendinopathies and acute and chronic knee ligament injuries, often require prolonged periods of time for recovery and in many cases turn out to be career ending. Anterior knee ligament injuries involving surgery necessitated

an average of 9 months before return to specialized training in a study by Ferretti et al. (35). In another study of severe ligament injuries, Ferretti et al. (37) reported that those who returned to playing did so after 11 months on average. Gerberich et al. (44) observed that 59% of all volleyball injuries they had treated were knee injuries, of which 97% required surgery.

## 4.2 Catastrophic Injuries

Only one source was found that referred to catastrophic injuries in volleyball. Rutherford et al. (82) identified four fatalities in volleyball between 1973 and 1980 from the National Electronic Injury Surveillance System (NEISS) data. No details are available on the nature of these casualties.

## 4.3 Injury Outcome

Data on long-term injury effects are very rare for volleyball. Ferretti et al. (35) reported that 35% of the ACL-injured players had to give up participating. Another study revealed a 37% dropout after knee ligament surgery (37). Long-term sequelae from other injury types in volleyball, such as back and shoulder injuries, are unknown and require the attention of future studies.

# 5. Injury Risk Factors

We discuss potential risk factors for injury in the sport of volleyball below and group them in the two categories recommended in the literature (65, 66). Intrinsic factors pertain to physical and psychological traits of the sport participant, whereas the extrinsic factors refer to environmental conditions, training methods, and equipment used.

**Table 24.10   Potential Injury Risk Factors in Volleyball**

| Intrinsic risk factors | Extrinsic risk factors |
|---|---|
| Physical characteristics | Exposure |
| • Age/maturity:<br>   During growth spurt<br>   At advanced age<br>• Gender<br>   Males more jumper's knee<br>   Males more shoulder<br>      entrapment<br>   Females more knee<br>      ligament injuries<br>• Age-gender interaction | • Level of competition<br>• Years in sport<br>• Specialization<br>• Number of training<br>   sessions per week |
| Functional characteristics | Training conditions |
| • Previous back problems<br>• Poor jumping technique<br>• Muscle imbalances in lower<br>   extremity | • Type of jump training (?) |
| Psychological characteristics | Environment |
| | • Floor type<br>• Low safety standards |

Virtually all volleyball injury studies that have included references to risk factors have been of the descriptive kind. The characteristics of the injured athletes, such as age, gender, experience, and specialization are listed, usually in percentages, and from this information the role of these characteristics as injury risk factors is hypothesized. Detailed comparisons of injured and uninjured volleyball players, or searches for predictor variables for *injury rate* and *time lost because of injury* have not been conducted in this sport. We summarized the available information below and listed the potential factors in Table 24.10.

## 5.1 Intrinsic Factors

### 5.1.1 Physical Characteristics

Current information on risk factors related to age, sex, and somatotype can be summarized in the following points, bearing in mind that these result from descriptive studies rather than from studies designed to analyze risk factors or injury predictors:

- The peak incidence of injuries is in the younger age groups (23, 44, 59).
- Rapid growth periods may be associated with higher incidence of injury (5, 13, 14, 26, 45, 48, 58).

- Injury risks also appear to increase in older participants, particularly Achilles tendinitis (78), and intervertebral disk alterations (6), but some studies did not find an age effect (76, 98).
- Females have been found to have more volleyball injuries in general (84), knee injuries of all kinds (23), stress fractures (48), and other overuse injuries (15) than males. However, some studies have found no sex differences in overall injury incidence with volleyball players (4, 15, 44, 60, 76).
- Specific injuries such as patellar apicitis and other forms of jumper's knee occur proportionally more in male volleyball players (27, 39, 58, 80), whereas knee ligament injuries in volleyball seem to be more likely to occur in female participants (35, 37). However, Gerberich et al. (44) reported that knee ligament injuries affected more males, whereas patellofemoral injuries were identified most often in females.
- The number of cases of suprascapular neuropathy resulting in weakening of the infraspinatus muscle has been found to be substantially higher in males (29).
- There may be an interaction between age and sex variables. Candela et al. (15) found that the proportion of overuse and acute injuries changed over age levels, with the women having more overuse injuries at higher age levels and the men having more acute injuries in the higher age groups.
- Somatotype, height, and weight have not been found to be related to volleyball injuries (27, 68, 76, 98).

### 5.1.2 Functional Characteristics

- Malalignment of the extensor mechanisms of the knee has often been suspected to underlie the jumper's knee condition (22, 49, 67, 83), but Ferretti (29, 31) found little evidence of abnormalities in the somatic characteristics of athletes with this condition.
- Muscle imbalances, particularly in the lower extremities, have been mentioned as potential risk factors by Gerberich et al. (44). In a sample of basketball and volleyball players, Sommer (86) found evidence of gluteal, hamstring, and abdominal imbalances, which they suspected may affect the jumping techniques and cause extra loading on the patella. However, the question remains whether these imbalances are the primary cause of the knee problems or whether they are in turn the result of poor training and jumping technique (29).

- History of injuries was not found to be related to the probability of suffering a volleyball injury (84), but Oudot et al. (76) suggested that players with previous back problems were more prone to sustain further back injury.

### 5.1.3 Psychological and Psychosocial Characteristics

Potential psychological risk factors in volleyball have received very little attention and study. One investigation by Williams et al. (96) did not find a relationship between high life stresses and injury risk in top intercollegiate male and female volleyball players.

## 5.2 Extrinsic Factors

### 5.2.1 Exposure

One aspect of exposure is the *frequency, length, and intensity* of training sessions and games per unit of time. Interacting with this is the level of competition, with presumably higher levels of intensity and technical demands at more advanced levels. Exposure can also be considered in a long-term sense under an assumption that wear and tear on the system can accumulate over years of involvement in the sport. The following points summarize what we know about exposure factors in volleyball:

- The length of consecutive playing may be a contributing factor (64, 84).
- Number of years of participation in the sport has not been shown to be a major factor by itself (29, 39, 45, 76).
- The length of training sessions appears to be less of a factor in volleyball injuries than the frequency of sessions, which is strongly implicated as a risk factor (25, 35, 39, 76).

There is evidence that the rate of occurrence of volleyball injuries is different for the various *positions on the court* and for the *assigned functions* of the players (50). The six court positions are numbered starting with the #1 serving position on the right side of the back row when facing the net, right forward #2, center forward #3, and so forth, up to center back #6. Playing at the net in the front row was found by Schafle et al. (84) to be three times as hazardous as playing in the back row. Blocking and spiking in positions 3 and 4 (center and left forward, respectively) accounted for nearly 68% of all the reported ankle injuries and for 69% of all injuries sustained in all six court positions. Ferretti

et al. (37) reported that traumatic knee ligament injuries were associated with jumping in attacking and blocking, with a majority in the #4 position where most of the spiking is performed.

Related to court position is the *specialization* of the players. A team is usually composed of one or two setters, two central blockers, and two or three spikers. Because the rules allow changing court positions by the players after the serve, with exception of back row players spiking ahead of the 3-meter line, the designated spikers will, where possible, assume the #4 position while the central blockers will take up position #3. Although Oudot et al. (76) concluded that function of the player as a spiker, blocker, or setter was not an influencing factor in the incidence of back injuries, Italian studies have shown that at top competitive levels there are substantial differences between incidences of knee and shoulder injuries for the various specializations (15, 35, 45).

### 5.2.2 Training Methods

Common training methods in volleyball intending to improve vertical height of jumping include weight training and plyometrics. The latter method attempts to simulate and exaggerate the volleyball spike take-off, in which a jump is immediately followed by a vertical take-off. In plyometrics the jumping from a landing phase is emphasized, and this creates enormous tensor stresses on the knee mechanisms within a fraction of a second's time.

- Although plyometrics were long suspected of being a source of risk of knee damage, no significant differences in jumper's knee incidence have been found between players who did plyometric training, those who used weight training, and those who did no specific knee strength training (29, 44).
- Training sessions with an emphasis on quadriceps training take a heavy toll on the knee structure, but some authors believe that it is more likely the quality of work than its length or frequency that affects injury risk (9, 37).
- The incidence of injury in female volleyball players has been found to relate markedly to the training technique followed, with those methods involving frequent strain and long duration of semi-squatting, kneeling, and throwing oneself to the ground posing a greater degree of risk (6, 98).

### 5.2.3 Environmental Conditions

In view of the fact that common mechanisms of volleyball injuries are landing and twisting in defensive moves, it has been suggested that there is a need to investigate the role of the types of surfaces the sport is being played on, and concurrently the nature of the footwear used on those surfaces (64).

- More injuries appear to occur when playing on concrete floors than on wooden or linoleum surfaces (45). Parquet type of floors (29, 39) and other wooden surfaces (91) are the preferred choice for playing and training.
- Playing alternately on wooden, concrete, and synthetic floors is associated with higher incidence of knee injuries than playing consistently on the same surface type (45).
- Participants playing on sand courts, such as in beach volleyball, seemed more prone to Achilles tendinitis than indoor players (78).

### 5.2.4 Equipment

Pace (77) regarded the knee protectors frequently used by volleyball players as a possible factor in the genesis of jumper's knee. However, Ferretti (29) argued against this on the basis that the syndrome is also frequently seen in sports such as basketball and high jumping where such knee cap guards are not used. Also, the condition was common before these devices became standard equipment in volleyball.

Safety measures on the playing court have reduced the number of serious traumatic injuries. Unmarked guide wires for the posts, absence of post padding, not regularly drying the floor, and lack of running space around the court have often been causes for accidents. Better regulations appear to have reduced these types of injuries.

## 6. Suggestions for Injury Prevention

Injury prevention in volleyball can be pursued along a variety of lines including the recommendation for changes in international rules of the sport, proposals for improved techniques for jumping and landing, the development and promotion of appropriate flexibility and strength exercises and prophylactic devices and practices, and environmental safety features.

The limited literature on risk factors and predictor variables of injuries in volleyball does not permit an empirically based list of suggestions for injury prevention. The many limitations of and variations in the design of volleyball studies leave much uncertainty about the incidence and causes of injury. Consequently, the list of suggestions in Table 24.11 should not be regarded as strongly based on research findings. Where they have resulted from published sources is indicated in the table. Following the example set by Adrian (1), the table is arranged in four categories, that is, items related to the participant, the sport, the environment, and the health support system.

## 7. Suggestions for Further Research

This chapter has summarized the available literature on injuries in the sport of volleyball up to 1993. Even though this sport is one of the most popular in the world today, it has not received its share of attention from medical and epidemiological researchers. Much more work needs to be completed before the many questions about injury incidence, risk factors, and prevention can be answered. There is a need for well-designed and thorough epidemiological research of volleyball injuries at the school and college/university levels, as well as at the amateur club and professional levels. To improve comparability of the results, researchers should carefully consider the study design and the injury definition. These have varied a great deal over previous investigations, resulting in widely varying findings that are often difficult to appreciate. Suggestions for the study design of epidemiological volleyball injury investigations are presented in Table 24.12.

It has become clear from this review that there is a paucity of information on injury rates, injury type, and injury location particularly at the school and college levels. Prospective epidemiological studies are called for that adhere to recognized standards such as those recommended by the American Orthopaedic Society for Sports Medicine. In addition, such studies should include methods to assess recurrence of injuries, gender differences, practice versus competition, injury severity, practice time loss and injury outcome, the role of specialization, and environmental conditions, because information on these variables is either lacking or equivocal.

**Table 24.11    Suggestions for Injury Prevention**

| Category and area | Examples/suggestions | Reference |
|---|---|---|
| **Participants** | | |
| Education | • As a routine part of any sport delivery program, participants should be educated in the areas of physical fitness, warm-up principles, training loads and progressive training concepts, injury risk factors, early injury reporting, injury self-care, and correct techniques for skill performance and conditioning.<br>• Coaching certification courses should include instruction in first aid, injury risk factors, injury recording and reporting, and injury prevention. | |
| Physical condition | • Fitness and ableness should be monitored and developed through appropriate progressive programs. | Ferretti & DiRosa, 1980 |
| Preventive exercise programs | • The literature has provided a number of training principles aimed at reducing the risk of knee, shoulder, and back injuries. | Bobbert, 1990; Zhang & Luo, 1986; Stacoff et al., 1987; Sommer, 1988; Bonsignore & Giombini, 1990; Rettagliata et al., 1990; Cerulli et al., 1990; Sturbois & Surowiecki, 1990; Bartolozzi et al., 1991; Frignani & Cremonini, 1990 |
| **The sport** | | |
| Technique | • Proper instruction in jumping and landing and hitting technique. | Dawel et al., 1989; Bobbert, 1990; Sturbois & Surowiecki, 1990 |
| | • A sound approach to jump training should be adopted. | Bobbert, 1990 |
| Age-appropriateness | • Modifications in training programs, particularly in jump training, for participants in their growing years. | Kujala et al., 1989 |
| Rules | • Change in rules pertaining to traversing the center line to reduce collision-type injuries. | Hell & Schoenle, 1985 |
| Equipment | • Prophylactic taping has been evaluated as ineffective. | Rovere et al., 1988; Fumich et al., 1981; Conteduca et al., 1990; Greene & Hillman, 1990 |
| | • The use of semirigid orthoses to stabilize weak or injured joints has been found to be more effective. | Fumich et al., 1981; Greene & Hillman, 1990 |
| | • The use of knee protectors does not appear to contribute to jumper's knee syndrome and reduces the impact of knee contact with the floors or players. | Ferretti, 1986 |
| **Environment** | | |
| Playing surface | • Extremely high (cement floor) and low (wet wooden or synthetic floor) friction conditions are conducive to injury and should be avoided. Wooden floors appear most suitable for the sport of volleyball. | Ferretti, 1986; Ferretti et al., 1984; Volpe et al., 1990 |
| | • Playing on a variety of floor types is more likely to produce injuries, particularly of the knee and ankle, than consistently playing on the same type of surface. | Giacomelli et al., 1986 |
| Facilities | • Playing areas for volleyball should be safe and suitable including sufficient surface area and margin around the court, padded posts and referee stand, no post guidewires, and sufficient lighting. | |
| **Health support system** | | |
| Medical exams | • A preparticipation medical examination is recommended for anyone entering competitive volleyball.<br>• Further medical evaluations should be undergone when changing participation levels and after each serious injury. For youngsters in their growth spurt and participants over the age of 40 a yearly medical examination is recommended. | |
| Injury reporting system | • National and/or regional volleyball associations should set up an injury reporting system for the documentation of volleyball injuries. | |

## Table 24.12 Guidelines for Further Research

| Research component | Guidelines |
| --- | --- |
| Injury definition | We recommend that the injury definition for a volleyball study include the following elements:<br>• occurred as a result of participation in volleyball practice or competition<br>• resulted in restriction of the player's participation in practice and/or competition for one or more days beyond the day of injury |
| Subjects | Large-scale studies involving males and females are required at school, university, amateur club, and professional levels. |
| Research design | The study design should be prospective longitudinal over an extended time period (minimally 2 years). A detailed initial questionnaire, pretesting, and medical examination are recommended. |
| Data collection | We suggest that injury information be collected using the interview technique where possible. When a sample is large or spread over a large area, the interview method should still be applied, but as follow-up to the injury report or questionnaire. The length of the recall period should be limited through frequent interviews (minimally monthly). Additional injury information from coach and medical personnel should be sought. |
| Research team | A multidisciplinary team comprising the following personnel: physician, health care professional (certified athletic trainer, licensed physical therapist, or registered nurse, all with a sport background); sport scientist; and epidemiologist/statistician is recommended. |

# References

1. Adrian, M.J. Action model to evaluate and reduce risk of catastrophic injuries. In: Adams, S.H.; Adrian M.J.; Bayless, M.A., eds. Catastrophic injuries in sports: Avoidance strategies. Indianapolis, IN: Benchmark Press; 1987:243-249.
2. Amorth, G.; Tosatti, E. Le dita da palla a volo [Volleyball finger]. Ortopedia e Traumatologia dell' Apparato Motore. 24:875-885; 1956.
3. Baacke, H. Development and status of volleyball. In Fédération Internationale de Volley-ball, ed. Coaches manual I. Lausanne: F.I.V.B.; 1989:Ch 2.
4. Backx, F.J.; Beijer, H.J.; Bol, E.; Erich, W.B. Injuries in high-risk persons and high-risk sports. A longitudinal study of 1,818 school children. Am. J. Sports Med. 19:124-130; 1991.
5. Backx, F.J.; Erich, W.B.; Kemper, A.B.; Verbeek, A.L. Sports injuries in school-aged children: An epidemiologic study. Am. J. Sports Med. 17:234-240; 1989.
6. Bartolozzi, C.; Caramella, D.; Zampa, V.; Dal Pozzo, G.; Tinacci, E.; Balducci, F. [The incidence of disk changes in volleyball players. The magnetic resonance findings]. Radiol MedTorino. 82:757-760; 1991.
7. Biedert, R.; Kentsch, A. [Arthroscopic revision of the subacromial space in impingement syndrome]. Unfallchirürg. 92:500-504; 1989.
8. Blazina, M.E.; Kerlan, R.K.; Jobe, F.W.; Carter, V.C.; Carlson, G.J. Jumper's knee. Orthop. Clin. N. Am. 4:665-678; 1973.
9. Bobbert, M.F. Drop jumping as a training method for jumping ability. Sports Med. 9:7-22; 1990.
10. Bonsignore, D.; Giombini, A. Possibilita terapeutiche nella spalla dolorosa del pallavolista mediante potenziamento isocinetico [Isokinetic exercise therapy in the treatment of shoulder pain in volleyball players]. J. Sports Traum. Rel. Res. 12:123-127; 1990.
11. Bracker, M.D.; Cohen, M.C.; Blasingame, J. Chronic shoulder pain in a volleyball player. Physician Sportsmed. 18:85-88; 1990.
12. Byra, M.; McCabe, J. Incidence of volleyball injuries. Volleyball Technical J. 7:55-57; 1982.
13. Caine, D.J.; Lindner, K.J. Preventing injury to young athletes, Part 1: Predisposing factors. Can. Assoc. Health, Phys. Educ. and Recr. J. 56:30-35; 1990.
14. Caine, D.J.; Lindner, K.J. Overuse injuries of growing bones: the young female gymnast at risk? Physican Sportsmed. 13:51-64; 1985.
15. Candela, V.; Faccini, P.; Colli, R. Traumatologia nella pallavolo. Indagine statistica su un gruppo di atleti di alto valore agonistico [Traumatology in volleyball. Statistical analysis of a group of elite Italian athletes]. J. Sports Traum. Rel. Res. 12:91-94; 1990.
16. Cerulli, G.; Caraffa, A.; Buompadre, V.; Bensi, G.; Stafisso, B. Patologie da pallavolo dell'arto superiore, aspetti di prevenzione [Pathology of injuries of the upper extremity in volleyball: preventive aspects]. J. Sports Traum. Rel. Res. 12:87-89; 1990.
17. Clarke, K.S.; Buckley, W.E. Women's injuries in collegiate sports: A preliminary comparative overview of three seasons. Am. J. Sports Med. 8:187-191; 1980.
18. Conteduca, F.; Russo, G.; delli Falconi, M. Aspetti preventivi nelle distorsioni del collo de piede [Prevention of ankle sprains]. J. Sports Traum. Rel. Res. 12:51-54; 1990.
19. Cooney, W.P. Sports injuries to the upper extremity. How to recognize and deal with some common problems. Postgrad. Med. 76:45-50; 1984.
20. Costa, G.; Perazzini, P.; Agueci, A.; Zorzi, C.; Giulini, G.; Conati, M. Aspetii patologici della spalla nello sport della pallavolo [Pathology of the shoulder in volleyball]. J. Sports Traum. Rel. Res. 12:77-79; 1990.
21. Curti, T.; D'Amato, M. Malattie vascolari dell'arto superiore nella pallavolo [Vascular illness in elite level volleyball]. J. Sports Traum. Rel. Res. 12:85-86; 1990.

22. Del Pizzo, W. Commentary to jumper's knee. Am. J. Sports Med. 11:62; 1983.

23. DeHaven, K.E.; Lintner, D.M. (1986). Athletic injuries: Comparison by age, sport, and gender. Am. J. Sports Med. 14:218-224; 1986.

24. Distefano, S. Neuropathy due to entrapment of the long thoracic nerve. A case report. Ital. J. Orthop. Traum. 15:259-262; 1989.

25. Falez, F.; Mariani, P.P.; Ferretti, A. Le lesioni legamentose della caviglia nei pallavolosti [Ankle ligament sprains in volleyballers]. J. Sports Traum. Rel. Res. 12:39-42; 1990.

26. Ferrari, G.P.; Turra, S.; Fama, G.; Gigante, C. Lesioni traumatiche della mano e del polso nello sport della pallavolo, eta evolutiva [Traumatic injury to the hand and wrist in volleyball, and its evolution]. J. Sports Traum. Rel. Res. 12:95-99; 1990.

27. Ferretti, A. Epidemiology of jumper's knee. Sports Med. 3:289-295; 1986.

28. Ferretti, A. Distorsione al ginocchio [Knee sprain]. Pallavolo. 17:39; 1981.

29. Ferretti, A.; Cerullo, G.; Russo, G. Suprascapular neuropathy in volleyball players. J. Bone Joint Surg. 69-A:260-263; 1987.

30. Ferretti, A.; Di Rosa, S.; eds. Traumatologica nella pallavollo. Rome: Societa Stampa Sportiva; 1980.

31. Ferretti, A.; Ippolito, E.; Mariani, P.; Puddu, G. Jumper's knee. Am. J. Sports Med. 11:58-62; 1983.

32. Ferretti, A.; Neri, M. Risultati dell'indagine epidemiologica sul ginocchio del saltatore [Results of the epidemiological investigation of the jumper's knee]. Pallavolo. 18:13-15; 1982.

33. Ferretti, A.; Neri, M.; Mariani, P.P.; Puddu, G. Considerazioni etiopatogenetische sul ginocchio del saltatore [Etiopathogenetic considerations in jumper's knee]. Ital. J. Sports Traum. 5:101-105; 1983.

34. Ferretti, A.; Papandrea, P.; Conteduca, F. Knee injuries in volleyball. Sports Med. 10:132-138; 1990a.

35. Ferretti, A.; Papandrea, P.; Conteduca, F.; Mariani, P.P. Knee ligament injuries in volleyball players. Am. J. Sports Med. 20:203-207; 1992.

36. Ferretti, A.; Papandrea, P.; Conteduca, F.; Mariani, P.P.; Puddu, G. Le lesioni capsulo-legamentose del ginocchio nei pallavolisti [Knee ligament injuries in volleyball players]. Ital. J. Sports Traum. 10:41-54; 1988.

37. Ferretti, A.; Papandrea, P.; Lucente, L.; Conteduca, F. Lesioni capsulo-legamentose acute e chroniche del ginocchio in giocatori dipallavolo. Analisi de 52 casi aperati [Acute and chronic injuries to the articular ligament of the knee in volleyball. Analysis of 52 cases]. J. Sports Traum. Rel. Res. 12:29-33; 1990b.

38. Ferretti, A.; Puddu, G. Sul dito de pallavolo (About volleyball fingers). Med dello Sport 6:325-328; 1977.

39. Ferretti, A.; Puddu, G.; Mariani, P.P.; Neri, M. Jumper's knee: An epidemiological study of volleyball players. Physician Sportsmed. 12:97-99; 101, 104, 106; 1984.

40. Frignani, R.; Cremonini, L. Patologia de rachide da sovraccarico funzionale (Spine overuse injuries). J. Sports Traum. Rel. Res. 12:11-14; 1990.

41. Fumich, R.M.; Ellison, A.E.; Guerin, G.J.; Grace, P.D. The measured effect of taping on combined foot and ankle motion before and after exercise. Am. J. Sports Med. 9:165-170; 1981.

42. Gangitano, R.; Pulvirenti, A.; Ardito, S. Lesioni traumatiche da pallavolo: Riliavi clinica-statistici [Volleyball injuries: Clinical and statistical findings]. Ital. J. Sports Traum. 3:31-44; 1981.

43. Garrick, J.G.; Requa, R.K. Injuries in high school sports. Pediatrics. 61:465-469; 1978.

44. Gerberich, S.G.; Luhmann, S.; Finke, C.; Priest, J.D.; Beard, B.J. Analysis of severe injuries associated with volleyball activities. Physician Sportsmed. 15:75-79; 1987.

45. Giacomelli, E.; Grassi, W.; Zampa, A.M. Le atlopatie nei pallavolisti [Athletes' diseases affecting volleyball players]. Med. dello Sport. 39:425-434; 1986.

46. Greene, T.A.; Hillman, S.K. Comparison of support provided by a semirigid orthosis and adhesive ankle taping before, during, and after exercise. Am. J. Sports Med. 18:498-506; 1990.

47. Guo, S.; Xu, C. [Entrapment injury of the suprascapular nerves—mechanisms of musculus infraspinatus atrophy in volleyball players]. Chinese J. Sports Med. 3:94, 98, 127-128; 1984.

48. Ha, K.I.; Hahn, S.H.; Chung, M.Y.; Yang, B.K.; Yi, S.R. A clinical study of stress fractures in sport activities. Orthopedics. 14:1089-1095; 1991.

49. Heckman, J.D.; Alkire, C.C. Distal patellar pole fractures: A proposed common mechanism of injury. Am. J. Sports Med. 12:424-429; 1984.

50. Hell, H.; Schoenle, C. Ursachen und Prophylaxe typischer Volleyballverletzungen [Causes and prevention of typical volleyball injuries]. Z. Orthop. 123:72-75; 1985.

51. Holzgräfe, M.; Klingerhofer, J.; Eggert, S.; Benecke, R. [Chronic neuropathy of the suprascapular nerve in high performance athletes]. Nervenarzt. 59:545-548; 1988.

52. Hoshikawa, Y.; Kurosawa, H.; Fukubayashi, T.; Nakajima, H.; Watarai, K. The prognosis of meniscectomy in athletes. The simple meniscus lesions without ligamentous instabilities. Am. J. Sports Med. 11:8-13; 1983.

53. Jacchia, G.E.; Gatti, U.; Gioregetti, A.; Capone, A. Traumatologia acuta del rachide nella pallavolo [Acute traumatology of the spine in volleyball]. J. Sports Traum. Rel. Res. 12:15-18; 1990.

54. Jerosch, J.; Castro, W.H.; Sons, H.U. [Secondary impingement syndrome in athletes]. Sportverletz Sportschäden. 4:180-185; 1990.

55. Julsrud, M.E. Osteochondrosis of the first metatarsal sesamoid in a volleyball player. Podiatric Sports Med. 1:34-36; 1983.

56. Kostianen, S.; Orava, S. Blunt injury of the radial and ulnar arteries in volleyball players. A report

of three cases of the antebrachial-palmar hammer syndrome. Brit. J. Sports Med. 17:172-176; 1983.

57. Kruger-Franke, M. [Isolated metacarpal fracture—a rare injury in volleyball]. Sportverletz Sportschäden, 4:99-100; 1990.

58. Kujala, U.M.; Aalto, T.; Österman, K.; Dahlström, S. The effect of volleyball playing on the knee extensor mechanism. Am. J. Sports Med. 17:766-769; 1989.

59. Kujala, U.M.; Kvist, M.; Österman, K. Knee injuries in athletes. Review of exertion injuries and retrospective study of outpatient sports clinic material. Sports Med. 3:447-460; 1986.

60. Lanese, R.R.; Strauss, R.H.; Leizman, D.J.; Rotondi, A.M. Injury and disability in matched men's and women's intercollegiate sports. Am. J. Public Health. 80:1459-1462; 1990.

61. Lanzetta, A. Spalla dolorosa ed instabilita nel volley [Shoulder pain and instability in volleyball]. J. Sports Traum. Rel. Res. 12:61-64; 1990.

62. Lanzetta, M.; Fox, U. Microaneurismi posttraumatici delle arterie periferiche in atleti di pallavolo: cas report [Post traumatic microaneurism of the ulnar artery in volleyball athlete: a case report]. J. Sports Traum. Rel. Res. 12:115-118; 1990.

63. Lindner, K.J.; Butcher, J.; Johns, D.P. Recall of competitive sport participation by urban grade 10 students. Can. Assoc. Physical Educ. Health Recr. J., Res. Suppl. 1:79-95; 1994.

64. Lund, P.M. Marathon volleyball: Changes after 61 hours play. Brit. J. Sports Med. 19:228-229; 1985.

65. Lysens, R.; de Weerdt, L.; Nieuwboer, A. Factors associated with injury proneness. Sports Med. 12:281-289; 1991.

66. Lysens, R.; Steverlynck, A.; van den Auweele, Y.; Lefevre, J.; Renson, L.; Claessens, A.; Ostyn, M. The predictability of sports injuries. Sports Med. 1:6-10; 1984.

67. Mariani, P.; Puddu, G.; Ferretti, A. Il ginocchio del saltatore (Jumper's knee). Ital. J. Orthop. Traum. 4:85-94; 1978.

68. Martens, M.A.; Wouters, P.; Burssens, A.; Mulier, J.C. Patellar tendinitis: pathology and results of treatment. Acta Orthop. Scan. 53:445-450; 1982.

69. Maurizio, E. La tendinite rotulea nel giocatore di pallavolo (Patellar tendinitis in volleyball players). Bollett Memorie della Soc Tosca Umbra do Chirurg. 24:443-453; 1963.

70. Melzer, C.; Wirth, J. [Complete rotator cuff lesions in athletes]. Sportverletz Sportschäden. 3:81-87; 1989.

71. Mollica, Q.; Gangitano, R.; Longo, G.; Salemi, M. Patologia musculo-tendinea della spalla [Musculo-tendinous pathology of the shoulder]. J. Sports Traum. Rel. Res. 12:71-75; 1990.

72. Montorsi, A.; Grandi, M.; Boschi, S.; Bedeschi, P. Lesions della mano nella pallavolo [Hand injuries in volleyball]. J. Sports Traum. Rel. Res. 12:81-84; 1990.

73. Moraldo, M.; Kirchner, H.G.; Düssen, G.A. Das Volleyballspiel aus orthopädischer Sicht [The volleyball game from the orthopedic point of view]. Deutsche Z. Sportmed. 32:286-290; 1981.

74. Mutoh, Y.; Mori, T.; Suzuki, Y.; Sugiura, Y. Stress fractures of the ulna in athletes. Am. J. Sports Med. 10:365-367; 1982.

75. Neugebauer, N.; Herzberger, M.; Rossak, K. Knorpelschäden im Femuropatellargelenk beim Volleyballspieler [Cartilage damage in the femuro-patellar joint in volleyball players]. Deutsche Z. Sportmed. 36:10; 1985.

76. Oudot, C.; Bence, Y.; Ziegler, G.; Ziegler, L.; Commandre, F. Volleyeur de haut-niveau. Rachis lombro-sacre. Résultats d'une enquête sur 157 cas [Elite volleyball players: lumbosacral pain. Results of an investigation of 157 cases]. Médecine Sport. 56:148-150, 152-156; 1982.

77. Pace, N. Ipotesi eziopatogenetische della gonalgia dei pallavolisti. Med dello Sport. 33:45-47; 1980.

78. Pace, N.; Lo Iacono, E.; Giacchetta, A.M.; Serafini, P.; Zanoli, S. Patologia tendinea del piede nella pallavolo [Pathology of Achilles tendinitis in volleyball]. J. Sports Traum. Rel. Res. 12:43-49; 1990.

79. Rettagliata, F.; Oliveri, M.; Sieni, G.; Gambaro, G.A. Il conflitto sub-acromiale nel volley [Subacromial impingement in volleyball]. J. Sports Traum. Rel. Res. 12:65-69; 1990.

80. Roels, J.; Martens, M.; Mulier, J.C.; Burssens, A. Patelar tendinitis (Jumper's knee). Am. J. Sports Med. 6:362-366; 1978.

81. Rovere, G.D.; Clarke, T.J.; Yates, C.S.; Burley, K. Retrospective comparison of taping and ankle stabilizers in preventing ankle injuries. Am. J. Sports Med. 16:228-233; 1988.

82. Rutherford, G.W.; Miles, R.B.; Brown, V.R.; et al. Overview of sports-related injuries to persons 5-14 years of age. Washington, DC: US Consumer Product Safety Commission; 1981.

83. Santilli, G. Patologia da sovraccarico funzionale dell'apparato locomotore. Med. dello Sport. 28:371-383; 1975.

84. Schafle, M.D.; Requa, R.K.; Patton, W.L.; Garrick, J.G. Injuries in the 1987 national amateur volleyball tournament. A.J. Sports Med. 18:624-631; 1990.

85. Shen, B. [Injuries of hand bones in adolescent volleyball players—an investigation based on findings of X-ray films of skeletal age]. Chinese J. Sports Med. 2:6-7, 67; 1983.

86. Sommer, H.M. Patellar chondropathy and apicitis, and muscle imbalances of the lower extremities in competitive sports. Sports Med. 5:386-394; 1988.

87. Stacoff, A.; Kälin, X.; Stüssi, E. Belastungen im Volleyball bei der Landung nach dem Block [Loads when landing after a volleyball block). Deutsche Z. Sportmed. 38:458-464; 1987.

88. Steinbruck, K. [Epidemiology of sports injuries. A 15 year analysis of sports orthopedic ambulatory care]. Sportverletz Sportschäden. 1:2-12; 1987.

89. Sturbois, X.; Surowiecki, R. Biomechanics and instability of the shoulder in volleyball. Hermes (Belgium). 21:423-430; 1990.

90. Van Soest, A.J.; Roebroeck, M.E.; Bobbert, M.F.; Huijing, P.A.; Van Ingen Schenau, G.J. A comparison

of one-legged and two-legged countermovement jumps. Med. Sci. Sports Exerc. 17:635-639; 1985.

91. Volpe, A.; Girotto, A.; Schiavon, R. Le plantalgie nella pallavolo [The foot in volleyball]. J. Sports Traum. Rel. Res. 12:55-59; 1990.

92. Volpi, P.; Vanni, C. Le lesioni meniscali del ginocchio nella pallavolo [Meniscus injury to the knee in volleyball]. J. Sports Traum. Rel. Res. 12:35-38; 1990.

93. Watson, F.M. Simultaneous interphalangeal dislocation in one finger. J. Trauma. 23:65; 1983.

94. Watson, A.W. Sports injuries during one academic year in 6799 Irish school children. Am. J. Sports Med. 12:65-70; 1984.

95. Whiteside, J.A.; Fleagle, S.B.; Kalenak, A. Fractures and refractures in intercollegiate athletes: An eleven-year experience. Am. J. Sports Med. 9:369-377; 1981.

96. Williams, J.M.; Tonymon, P.; Wadsworth, W.A. Relationship of life stress to injury in intercollegiate volleyball. J. Human Stress. 12:38-43; 1986.

97. Zaricznyj, B.; Shattuck, L.J.; Mast, T.A.; Robertson, R.V.; D'Elia, G. Sports-related injuries in school-aged children. Am. J. Sports Med. 8:318-323; 1980.

98. Zhang, S.; Luo, Y. [The pathogenesis of patellar strain in women volleyball players]. Chinese J. Sports Med. 5:98-102; 1986.

# 25

# Wrestling

*Randall R. Wroble*

## 1. Introduction

Currently wrestling is a popular sport at the youth, high school, college, and senior level. Part of its popularity relates to the opportunity for participation by men and boys of all sizes. Wrestling has evolved into three distinct styles. In the United States, high school and collegiate athletes practice what is termed American Folkstyle. Competitions are also held in Freestyle wrestling, which is practiced throughout the rest of the world, and in Greco-Roman wrestling, another international style that allows holds only above the waist. Each style of wrestling requires similar training methods but match length differs by level and by style.

Because the competitive season is long, and practices are frequent, long, and intense, the number of exposures for an individual wrestler is high. Wrestlers appear to be at risk in the same way that other contact sports athletes are at risk. But unlike many other sports, contact in wrestling occurs virtually 100% of the time. Consequently, the effective exposure period is increased. Secondly, wrestling is also a collision sport. Collisions occur when a wrestler "shoots" or attempts a takedown.

In many studies that have examined injury rates in sports, the number of injuries in wrestling is significantly high. Furthermore, in a small number of long-term follow-up studies, former wrestlers had a significant number of health problems. These facts alone mandate that more knowledge be available about the injury problem in wrestling in terms of incidence and severity. Only in this way can preventive measures be implemented.

The goal of this review was to examine work done on wrestling injuries in order to start the sequence of injury prevention described by van Mechelen (57). In this sequence, the magnitude of the problem is first established by determining

injury rates, types of injuries, and time loss caused by these injuries. More detailed research determines the etiology and mechanism of these injuries. The next step is the introduction of various preventive measures. Finally, further studies are done to assess the effectiveness of these measures.

To carry out the present study, we searched the English language literature from 1975 to 1992 using Medline and Sport Discus. Furthermore, we retrieved research cited in other clinical reports and data collected but not published by the National Collegiate Athletic Association (NCAA) (38). As with all reviews of sports injuries, problems occur in comparing studies because of lack of consistency regarding injury definition, study design, data collection methodology, sample sizes, and study populations.

## 2. Incidence of Injury

### 2.1 Injury Rates

Some of the earliest epidemiological work in wrestling was done in the 1950s and 1960s in a series of theses (2, 9, 28, 40), Table 25.1. Although these efforts are flawed because of poor injury definitions and data collection by questionnaire, the questions raised in these studies were many and varied. The injury rates reported for high school and college wrestlers were generally lower than in the newer series discussed below.

More recent injury data are shown in Table 25.2. Injury rates per 100 wrestlers range from 16.4 to 288. The differences in study population, injury definition, exposure, study design, and data collection methods are significant. Although the studies of National High School Injury Registry (NHSIR) (39), Garrick (17), Estwanik (15), Powell (41), and the NCAA (38) required time loss as a criterion

**Table 25.1  Injury Rates, Early Studies 1951-66**

| Study | Level | Study design[a] | Data collection method[b] | Duration | # of injuries | # of wrestlers | # of teams | Rate |
|-------|-------|-----------------|----------------------------|----------|---------------|----------------|------------|------|
| Konrad, 1951 | H.S. | P | Q | 1 season | 735 | 4,835 | 176 | 15.2/100 wr. |
| Patacsil, 1955 | H.S. | P | Q | 1 season | 80 | 907 | 18 | 8.8/100 wr. |
| Patacsil, 1955 | C | P | Q | 1 season | 120 | 711 | 20 | 16.9/100 wr. |
| | | | | | | | | Range = 8.8-16.9 |
| Acksel, 1966 | H.S. | R | Q | 1 season | 289 | 2,032 | 49 | 14.2/100 wr. |
| Brown, 1951 | H.S. | R | Q | 1 season | 68 | 201 | — | 33.8/100 wr. |
| | | | | | | | | Range = 14.2-33.8 |

[a]R = retrospective, P = prospective.

[b]I = interview, Q = questionnaire.

**Table 25.2  Injury Rates, 1978-Present**

| Study | Level | Study design[a] | Data collection method[b] | Duration | # of injuries | # of wrestlers | # of teams | Rate[c] | Rate[d] |
|-------|-------|-----------------|----------------------------|----------|---------------|----------------|------------|---------|---------|
| **High school** | | | | | | | | | |
| Garrick, 1978 | H.S. | P | I | 2 seasons | 176 | 234 | 4 | 75 | |
| Estwanik, 1983 | H.S. | P | Q | 2 seasons | 248 | 1,091 | 49 | 22.7 | |
| Zaricznyj, 1980 | Y, H.S.[e] | P | I | 1 year | 27 | 165 | — | 16.4 | |
| NHSIR, 1989 | H.S. | P | I | 1 season[f] | 690 | 1,387 | 47 | 50 | |
| | | | | | | | | Range = 16.4-75 | |
| NHSIR, 1989 | H.S. | P | I | 2 seasons[g] | — | — | 47[h] | | 7.6 |
| | | | | | | | 47[i] | | |
| **College** | | | | | | | | | |
| Powell, 1981 | C | P | I | 5 seasons | 2,129 | 2,255 | 87 | 94 | 9.5 |
| NCAA, 1993 | C | P | I | 8 seasons | 5,999 | — | 343 | | 9.41 |
| Roy, 1979 | C | R | I | 3 seasons | 332 | 115 | 1 | 288 | |
| Jackson, 1980 | C | R | I | 2 seasons | 17 | 89 | 2 | 19.1 | |
| Wroble, 1986 | C | R | I | 8 seasons | 847 | 464 | 1 | 176 | |
| Snook, 1982 | C | R | I | 5 seasons | 90 | 129 | 1 | 69.8 | |
| | | | | | | | | Range = 19.1-288 | |
| **International** | | | | | | | | | |
| Lok, 1975 | I | R | I | 1 season | 31 | 128 | 1 | 24.2/100 wr. | |

[a]P = prospective, R = retrospective.

[b]I = interview, Q = questionnaire.

[c]Injuries/100 wrestlers.

[d]Injuries/1,000 athlete exposures.

[e]Includes ages 5-18.

[f]Data from 1987-88 only.

[g]Data includes 1987-88 and 1988-89 seasons.

[h]1987-88.

[i]1988-89.

for injury, the other studies did not. Roy's study merely required that the athlete consult the team physician (46). Furthermore, he included skin infections as injuries. These are not included in most series. In the other study with high injury rate (61), time loss was also not required for the definition of injury. Lower injury rates were found in studies in which college athletes had to report to a student health service (25), pre-high school athletes were included and an accident report was required(63), a questionnaire was filled out by coaches (15), and in a study of international wrestling in which the definition of injury was not specified (31).

Injury rates in wrestling expressed by exposure are available only in three large studies (38, 39, 41). Each study defined injury as requiring that participation be restricted for one or more days. Athlete exposure was defined as each opportunity for an athlete to get hurt: one athlete participating in one practice or one match constitutes one exposure. Data for high school wrestlers showed an injury rate of 7.6 injuries per 1,000 athlete exposures (22, 39). This number can be contrasted with the results of two studies done of college wrestlers performed with identical methodology, which reported injury rates of 9.5 (41) and 9.4 (38) injuries per 1,000 athlete exposures.

The majority of studies have involved high school (15, 17, 39, 63) and collegiate (25, 38, 41, 46, 49, 59) wrestlers. When calculated by athlete exposure, college injury rates are approximately 25% higher than those seen at the high school level. When calculated by injuries per 100 wrestlers however, the college injury rate appears much higher. This may reflect in part the difference in intensity of competition between the two levels. College wrestling is a much more aggressive sport than high school wrestling. Training sessions and matches occur more frequently. On the other hand, the methodologic differences between the high school and college studies may account for some of the difference. In general, time loss criteria were not required for an injury to be recorded in most of the college studies. Further, scrutiny over the collegiate level athlete is generally more thoroughly and easily accomplished than at the high school level.

Lorish et al. studied injuries in two youth wrestling tournaments (32). Logistic regression indicated that older age was associated with higher injury rate (Table 25.5). Patacsil examined injury rates by grade in high school or grade in college (40). He demonstrated a trend toward higher injury rates in the juniors and seniors in both high school and college. Because the match injury rate is so much higher than practice injury rate (see section 2.3) and upper class wrestlers are more likely to participate in matches than the underclassmen by virtue of their relative skill levels, it is perhaps not surprising that the upper class wrestlers should have higher injury rates. Strauss and Lanese compared four wrestling tournaments (52). In the youth tournament (3-minute matches) injury rates were lower than at the high school level (6-minute matches) and at the collegiate level (6- or 8-minute matches) (Table 25.5).

Conversely, Hartmann demonstrated no variation in injury rate by age in a youth tournament (20). However, only 21 injuries were reported in this tournament. Also, Wroble et al. were unable to discern any variation in injury rate among collegiate wrestlers when considering their age or years of wrestling experience (61).

## 2.2 Reinjury Rates

Table 25.3 shows the percentage of reinjuries. High school reinjuries ranged from 16.2 per 100 injuries

**Table 25.3  Percent Comparison of Reinjury**

| Study | Study design[a] | Level | Participants | Injuries | Reinjuries | Percentage[b] |
|---|---|---|---|---|---|---|
| Patacsil | P | H.S. | 907 | 80 | 9 | 11 |
| Patacsil | P | C | 711 | 120 | 23 | 19 |
| Requa, 1981 | P | H.S. | 234 | 176 | 28 | 16.2 |
| Strauss, 1982 | P | Y, H.S., C | 1,049 | 102 | 40 | 39 |
| NHSIR | P | H.S. | — | — | — | 9[c] |
| NCAA | P | C | — | 1,054 | 193 | 18.3[d] |
| | | | | | | Range = 9-39 |
| Wroble, 1986, knee | R | C | 136 | 65 | 136 | 48 |
| Wroble, 1986, neck | R | C | 464 | 41 | 19 | 46 |
| Wroble, 1986, back | R | C | 464 | 41 | 17 | 41 |

[a]R = retrospective, P = prospective.

[b]Percent of total injuries.

[c]Projection from 2-year study.

[d]Data from 1992-93 season only.

to 9 per 100 injuries. The difference may reflect the more intense observation applied to injuries in the former study (17, 18, 39, 42). A similar proportion of reinjuries was found at the college level (38). Those studies that applied a liberal definition of injury not requiring time loss and thus documenting any wrestler who presented with recurrent symptoms as having a reinjury showed a high percentage of reinjuries (52, 59, 61).

## 2.3 Practice Versus Competition

The competitive wrestling season is typically a long one, 5 to 6 months. Wrestlers train 5 to 7 days a week, and during more intense parts of the season, up to 2 or 3 times per day. Each of these sessions may last 1-1/2 to 2 hours. The amount of exposure to competition is much less but significantly more intense. A high school wrestler may compete in 30 to 40 6-minute matches a year, a college wrestler in 40 to 50 7-minute matches.

Practice and competition injury rates have been studied. In every instance, the percentage of injuries that occurred during practice is greater than 60% of the total number of injuries and reached as high as 89% in Roy's study (46), Table 25.4. When injury rate by athlete exposure is calculated, however, the situation is reversed. Practice results in a range of injury rates of 6.45 to 7.8 injuries per 1,000 athlete exposures, and matches result in a range of injury rates of 11.6 to 31.3 injuries per 1,000 athlete exposures.

The tournament studies shown in Table 25.5 show injury rates per 100 matches or per 100 wrestlers. The injury rate per 100 matches increases from youth tournaments to high school tournaments and finally to college tournaments. In the single study of international wrestling the differ-

ence in injury rate between Freestyle and Greco-Roman wrestling was striking, being more than twice as high in Freestyle than in Greco-Roman (13). The authors offer no explanation for this finding.

## 2.4 Weight Class

Wrestling at all levels is contested at several weight classes, ensuring that athletes are size matched. Each wrestler is required to attain a specific body weight corresponding to the weight class prior to competing in a match.

Several authors have examined the relationship between weight class and injury (shown in Table 25.6). Because the number of weight classes and the actual weight assigned to each class varied over the time of this survey and from level to level of wrestling, for the purposes of this review weight classes are divided into lower, middle, upper, and heavyweight.

It is difficult to interpret injuries by weight class as a percentage of total injuries in a study because the distribution of wrestlers across the classes is unknown. Despite this, the two largest studies that report weight class data show injuries only as a percentage of the total, revealing proportions of injuries that are relatively equal between lower, middle, and upper weight classes (22, 38). Three studies did provide injury rates (13, 32, 35). These studies showed the injury rate in the upper weight classes to be slightly higher. In Wroble and Mysnyk, et al.'s study of knee injuries in college wrestlers, injury rates were almost identical in lower, middle, and upper weights (61). Hartmann (20), Kersey and Rowan (26), and Strauss and Lanese (52) reported no difference in injury rates by weight class although no data was supplied.

### Table 25.4  Practice vs. Competition Injury Rates

| Study | Level | Study design[a] | Participants | Practice injuries | Percentage[b] | Practice rate[c] | Competition injuries | Percentage[b] | Competition rate[c] |
|---|---|---|---|---|---|---|---|---|---|
| NHSIR | H.S. | P | — | 816 | 68 | 6.45 | 421 | 32 | 11.6 |
| NCAA | C | P | — | 4,009 | 67 | 7.1 | 1,990 | 33 | 31.3 |
| Powell | C | P | 2,255 | 1,582 | 74 | 7.8 | 547 | 26 | 27.0 |
| Garrick, 1978 | H.S. | P | 234 | 114 | 65 | — | 62 | 35 | — |
| Zaricznyj | Y, H.S. | P | 165 | 17 | 63 | — | 10 | 27 | — |
| | | | | Range | 63-74 | 6.45-7.8 | | 26-35 | 11.6-31.3 |
| Roy | C | R | 115 | 295 | 89 | — | 37 | 11 | — |

[a]R = retrospective, P = prospective.

[b]Percent of total injuries.

[c]Injuries/1,000 athlete-exposures.

**Table 25.5  Practice vs. Competition in Tournament Studies**

| Study | Level | Data collection methods[a] | Study design[b] | Duration | # of injuries | # of wrestlers | # of matches | Injuries/ 100 matches | Injuries/ 100 wrestlers |
|---|---|---|---|---|---|---|---|---|---|
| Youth | | | | | | | | | |
| Hartmann, 1978 | Y[c] | I | P | 1 tourn. | 21 | — | 190 | 11 | — |
| Strauss,[d] 1982 | Y | I | P | 1 tourn. | 11 | 291 | 525 | 2.1 | 3.8 |
| Lorish, 1992 | Y[e] | I | P | 2 tourn. | 221 | 1,742 | 7,196 | 3.1 | 12.7 |
| | | | | | | | | | 9.7[f] |
| | | | | | | | | | 22.1[g] |
| | | | | | | | Range | 2.1-11 | 3.8-12.7 |
| High school | | | | | | | | | |
| Strauss,[d] 1982 | H.S. | I | P | 4 tourn. | 58 | 520 | 676 | 8.6 | 11.1 |
| College | | | | | | | | | |
| Strauss,[d] 1982 | C | I | P | 2 tourn. | 33 | 238 | 406 | 8.1 | 13.9 |
| Kersey, 1983 | C | I | P | 1 tourn. | 110 | 353 | 493 | 22 | 31.2 |
| McGuine, 1989 | C | I | P | 1 tourn. | 129 | 341 | 628 | 21 | 38 |
| | | | | | | | Range | 8.1-22 | 13.9-38 |
| International | | | | | | | | | |
| Estwanik, 1978 | I (freestyle) | I | P | 1 tourn. | 83 | 313 | 1,141 | 7.1 | 26 |
| | I (greco-roman) | I | P | 1 tourn. | 15 | 146 | 499 | 3.0 | 10 |
| | | | | | | | Range | 3.0-7.1 | 10-26 |

[a] I = interview, Q = questionnaire.

[b] P = prospective.

[c] Ages 7-12.

[d] 4 tournaments: 1 youth, 1 H.S., 2 college.

[e] Ages 6-16.

[f] Injury rate for 6- to 8-year-olds.

[g] Injury rate for 14- to 16-year-olds.

**Table 25.6  Injuries by Weight Class**

| Study | Study design[a] | Level | Lower weight classes # injuries | Rate | %[b] | Middle weight classes # injuries | Rate | %[b] | Upper weight classes # injuries | Rate | %[b] | Heavy weight class # injuries | Rate | %[b] |
|---|---|---|---|---|---|---|---|---|---|---|---|---|---|---|
| Lorish, 1992 | P | Y, H.S. | 71 | 10.2[c] | | 81 | 10.4[c] | | 38 | 14.3[c] | | | | |
| McGuine, 1989 | P | C | 29 | 30[c] | | 35 | 32[c] | | 44 | 32[c] | | | | |
| Estwanik, 1978 | P | I | 17 | 19.3[c] | | 31 | 27.4[c] | | 35 | 31.5[c] | | | | |
| | | Range | 10.2-30 | | | 10.4-32 | | | 14.3-32 | | | | | |
| Hoffman | P | H.S. | 184 | | 26.7 | 228 | | 33.1 | 226 | | 32.7 | 33 | | 4.8 |
| NCAA[d] | P | C | 1,701 | | 28.2 | 2,159 | | 35.8 | 1,689 | | 28.0 | 477 | | 7.9 |
| Wroble,[e] 1986 | R | C | 42 | 7[c] | | 52 | 8.0[c] | | 37 | 8[c] | | 5 | 4[c] | |

[a] R = retrospective, P = prospective.

[b] Percentage of total injuries.

[c] Injuries/100 wrestlers.

[d] Injury totals for 8 seasons.

[e] Knee injuries only.

## 3. Injury Characteristics

### 3.1 Injury Onset

Wrestlers maintain a high level of training and fitness throughout the entire wrestling season. With this large volume of training, overuse or gradual onset injuries can and do occur. They are overshadowed both in frequency and in severity by their acute counterparts. Thus it is not surprising that these injuries have not been reported well.

In fact, none of the large studies include a category for this type of injury.

With the exception of skin infections and a minuscule number of other injuries, sudden onset injuries are the ones reported in all the large surveys of wrestling injuries.

## 3.2 Injury Type

The vast majority of reports and statistics regarding wrestling injuries deal with those concerning the musculoskeletal system. However, wrestling does present a different set of problems: dermatologic and systemic illnesses. Dermatologic illnesses are bacterial such as impetigo or folliculitis, viral such as herpes simplex (called herpes gladiatorum in wrestlers), and fungal such as tinea corporis (ringworm) and athlete's foot. Systemic illnesses are typified by viral upper respiratory infections.

Table 25.7 shows the results of studies that tabulate injury by type. All studies show sprain injuries to be the most common. Tendinitis/strains, fractures, and contusions are also relatively common. In studies in which infectious diseases are counted, their proportion is also high.

Whiteside et al. integrated student health records, X rays, and National Athletic Injury Reporting System (NAIRS) reports over an 11-year period at a large university to compile data on all fractures sustained in their athletes (58). They documented 14 fractures in 899 wrestlers during this period (1.5 per 100 wrestlers).

## 3.3 Injury Location

A detailed breakdown of injury location is shown in Table 25.8. As far as musculoskeletal injuries by body region, upper extremity injuries occur with slightly lower frequency than lower extremity injuries. Injuries to the head, spine, and trunk occur most commonly across all studies. Note that each author has used a slightly different schema for injury location. Only a small number of studies included a breakdown of dermatologic problems. Furthermore, some studies included skin injuries, but by their location on the body rather than as a separate category. Injuries to the ears and ribs have a relatively high proportion. As borne out by a wide range of studies, injuries to the neck occur in substantial numbers. In the upper extremity, injuries to the shoulder dominate. In the lower extremity and in the body overall, the knee is most frequently injured. Ankle injuries and more specifically ankle sprains, appear to be the next most commonly injured area in the lower extremity.

### 3.3.1 Head/Spine/Trunk

Wrestling injuries in these locations make up 30.8 to 51.8% of the total number of injuries in wrestling in prospective studies (24.3-45.4% in retrospective studies). In 9 of 13 prospective studies this was the most frequently injured body region.

Injuries to the head, mainly concussions, occur by head-head or head-knee collisions during takedowns. Concussions are also produced by contact with the wrestling mat. The proscription of slamming an opponent to the mat makes serious head injury less likely via this mechanism. A common mechanism for a neck injury occurs during a takedown. In this, the wrestler drives into his opponent with his neck, hyperextending it while "shooting." This can cause sprains, strains, and neurologic trauma such as stingers.

Wroble and Albright reviewed injuries over an 8-year period on a college wrestling team (59). The neck was the second most frequent anatomic location injured. The vast majority of these 104 injuries were sprain/strain injuries and neurogenic pain syndromes such as stingers. Estwanik (14) also noted the predominance of sprains and nerve injuries.

Ear injuries, specifically the auricular hematoma or cauliflower ear, result from direct trauma to the ear, either on impact with another wrestler's head or knee, or by abrasive friction-causing forces as when wrestlers "tie-up" head-to-head. Most of these injuries occur when the wrestler is not wearing headgear. However these can and do occur with headgear on (47). The wrestler begins to sweat and the headgear can then slide and cause the hematoma by abrading the external ear.

Schuller et al. sent questionnaires to all Division I NCAA wrestling programs regarding headgear use and received responses from 537 wrestlers (about 20% of the total college wrestlers) (47). Only 189 of the 537 wrestlers (35.2%) wore their headgear all the time. Of those who wore headgear, 25.5% developed hematoma. Of those who did not wear headgear, 51% developed hematoma. There were 38.7% of wrestlers left with a permanent ear deformity. Approximately one fourth of those with deformity incurred their injury while they were wearing headgear. A response by coaches in the same study indicated that 82% of coaches don't require wearing headgear at practice. In an early high school study only 2 of 49 coaches (4.1%) required their wrestlers to wear headgear (2).

Lower back injuries commonly take place during takedowns. While sparring for position, wrestlers

**Table 25.7  Injury Type (Percent of Total Injuries)**

| Study | Study design[a] | Level | Participants | Injuries | Abrasion | Concussion | Contusion | Dislocation | Fx.[c] | Infection | Laceration | Tendinitis/strain | Sprain | Bursitis | Meniscus tear | Neuro-trauma | Other |
|---|---|---|---|---|---|---|---|---|---|---|---|---|---|---|---|---|---|
| NHSIR, 1988-1989 | P | H.S. | — | — | | | | | 7 | | | 23 | 30 | | | 14 | |
| Garrick, 1981 | P | H.S. | 234 | 176 | | | 5.6 | | 3.8 | | 0.9 | 24.8 | 29.1 | | | | |
| NCAA, 1993 | P | C | — | 1,055 | 0.28 | 2.2 | 5.0 | 6.5 | 3.7 | 22.3 | 3.0 | 14.7 | 28.8 | 0.85 | 5.0 | 2.3 | 5.2 |
| | | | | | .03[b] | .24[b] | .55[b] | .72[b] | .40[b] | 2.45[b] | .33[b] | 1.61[b] | 3.17[b] | .09[b] | .55[b] | .25[b] | .56[b] |
| Estwanik, 1978 | P | I | 459 | 98 | | | 17.3 | | 2.0 | | 11.2 | 10.2 | 42.8 | 4.1 | | 3.1 | 8.2 |
| NCAA, 1985-93 | P | C | — | 5,999 | | | | | | | | 17.25 | 28 | | | | |
| | | | | | | | | | | | | 1.65[b] | 2.7[b] | | | | |
| | | | | Range | | | 5.0-17.3 | | 2.0-7 | | 0.9-11.2 | 10.2-24.8 | 28.0-42.8 | 0.85-4.1 | | 2.0-3.1 | 5.2-8.2 |
| Roy, 1979 | R | C | 115 | 332 | | 0.3 | 17.2 | | 1.5 | 16.9 | 3.6 | 19 | 23.8 | 1.2 | 1.8 | 2.1 | 12.3 |
| Snook, 1982 | R | C | 90 | 129 | 1.1 | 1.1 | | 20 | 4.4 | 16.7 | 3.3 | 3.3 | 42.2 | 1.1 | 3.3 | 1.1 | 3.3 |
| | | | | Range | .03-1.1 | .03-1.1 | | | 1.5-4.4 | 16.7-16.9 | 3.3-3.6 | 3.3-19.0 | 23.8-42.2 | 1.1-1.2 | 1.8-3.3 | 1.1-2.1 | 3.3-12.3 |

*Note.* All data collected through interview method.

[a]P = prospective, R = retrospective.

[b]Per 1,000 athlete exposures.

[c]Fx = fracture.

**Table 25.8a   Injury Location, Percent of Total Injuries**

| Study | Konrad | Patacsil H.S. | Patacsil C | Estwanik 1978 | Estwanik 1983 | Kersey | McGuine | Lorish | Strauss 1982 | Requa | Powell | NCAA 1985-92 | NCAA 1992-93 | NHSIR | Range |
|---|---|---|---|---|---|---|---|---|---|---|---|---|---|---|---|
| Study design[a] | P | P | P | P | P | P | P | P | P | P | P | P | P | P | |
| **Skin** | 21.6 | | | | | | | 6.8 | | | | | | | **6.8-26** |
| **Head/spine/trunk** | **39.5** | **47.2** | **30.8** | **49** | **31.9** | **40** | **51.8** | **43.9** | **48** | **37.5** | **31.9** | | **35.0** | **32.5** | **30.8-51.8** |
| Head | | 1.2 | 3.3 | 5.1 | | | | 6.3 | | | | | 4.9 | | 1.2-6.3 |
| Face/mouth | | 2.5 | 1.7 | 9.2 | | | | 2.3 | | | | | 7.6 | | 1.7-9.2 |
| Ear | 23.4 | 16.2 | 5.0 | 7.1 | | | | 0.9 | | 3.6 | | | 1.7 | | 1.7-23.4 |
| Nose | 1.2 | 2.5 | 2.5 | | 16.1 | 36.4 | 43.3 | 1.8 | 29.4 | | | | 0.7 | | 0.7-2.5 |
| Eye | | 3.7 | 1.7 | | | | | 4.1 | | | 20.4 | | 1.8 | 15.6 | 1.7-4.1 |
| Teeth | | 2.5 | 0.8 | | | | | | | | | | 0.2 | | 0.2-2.5 |
| Neck | 3.6 | 8.7 | 0.8 | 8.2 | | | | 14.9 | | | | | 5.9 | | 0.8-14.9 |
| Upper back | | 2.5 | 2.5 | | | | | 1.4 | | | | | 2.1 | | 1.4-2.5 |
| Lower back | 4.7 | 1.2 | 3.3 | 5.1 | 8.1 | 3.6 | | 7.7 | 18.6 | 33.9 | | | 4.9 | | 1.2-8.1 |
| Rib/chest | 6.6 | 6.2 | 9.2 | 14.3 | 7.7 | | 8.5 | 4.1 | | | 11.5 | | 4.5 | 16.9 | 3.6-14.3 |
| Abdomen | | | | | | | | 0.4 | | | | | 0.7 | | 0.4-0.7 |
| **Upper extremity** | **9.3** | **22.4** | **35.8** | **22.4** | **37.1** | **20.8** | **22.4** | **33** | **20.6** | **29.1** | **21.4** | | **26.95** | **33.7** | **9.3-37.1** |
| Shoulder | 3.5 | 7.5 | 20.8 | 16.3 | 14.9 | 12.7 | | 16.7 | | | | 14.1 | 13.3 | | 3.5-20.8 |
| Arm | 0.8 | | 1.7 | | | | | 1.4 | | 23.2 | | | 1.8 | | 0.8-1.8 |
| Elbow | 1.0 | 3.7 | 8.3 | 5.1 | 9.3 | 5.4 | | 3.6 | | | 10.9 | | 4.2 | 16.5 | 1.0-9.3 |
| Wrist | 2.8 | | | 1.0 | | | 22.4 | 2.7 | 20.6 | | | | 0.85 | | 0.85-2.8 |
| Forearm | | | | | | | | | | | | | 2.6 | | |
| Hand/finger | 1.2 | 11.2 | 5.0 | | 12.9 | 2.7 | | 8.6 | | 5.9 | 10.5 | | 4.2 | 17.2 | 1.2-17.2 |
| **Lower extremity** | **7.5** | **29.9** | **31.6** | **26.4** | **20.9** | **24.5** | **24.8** | **15.4** | **31.4** | **33.3**[b] | **41.8** | | **34.9** | **28.6** | **7.5-41.4** |
| Pelvis/hip | | 2.5 | | 1.0 | | | | 1.8 | | | | | 1.8 | | 1.0-2.5 |
| Thigh | | 2.5 | 1.7 | 7.1 | | | | | | 1.2 | 5.3 | | 3.1 | 5.9 | 1.7-7.1 |
| Knee | 1.2 | 13.7 | 18.3 | 11.2 | 14.1 | 20 | 24.8 | 7.7 | 19.6 | | 26.0 | 21.1 | 19.5 | 14.2 | 1.2-26.0 |
| Leg | | | 0.8 | | | | | 0.9 | 31.4 | | | | 1.7 | | 0.8-1.7 |
| Ankle | 6.3 | 8.7 | 10 | 5.1 | 6.8 | 4.5 | | 3.2 | | 5.4 | | | 7.3 | | 3.2-10 |
| Heel/foot/toe | | 2.5 | 0.8 | 2.0 | | | | 1.8 | | | 10.5 | | 1.5 | 8.5 | 0.8-2.5 |
| Other | 21.4 | | 1.7 | 2.0 | 10.1 | 14.5 | | 0.9 | | | 4.9 | | 3.2 | 4.9 | |
| Total # of injuries | 735 | 80 | 120 | 98 | 248 | 110 | 129 | 221 | 102 | 168 | 2,129 | 4,992 | 1,055 | 690 | |
| Total # of participants | 4,835 | 907 | 711 | 459 | 1,091 | 353 | 341 | 1,742 | 1,059 | 234 | 2,255 | — | — | 1,387 | |

[a]P = prospective, R = retrospective.

[b]Total consists of 7.1% injuries described as lower extremity, other.

**Table 25.8b   Injury Location, Percent of Total Injuries**

| Study | Lok | Roy | Estwanik 1980 | Snook | Brown | Acksel | Wroble, Albright 1986 | Range |
|---|---|---|---|---|---|---|---|---|
| Study design[a] | R | R | R | R | R | R | R | Range |
| **Skin** | | 16.9 | | 16.7 | 15.9 | | | 15.9-16.9 |
| **Head/spine/trunk** | 25.7 | 34.2 | 24.5 | 24.3 | 36.2 | 45.35 | 40.6 | 24.3-45.35 |
| Head | | 3.3 | | 1.1 | | 3.8 | 3.1 | 1.1-3.8 |
| Face/mouth | | 2.7 | | 3.3 | | 1.0 | 8.2 | 1.0-8.2 |
| Ear | | 6.9 | 7.6[b] | 2.2 | 24.6 | 17.3 | 5.4 | 2.2-24.6 |
| Nose | 3.2 | 1.8 | 5.7[c] | 1.1 | | 0.7 | | 0.7-3.2 |
| Eye | | | | 1.1 | | | | |
| Teeth | | 0.3 | | | | 2.1 | 2.4 | 0.3-2.4 |
| Neck | 6.4 | 8.4 | | 5.5 | | 3.5 | 12.0 | 3.5-12.0 |
| Upper back | | 1.5 | | | | | 4.7 | 3.9-8.3 |
| Lower back | | 2.4 | 6.2 | 3.3 | | 8.3 | | 5.0-16.1 |
| Rib/chest | 16.1 | 6.9 | 5.0 | 6.7 | 11.6 | 8.3 | 4.8 | 5.0-16.1 |
| Abdomen | | | | | | 0.35 | | |
| **Upper extremity** | 29 | 19.5 | 26.2 | 31.1 | 26.1 | 32.8 | 20.5 | 19.5-32.8 |
| Shoulder | 22.6 | 8.4 | 16.2 | 17.8 | | 10.7 | 11.4 | 8.4-22.6 |
| Arm | | | | | | 1.4 | 4.6[d] | |
| Elbow | 3.2 | 3.9 | 5.0 | 7.8 | | 7.3 | | 3.2-7.8 |
| Wrist | 3.2 | | | | 26.1 | 4.8 | | 3.2-4.8 |
| Forearm | | 0.3 | | 5.5 | | | | |
| Hand/finger | | 6.9 | 5.0 | | | 8.6 | 4.5[e] | 5.0-8.6 |
| **Lower extremity** | 45.1 | 28.6 | 42.3 | 27.7 | 21.7 | 21.45 | 38.7 | 21.45-45.1 |
| Pelvis/hip | 3.2 | 1.2 | | | | 2.1 | 3.9 | 1.2-3.2 |
| Thigh | 3.2 | 1.5 | | 3.3 | | 0 | | 0-3.3 |
| Knee | 29.0 | 15.4 | 38.4 | 20 | | 9.3 | 25.4 | 9.3-29 |
| Leg | | 2.4 | | | 21.7 | 9.7 | 8.1 | |
| Ankle | 9.7 | 6.0 | 3.9 | 4.4 | | 9.7 | | 3.9-9.7 |
| Heel/foot/toe | | 2.1 | | | | 0.35 | 1.3 | .35-2.1 |
| Other | | 0.3 | 7.1 | | | 0.35 | | |
| **Total # of injuries** | 31 | 331 | 666 | 90 | 69 | 289 | 866 | |
| **Total # of participants** | 128 | 115 | — | 129 | 201 | 2,032 | 464 | |

[a]P = prospective, R = retrospective.

[b]Ear only.

[c]Total less ear.

[d]Includes forearm.

[e]Includes wrist.

pull and push against each other with the lumbar spine in mild hyperextension. This extension, coupled with twisting, results in injuries. Extension against resistance, as in lifting an opponent off the mat, and hyperflexion, as when rolling, are also mechanisms that account for low-back sprain or strain. On the other hand, low-back injury may result not only from a single episode but also from overuse. Low-back injuries are less frequent and are generally less severe than corresponding cervical injuries. Wroble and Albright reviewed 41 low-back injuries over an 8-year period (59). Virtually all were sprains and strains.

Rossi and Dragoni reviewed the X rays of 3,132 athletes (ages 15 to 27) who were evaluated for low-back pain over a 26-year period (45). They found that wrestlers with back pain had a 29.8% incidence of spondylolysis (17 of 57 wrestlers).

Hellstrom et al. (21) and Sward et al. (55) published two cross-sectional studies in which they reviewed back pain and X ray changes in randomly selected Swedish wrestlers aged 17 to 25. They defined low-back pain as pain lasting one week or recurrent pain. Pain was defined as severe only if they were unable to train. Twenty of 29 wrestlers (69%) exhibited low-back pain, but only 10 of the 29 (34%) had severe low-back pain. Seventeen of 30 wrestlers (56.7%) were found to have X ray abnormalities, including scoliosis, spondylolysis, spina bifida occulta, abnormal configuration of vertebrae, decreased disc height, Schmorl's nodes, and apophyseal injuries.

Estwanik also noted that 25% of his wrestlers presenting with back pain had spondylolysis or spondylolisthesis (14). Fifty-eight percent of his patients were diagnosed with lumbar strain.

Injuries to the rib cage result from direct trauma during takedowns when the opponent's head or shoulder strikes the anterior chest with considerable force. Another mechanism occurs when direct pressure is applied during a bear hug. When the opponent lifts or throws a wrestler while in this position, the force generated by the opponent's hand can be enough to cause chest wall injury.

Injuries to the ribs and chest comprise 3.6 to 14.3% of total injuries in prospective studies. Most of these injuries are contusions or costochondral sprains, but rib fractures are also common.

Dental injuries were reported in relatively small numbers in Table 25.8. One other study addressed this question. Lee-Knight et al. reviewed dental injuries at the Canada Games (30). In this 7-day Freestyle competition 101 wrestlers aged 14 to 21 sustained only one dental injury.

Ocular trauma was found at very low rates in the large epidemiologic studies cited above. However, Marton et al. reported on eye trauma in college athletes over a 10-year period (33). This study included 2,750 varsity athletes in 10 sports. One hundred fifty-two injuries occurred in wrestling. Wrestling had the highest average injury rate per year of 18.4%. Lacerations and corneal abrasions were the most common injuries.

### 3.3.2 Upper Extremity

Upper extremity injuries account for 9.3 to 37.1% of all wrestling injuries in prospective studies (19.5-32.8% in retrospective studies), Table 25.8. In 8 of 13 prospective studies, this was the least frequently injured body region. The shoulder, which is second only to the knee in injury rate, is injured via three principal mechanisms. When being thrown to the mat from a standing position, a wrestler may attempt to brace his fall with his extended arm, imparting force to the shoulder girdle. If he is unable to extend his arm, the fall may be taken directly on the shoulder. Falls onto an extended arm are the cause of many of elbow, wrist, hand, and finger injuries as well. A third important mechanism of shoulder injury occurs during the takedown maneuver. When the wrestler attacks his opponent's legs and gets caught in a position with the body overextended and the head down, the arm is elevated above the head. The opponent's body is positioned above the attacker's shoulder. As the opponent throws his hips back and increases the weight upon the wrestler's shoulder, hyperflexion and external rotation ensues, causing anterior subluxation.

Surprisingly little detail is available about shoulder injuries in wrestling. The most common problems found in the University of Iowa study were anterior shoulder instability (subluxation/dislocation) and acromioclavicular (AC) sprains (59).

Elbow injuries are sustained less frequently than shoulder injuries but appear to be more severe. Estwanik reported that almost half of his wrestlers with injured elbows missed an entire season (15). Eight of the 23 elbow injuries were dislocations. The most common elbow injury, however, is the hyperextension abduction sprain affecting the ulnar collateral ligament and the anterior capsule.

### 3.3.3 Lower Extremity

Overall, lower extremity injuries comprise 7.5 to 41.1% of wrestling injuries in prospective studies (21.4-45.1% in retrospective studies) (Table 25.8). In 8 of 13 prospective studies, the lower extremities were the second most frequently injured body region. The knee and ankle make up the majority.

Knee injuries are detailed in Table 25.9, ranging from 7.6 to 26% of the total number of injuries in prospective studies (15.4-38.4% in retrospective studies). In the only study with the percentage of knee injuries below 10%, Lorish described injuries in tournaments to wrestlers aged 6 to 16 years (32). A liberal injury definition was used that required only that medical attention be sought.

In one prospective study in which injury severity was well delineated, 56% of knee injuries were significant, resulting in a 7-day or greater time loss (41, 46, 61). In two retrospective studies, 39% and 46% of injuries had significant time loss. The most common type of knee injury was the sprain, 30 to 65% of the total number of knee injuries. Meniscal injuries were also common. Note the relatively high proportion of lateral to medial meniscal tears. In the two studies that broke this down, lateral meniscus injuries represented 46% of the total number of meniscal injuries (14, 61). Baker et al. also noted 45% lateral versus medial meniscectomy in their study of 56 meniscectomies in wrestlers (4).

Takedowns are involved in the majority of knee injuries of all types. Usually the wrestler on the defense sustains the injury. Meniscus injuries occur most commonly via a twisting injury to a weight-bearing extremity. Collateral ligament sprains

**Table 25.9    Knee Injuries**

| Study | Study design[a] | Injuries/ total (%) | Significant injuries/ total (%) | Sprains (% of total) | Lateral meniscus/ medial meniscus (ratio) |
|---|---|---|---|---|---|
| Powell | P | 553/2,129 (26) | 308/553 (56) | | |
| Kersey | P | 22/110 (20) | | | |
| Lorish | P | 17/221 (7.6) | | | |
| Requa & Garrick | P | 33/176 (18.7) | | | |
| Estwanik, 1978 | P | 11/98 (11.2) | | | |
| Estwanik, 1983 | P | 35/248 (14) | | | |
| NCAA | P | 1,257/5,999 (20.9) | | | |
| NHSIR | P | 98/690 (14.2) | | | |
| | | Range 7.6-26% | | | |
| Wroble, 6-year data, 1986 | R | 136/504 (27) | 63/136 (46) | 51 (37) | 12/14 (.46) |
| Roy | R | 51/332 (15.4) | 20/51 (39) | 33 (65) | |
| Estwanik, 1980 | R | 256/666 (38.4) | | 77 (30) | 41/48 (.46) |
| Snook | R | 18/90 (20) | | | |
| Lok | R | 9/31 (29) | | | |
| | | Range 15.4-38.4% | Range 39-46% | Range 30-65% | |

[a]R = retrospective, P = prospective.

occur when a varus or valgus force is applied to the weight-bearing extremity of a defending wrestler. These mechanisms far more commonly cause injury than application of holds that intentionally apply twisting forces. The latter techniques are considered illegal and are penalized.

Prepatellar bursitis was discussed in detail by Mysnyk et al. (37). Twenty-eight cases were documented, representing 21% of all knee injuries. Fifty percent of these were recurrent injuries. Eight cases of septic bursitis were reported. The mechanism of injury may be a single traumatic event or chronic repetitive trauma.

Anterior cruciate ligament injuries were noted in only 4 of 136 knee injuries in one series (61) and in 14 of 256 cases in another (14). Stanish presented two cases of isolated posterior cruciate ligament rupture in Canadian National Team members (51). He described the mechanism as forced flexion and internal rotation, which occurs in several wrestling maneuvers.

Ankle injuries are moderately frequent, the most common being the anterior talo-fibular ligament sprain. Most occur during takedowns. When a wrestler attempts to throw his opponent, he rises onto his toes and twists. A momentary loss of balance may then cause him to "roll over" his ankle into an inverted position. The second mechanism occurs to a defensive wrestler during a takedown. When his opponent has lifted one of his legs, all his support remains on a single foot. As his opponent attempts to bring him to the mat by various combinations of changes in directions or trips, inversion stress can occur.

In a 2-year study of seven college wrestling teams, ankle injuries made up 11.2% of all wrestling injuries (16). In this same report, the authors describe the results of the first year of the Seattle High School injury study. Ankle injuries made up 6 of 105 (6%) of wrestling injuries in that portion of the study.

### 3.3.4 Skin/Systemic Illnesses

Only a few studies have reported the details of skin infections. Roy stated that of 332 injuries, 56 were skin infections—staphylococcus, herpes simplex, or a combination of the two (46). Konrad (28) reported that skin infections comprised 21.6% of all injuries! In this retrospective questionnaire-based study, Konrad noted that bacterial skin infections decreased in programs where mats were disinfected daily. In the 41 schools in which mat disinfection was not practiced, 123 infections occurred (three infections per school). In those schools that practiced daily mat disinfection, only 26 infections occurred (0.4 infections per school). Shelley reported a case of herpetic arthritis in a wrestler with severe herpes gladiatorum (48).

Table 25.10 summarizes results of studies of herpes infections in wrestlers. Belongia et al. (8) investigated a herpes outbreak at a wrestling camp. The anatomic distribution of lesions reflects the areas of exposed skin where wrestler to wrestler contact is possible. The camp was divided into three practice groups by weight. In the first two practice groups, infection rates were 25 and 37%. In the third practice group, 67% of the wrestlers were

**Table 25.10    Studies of Herpes Infections in Wrestlers**

| Study | Level | Study design[a] | Data collection method[b] | Duration | Participants | # infections | Percentage infected | Anatomic location | | |
|-------|-------|---------|--------|----------|--------------|--------------|---------------------|------|-----|-------|
| | | | | | | | | Head | Ext | Trunk |
| Belongia | H.S. | R | I | 1 camp | 175 | 60 | 34 | 73 | 42 | 28 |
| Becker, 1988 & 1992 | C | R | I | 1 season, 4 teams | 48 | 9 | 18.5 | 78 | 11 | 22 |
| Becker, 1988 | C | R | Q | 1 season | 2,625 | 199 | 7.6 | | | |
| | H.S. | R | Q | 1 season | 2,354 | 62 | 2.6 | | | |

[a]R = retrospective.

[b]I = interview, Q = questionnaire.

infected. Fifty-seven percent of the infections occurred on the right side only, 8% on the left side only, and 35% on both the right and left sides. This reflects the standard positioning during wrestling in which the right side of the face is in contact with the right side of the opponent's face. They found no difference in the attack rate in wrestlers with previous herpes labialis and concluded that there was no protective effect. They also found that the risk of transmitting infection was the same with or without headgear and determined that transmission was via skin-to-skin contact and not via saliva.

In the first part of their study, Becker et al. (7) interviewed members of four college teams regarding herpes gladiatorum. They required the diagnosis of herpetic infection be made by culture or by a physician. Seven of the nine infected wrestlers noted contact with an opponent who had a cold sore or a facial rash. Conversely only 6 of 39 uninfected wrestlers had contact with an opponent with similar findings. They found prior oral herpes simplex infection to be protective and in fact documented a relative risk of 9.4 in those with no prior herpes labialis.

Becker et al. (7) also surveyed 163 NATA members (11% response rate). Sixty-five percent of the college teams reported infections, whereas only 25% of high school teams had a history of herpes. At the high school level bacterial and fungal infections occurred in rates nearly equal to those in college. Of college teams, 58.5% had documented cases of impetigo, and 60.6% had one or more wrestlers with a fungal infection. The impetigo rate was 44.3% and the fungal rate was 52.2% among high school teams.

Systemic infections occur frequently in wrestlers but have not been described extensively. When wrestlers are in hard training, they are exposed to pathogens from other wrestlers at a time when their bodies are stressed, not well equipped to deal with them, and if poorly nourished, perhaps mildly immunocompromised.

Strauss et al. studied a college wrestling team over an 8-week period during the middle of the competitive season (53). During this time period 92% of the wrestlers sustained a respiratory illness. Dermatologic illnesses were found in 46%, gastrointestinal problems in 8%, and other illnesses in 38%. Furthermore, 43% of these athletes missed one or more days of practice because of illness.

## 4. Injury Severity

### 4.1 Time Loss

Several large studies have assessed the proportion of injuries by the number of days missed from competition. In general, injuries are classified as minor if time loss is less than or equal to 7 days, moderate if time loss is 8 to 21 days, and major if greater than 21 days. The moderate and major injury groups are often lumped together and then are referred to as significant injuries. The breakdown of injuries by time loss is shown in Table 25.11. Note the similarity in rates of minor and significant injuries between studies. Minor injuries occurred in all studies at rates of 58 to 68%.

Note that the severity of neck, back, and knee injuries was substantially higher than those found in the overall injury group. Wroble and Albright (59) noted that the average time lost from wrestling for all neck injuries was 10.7 days. Neurogenic pain syndromes tended to be more severe, with an average number of days lost of 17.9. Sprain or strain injuries resulted in an average loss of 6.3 days. There were 38.5% of injuries that caused time

**Table 25.11    Time Loss**

| Study | Study design[a] | Minor[b] (%) | Moderate[c] (%) | Major[d] (%) |
|---|---|---|---|---|
| NHSIR | P | 469 (68) | 117 (17) | 104 (15) |
| Garrick, 1981 | P | 111 (65)[e] | 48 (29)[f] | 11 (6)[g] |
| Powell | P | 1,234 (58) | 486 (23) | 409 (19) |
|  |  |  | Range 17-29% | 6-19% |
| NCAA | P | 3,714 (61.5)[h] | 2,325 (38.5)[i] | |
|  |  | Range 58-68% | | |
| Roy | R | 106 (65) | 38 (23) | 19 (12) |
| Wroble, 1986, back | R | 15 (55) | 12 (45) | |
| Wroble, 1986, neck | R | 38 (49) | 40 (51) | |
| Wroble, 1986, knee | R | 48 (43) | 63 (57) | |

[a]R = retrospective, P = prospective.

[b]7 days or less.

[c]8 to 21 days.

[d]More than 21 days.

[e]4 days or less.

[f]5 to 19 days.

[g]More than 19 days.

[h]6 days or less.

[i]More than 6 days.

loss greater than one week. The average number of days lost for low-back injuries was 5.3 days. Of the back injuries, 31.6% resulted in a time loss of 7 or more days (59).

In the Seattle study (18) four athletic trainers were placed in high schools for a 2-year period and injury rates monitored. Injury severity remained the same between the first and second year with nearly identical proportions of minor and significant injuries, although a 24% decrease in wrestling injury rate was seen.

Injury severity has also been measured by how often athletes require surgery for their injuries. Hoffman showed that of 690 high school wrestling injuries, 21 (3%) required surgery (22). In one year data presented by the NCAA, 73 of 1,053 injuries (6.9%) required surgery (38). The rate of knee surgery in the University of Iowa study (61) was much higher, with 30 surgeries performed for 136 injuries recorded (22%). This supports the notion that knee injuries are generally more severe.

## 4.2 Catastrophic Injuries

Fortunately, catastrophic injuries in wrestling are rare. Understandably, the majority of catastrophic injuries in wrestling occur to the head and cervical spine. Reports of these types of injuries are summarized in Table 25.12. Laudermilk reviewed data from the National Center for Catastrophic Sports Injury Research (29). Information for this study was obtained from clipping services, individuals, and from the National Federation of State High School Sports Associations. The athletic director, coach, and physician of the injured wrestler were then contacted. Serious injuries were defined as those with no permanent disability. Nonfatal injuries caused severe permanent disabilities. Fifty percent of the injuries were found to involve the cervical spine, spinal cord, or head. Other causes were cardiac arrhythmia, cardiomyopathy, respiratory arrest, pulmonary embolism, and unspecified cardiac disease. Forty-two percent of the injuries occurred during takedowns and 71% occurred during matches.

Clarke sent surveys to state high school associations and to individual colleges (10). He defined a catastrophic injury as causing permanent paralysis or death. Eight injuries were found, all at the high school level. All resulted in permanent spinal cord injury, none in death. Thirteen other spinal cord injuries were reported in a series of case reports, one retrospective study, and two case series (1, 27, 44, 62). All but two were cervical fractures or fracture/dislocations. One patient fully recovered, 10 had permanent paralysis, and 2 patients died. Various case reports summarized in Table 25.12 have appeared in literature describing other catastrophic injuries (3, 5, 11, 12, 34, 43, 56).

## 4.3 Clinical Outcome/Residual Symptoms

Two investigations studied the long-term consequences of wrestling injuries. Mysnyk et al. (36) interviewed 542 males 30 or more years of age (average 44.1 years) at the 1986 NCAA Wrestling Championships. Three hundred and seven former wrestlers were compared to a control group who competed in no sports or only in noncontact sports. Forty-two percent of ex-wrestlers had current musculoskeletal problems whereas only 24% of controls did so. Neck problems occurred nearly three times as frequently and knee problems occurred nearly four times as frequently among ex-wrestlers. These data emphasize the significance of long-term consequences of injuries in wrestlers but are biased by the fact that of the 307 ex-wrestlers, only 91 competed solely in wrestling. The other 216 played additional sports, usually

**Table 25.12   Catastrophic Injuries**

| Study | Level | Study design[a] | Data collection methods[b] | Duration | # of injuries | Rate | Condition |
|---|---|---|---|---|---|---|---|
| Laudermilk | J.H.S., H.S. | R | Q | 5 seasons | 24 (8 serious, 6 nonfatal, 10 fatal) | 1.07/100,000 wrestlers | 12 cervical/head 12 cardiac/systemic |
| Clarke | H.S., C | R | Q | 3 years | 8 H.S. 0 C | | 8 permanent SCI[c] |
| Acikgoz | H.S., I | C.S. | I | | 4 | | 4 SCI (1 full recovery, 2 permanent, 1 fatal) |
| Wu | H.S. | C.S. | I | | 3 | | 3 SCI (3 permanent) |
| Kewalramani | | R | I | | 5 | | 5 SCI (5 permanent) |
| Rontoyannis | H.S. | C | | | 1 | | 1 SCI (1 fatal) |
| Rogers | H.S. | C | | | | | Stroke |
| Cohn | H.S. | C | | | 1 | | 11th cranial nerve injury |
| Croyle | H.S. | C | | | 1 | | Pulmonary embolism |
| Baratta | Y | C | | | 1 | | Axillary art. disruption w/shoulder disl. |
| McCormack | H.S. | C | | | 1 | | Ruptured diaphragm |
| Tudor | H.S. | C | | | 1 | | Pott's puffy tumor, sinusitis, osteomyelitis, and epidural abscess |
| Annenberg | H.S. | C | | | 1 | | Femoral art. pseudoaneurysm |

[a]R = retrospective, C.S. = case series, C = case report.

[b]I = interview, Q = questionnaire.

[c]Spinal cord injury. Permanent refers to residual paralysis.

football. Also, the authors did not exclude ex-wrestlers who had nonwrestling injuries, either while in other sports in high school or later in life.

Questionnaires, physical exams, and radiographs were used to compare 32 former top-ranked Swedish wrestlers (ages 39 to 62) versus a group of historic controls (19). Seventy-one percent stated that they had some residual physical problems, 37% had neck problems, and 59% had low-back problems. The control group had only 31% low-back problems, a statistically significant difference. Compared with controls, wrestlers had a higher incidence of reduced spine mobility, pain during motion of the spine, and positive straight leg raising tests. Radiographic findings were no different from controls. The ex-wrestlers with back pain had less interference with work than the control group. The authors concluded that although retired wrestlers had more low-back pain than untrained men of the same age, they had a higher tolerance for low-back pain and thus functioned at a higher level.

# 5. Injury Risk Factors

Table 25.13 summarizes injury risk factors. Note that many of these factors are intuitively obvious. Even those that appear to have a positive relationship are often derived from retrospective studies or case series and thus do not have the same value as if they were obtained from prospective work. These risk factors, however, may be important in design and analysis of future epidemiologic studies of wrestling.

## 5.1 Intrinsic Factors

### 5.1.1 Physical Characteristics

There is a slight trend for wrestlers at the higher weights to be injured more frequently (Table 25.6). This is perhaps due to the greater force that can be exerted by athletes of greater size. The relationship of age to injury is also interesting. Very young wrestlers tend to be injured less frequently than

**Table 25.13  Injury Risk Factors in Wrestling**

| Intrinsic risk factors | Extrinsic risk factors |
| --- | --- |
| **Physical factors**<br>• Weight (?)<br>• Age (+)<br>• Weight loss (?)<br>• Skill (?)<br>• Previous injury (+)<br>• Varsity status (+)<br><br>**Motor/fitness factors**<br>• Fatigue (?)<br>• Timing in match (?)<br>• Matches/day(?)<br><br>**Psychosocial factors**<br>• Noncompliance (+) | **Exposure**<br>• Level of competition (+)<br>• Takedowns (+)<br>• Position on mat (+)<br><br>**Training conditions**<br>• Inadequate supervision (?)<br>• Inadequate technique (?)<br>• Abrasive shirts (+)<br>• Unwashed workout clothing (?)<br>• Poor nutrition/dehydration (?)<br><br>**Environment**<br>• Time in season (+)<br>• Mat condition (?)<br>• Mat cleanliness (+)<br>• Temperature, humidity of<br>  wrestling room (?)<br><br>**Protective equipment**<br>• Head gear (+)<br>• Knee pads (+)<br>• Mouth guards (?)<br>• Shoes (?) |

*Note.* The + sign indicates a positive relationship as suggested by current research. The question mark signifies that either the findings have been ambiguous or that no empirical data are available.

their older counterparts (section 2.1). This is probably a factor of their physical maturity, size, and strength. Also, a trend is noted toward more injuries in the senior members of college and high school teams (section 2.1), perhaps because the senior level team members compete more often in matches, which are clearly high-risk activities.

The principle of the weight class system is to reduce the risk of injury by eliminating vast discrepancies in size and strength between opponents. But, rapid and drastic weight loss performed to "make weight" may itself be a risk factor for injury, given the adverse physiologic changes induced by dehydration and fasting. Nonetheless Horswill has stated that a wrestler who loses fat may enhance power and strength capacities relative to body weight (23, 24). This suggests that the wrestler who practices rapid weight loss can compete against a relatively weaker opponent. This in turn may be reflected in increased injury rates in the weaker of the two wrestlers.

Wroble and Moxley demonstrated that among high school wrestlers, those with the lowest body weights, even lower than the recommended minimum, tend to have a slightly higher chance of success than those who wrestle at a higher percent

body fat (60). Although the more successful wrestlers might be subject to a lower injury rate, this relationship has also not been clearly elucidated. In fact, McGuine showed that the injury rate in placers was equal to the injury rate in nonplacers in his study of the 1985 Northern Open (35). In contrast, Requa and Garrick stated that 70% of the match-related injuries in their study occurred in the wrestler who was behind at the time (42).

Reinjury rates in wrestling have been noted to be high. For example, in the Iowa study a wrestler had a 30% chance of sustaining a first time knee injury. Once the knee was injured, the chance of a second injury rose to 57% (61).

Two studies compared days lost for similar injuries in varsity and reserve wrestlers. Roy (46) stated that varsity wrestlers tended to return to practice far earlier than did reserve wrestlers. In studying knee injuries, for all diagnoses except two, reserve wrestlers lost more time per injury than varsity wrestlers (61). These differences could be explained by the fact that the reserve wrestlers were not as skilled and therefore sustained more severe injuries. A second factor is that varsity wrestlers may be more highly motivated to return to action because of the pressing need to return for the next varsity match.

### 5.1.2 Motor Functional Characteristics

As fatigue may play a role in injuries, the timing of injuries in matches and in tournaments has been evaluated. If injury rates rise in the third period compared with the first and second periods, this may in part be due to fatigue. Bear in mind, however, that since wrestling matches terminate immediately after a fall, not all wrestling matches last the full three periods. Thus, the amount of exposure in the second and third periods is lower, skewing injury rates.

Hartmann (20) and Wroble, Mysnyk, et al. (61) stated that no relation existed between injury rates and timing in the match in their studies. The injury definitions and data collection methodology vary widely among the studies shown in Table 25.14. Although the first period of a match provides the greatest exposure there is a slightly lower injury risk. An explanation for this may be that the wrestlers are freshest and not fatigued in the first period. The second period appears to have the highest injury rate, which may be accounted for by a balance between initiation of fatigue and exposure still being relatively high. In the third period, fatigue would be most important, but exposure time is less.

**Table 25.14    Injuries by Timing in Match**

| Study | Study design[a] | Level | # of injuries 1st period (%) | 2nd period (%) | 3rd period (%) |
|---|---|---|---|---|---|
| Strauss, 1982 | P | H.S. | 12 (25.5) | 22 (47) | 13 (27.5) |
| Konrad | P | H.S. | 35 (43) | 23 (28) | 24 (29) |
| Patacsil | P | H.S. | 13 (50) | 8 (31) | 5 (19) |
| Patacsil | P | C | 5 (29) | 10 (59) | 3 (12) |
| Strauss, 1982 | P | C (Ohio Open) | 3 (25) | 7 (58) | 2 (17) |
| Strauss, 1982 | P | C (Big Ten) | 3 (25) | 6 (50) | 3 (25) |
| Kersey | P | C | 21 (19.1) | 31 (28.2) | 58 (52.7) |
| NCAA | P | C | 54 (19.4) | 135 (48.6) | 89 (31.6)[b] |
| | | Range | 19.1-50% | 28-59% | 12-52.7% |
| Acksel | R | H.S. | 31 (28.7) | 41 (37.3) | 38 (34.5) |

[a]R = retrospective, P = prospective.

[b]Includes 1 overtime injury.

If more injuries occur as the number of matches in a day increases, fatigue may play a role. A warning is that multiple matches in a day are always wrestled in a tournament setting. Thus, as more matches are wrestled, the competition becomes more challenging and opponents more closely matched, which may affect injury rates.

Strauss and Lanese (52) studied two large wrestling tournaments (one high school, one college). They compared injury rates in the first, second, and aggregate of the third and later matches and concluded that injury rates seemed to be similar in all categories. McGuine (35) reviewed the injuries in a large one-day collegiate wrestling tournament in which wrestlers competed in two to seven matches. He found that injury rate did not increase after the wrestler had competed in several matches. There was a trend, however, for a decreased incidence of injury after the wrestlers had competed in three matches. The injury rate for the first three rounds was 10.5% but only 5.2% in the fourth round or greater. Kersey and Rowan (26) examined the results of successive matches in a three-day, six-round tournament, the 1980 NCAA Championships. Injury was defined as any stoppage of competition. In the first three rounds the injury rate was 12.0% and in the final three rounds it was 9.7%.

### 5.1.3 Psychosocial Characteristics

A factor that is rarely mentioned but appears significant in wrestling is compliance. Wroble,

Mysnyk, et al. (61) retrospectively studied compliance concerning knee injuries in college wrestlers. In their study a compliance rating was given to each wrestler by the head trainer indicating how well the wrestler followed medical advice. They found that only 7 of 24 (29%) of the compliant wrestlers had a recurrence of their knee injury, but 13 of 21 (62%) of the less compliant wrestlers had a recurrent knee injury.

### 5.2 Extrinsic Factors

#### 5.2.1 Exposure

The intensity of the wrestling exposure in large part determines the risk of injury. For example, at successively higher and thus more competitive levels, injury rates increase. Match injury rates are always higher than practice injury rates.

The more explosive, collision-oriented maneuvers involved in takedowns result in higher injury rates as well. Takedowns make up a significant portion of every match, and because of their importance, 50% of practices may be devoted to this activity. A variety of authors have noted the frequency of takedown injuries among their overall number of injuries in each study (Table 25.15).

Studies of college wrestlers have generally shown takedown injuries to be slightly more common compared to high school wrestlers. The single study with a low frequency of takedown injuries included all injuries for which timeout was called during the matches, thereby slanting it toward minor injuries (26). In all levels of wrestling, injury timeout may be requested by a wrestler at anytime.

**Table 25.15    Takedown Injuries**

| Study | Level | Takedown injuries (% of total) |
|---|---|---|
| Hoffman | H.S. | 304 (44.1) |
| Requa | H.S. | 88 (50) |
| Strauss, 1982 | H.S. | 20 (42) |
| | | Range 42-50% |
| Estwanik, 1980 | H.S. | 71 (59.7)[a] |
| | | 36 (63)[b] |
| NCAA | C | 369 (51.1) |
| Kersey | C | 27 (24.5) |
| Strauss, 1982 | C | 19 (68) |
| Snook | C | 58 (64) |
| | | Range 24.5-68% |
| Wroble, 1986 | C | 47 (71)[a] |
| Estwanik, 1978 | I | 40 (75.5) |

[a]Knee injuries only.

[b]Shoulder injuries only.

The referee is then required to stop the match temporarily. Knee injuries occurred more commonly during takedowns in both high school (14) and college (61).

In the only study that evaluated wrestling at the international level, Estwanik et al. (13) studied injuries at the 1976 Olympic trials. Takedowns accounted for 75% of the injuries. This high frequency is perhaps accounted for by the difference in styles, because in Freestyle and Greco-Roman wrestling a greater percentage of time is spent in the standing neutral position than in high school or college wrestling.

It appears to be a risk factor to take a defensive role when in a standing position. During takedown injuries, 60% of the time the defensive man was injured (61).

In a few studies, the position of the wrestler at the time of injury has been analyzed. Injury rates are higher for the wrestler in the down or disadvantage position in both college and high school studies (Table 25.16). This may reflect disparity in skill of the wrestlers as the wrestler of higher ability will more often be in the position of advantage. Certainly the wrestler on top has more of an ability to apply leverage and potentially injurious holds to the wrestler he is dominating.

### 5.2.2 Training Conditions

No analytical data is available on training conditions as risk factors in wrestling. But, a number of intuitive observations can be made.

Inadequate supervision of a wrestling team may increase injury risk by lack of monitoring potentially dangerous situations and techniques and the inability to discourage horseplay.

**Table 25.16   Injuries by Position**

| Study | Study design[a] | Level | # of injuries (% of total) | |
| | | | Advantage | Disadvantage |
| --- | --- | --- | --- | --- |
| Requa | P | H.S. | 13 (15) | 75 (85) |
| Patacsil | P | H.S. | 11 (29) | 27 (71) |
| NCAA | P | C | 56 (20) | 224 (80) |
| Kersey | P | C | 29 (35) | 54 (65) |
| Patacsil | P | C | 12 (24) | 38 (76) |
| | | Range | 15-35% | 65-85% |
| Acksel | R | H.S. | 47 (26) | 137 (74) |
| Wroble[b] | R | C | 4 (25) | 12 (75) |

[a]P = prospective, R = retrospective.

[b]Knee injuries only.

Inadequate wrestling technique may increase injury risk. One good example is how shoulder injuries occur during takedowns. If a wrestler gets caught in the overextended position with his shoulder sharply forward flexed and externally rotated, subluxation or anterior sprains commonly occur. If proper technique is used and this situation avoided, injuries would likely decrease.

Dermatologic problems stem from the close body contact integral to the sport in combination with warm conditions, humidity, sweaty workout clothes, and mat contact. Contact with an opponent with a cold sore or facial rash is also a risk factor.

Strauss et al. (54) identified that abrasive shirts were a risk factor in spreading herpes gladiatorum. In following a collegiate wrestling team for 3 years they found that variation in herpes episodes coincided with changes in shirts. In the first year of the study, wrestlers wore 100% cotton shirts, and 9.8 episodes per 100 wrestlers were identified. In the second year when 50% cotton/50% polyester shirts were used, 73.8 episodes per 100 wrestlers were documented. Because of the herpes experience in the second year the shirts were changed, and after going back to 100% cotton shirts, rates were decreased to 50 episodes per 100 wrestlers. Statistical significance of these findings was not calculated.

Systemic illnesses are endemic for these reasons in addition to the fact that the hot, sweaty wrestler often emerges to a cold, wintery evening after practice. Also, poor nutrition and dehydration have been suggested to compromise the immune status of wrestlers who are cutting weight.

### 5.2.3 Environment

The overall pattern of training during the season may affect injury rates. Patacsil (40) found that the majority of injuries, 123 out of 200 (61.5%), occurred in the first half of the season. In a later study of six college wrestling seasons, more than three times as many injuries occurred during the first month as any other month during the wrestling season (61).

Early in the season, more wrestlers are vying for starting roles and more are preparing for the first tournaments of the year. Wrestle-offs for spots on the team also occur during the first month of the season. Intensity may then diminish because many wrestlers resolve themselves to nonstarting status and don't push themselves hard. Early season tournaments may present an increased risk. Wrestlers' conditioning has not reached optimum levels. With multiple matches in a day it is easy for a minor injury to become a significant injury.

The condition of the wrestling room is important. If mats are in poor condition, their ability to absorb shock may deteriorate and thus increase injury risk when wrestlers land on them. A second major item is the cleanliness of the mats. Without daily disinfection, counts of microorganisms on the mat would theoretically increase and so increase the chance of transmission of dermatologic infections from mat to wrestler. Unpadded walls, obstacles such as columns or bleachers, inadequate space, and extreme heat or humidity are obviously detrimental.

### 5.2.4 Protective Equipment

The amount of protective gear worn in wrestling is minimal. Headgear has been investigated, and not wearing headgear is a risk factor in sustaining auricular hematoma. Nonetheless, these injuries do occur with headgear on (47). This suggests that proper fit and in fact proper choice of headgear are also important. The role of knee pads, shoes, and mouth guards has not been evaluated, but in other sports they have been effective in preventing injuries.

**Table 25.17   Suggestions for Injury Prevention in Wrestling**

| Preventive measure | Examples/suggestion |
| --- | --- |
| **The wrestler** | |
| Proper warm-up | Begin by movements to increase muscle temperature, then stretching to increase range of motion. |
| Strength training (5.1.2) | Maximize muscular power and endurance with sport-specific program. |
| Cardiovascular conditioning | Fatigue suggested to increase injuries in some studies but not others (Table 25.13). |
| Correct technique (3.3.2) | Shoulder injuries caused by poor technique. |
| Size/ability matching | No gross discrepancy in practice partners. |
| Limits on weight reduction (3.3.4, 5.2.2) | Horswill (23, 24) recommends limits of 5% body fat: no firm data available. |
| Proper hygiene (5.1.1) | Dermatologic illness transmitted skin to skin (8). Daily washing of workout clothes/after practice shower. |
| Adherence to rules | High school and college rules ban holds that exert potentially injurious forces to the spine and extremities. |
| **The sport** | |
| Adequate supervision (coach/wrestler ratio) | Optimal ratio not defined. Minimize horseplay, monitor dangerous techniques. |
| Coaching education/certification | Courses should include medical components. Enhance relationship with health care team. |
| Officials education/certification | |
| Require use of proper headgear (3.3.1, 5.2.4) | Shown to decrease injury when worn (47). Not mandated by most coaches at practice (2). Four strap type best. |
| Mouthguards (3.3.1, 5.2.4) | Dental injuries uncommon but often irreversible. |
| Early start of practice/delayed start of competition (5.2.3) | Injuries more common in early competition (40, 61). |
| **External environment** | |
| Removal or padding of hazards (5.2.3) | Already mandatory for matches. Enact for practice. |
| Adequate space (5.2.3) | Snook suggests 50 sq. ft. per pair of wrestlers (50). If not available, group wrestlers and provide off-mat activities such as strengthening or conditioning for other groups. |
| Appropriate temp/humidity (5.2.3) | Avoid dehydration/heat injury, optimal temperature not known. |
| Quality mats (3.3.1, 5.2.3) | Need optimum biomechanical properties (not as yet defined). Resurface if worn or damaged. |
| Mat disinfection (3.3.4, 5.2.3) | Shown to decrease bacterial infections (28). |
| Nonabrasive shirts (5.2.2) | Strauss (54) showed increased herpes infection with abrasive shirts. |
| **Health support system** | |
| Preseason evaluation-physical exam, body composition, muscle/fitness testing | Identify conditions that preclude competition and abnormalities that predispose to injury; allow optimal weight reduction planning. |
| Medical coverage | Physician and trainers at all competitions. At minimum, trainers available for practices. |
| Emergency protocols | Well defined so they can be implemented in any competitive environment. |
| Skin hygiene (3.3.4, 5.2.2) | Soap shower after practice, adequate drying of skin. Exclusion of infected wrestlers/occlusive coverage. Coaches to perform routine exams; wrestler/coach education. |
| Precise treatment protocols | This will reduce the incidence of reinjury and long-term sequelae (for example, neck, 59). Monitor noncompliance (61). |
| Strict return criteria | |
| Proper rehabilitation | |

# 6. Suggestions for Injury Prevention

The suggested preventive measures are summarized in Table 25.17 with reference to chapter section(s) from which they have been generated. The recommended suggestions are grouped under the following subsection headings: The wrestler, the sport of wrestling, external environment, and health support system.

As is apparent from the discussion of available studies, very few, if any, studies on wrestling are rigorous enough to draw definitive conclusions about risk factors. Given that, it is still possible to suggest measures that reflect the best and most current information in the literature. Naturally, these suggestions await confirmation in well-controlled prospective studies.

# 7. Suggestions for Further Research

In this review of wrestling injury reports, we have found that there is no consistent injury definition. An encouraging factor, however, is that most recent studies have adopted the definitions used by NAIRS. All future studies should use their criteria for minor and significant injuries as well as using time loss as the major component for determining reportability of an injury. Because wrestling doesn't have a method for reporting dermatologic and systemic illnesses, a logical and consistent approach to these problems must be developed. It is apparent that there is inconsistency in whether these are reported at all.

The majority of work on wrestling epidemiology has been done at the high school and college levels. Athletes in fairly large numbers compete at the youth level and also at the international level. Work needs to be done at these levels to determine injury rates and risk factors.

Although wrestling is no different from any other sport in that a prospective study design is most effective in gaining information, the best prospective studies are generated after initial work has been reviewed. The groundwork has been laid in wrestling. Adequate hypotheses can be generated about many aspects of the sport from which to design excellent prospective studies.

Data collection methods, while being efficient, should also sacrifice the least accuracy. The interview method with a person in charge of data collection on-site is the most accurate. One method that would lend itself to wrestling is video analysis. In most competitions every match is videotaped. This allows accurate evaluation, particularly about mechanism of injury. Bout sheets from tournament matches also show detailed information about timing and type of injury in a match. These could be exploited in an epidemiologic study.

**Table 25.18  Suggestions for Further Research**

| Research component | Research direction/questions |
| --- | --- |
| Incidence of injury | |
| Injury rates | Using a consistent injury definition, such as NAIRS, study injury rates using exposure data. Explore injury rates in youth and international wrestling. Develop a method for reporting dermatologic/systemic illnesses. |
| Reinjury rates | Study reinjury rates with rigorous definitions. |
| Practice vs. competition | Video analysis should be used for documenting match injury. Effect of rule changes on competition injury rates should be examined. |
| Weight class | Injury data currently available by wt class has no denominator. We need to know the number of wrestlers in each class. |
| Injury characteristics | |
| Injury onset | Define and record gradual onset injuries. Compare rates vs. acute onset. Do unreported overuse injuries lead to acute injuries? |
| Injury type/location | Standardize schema for recording injury type. Perform detailed studies of knee, neck, and shoulder injuries. |
| | Study skin problems. Is there a protective effect of previous herpes labialis infection? What is the role of acyclovir prophylaxis? What are the long-term sequelae of herpes gladiatorum? What is the most effective mat washing technique? |
| Injury severity | |
| Time loss | Develop a standardized schema for reporting time loss and study time loss in reference to level of competition. |
| Catastrophic injury | What is the risk of catastrophic injury, and does it vary by level of competition? |
| Clinical outcome | Larger and better studies need to document the long-term effects of wrestling injuries and of repetitive bouts of rapid weight loss. |

| Research component | Research direction/questions |
|---|---|
| **Risk factors** | |
| **Intrinsic** | |
| Weight loss, success | How do weight loss and injuries interact? How do success and injury rates interact? |
| Fatigue | Use match data with bout sheets containing time of injury to find accurate injury rates by period. This may be related to fatigue. Since match length has changed over time, a retrospective study may even be helpful. Even now, consolation and championship matches are of different lengths. Are their injury rates different? |
| Compliance | Why are wrestlers noncompliant with medical advice? Are they different from other athletes in similar sports? Is the psychological profile of the wrestler different enough so that he has an increased or decreased risk compared to other athletes? |
| **Extrinsic** | |
| Coaching experience/ coach-wrestler ratio | Is there a relationship between coaching experience and injury rates? What is the optimal coach-wrestler ratio? |
| Mats | What are the frictional and shock-absorbing properties of mats, and how do these vary with the age and material of the mat? |
| Protective equipment | What is the role of headgear in preventing and in producing auricular hematoma? What type of headgear is most effective? |
| | How effective are mouthguards in preventing dental injuries? |
| | Do knee pads reduce the incidence of prepatellar bursitis? |
| | Would wrestling shoes that more effectively control inversion/eversion prevent ankle sprains? |
| Health support system | Does the presence of an athletic trainer decrease injury rate or injury severity? |
| **Injury prevention** | Introduce measures designed to reduce injury risk. Prospectively evaluate the effectiveness of these measures. |

The multidisciplinary approach to putting together an epidemiologic team would work most effectively for wrestling, combining the talents of the athletic trainer, team physician, coach or school administrator, statistician, and epidemiologist.

Suggestions and questions appropriate for further research studies as derived from the literature reviewed in this chapter are shown in Table 25.18. They are grouped in reference to the chapter section from which they have been derived.

# References

1. Acikgoz, B.; Ozgen, T.; Erbengi, A.; Peker, S.; Bertan, V.; Saglam, S. Wrestling causing paraplegia. Paraplegia. 28:265-268; 1990.

2. Acksel, G.J. A study of interscholastic wrestling injuries in the state of Missouri during the 1965-66 season. Thesis, Eastern Illinois University; 1966.

3. Annenberg, A.J.; Vaccaro, P.S.; Zuelzer, W.A. Traumatic pseudoaneurysm in a wrestler. Annals of Vascular Surgery. 4:69-71; 1990.

4. Baker, B.D.; Peckham, A.C.; Pupparo, F.; Sanborn, J.C. Review of meniscal injury and associated sports. American Journal of Sports Medicine. 13:1-4; 1985.

5. Baratta, J.B.; Lim, V.; Mastromonaco, E.; Edillon, E.L. Axillary artery disruption secondary to anterior dislocation of the shoulder. Journal of Trauma. 23:1009-1011; 1983.

6. Becker, T.M. Herpes gladiatorum: A growing problem in sports medicine. Cutis. 50:150-152; 1992.

7. Becker, T.M.; Kosdi, R.; Bailey, P.; Lee, F.; Levandowski, R.; Nahmias, A.J. Grappling with herpes: Herpes gladiatorum. American Journal of Sports Medicine. 16:665-669; 1988.

8. Belongia, E.A.; Goodman, J.L.; Holland, E.J.; Andras, C.W.; Homann, S.R.; Mahanti, R.L.; Mizener, M.W.; Erice, A.; Osterholm, M.T. An outbreak of herpes gladiatorum at a high-school wrestling camp. New England Journal of Medicine. 325:906-910; 1991.

9. Brown, R.G. Nature and frequency of injuries occurring in Oregon high school interscholastic sports. Thesis, University of Oregon; 1951.

10. Clarke, K.S. A survey of sports-related spinal cord injuries in schools and colleges, 1973-1975. Journal of Safety Research. 9:140-146; 1977.

11. Cohn, B.T.; Brahms, M.A.; Cohn, M. Injury to the eleventh cranial nerve in a high school wrestler. Orthopedic Review. 15:590-595; 1986.

12. Croyle, P.H.; Place, R.A.; Hilgenberg, A.D. Massive pulmonary embolism in a high school wrestler. JAMA. 241:827-828; 1979.

13. Estwanik, J.J.; Bergfeld, J.A.; Canty, T. Report of injuries sustained during the United States Olympic Wrestling Trials. American Journal of Sports Medicine. 6:335-340; 1978.

14. Estwanik, J.J.; Bergfeld, J.A.; Collins, H.R.; Hall, R. Injuries in interscholastic wrestling. Physician and SportsMedicine. 8(3):111-121; 1980.

15. Estwanik, J.J.; Rovere, G.D. Wrestling injuries in North Carolina high schools. Physician and SportsMedicine. 11(1):100-108; 1983.

16. Garrick, J.G. Ankle injuries: Frequency and mechanism of injury Athletic Training. 10:109-111; 1975.

17. Garrick, J.G.; Requa, R.K. Injuries in high school sports. Pediatrics. 61:465-469; 1978.
18. Garrick, J.G.; Requa, R.K. Medical care and injury surveillance in the high school setting. Physician and SportsMedicine. 9(2)115-120; 1981.
19. Granhed, H.; Morelli, B. Low back pain among retired wrestlers and heavyweight lifters. American Journal of Sports Medicine. 16:530-533; 1988.
20. Hartmann, P.M. Injuries in preadolescent wrestlers. Physician and SportsMedicine. 6(11):79-82; 1978.
21. Hellstrom, M.; Jacobsson, B.; Sward, L.; Peterson, L. Radiologic abnormalities of the thoracolumbar spine in athletes. ACTA Radiologica. 31:127-132; 1990.
22. Hoffman, H.S.; Powell, J.W. Analysis of NATA high school injury registry data on wrestling. Athletic Training. 25:125; 1990.
23. Horswill, C.A. Applied physiology of amateur wrestling. Sports Medicine. 14:114-143; 1992a.
24. Horswill, C.A. When wrestlers slim to win. Physician and SportsMedicine. 20(9):91-104; 1992b.
25. Jackson, D.S.; Furman, W.K.; Berson, B.L. Patterns of injuries in college athletes: A retrospective study of injuries sustained in intercollegiate athletics in two colleges over a two-year period. Mt. Sinai Journal of Medicine. 47:423-426; 1980.
26. Kersey, R.D.; Rowan, L. Injury account during the 1980 NCAA wrestling championships. American Journal of Sports Medicine. 11:147-151; 1983.
27. Kewalramani, L.S.; Krauss, J.F. Cervical spine injuries resulting from collision sports. Paraplegia. 19:303-312; 1981.
28. Konrad, I.J. A study of wrestling injuries in high schools throughout seven midwest states. Thesis, Michigan State College; 1951.
29. Laudermilk, J.I. Catastrophic injuries in junior high and high school wrestling: A five-season study. Thesis, University of North Carolina, Chapel Hill; 1988.
30. Lee-Knight, C.T.; Harrison, E.L.; Price, C.J. Dental injuries at the 1989 Canada Games: An epidemiological study. Journal of the Canadian Dental Association. 58:810-815; 1992.
31. Lok, V.; Yuceturk, G. Injuries of wrestling. Journal of Sports Medicine. 2:324-328; 1975.
32. Lorish, T.R.; Rizzo, T.D.; Ilstrup, D.M.; Scott, S.G. Injuries in adolescent and preadolescent boys at two large wrestling tournaments. American Journal of Sports Medicine. 20:199-202; 1992.
33. Marton, K.; Wilson, D.; McKeag, D. Ocular trauma in college varsity sports. Medicine and Science in Sports and Exercise. 19:S53; 1987.
34. McCormack, D.L.; Bliss, W.R. Rupture of the diaphragm in a wrestling match. Journal of the Iowa Medical Society. 73:406-408; 1983.
35. McGuine, T.A. Injury frequency during a one-day collegiate wrestling tournament. Athletic Training. 24:227-229; 1989.
36. Mysnyk, M.C.; Albright, J.P. Relative risks and long-term impact of injuries from amateur football and wrestling competition. Hawkeye Sports Medicine Symposium, Iowa City, Iowa; May 20, 1988.
37. Mysnyk, M.C.; Wroble, R.R.; Foster, D.T.; Albright, J.P. Prepatellar bursitis in wrestlers. American Journal of Sports Medicine. 14:46-54; 1986.
38. National Collegiate Athletic Association Injury Surveillance System. 1992-93 Wrestling Summary, Shawnee Mission, Kansas; 1993.
39. National High School Injury Registry, reported in Athletic Training, 23:383-388; 1988 and 24:360-373; 1989.
40. Patacsil, J. An analytical survey of the incidence of injuries sustained in intercollegiate and interscholastic wrestling. Thesis, Purdue University; 1955.
41. Powell, J.W. National athletic injuries/illness reporting system: Eye injuries in college wrestling. International Ophthalmology Clinics. 21:47-58; 1981.
42. Requa, R.; Garrick, J.G. Injuries in interscholastic wrestling. Physician and SportsMedicine. 9(4):44-51; 1981.
43. Rogers, L.; Sweeney, P.J. Stroke: A neurologic complication of wrestling. American Journal of Sports Medicine. 7:352-354; 1979.
44. Rontoyannis, G.P.; Pahtas, G.; Dinis, D.; Pournaras, N. Sudden death of a young wrestler during competition. International Journal of Sports Medicine. 9:353-355; 1988.
45. Rossi, F.; Dragoni, S. Lumbar spondylolysis: Occurrence in competitive athletes. Updated achievements in a series of 390 cases. Journal of Sports Medicine and Physical Fitness. 30:450-452; 1990.
46. Roy, S.P. Intercollegiate wrestling injuries. Physician and SportsMedicine. 7(11):83-91; 1979.
47. Schuller, D.E.; Dankle, S.K.; Martin, M.; Strauss, R.H. Auricular injury and the use of headgear in wrestlers. Archives of Otolaryngology Head and Neck Surgery. 115:714-717; 1989.
48. Shelley, W.B. Herpetic arthritis associated with disseminate herpes simplex in a wrestler. British Journal of Dermatology. 103:209-212; 1980.
49. Snook, G.A. Injuries in intercollegiate wrestling. A five-year study. American Journal of Sports Medicine. 10:142-144; 1982.
50. Snook, G.A. Wrestling. In: Schneider, R.C.; Kennedy, J.C.; Plant, M.L., eds., Sports injuries: Mechanisms, prevention and treatment. Baltimore: Williams and Wilkins; 1985.
51. Stanish, W.D.; Rubinovich, M.; Armason, T.; Lapenskie, G. Posterior cruciate ligament tears in wrestlers. Canadian Journal of Applied Sports Science. 11:173-177; 1986.
52. Strauss, R.H.; Lanese, R.R. Injuries among wrestlers in school and college tournaments. JAMA. 248:2016-2019; 1982.
53. Strauss, R.H.; Lanese, R.R.; Leizman, D.J. Illness and absence among wrestlers, swimmers, and gymnasts at a large university. American Journal of Sports Medicine. 16:653-655; 1988.
54. Strauss, R.H.; Leizman, D.J.; Lanese, R.R.; Para, M.F. Abrasive shirts may contribute to herpes gladiatorum among wrestlers. New England Journal of Medicine. 320:598-599; 1989.

55. Sward, L.; Hellstrom, M.; Jacobsson, B.; Peterson, L. Back pain and radiologic changes in the thoracolumbar spine of athletes. Spine. 15:124-129; 1990.

56. Tudor, R.B.; Carson, J.P.; Pulliam, M.W.; Hill, A. Pott's puffy tumor, frontal sinusitis, frontal bone osteomyelitis, and epidural abscess secondary to a wrestling injury. American Journal of Sports Medicine. 9:390-391; 1981.

57. van Mechelen, W.; Hlobil, H.; Kemper, H.C.G. Incidence, severity, aetiology and prevention of sports injuries: A review of concepts. Sports Medicine. 14:82-89; 1992.

58. Whiteside, J.A.; Fleagle, S.B.; Kalenak, A. Fractures and refractures in intercollegiate athletes: An eleven-year experience. American Journal of Sports Medicine. 9:369-377; 1981.

59. Wroble, R.R.; Albright, J.P. Neck and low back injuries in wrestling. Clinic in Sports Medicine. 5:295-325; 1986.

60. Wroble, R.R.; Moxley, D.P. Weight loss patterns and success rates in high school wrestlers. Medicine and Science in Sports and Exercise. 26:S120; 1994.

61. Wroble, R.R.; Mysnyk, M.C.; Foster, D.T.; Albright, J.P. Patterns of knee injuries in wrestling: A six-year study. American Journal of Sports Medicine. 14:55-66; 1986.

62. Wu, W.Q.; Lewis, R.C. Injuries of the cervical spine in high school wrestling. Surgical Neurology. 23:143-147; 1985.

63. Zaricnzyj, B.; Shattuck, L.J.M.; Mast, T.A.; Robertson, R.V.; D'elia, G. Sports-related injuries in school aged children. American Journal of Sports Medicine. 8:318-324; 1980.

# 26

# Injury Prevention

*John Weaver, Craig K. Moore, and Warren B. Howe*

## 1. Introduction

Sport is not without risk, whether the individual participant is an elite athlete or involved only in recreational athletic pursuits. Sports injuries cause significant discomfort and disability, reduce productivity, and are responsible for substantial medical expenses (13). Although it is impossible to eliminate all injuries, attempts to reduce them are obviously warranted. That this compendium of epidemiologic information about sports injuries should lead to suggestions for prevention of those injuries is not surprising. Indeed, epidemiology and prevention are inextricably linked, the former being meaningless without the latter, and the latter approaching impossibility without consideration of the former.

It is essential to consider injury prevention in an organized fashion, so as not to miss important factors. Several schemata for organizing preventive efforts have been described. Cross (5) proposed that injury-related factors be termed either intrinsic (within the body of the participant) or extrinsic (acting upon the body from without). Hierarchical models have also been suggested, in which factors are listed as either primary, secondary, or tertiary. The public health model (6) of such a hierarchical system is not particularly helpful in organizing injury prevention efforts. Kannus' sports injury model (11), in which "primary" refers to factors at the individual level, "secondary" refers to factors operating at the group or team level, and "tertiary" focuses on factors at the societal level, is useful. Many models seem to combine Cross' and Kannus' concepts with success.

Adrian's "action model" (1) combines the above approaches to create a very workable mechanism for organizing a review of injury prevention. Injury prevention factors are considered first from the standpoint of the player, then the sport, then the environment, and finally the health support system. Using this framework, each chapter in this book has presented sport-specific suggestions for preventive strategies based on the epidemiology reviewed. In similar fashion, this chapter seeks to extract the principles of injury prevention applicable to sport participation in general, and to summarize the preventive suggestions, which have broad application across sports, made in the preceding chapters. References to literature cited in previous chapters will not be repeated here, and we refer the reader to those earlier chapters for the specifics from which these generalizations are made. It is important for the reader to understand that in most cases there has been no objective assessment of the actual preventive value inherent in these suggestions, although they are based on sound inference and the accumulated experience of many experts over many years.

## 2. Suggestions for Injury Prevention

### 2.1 Players

#### 2.1.1 Anatomical

Muscle tightness has been correlated with an increased incidence of strain injuries to muscles and tendons (7). The use of stretching and warm-up exercises to promote suppleness and flexibility may serve a preventive function. To be effective, and not harmful in themselves, such exercises should be done in a static, rather than ballistic manner. Static stretching, combined with contraction of the antagonist muscles to relax the muscles further, has also been recommended. Stretching exercises are most effective at the end of a workout, when the muscles and connective tissue are warm and well perfused. They are less valuable as warm-up exercises, although they are commonly used, without ill effect, for that purpose (2).

The use of braces or taping to stabilize weak or unstable joints after injury, during the return-to-play, or rehabilitation phase is widely practiced. For some joints, notably the knee and ankle, external support is frequently recommended in the absence of joint abnormality as a prophylactic action against injury. Significant controversy exists about the benefit, and studies supporting both sides of the argument can be found in respected publications. Taping and bracing may function more by improving proprioception and thereby stimulating earlier recruitment of supportive muscles rather than by actual physical support of a joint. It is critically important to understand that no tape application or brace can guarantee protection from either new injury or exacerbation of a preexisting trauma. The decision to tape or brace the injured athlete in an attempt to allow earlier return to participation than might be possible otherwise is difficult. It can only be justified in those cases in which the risk of complicating the underlying injury is small or absent, and the athlete fully understands the potential risks and benefits of the proposed action.

Ankle stabilizing braces are probably more effective than taping and are more cost-effective (15). Functional knee braces are probably effective when properly selected and fitted to the athlete undergoing post-operative or injury rehabilitation (9). The efficacy of prophylactic knee bracing in contact sports is not proven, and the subject remains open to study (14).

### 2.1.2 Physiological

Conditioning programs for athletes are designed to improve the "Five S's" necessary for performance: Strength, Stamina, Suppleness (flexibility), Synergy (balance), and Skill. They also serve to prepare the athlete for the environment expected in competition. A common thread in the literature of sports medicine and coaching is the importance of both general and sport-specific conditioning to attain successful performance and avoid injury.

Since the sports participant spends more time in preparation than in actual competition, avoidance of "overuse" injuries is a critical part of designing and monitoring the conditioning program, particularly in the endurance sports such as running. By employing gradual increases in intensity, speed, and duration of activity and carefully addressing early or subtle signs of injury, such injuries can usually be avoided or their long-term

effect minimized. A common rule that may be employed is the caution not to increase more than one parameter (intensity, speed, or duration) at a time. Attempting to quantitate progression by specific percentages of increase at defined intervals of time is attractive, but may produce unrealistically slow progress in early training, and dangerously increased loads as training approaches maximum.

The most ominous result of overtraining is "staleness," a term used by Martin and Coe (12) to describe that point of cellular injury combined with fuel exhaustion that results in breakdown of body defenses, and neurological and endocrine disturbances. Staleness is the consequence of long term overtraining, and may require weeks, months, or years to overcome. It is sometimes a career ending insult. Warning signs of overtraining and staleness are listed in Table 26.1.

Once overtraining or staleness is acknowledged, rest is the treatment; not necessarily idle rest, but therapeutic rest. This may involve cutting back, possibly stopping training for a time, or perhaps switching to an alternative activity. Clearly it is preferable to prevent this complication of training by programming adequate rest, variations in training activity, cross-training programs, and being alert to early symptoms. The athlete who carefully maintains a training log or journal will profit from the insights it reflects, and may be much more sensitive to early indications of overuse or overtraining.

**Table 26.1  Warning Signs of Overtraining and Staleness**

Training related
  Unusual muscle soreness the day after training
  Progressive increase in soreness with continued training
  Performance plateau or decrement despite increased training
  Inability to complete previously manageable training load
  Elevated effort sense or delay in recovery
  Thoughts of quitting or skipping training

Lifestyle related
  Increased tension, depression, anger, fatigue, confusion, inability to relax
  Decreased vigor in completing daily activities
  Loss of pleasure in previously pleasurable things
  Poor sleep quality/quantity

Health related
  Swelling of lymph nodes, constipation, diarrhea
  Increased frequency of illness (fever, head colds, etc.)
  Increased blood pressure, morning pulse
  Weight loss
  Loss of appetite

Athletes should follow a prescribed regimen of activity immediately before and after practice or competition. Warm-up and cool-down are uniformly viewed as important in preventing injury related to activity. Attention to the content of the warm-up and cool-down periods, and to the proper execution of the exercises is important (8).

Proper nutrition provides the energy needed for performance and the materials necessary for injury repair. Although improper nutrition is not, strictly speaking, an injury, the effects of disordered eating practices can be devastating, even fatal. Surveillance of athlete nutrition by serial weight measurement and coach attention, especially in activities such as dance, gymnastics, rowing, and wrestling, with early referral for medical evaluation if a problem is suspected, is certainly appropriate.

Adequate hydration is critical, especially in warm climates. The thirst mechanism lags behind the body's need for water replacement, and fluid intake should be scheduled and monitored. Although studies indicate that fluids containing carbohydrate (5-7%) and dilute sodium are better absorbed and utilized during exercise, cool water is probably adequate for most athletic activity lasting less than 90 minutes (10).

### 2.1.3 Psychological

Psychological stress in sport can precipitate injuries in athletes. It is important to recognize that the stress that motivates can become excessive and lead to increased susceptibility to injury. Attention and focus are not only necessary for successful performance, but for avoiding dangerous situations and injury; stress may interfere with concentration at critical times. Recognition of this can help athlete and coach to take action to minimize the effects of stress. Insofar as possible, the total psychological profile of the athlete must be understood, including possible stress from work, family, school, personal relationships, and finances.

### 2.1.4 Educational

As part of the athlete's preparation, certain educational efforts may be valuable in reducing injury risk or in improving the outcome after injury. The athlete should learn general preventive measures, including the importance of preparticipation medical evaluation in which he or she interacts constructively with medical personnel to develop an accurate clinical understanding of the proposed participation. Coincident with medical evaluation, athletes can learn the role of medical personnel and how to access them, and gain knowledge of the risk factors likely to be involved in the sport. Athletes who learn, early in their careers, that prompt treatment of minor illness or injury maximizes, rather than decreases, performance and participation time will probably enhance their success. The appropriate application of self-care techniques, such as the use of ice, mild analgesics, padding and bandaging, and so forth, can be taught as dictated by events as the athlete acquires experience. All athletes should be familiar with general and sport-specific principles of hygiene. An understanding of basic nutrition, including hydration, and any nutritional variations that may help or hinder specific sports success or safety is advisable. The impact of environmental variables and adjustments for them required for performance and safety should be communicated.

All athletes should understand the principles of conditioning, both general and sport-specific, including in-season and off-season regimens. They should pursue knowledge of and skill in the techniques specific to their sport, and accept that advanced skills and higher levels of competition should wait until training and experience have built a good foundation. If the chosen sport requires certain protective equipment, the athlete must know how to use, fit, and maintain it properly. Certain precautionary measures, such as water safety and head and spine injury prevention, are well suited to didactic training. The lessons should be reinforced by practical application in training situations and timely reminders from the coach.

## 2.2 Sport

### 2.2.1 Techniques

In training the athlete, the coach should monitor the correct and safe execution of sport skills, especially those identified as "critical" to success in the sport. Although "repetition is the mother of learning," overuse must be carefully avoided by employing variable training routines, doing cross-training, limiting practice length and/or frequency, and, where appropriate, using mental drills or performance imaging to substitute for repetitive performance. It is important to avoid sudden changes in practice intensity, terrain, or style.

Practice content should be modified to take factors such as age, maturity (physical and emotional), rate of maturation, physical characteristics such as size and build, level of conditioning, and competitive level into account. In heavy contact or "collision" sports, some authorities recommend avoiding "hard contact" practices.

As the ability of any athlete grows, the potential relationship between improved performance, higher physical expectation and demand, and increased risk of injury must be recognized.

### 2.2.2 Rules

Rules, which should be uniform across geographic boundaries, are the starting point for safety promotion in competition. Many have their origin rooted in recognition of and attempts to minimize a potential hazard to participating athletes. They should set the basic preconditions for participation, including requirements for preparticipation evaluation and medical clearance when returning from injury or illness. Rules should speak to required protective and safety equipment, such as shin guards in soccer. In addition, they should prohibit activity with a high likelihood of injury, such as head or face blows in karate or spearing or grabbing the face mask in football.

Rules can and should be modified based on the skill and maturity levels of the participants. Thus, elements of a sport appropriate to the players' developmental level can be emphasized, as in limiting pitching or utilizing a batting tee in youth baseball. Rules can set preconditions for advancement to more difficult, and more dangerous, competitive levels or skills, thus providing some assurance that an athlete is not attempting too much too soon.

For performance-graded sports, it has been suggested that judging be based on accuracy of execution rather than difficulty of the attempted skill, especially at less elite levels of competition.

### 2.2.3 Officiating

Rules have little impact on safe participation without qualified officials with authority to enforce them. The focus on safety by sports officials must be paramount. In those sports where officials have both a scoring function and a safety function, the latter must take precedence. Rules against dangerous play must be rigidly enforced.

Officials must understand risk factors for injury that may be inherent in the sport being supervised. The more they understand about the demands placed upon the participants' physical and emotional being, the more likely they are to intervene successfully and in timely fashion to prevent injury. Development and application of mechanisms to certify officials in all sports are worthy goals; an official's level of experience should match the level of sport being officiated.

### 2.2.4 Equipment

The equipment used in sport has the potential for causing or contributing to injury. It should be designed to minimize potentially dangerous construction, such as sharp points on surfboards. If certification standards for the equipment exist, any such devices must conform to those standards and be certified. No modifications of certified equipment should be allowed. The risk of loose or "runaway" equipment in sports such as skiing is well recognized, and should be taken into account in design. Insofar as possible, equipment should be designed to require a minimum of maintenance, and to make the presence of poor maintenance or damage easily apparent.

Equipment should fit the conditions for which it is employed. Thus, shoe design should match the specific type of surface being played on to provide optimal traction and support. Clothing should match the environment to be encountered. Some equipment, such as the vaulting pole, must be carefully matched to the individual using it.

Appropriate equipment improperly used may increase risk of injury. The purpose of the football helmet, for instance, is not to allow use of the head as a battering ram. The user must understand proper use of the equipment, as well as its maintenance, proper fit, and adjustment. The coach should caution against misuse of the equipment.

As sports evolve, there is often tension between the traditions of the sport and the development of equipment to improve safety or performance. One can recall that the advent of batting helmets in baseball or face masks in ice hockey caused concern that these were unwarranted intrusions into the nature of the sport. Such unease will undoubtedly attend many innovations as yet undiscovered.

Protective equipment, some specified by rule and some improvised by individual athletes, is recognized in all sports. Custom fitting of padding is necessary to shield points of repetitive contact and impact. Helmets are common in sports with significant risk of head injury; they should be certified for the use intended and must be properly fitted. Protection of critical sense organs, the eye and the ear, by appropriately designed shields, has become routine in most sports where threat to these exists.

Taping and bracing for performance (functional taping/bracing) is common in many sports, both on a prophylactic and therapeutic basis. A more extensive discussion of taping and bracing appeared earlier in this chapter.

### 2.2.5 Coaching

The coach occupies a critical position in the organizational structure of preventive efforts. As supervisor of the athlete's participation in practice and competition, he or she must recognize potentially risky situations, and either avoid them or develop strategies to minimize their danger. The athlete must be guided in matching competence to imposed demand, and should be prevented from attempting skills or competitive levels for which skill, maturity, strength, or similar requirements are not adequate.

Coaches should design safe and effective training programs for their athletes, incorporating gradual progression to greater imposed demand, and adjusting routines for individual differences. Within training programs, coaches should design safe practice sessions, building in variations in activity and avoiding endless repetition to maintain athletes' interest and concentration and avoid overuse injuries. Because they are usually keen observers of their charges' abilities, coaches are often the first to spot the changes in performance that may signal injury or impending staleness. They should learn to trust their instincts and encourage evaluation by trainer or physician in these situations.

Regardless of the performance level involved, coaching competence is critical for injury prevention. Coaches must be educated in general principles of sport and fitness, and understand the specific sport and its potential risks. It is entirely appropriate for coaches to take courses in injury prevention, injury recognition, first aid, basic life support, and rehabilitation principles; some sponsoring organizations require this for coaches. Some youth sport organizations, such as Little League Baseball, make short videotapes on such subjects, keyed to the particular sport, available for training coaches and leaders. Where they exist, mechanisms for achieving and requiring coaching certification and recertification should be employed to upgrade and assure competence. If such mechanisms do not exist, they should be developed.

Coaches must appreciate and honor the unique position of trust they have in the minds of the athletes, recognizing that out of loyalty and desire to please, the athlete may be placed under excessive pressure or demand by a coach. Bowerman has said, "Coaches have to know that everyone has a zone of stress that will prompt athletes to improve and a zone of just a little more stress that will prompt them to disintegrate (4)." The fine line between presenting appropriate challenges and excessively stressing an athlete is usually difficult to discern, but the coach should try to find it. Coaches should recognize the potential for conflict between the desire to win and welfare of the athlete, and continually attempt to minimize that conflict.

## 2.3 Environment

### 2.3.1 Facility

The facility where sport occurs impacts the safety of participation. It must be designed to present as little hazard as possible to participants, in addition to providing for maximal performances. Fences should be of appropriate height, location, and construction. Field layout, such as placement of dugouts in baseball or venues in track and field, should protect inactive athletes from injury by missile impact or collision with other participants. Competitive surfaces should suit the proposed usage, and must be maintained well to avoid uneven spots and to cushion impacts. Lighting, both natural and artificial, must be considered not only from the standpoint of utility, but for its potential for interfering with vision at times critical for safety. Painting and decor should be designed as much on the basis of safety as on "eye-appeal" and aesthetics. Potential obstructions on the playing field should be eliminated where possible. Those that are mandatory, such as goals and bases, should be designed to minimize the potential for harm to players upon impact, either by padding or breakaway construction. The periphery of the playing field, where obstructions such as benches, crowd restraints or equipment are often present, should receive as careful attention as the playing field itself. Locker rooms and surfaces of approach paths to the playing field should be evaluated from the perspective of safety to prevent falls for athletes in competitive footwear.

If facilities are used for multiple sports, especially when simultaneous use by different sports occurs (such as when skiers and snowboarders share the same hill or swimmers and divers the same pool), care must be taken to avoid dangerous interactions of participants.

### 2.3.2 Weather

The most important weather factors requiring preventive thought are heat and cold. Hot, humid weather should be recognized as carrying the threat of heat illness and/or dehydration and therefore serious injury to participants. The wet-bulb thermometer should be employed to help recognize potentially dangerous conditions, and to guide when participation should be carefully monitored, postponed, or significantly modified. Cool water or hydrating solutions of dilute carbohydrate/electrolyte must be readily available and its use encouraged, remembering that thirst is not an adequate guide to the need for fluid replacement during physical activity.

Cold weather requires alertness to the possibility of hypothermia. Clothing for sports participation in the cold should be designed to be worn in layers so that insulation can be easily matched to conditions. Warming facilities should be available for participants between bouts of activity. Athletes should know signs of hypothermia and frostbite, and where necessary, evaluate each other for early signs of those problems.

## 2.4 Health Support System

### 2.4.1 Preparticipation Evaluation

A preparticipation evaluation (PPE) of athletes is frequently required by school systems and other authorities that organize sports participation. Such an evaluation is usually recommended for all sports participants, according to the authors of several chapters in this volume. The stated goals and potential benefits of the PPE, in addition to fulfilling administrative and legal necessities, seem to fall into three categories: (a) detection of the potential for sudden death during participation, (b) detection of factors that may predispose to new injury or worsening of preexisting injury, and (c) detection of impediments to the athlete's performance. The obvious hope is that detection of these factors can lead to prevention of death or injury, and improvement in performance.

Nontraumatic sudden death during sports participation is a rare event, usually involving a young and vigorous person who, until the event, seemed perfectly healthy. The most common cause is cardiovascular catastrophe, with other causes such as heat injury or severe allergic reactions being much less common. Recent head injury may set the stage for sudden death due to the "second-impact syndrome" precipitated by relatively minor head trauma. Some cases of sudden death, even when exhaustively investigated, seem inexplicable. The PPE can probably spotlight some athletes who may be victims, so that with counseling they may be directed toward safer pursuits. The detection of the Marfan syndrome, hypertrophic cardiomyopathy or significant congenital cardiac disease, is an obvious example. Athletes who have a history of heat illness, or factors such as sickle cell trait that may predispose to heat intolerance, may be detected, as can those with severe allergic responses to exercise such as anaphylaxis. However, many, perhaps most, of the participants at high risk will not be detected by reasonable, cost-effective means.

Various physical factors have been reported to increase the risk of an athlete being injured, and these may be detected during the PPE. "Tightness" has been linked to a tendency toward muscular strains and tendon injuries, and "laxity" has been associated with sprains and dislocations. Physical immaturity may be a risk factor when a child is matched in competition with one more mature. Compared with adults, the immature athlete's less efficient ability to thermoregulate may increase risk in hot environments or during endurance events. The growth spurt of adolescence may be associated with heightened risk of injury. Perhaps the most telling association suggesting increased injury risk is a history of recent or unrehabilitated injury. It has been suggested that tendencies toward risk-taking behavior, illicit drug use, unsafe sexual activity, or eating disorders might be detected during the PPE and allow earlier intervention. Discovery of any of these factors offers the opportunity for intervention in the form of counseling, appropriate training or rehabilitation, or direction toward an alternative activity.

The PPE may allow detection of defects in the "Five S's" of muscle characteristics previously enumerated. Similarly, metabolic abnormalities, including diseases such as diabetes, hypertension, and more pervasive problems such as obesity, may be identified. The potential participant found to have a problem in these areas can be counseled and guided to correct or improve the situation, with the desire for involvement in the sporting activity serving as a useful goad to positive action.

Although almost universally recommended, and we believe appropriately so, the limitations of the PPE must be recognized. It will not weed out all for whom participation will pose a high risk, and it will not prevent all potential injuries. It should consist of a carefully elicited history, examination by a skilled sports clinician, and appropriate application of cost-effective supplemental laboratory and other studies where specifically indicated. Once completed, its results should be applied in a thoughtful fashion, rather than by inflexible rule, to provide guidance for the participant. Very few persons will be "disqualified" by virtue of the PPE; many may be influenced toward safer participation.

A recent monograph produced through the collaboration of five national medical associations concerned with sports medicine elaborates on the content, conduct, and interpretation of the PPE well, and is a recommended guide (3).

### 2.4.2 Practice/Game Services

Skilled medical personnel should be on-site for athletic events during which there is a significant likelihood of severe or significant injury. In some cases this will be a physician, but in many cases, particularly in more rural areas, paramedics or emergency medical technicians undertake such responsibilities. Certified athletic trainers are becoming more numerous, and fill a unique and valuable niche because they are knowledgeable about injury recognition, diagnosis, and treatment specifically from the viewpoint of sports participation. Once an injury is identified, prompt referral to the most appropriate level of medical care is recommended.

Although "game" situations seem to give rise to a disproportionate number of injuries compared with the actual time of exposure, exposure in practice is also significant, with hours being spent there for each minute spent in competition. Coping with practice emergencies, when full medical coverage is seldom available, must be part of the coach's training and planning process. Coaches and other supervisory personnel present at practice should have up-to-date first aid and resuscitation training. The ability to call for help quickly must be available; the use of the cellular phone is highly recommended. At both practice and competition, appropriate medical and safety equipment must be present, with needs determined by the risks of the sport involved.

### 2.4.3 Monitoring Programs

Monitoring of ongoing sporting activity for injury occurrence and its treatment must be carried out systematically. Early recognition of injury is important, and is improved by the day-to-day presence of medically competent personnel, especially athletic trainers. A useful technique for increasing an athlete's self-awareness is to encourage each one to maintain a training log or journal that may alert one to a developing problem, or allow reconstruction of causal factors after an injury has occurred. Records of injury occurrence and therapy should be kept routinely, so that adherence to therapeutic or rehabilitation programs can be kept

under surveillance and communicated to those involved in the athlete's care. Expediency in treatment should be avoided, and rehabilitation to preinjury status prior to return to competition should be achieved.

## 3. Suggestions for Further Research

In 1987, vanMechelen (16) described a "sequence of sports injury prevention" that consists of a recurring four-step cycle of activity. The steps are as follows:

1. Descriptive: establish the extent of the injury problem.
2. Analytical: establish etiology and mechanisms of injury.
3. Intervention: introduce preventive measures.
4. Clinical trial: assess effectiveness by repeating (1).

This seems an entirely rational way to organize efforts at reducing injury incidence, and is the instinctive way most efforts at problem-solving occur. At present, there is a paucity of data relating to steps (1) through (4), and progressively less data as one moves through the sequential steps.

The key to making this system work is organized data collection and analysis. Unfortunately, this is exceedingly difficult and, as reflected in this volume repeatedly, is handicapped by procedural problems. Therefore, one of the priorities in sports injury prevention must be to achieve standardization in terminology and uniformity in definitions so studies can be accurately compared. Investigators should define "injury," "severity," "recovery," "participation," and other variables in similar fashion, and it would be helpful if there were broad agreement on the information to be collected and displayed in particular types of studies. There must be agreement on quantitation of exposure rates, so that presently unreliable denominator information can be made useful.

Once procedural details are standardized, attention to individual sports by interested investigators can be expected to be much more effective at eliciting useful information. For each sport, there are many factors that might be investigated. Some suggestions might include the following:

1. Forces on body in various sports/events (e.g., biomechanics, kinesiology)
2. Role of reinjury in injury statistics

3. Factors that may predict injury
    a. Intrinsic (e.g., physiological, biomechanical, age/maturity, psychological)
    b. Extrinsic (e.g., environmental factors, equipment, coaching)
4. Impact of interventions on injury statistics (e.g., spearing rules in football, prophylactic knee bracing, skiing studies, preparticipation evaluation)
5. Occurrence statistic studies
6. Economic impact studies (e.g., time loss, medical care costs, economic impact of prevention suggestions)
7. Use of noncontact practice programs in preparation for contact sport participation
    a. Do they improve injury statistics?
    b. Do they produce effective team performance?

One would hope that eventually sports injury research will proceed from amassing data in search of questions to answer, its present state, to the more specific process of asking questions and designing studies to answer them.

## 4. Food for Thought and Contemplation

In trying to summarize suggestions for prevention of injury across the many sports extant, there are at least three recurring questions that eventually will require answers; these serve as an appropriate conclusion to this chapter.

What about the perception that some efforts at prevention seem to open up new problems? One thinks immediately of the hard shell football helmet that improved head protection but led to "spearing" and a substantial rise in catastrophic neck injuries. Another example is the improvement in ski boots that diminishes ankle fractures, only to increase tibial fractures and knee injuries. The effect of preventive efforts may not be entirely straightforward, and untoward results can be expected. At the very least, this consideration should invite comprehensive evaluation and due caution in introducing "improvements for safety."

The expense and logistics required for the many injury-reporting and surveillance systems suggested seems potentially staggering. Are they, in fact, worth the trouble and expense? How can that be determined in an objective manner? If found to be worthwhile, how can they be financed?

Finally, will injury prevention efforts eventually impinge on the basic nature of some sports? Some conflicts are already apparent, such as recommendations recently made that soccer goals be padded, a move that would significantly alter the basic actions and strategies in the game. Is there a point at which the pursuit of risk reduction should be abandoned in favor of preserving the traditions and basic elements of the game, knowing that, ultimately, sport cannot be pursued without risk, and the risk may be part of the sport's allure to participants?

Regardless of the eventual answers to these questions, and the others that will undoubtedly occur to those interested, there seems little doubt that there will be continual pressure to improve safety in sport. If the goal is pursued with an emphasis on accurate data collection, careful analysis, and cautious institution of indicated changes, the results will be worth the effort expended.

## References

1. Adrian, M. Action model to evaluate and reduce risk of catastrophic injuries. In: Adams, S.H.; Adrian, M.J.; Bayless, M.A., eds. Catastrophic injuries in sports: Avoidance strategies. Indianapolis: Benchmark Press; 1987:243-249.
2. Alter, M.J. Sport stretch. Champaign, IL: Leisure Press; 1990.
3. American Academy of Family Physicians; American Academy of Pediatrics; American Medical Society for Sports Medicine; American Orthopaedic Society for Sports Medicine; American Osteopathic Academy of Sports Medicine. Preparticipation Physical Evaluation (PPE). AAFP et al.; 1992.
4. Bowerman, W.; quoted in Runners' World, June 1987, p. 9.
5. Cross, M.J. General prevention of injuries in sport. In: Renstrom, P.A.F.H., ed. Sports injuries: Basic principles of prevention and care. Oxford: Blackwell Scientific Publications; 1993:334-342.
6. Duncan, D.F. Epidemiology: Basis for disease prevention and health promotion. New York: MacMillan; 1988.
7. Ekstrand, J.; Gillquist, J. Avoidability of soccer injuries. Int. J. Sports Med. 4:124-128; 1983.
8. Ekstrand, J.; Gillquist, J.; Moller, M.; Oberg, B.; Liljedahl, S. Incidence of soccer injuries and their relation to training and team success. Am. J. Sports Med. 11:63-67; 1983.
9. France, E.P.; Cawley, P.W.; Paulos, L.E. Choosing functional knee braces. Clin. Sports Med. 9:743-750; 1990.

10. Gisolfi, C.V.; Duchman, S.M. Guidelines for optimal replacement beverages for different athletic events. Med. Sci. Sports Exerc. 24:679-687; 1992.

11. Kannus, P. Types of injury prevention. In: Renstrom, P.A.F.H., ed. Sports injuries: Basic principles of prevention and care. Oxford: Blackwell Scientific Publications; 1993:16-23.

12. Martin, D.E.; Coe, P.N. Training distance runners. Champaign, IL: Human Kinetics; 1991.

13. Pritchett, J.W. High cost of high school football injuries. Am. J. Sports Med. 8(3):197-199; 1980.

14. Requa, R.K.; Garrick, J.G. Clinical significance and evaluation of prophylactic knee brace studies in football. Clin. Sports Med. 9:853-869; 1990.

15. Rovere, G.D.; Clarke, T.J.; Yates, C.S.; Burley, K. Retrospective comparison of taping and ankle stabilizers in preventing ankle injuries. Am. J. Sports Med. 16:228-233; 1988.

16. van Mechelen, W.; Hlobil, H.; Kemper, H. Incidence, severity, aetiology and prevention of sports injuries. Sports Med. 14:82-99; 1992.

# 27

# Guidelines for Evaluating Future Research in the Epidemiology of Sport Injuries

*Lawrence Hart*

As the fledgling science of sports medicine grows and becomes more sophisticated, we are learning more about the natural history and outcome of injuries that can occur in particular sports. By bringing together the relevant literature on the epidemiology of sport injuries, this book provides a usable compendium of facts for clinicians and sport scientists. At the same time, it draws attention to areas in which considerably more work needs to be done before we will be in a position to address some essential questions on the incidence, causes, treatment, and prognosis of the more common conditions that interrupt activity and promote morbidity.

The bottom line in each of the foregoing sport-specific chapters has focused on defining priorities for future research and, in time, it is likely that many of these will be addressed. The challenge, therefore, will be to determine the robustness of individual studies so that the emerging literature might be harnessed in a way that makes it relevant and applicable in the clinical domain. The tenets and practices of what has become known as *critical appraisal* can assist in this endeavor, and the purpose of this chapter will be to provide an approach to some of these concepts.

## Critical Appraisal

Critical appraisal, in its broadest sense, refers to the application of certain rules of evidence to published data in order to determine their validity and applicability (25). The process is directed toward the efficient extraction of relevant and methodologically robust data in order to address a pertinent clinical or research question. By providing a mechanism for excluding less rigorous (and often anecdotal) studies on the subject of interest, critical appraisal strategies also help the clinician or researcher to reduce the volume of material that might previously have required closer scrutiny.

As approaches to critical appraisal have become increasingly refined, their application in the clinical domain has been formalized under the rubric of "evidence-based medicine" (EBM). The objective of EBM is to offer a sound and rational approach to clinical practice. This new paradigm stresses the careful examination of research evidence and cautions against the exclusive use of intuition, unsubstantiated pathophysiologic rationale, and unsystematic clinical experience when making crucial clinical decisions (7, 23). An EBM exercise usually begins with a critical appraisal component in which a clear definition of a presenting problem provides direction to a focused literature search. This allows the physician to arrive at a clinical decision based on studies that have met predetermined methodologic criteria.

To promote critical appraisal and EBM, various journals, such as the Annals of Internal Medicine (through the ACP Journal Club) and the Clinical Journal of Sport Medicine (through the Sport Medicine Journal Club) have utilized a structured abstract format with accompanying commentaries (11). Papers are selected for abstraction on the basis of their methodologic rigor and clinical relevance, and the commentary is designed to highlight these attributes and place a particular study in the context of its broader literature.

In keeping with the major themes in preceding chapters, this review will focus on critical appraisal criteria for causation and prognosis. However, it will also summarize guidelines for assessing articles on therapy and diagnostic testing (in which aspects of epidemiologic methods can be applied). Principles for appraising scientific overviews and meta-analyses will be dealt with as well. Table 27.1 provides an outline of the different categories that are covered. Other concepts of epidemiology and particular elements of study design have already been dealt with by Caine et al. in Chapter 1 and will not be explored further in this presentation.

## What to Look for in Particular Studies

### 1. Studies on Causation

Although cause-effect relationships are often inferred in the sports medicine literature, most of these associations are based on evidence that is insufficient to advance the case for true causation. It is often overlooked that in sports medicine, as in other areas of clinical investigation, cause-effect relationships are extremely difficult to prove. Nonetheless, it is possible to increase the likelihood of a cause-effect relationship by means of accumulated empiric data to the point at which, for practical purposes, cause can be assumed. In contrast, evidence against causation can be gathered until it becomes clear that a cause-effect relationship becomes implausible (6).

What appears to be important, therefore, is to identify the evidence that, when present, will help to support the likelihood of causation. In most instances, the strength of the research design will provide useful clues (9, 25). A good randomized controlled trial (RCT) is recognized as the most powerful way to determine cause-effect relationships in clinical studies but, for a variety of practical reasons, it is often not possible to utilize this design to address certain research questions (2, 14). Instead, one or another of the observational study designs (such as cohort studies, case-control studies, cross-sectional studies or case series) might be used. These are more prone to biases and usually provide much weaker evidence for causal relationships.

**Table 27.1    Critical Appraisal Criteria**

| | Purpose of study | | | |
|---|---|---|---|---|
| Causation | Prognosis | Therapy | Diagnosis | Review |
| Was the type of study strong? (RCT > cohort > case control > survey) | Was an inception cohort assembled? | Was the assignment of patients to treatments really randomized? | Was the test compared blindly with a gold standard? | Were the questions clearly stated? |
| Was the assessment of exposure and outcome free of bias? (e.g., blinded assessors) | Were baseline features measured reproducibly? | Were clinically important outcomes assessed objectively? | Was there an adequate spectrum of disease among patients tested? | Were the criteria for selecting articles for review explicit? |
| Was the association both significant and clinically important? If not, was power considered? | Were the outcome criteria clinically important and reproducibly measured? | Was the treatment feasible to use in your practice? | Was the referral pattern described? | Was the validity of the primary studies assessed? |
| Was the association consistent across studies? | Was follow-up at least 80%? | Was there at least 80% follow-up of subjects? | Was the description of the test clear enough to reproduce it? | Was the assessment of primary studies reproducible? |
| Was the "cause" shown to precede the "effect"? | Was there adjustment for extraneous prognostic factors? | Were both statistical and clinical significance considered? | Was the test reproducible (observer variation)? | Was variability in the results of studies analyzed? |
| Was there a dose-response relationship? | | If the study was negative, was power assessed? | Was the contribution of the test to the overall diagnosis assessed? | Were the findings of the primary studies combined appropriately? |

*Note.* Adapted from Sackett, D.L., Haynes, R.B., Guyatt, G.H., Tugwell, P. (25). Clinical Epidemiology. A basic science for clinical medicine (pp. 366-367). Boston: Little Brown and Company.

However, regardless of the study design that is selected, it is important that the strongest possible one has been used in a given circumstance. Moreover, when cohort or case-control studies are performed, it is essential that the determination of outcomes, in the former, and the clear distinction between cases and controls, in the latter, are free from discernible bias (25). The case for causation in observational studies needs to be very carefully evaluated, and it is fortunate, therefore, that recognized criteria can be applied to facilitate this sort of exercise (4, 6, 25). These include temporality (i.e., the recognition that cause precedes effect); strength of association (i.e., the observation that a large relative risk or odds ratio is better evidence for a causal relationship than a weak association); the presence of dose-response relationships (i.e., varying amounts of dose are related commensurately with varying amounts of effect); reversibility (i.e., a reduction in exposure is associated with lower rates of a particular condition); consistency (i.e., the assertion that causal associations are strengthened when several studies, conducted at variable times and in different settings, all arrive at essentially the same conclusion); biologic plausibility (i.e., the recognition that cause and effect are consistent with prevailing knowledge of the condition of interest); specificity (i.e., a single cause and effect); and analogy (i.e., cause-effect relationships have already been demonstrated for a similar condition).

An assessment of causation becomes more complex in instances in which multiple factors might be contributing to an overall effect. For example, if one considers the possible intrinsic and extrinsic factors that have been implicated in one or another of the overuse syndromes, it is evident that a single or more dominant factor is often very difficult to identify. In a recent article, Meeuwisse has proposed a model that accommodates a multifactorial assessment of causation in athletic injuries (20). It is his contention that such an approach will promote a better understanding of injury causation and might thereby assist in the more rational development of treatment or prevention guidelines.

## 2. Studies on Risk and Prognosis

Though risk and prognosis have similar attributes (and both are usually assessed by way of cohort studies), they occupy different time frames in the natural history of a given condition. Risk factors predate the onset of the condition in question and prognostic factors predict outcome once the condition has already been acquired.

In addition to predicting the occurrence of a disease or injury, risk factors are helpful in the diagnostic process and can also be applied in recommendations on disease or injury prevention. Because the presence of risk factors increases the probability that a particular condition is present, diagnosis can occur earlier and with greater certainty. If a risk factor is also recognized as a cause of a particular condition, then its elimination can be used to prevent future occurrences (6).

It needs to be acknowledged that risk factors need not be, and often are not, causes of disease or injury. A risk factor may merely be a marker of a particular condition and, by virtue of an association with some other determinants of the same condition, it may be confounded with a causal factor. For example, it has been suggested that distance runners who "sometimes stretch" are at increased risk for musculoskeletal injuries (13, 27). However, this does not necessarily mean that "sometimes stretching" actually *causes* injury. Several other factors may potentially provoke the same spectrum of morbidity. In effect, we know relatively little about risk factors for sport-related injuries, and the studies that exist have focused mostly on running injuries (1, 8, 15, 17, 18, 19, 27).

When assessing articles on prognosis, several factors need to be considered (6, 10, 16, 25). The most important of these is to determine whether an inception cohort was assembled. This refers to a group of study subjects who have been identified at an early and uniform point in the conduct of a study (i.e., at zero time). If the study has not identified an inception cohort, the subsequent course will lack precision and the outcome will likely be unpredictable. It is generally considered that the absence of an identifiable inception cohort constitutes a fatal flaw in the methodology of prognosis studies.

It is also essential that the pattern whereby subjects were entered into the study be satisfactorily described. This provides information on the nature of the participants and permits a judgment on the generalizability of the results. Moreover, knowledge of the referral pattern makes it easier to judge whether various biases (25) have been avoided.

Follow-up is the next important component of a prognosis study. All members of the inception cohort should be accounted for at the end of the study and the reasons for any "dropouts" should be clearly documented. Attrition usually does not occur without good reason, and may be associated with prognostic outcomes that need to be carefully considered when drawing inferences from the study's conclusions (25).

Objective outcome criteria should be developed and used in prognosis studies and outcome assessments should be blinded. Without blinding, studies are more prone to a diagnostic-suspicion bias (whereby an investigator who knows that a study subject has an attribute of presumed importance will look much more carefully for the prognostic outcome of interest) or an expectation bias (in which prior knowledge of a particular attribute may influence subsequent clinical judgment). Adjustment for extraneous prognostic factors is a further criterion that should be appraised. For example, in the Ontario Cohort Study of Running Related Injuries, it appeared that taller runners may have been more prone to injury than their shorter counterparts. However, once the data were subjected to more robust interpretation (by multivariate, rather than univariate, analysis), the height factor did not feature as a significant risk factor (27).

### 3. Choosing the Best Therapy

In their day-to-day practice, most clinicians are required to make judgments on whether a proposed treatment does more good than harm. It is in this area, perhaps more than in any other, that the strength of the studies used to arrive at such decisions is of the utmost importance. A well-conducted RCT is generally recognized as the gold standard for determining the efficacy of any therapeutic intervention (24, 25). Usually, a large RCT with clear-cut results and a low risk of error will provide the best evidence for invoking a specific treatment strategy (10, 22).

The following six guides are recommended when attempting to differentiate useful from useless or even harmful therapy (5, 25): (a) establish whether the assignment of patients to treatments was really randomized, (b) determine whether all clinically relevant outcomes were reported, (c) decide on the applicability of a particular therapy to the patients that you see (i.e., determine whether the study patients were recognizably similar to your own), (d) assess whether both clinical and statistical significance were considered and documented, (e) decide whether the therapeutic maneuver is feasible in your practice, and (f) determine whether complete follow-up of study patients has occurred (i.e., were all the patients who entered the study accounted for at its conclusion?).

### 4. Selecting a Diagnostic Test

When appraising the clinical usefulness of a diagnostic test, it is important to determine whether there has been an independent, blind, comparison with a gold standard of diagnosis. The following methodologic questions should also be addressed (3, 25): (a) Does the patient sample used to evaluate the test include a spectrum of those with mild and severe, and treated and untreated disease and also those with different but commonly confused conditions? (b) Was the study's setting and the filter through which patients passed adequately described? (c) Were the reproducibility of the test and its interpretation determined? (d) Was the term "normal" described for the test in question? (e) If applicable, has the individual contribution of the test to the overall validity of a cluster or sequence of tests been determined? (f) Has the test been sufficiently described to facilitate its replication? and (g) Has the test utility been determined?

### 5. Assessing Reviews, Overviews, and Meta-Analyses

Review articles have long been regarded as a time efficient resource for covering a particular topic of interest, but it is well recognized that they may vary in their quality and comprehensiveness. Recently, attempts have been made to refine and redefine the traditional review article. In general terms, a *review* can be regarded as any synthesis of the results and conclusions of two or more publications on a given topic. When strategies have been used comprehensively to identify and extract all of the available literature on the topic, the term *overview* is invoked. When the overview also utilizes a recognized statistical technique to bring together the results of several studies into a single estimate, the resulting publication is termed a *meta-analysis* (21, 25). Although meta-analyses are still extremely rare commodities in the sports sciences, reviews and overviews are commonplace and often provide a basis for drawing inferences on causation, prognosis, and clinical management.

When subjecting a "quality filter" to any articles of this sort, the following issues should be addressed: (a) Were the questions and methods clearly stated? (b) Were the search methods used to locate relevant studies comprehensive? (c) Were explicit methods used to determine which articles to include? (d) Was the methodologic quality of the primary studies evaluated? (e) Were the selection and assessment of the primary studies reproducible and free from bias? (f) Were differences in individual study results adequately explained? (g) Were the results of the primary studies combined appropriately? and (h) Were the reviewer's conclusions supported by the data cited? (10, 21, 25).

Many of these guidelines focus specifically on the qualities of the individual articles that contribute to the review and, unless there is confidence that these component studies are methodologically robust and free of bias, the message conveyed by the review itself may turn out to be inconclusive. Moreover, a good review will expand on areas of potential (or real) disagreement between different studies on the same topic and will provide enough detail on the primary studies to enable the reader to critically evaluate the rationale for the reviewer's conclusions. Any review that overinterprets the available data or provides a recommendation without defending it on the basis of sound evidence should be regarded with scepticism.

Each of the sport-specific chapters in this book is presented as an overview. Meta-analysis may have been the preferred format but this was thought to be impractical given the inherent limitations in sizeable segments of the available literature on sport injuries.

### 6. The Critical Appraisal of Other Types of Studies

Sets of critical appraisal guidelines have also been proposed for studies on screening, quality of care, and economic analyses and can be reviewed through their original sources (25).

## Quality of the Sports Medicine Literature

When scanning the sport-specific chapters in this book, it is evident that the number and quality of studies for specific sports vary considerably. There are many instances in which the data necessary to make causal or prognostic inferences are just not available either because an essential area has not been explored or because an appropriate question has been addressed by way of a study design that lacks sufficient rigor and therefore prevents valid inferences on its conclusion(s). These problems are not unique to this sampling of the sports medicine literature.

To obtain a general impression of the robustness of sports medicine research, a study has been reported in which a selection of the literature, over a specified 12-month period, was critically appraised (12, 26). Of the 756 papers that were reviewed, according to specific criteria, 606 (80%)

were original research studies. Of these, 182 had used an epidemiologic approach and of those that did, only 8% were RCTs. Thirty-seven percent used a cohort study design, 35% were cross-sectional studies, 13% were case series, and 7% used case-control methodology. The most commonly identified pitfalls in this literature sample were the following: overinterpretation of numerator-based case series data (implying nonrecognition of the limitations of this design), inadequate attention to power (i.e., sample size) considerations in study design, and the frequent lack of randomization or the exclusion of a control group in studies in which such elements of methodology were deemed to be essential.

These observations appear to corroborate the general trends in the sport-specific chapters in this book. They also reflect prevailing standards in other subspecialty literatures in which observational studies inevitably outnumber RCTs (and a proportion of these are much less robust than what might be considered ideal). Given this reality, we need to be especially mindful of the potential strengths and weaknesses inherent in specific designs and what inferences might safely be drawn from them. The introductory chapter of *Epidemiology of Sport Injuries* contains a broader exploration of the attributes of study design, and for further information on this topic the reader is referred, in particular, to texts by Sackett et al. (25) and Fletcher et al. (6) and to comprehensive reviews by Casperson (2) and by Walter and Hart (26).

## Conclusions

Each of the sport-specific chapters in this book has ended with suggestions for future studies and it is to be anticipated that many of the potential research topics will be explored over the next several years. However, regardless of the scope and ingenuity of the projects that are about to be undertaken, the definitive measure of their success will be the extent to which their findings are valid and applicable in the day-to-day care of injured athletes. Ultimately, the caregiver, rather than the researcher, will have to make informed management decisions based on complex and sometimes conflicting bodies of emerging knowledge.

By providing a framework for filtering and sorting this new information according to prescribed criteria, critical appraisal techniques can, and should, be used to assist with decision making that is based on the robust conclusions of methodologically sound studies rather than on the anecdotal or even authoritarian dictates of poor research.

# References

1. Blair, S.N.; Kohl, H.W. Rates and risks for running and exercise injuries: studies in three populations. Res. Q. Exercise Sport. 58:221-228; 1987.

2. Casperson, C.J. Physical activity epidemiology: concepts, methods, and applications to exercise science. Exercise and Sport Sciences Reviews. 17:423-473; 1989.

3. Department of Clinical Epidemiology and Biostatistics, McMaster University, Hamilton, ON. How to read clinical journals: II. To learn about a diagnostic test. Can. Med. Assoc. J. 124:703-710; 1981.

4. Department of Clinical Epidemiology and Biostatistics, McMaster University, Hamilton, ON. How to read clinical journals: IV. To determine etiology or causation. Can. Med. Assoc. J. 124:985-990; 1981.

5. Department of Clinical Epidemiology and Biostatistics, McMaster University, Hamilton, ON. How to read clinical journals: V. To distinguish useful from useless or even harmful therapy. Can. Med. Assoc. J. 124:1156-1162; 1981.

6. Fletcher, R.H.; Fletcher, S.W.; Wagner, E.H. Clinical epidemiology: The essentials. 2nd edition. Baltimore: Williams & Wilkins; 1988.

7. Hart, L.E. Evidence-based medicine. Clin. J. Sport Med. 4:198; 1994.

8. Hart, L.E. Exercise and soft tissue injury. Balliere's Clinical Rheumatology. 8:137-148; 1994.

9. Hart, L.E. Making the case for causation. Clin. J. Sport Med. 4:276; 1994.

10. Hart, L.E. The role of evidence in promoting consensus in the research literature. In: Bouchard, C.; Shephard, R.J.; Stephens, T., eds. Physical activity, fitness, and health: International proceedings and consensus statement. Champaign, IL: Human Kinetics Publishers; 1994:89-97.

11. Hart, L.E.; Meeuwisse, W.H. Evaluating methodology in the sport medicine literature. Clin. J. Sport Med. 4:64; 1994.

12. Hart, L.E.; Walter, S.D. Critical appraisal of a selection of the sports medicine literature. Med. Sci. Sport Exercise 22(2) (Suppl.):S116; 1990.

13. Hart, L.E.; Walter, S.D.; McIntosh, J.M.; Sutton, J.R. The effect of stretching and warmup on the development of musculoskeletal injuries in distance runners. Med. Sci. Sport Exercise. 21(2)(Suppl.):S59; 1989.

14. Horwitz, R.I. The experimental paradigm and observational studies of cause-effect relationships in clinical medicine. J. Chron. Dis. 40:91-99; 1987.

15. Koplan, J.P.; Powell, K.E.; Sikes, R.K.; et al. An epidemiologic study of the benefits and risks of running. JAMA. 248:3118-3121; 1982.

16. Laupacis, A.; Wells, G.; Richardson, W.S.; Tugwell, P. Users' guide to the medical literature: how to use an article about prognosis. JAMA. 272(3):234-237; 1994.

17. Macera, C.A. Lower extremity injuries in runners: advances in prediction. Sports Medicine. 13:50-57; 1992.

18. Macera, C.A.; Pate, R.R.; Powell, K.E.; et al. Predicting lower extremity injuries among habitual runners. Arch. Intern. Med. 149:2565-2568; 1989.

19. Marti, B.; Vader, J.P.; Minder, C.E.; Abelin, T. On the epidemiology of running injuries: the 1984 Bern Grand-Prix Study. Amer. J. Sport Med. 16:285-294; 1988.

20. Meeuwisse, W.H. Assessing causation in sport injury: a multifactorial model. Clin. J. Sport Med. 4:166-170; 1994.

21. Oxman, A.D.; Guyatt, G.H. Guidelines for reading literature reviews. Can. Med. Assoc. J. 138:697-703; 1988.

22. Sackett, D.L. Rules of evidence and clinical recommendations on the use of antithrombotic agents. Chest. 95:2S-4S; 1989.

23. Sackett, D.L. Evidence-based medicine: a new approach to teaching the practice of medicine. JAMA. 268(17):2420-2425; 1992.

24. Sackett, D.L. The Cochrane collaboration. ACP J. Club. May/June, A-11; 1994.

25. Sackett, D.L.; Haynes, R.B.; Guyatt, G.H.; Tugwell, P. Clinical epidemiology: A basic science for clinical medicine. 2nd ed. Boston: Little, Brown; 1991.

26. Walter, S.D.; Hart, L.E. Application of epidemiological methodology to sports and exercise science research. Exercise and Sport Sciences Reviews. 18:417-448; 1990.

27. Walter, S.D.; Hart, L.E.; McIntosh, J.M.; Sutton, J.R. The Ontario cohort study of running-related injuries. Arch. Intern. Med. 149:2561-2564; 1989.

# Editors

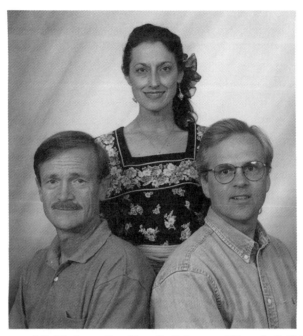

Koenraad J. Lindner, Caroline G. Caine, and Dennis J. Caine

**Dennis J. Caine** is an internationally recognized authority on the epidemiology of injury in sports. His research and writing—much of it on pediatric sports injuries—has been published in many journals. Most notably, his articles on gymnastics injuries resulted from his leadership in two longitudinal epidemiological studies. A frequent speaker on the subject at conferences and meetings held around the world, he is an associate professor in the Department of Physical Education, Health and Recreation at Western Washington University (WWU). Dennis holds a PhD in lifespan human growth and motor development from the University of Oregon. He is a member of the International Society for the Advancement of Kinanthropometry and serves on the Editorial Review Board of the *Clinical Journal of Sport Medicine*.

**Caroline G. Caine** brings expertise in dance science, experience as a writer and editor, and interest in sport science to this book. In addition to having taught dance at the university level for 20 years, Caroline has enjoyed a lengthy career in professional performance and choreography both in the United States and Canada. She was editor of the book *The Dancer as Athlete* and the coauthor of papers on kinanthropometry in dancers and epidemiology of gymnastics injuries. She also initiated

and coordinated the International Symposium on the Scientific Aspects of Dance (an associate program of the 1984 Olympic Scientific Congress). A recipient of many academic awards and honors, Caroline holds a PhD in dance and the related arts from Texas Woman's University in Denton. She is currently assistant to the dean and an adjunct dance faculty member in the College of Fine and Performing Arts at WWU.

**Koenraad J. Lindner** has been a lecturer in the Physical Education and Sports Science Unit at the University of Hong Kong since 1992. Prior to this appointment, he was a teacher and researcher at the University of Manitoba for 18 years. At the forefront of research on sports injuries, he was the principal investigator for a three-year longitudinal study sponsored by Sport Canada on injuries incurred in gymnastics. He is also the author of numerous articles and book chapters on sports injuries. Koenraad received the Canadian Association for Health, Physical Education and Recreation Fellow Award as well as the University of Manitoba Merit Award, presented for excellence in teaching, service, and research. He is a board member of the Hong Kong Association for Sports Medicine and Sports Science.